Essentials of Psychosomatic Medicine

Edited by

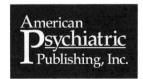

James L. Levenson, M.D.

Chair, Consultation-Liaison Psychiatry, and Vice-Chair, Psychiatry
Professor of Psychiatry, Medicine, and Surgery
Virginia Commonwealth University
Richmond, Virginia

American Psychiatric Publishing, Inc.

Washington, DC
London, England

Copyright © 2007 American Psychiatric Publishing, Inc.
ALL RIGHTS RESERVED

WM
90
E78
2007

Manufactured in the United States of America on acid-free paper
09 08 07 06 05   5 4 3 2 1
First Edition

Typeset in Adobe's Janson Text and Frutiger 55 Roman

American Psychiatric Publishing, Inc.
1000 Wilson Boulevard
Arlington, VA 22209-3901
www.appi.org

Library of Congress Cataloging-in-Publication Data
Essentials of psychosomatic medicine / edited by James L. Levenson.
    p. ; cm.
  Includes bibliographical references and index.
  ISBN 1-58562-246-X (pbk. : alk. paper)
  1. Medicine, Psychosomatic. 2. Mind and body. I. Levenson, James L.
  [DNLM: 1. Psychophysiologic Disorders. 2. Psychosomatic Medicine.
WM 90 E78 2007]
  RC49.E872 2007
  616.001'9—dc22
                                                        2006023465

British Library Cataloguing in Publication Data
A CIP record is available from the British Library.

Essentials of Psychosomatic Medicine

Contents

Contributors

Sharon L. Alspector, M.D.
Assistant Clinical Professor of Psychiatry, Columbia University College of Physicians and Surgeons, New York, New York

Lesley M. Arnold, M.D.
Associate Professor of Psychiatry and Director, Women's Health Research Program, Department of Psychiatry, University of Cincinnati College of Medicine, Cincinnati, Ohio

Iram Ashraf, B.Sc.
Research Analyst, University Health Network Women's Health Program, Toronto, Ontario, Canada

Charles H. Bombardier, Ph.D.
Professor, Department of Rehabilitation Medicine, University of Washington, Seattle, Washington

Brenda Bursch, Ph.D.
Associate Professor of Psychiatry and Biobehavioral Sciences, and Pediatrics, David Geffen School of Medicine at UCLA, Los Angeles, California

Alan J. Carson, M.Phil., M.D., M.R.C.Psych.
Consultant Neuropsychiatrist and part-time Senior Lecturer, Department of Clinical Neurosciences, Western General Hospital, University of Edinburgh, Edinburgh, United Kingdom

Michael R. Clark, M.D., M.P.H.
Associate Professor and Director, Adolf Meyer Chronic Pain Treatment Programs, Department of Psychiatry and Behavioral Sciences, Johns Hopkins Medical Institutions, Baltimore, Maryland

Kathy Coffman, M.D.
Attending Psychiatrist, Cedars–Sinai Medical Center, Los Angeles, California

Lewis M. Cohen, M.D.
Professor of Psychiatry, Tufts University School of Medicine, Boston, Massachusetts;

Director of Renal Palliative Care Initiative, Baystate Medical Center, Springfield, Massachusetts

Wendy Cohen, M.D.
Clinical Assistant Professor of Psychiatry, Virginia Commonwealth University, Richmond, Virginia

Francis Creed, M.D., F.R.C.P., F.R.C.Psych., F.Med.Sci.
Professor of Psychological Medicine, Division of Psychiatry, University of Manchester, United Kingdom

Niccolò D. Della Penna, M.D.
Fellow, Department of Psychiatry and Behavioral Sciences, The Johns Hopkins School of Medicine, Baltimore, Maryland

Mary Amanda Dew, Ph.D.
Professor of Psychiatry, Psychology, and Epidemiology; Director of Quality of Life Research, Artificial Heart Program, Western Psychiatric Institute and Clinics, University of Pittsburgh Medical Center, Pittsburgh, Pennsylvania

Chris Dickens, M.B.B.S., Ph.D.
Senior Lecturer in Psychological Medicine, Department of Psychiatry, Manchester Royal Infirmary, Manchester, United Kingdom

Andrea F. DiMartini, M.D.
Associate Professor of Psychiatry and Surgery, and Liaison to the Starzl Transplant Institute, Western Psychiatric Institute and Clinics, University of Pittsburgh Medical Center, Pittsburgh, Pennsylvania

Jesse R. Fann, M.D., M.P.H.
Associate Professor, Department of Psychiatry and Behavioral Sciences, and Adjunct Associate Professor, Departments of Rehabilitation Medicine and Epidemiology, University of Washington, Seattle; Associate in Clinical Research, Fred Hutchinson Cancer Research Center; Director, Psychiatry and Psychology Consultation Service, Seattle Cancer Care Alliance, Seattle, Washington

Michael J. Germain, M.D.
Associate Professor of Medicine, Tufts University School of Medicine, Boston, Massachusetts; Medical Director, Renal Transplantation Service, Baystate Medical Center, Springfield, Massachusetts

Ann Goebel-Fabbri, Ph.D.
Instructor in Psychology, Department of Psychiatry, Harvard Medical School; Psychologist, Behavioral and Mental Health Research Section, Joslin Diabetes Center, Harvard Medical School, Boston, Massachusetts

Donna B. Greenberg, M.D.
Director, Psychiatric Oncology Service, Massachusetts General Hospital Cancer Center; Associate Professor of Psychiatry, Harvard Medical School, Boston, Massachusetts

Judy A. Greene, M.D.
Clinical Fellow in Psychiatry, Department of Psychiatry, Beth Israel Deaconess Medical Center, Boston, Massachusetts

Alan M. Jacobson, M.D.
Senior Vice President, Strategic Initiatives Division, Joslin Diabetes Center, Harvard Medical School; and Professor of Psychiatry, Harvard Medical School, Boston, Massachusetts

Richard Kennedy, M.D.
Assistant Professor, Department of Psychiatry and Department of Physical Medicine and Rehabilitation, Virginia Commonwealth University, Richmond, Virginia

James L. Levenson, M.D.
Chair, Consultation-Liaison Psychiatry, and Vice-Chair, Psychiatry; Professor of Psychiatry, Medicine, and Surgery; Virginia Commonwealth University, Richmond, Virginia

Norman B. Levy, M.D.
Clinical Professor of Psychiatry, State University of New York Downstate Medical Center; Director of Psychiatry, Kingsboro Psychiatric Center, Brooklyn, New York

Mary Jane Massie, M.D.
Attending Psychiatrist, Memorial Sloan-Kettering Cancer Center; Professor of Clinical Psychiatry, Weill Medical College of Cornell University, New York, New York

Sarah E. Munce, M.Sc.
Graduate student, University of Toronto, University Health Network Women's Health Program, Toronto, Ontario, Canada

Gail Musen, Ph.D.
Assistant Investigator, Behavioral and Mental Health Research Section, Joslin Diabetes Center; Instructor in Psychiatry, Department of Psychiatry, Harvard Medical School, Boston, Massachusetts

Lynn Myles, B.Sc., M.D., F.R.C.S.Ed.
Consultant Neurosurgeon, Department of Clinical Neurosciences, Western General Hospital, University of Edinburgh, Edinburgh, United Kingdom

Kevin W. Olden, M.D.
Levy Professor of Medicine and Psychiatry and Chief, Division of Gastroenterology, University of Arkansas School of Medicine, Little Rock, Arkansas

Patrick G. O'Malley, M.D., M.P.H.
Professor of Medicine, Uniformed Services University of the Health Sciences, Bethesda, Maryland

Pauline S. Powers, M.D.
Professor of Psychiatry and Behavioral Medicine, Department of Psychiatry and Behavioral Medicine, College of Medicine, University of South Florida, Tampa, Florida

John Querques, M.D.
Assistant in Psychiatry, Massachusetts General Hospital; Instructor in Psychiatry, Harvard Medical School, Boston, Massachusetts

Carlos A. Santana, M.D.
Associate Professor, Department of Psychiatry and Behavioral Medicine, College of Medicine, University of South Florida, Tampa, Florida

Robert K. Schneider, M.D.
Associate Professor of Psychiatry, Internal Medicine, and Family Practice; Chair, Division of Ambulatory Psychiatry: Virginia Commonwealth University, Richmond, Virginia

Peter A. Shapiro, M.D.
Associate Professor of Clinical Psychiatry, Columbia University College of Physicians and Surgeons; Associate Director, Consultation-

Liaison Psychiatry Service; Director, Transplantation Psychiatry Service, Columbia University Medical Center, New York–Presbyterian Hospital, New York, New York

Michael C. Sharpe, M.A., M.D., F.R.C.P., F.R.C.Psych.
Professor of Psychological Medicine and Symptoms Research, School of Molecular and Clinical Medicine, University of Edinburgh, Edinburgh, United Kingdom

Felicia A. Smith, M.D.
Assistant in Psychiatry, Massachusetts General Hospital; Instructor in Psychiatry, Harvard Medical School, Boston, Massachusetts

Caitlin R. Sparks, B.A.
Senior Research Assistant, Behavioral and Mental Health Research Section, Joslin Diabetes Center, Harvard Medical School, Boston, Massachusetts

Theodore A. Stern, M.D.
Chief, Psychiatric Consultation Service, Massachusetts General Hospital; Professor of Psychiatry, Harvard Medical School, Boston, Massachusetts

Donna E. Stewart, M.D., F.R.C.P.C.
Professor and Chair of Women's Health, University of Toronto, University Health Network Women's Health Program, Toronto, Ontario, Canada

Nada L. Stotland, M.D., M.P.H.
Professor of Psychiatry and Obstetrics/Gynecology, Rush Medical College, Chicago, Illinois

Margaret Stuber, M.D.
Professor of Psychiatry and Biobehavioral Sciences, David Geffen School of Medicine at UCLA, Los Angeles, California

Edward G. Tessier, Pharm.D., M.P.H.
Lecturer, School of Nursing, University of Massachusetts Amherst, Amherst, Massachusetts

Glenn J. Treisman, M.D., Ph.D.
Associate Professor, Department of Psychiatry and Behavioral Sciences and Department of Medicine, The Johns Hopkins School of Medicine, Baltimore, Maryland

Paula T. Trzepacz, M.D.
Medical Director, U.S. Neurosciences, Lilly Research Laboratories, Indianapolis, Indiana; Clinical Professor of Psychiatry, University of Mississippi Medical School, Jackson, Mississippi; Adjunct Professor of Psychiatry, Tufts University School of Medicine, Boston, Massachusetts

Adam Zeman, M.A., D.M., M.R.C.P.
Professor of Cognitive and Behavioural Neurology, Peninsula Medical School, Exeter, United Kingdom

Preface

James L. Levenson, M.D.

WHAT IS PSYCHOSOMATIC Medicine? In the past, Psychosomatic Medicine has had ambiguous connotations, alternatively "psychogenic" or "holistic," but it is the latter meaning that has characterized its emergence as a contemporary scientific and clinical discipline (Lipowski 1984). In this book, it refers to a specialized area of psychiatry whose practitioners have particular expertise in the diagnosis and treatment of psychiatric disorders and difficulties in complex medically ill patients (Gitlin et al. 2004).

We treat and study three general groups of patients: those with comorbid psychiatric and general medical illnesses complicating each other's management, those with somatoform and functional disorders, and those with psychiatric disorders that are the direct consequence of a primary medical condition or its treatment. Psychosomatic Medicine practitioners work as hospital-based consultation-liaison psychiatrists (Kornfeld 1996), on medical-psychiatric inpatient units (Kathol and Stoudemire 2002), and in settings in which mental health services are integrated into primary care (Unutzer et al. 2002). Thus the field's name reflects the fact that it exists at the interface of psychiatry and medicine.

Psychosomatic Medicine is the newest psychiatric subspecialty formally approved by the American Board of Medical Specialties. There have been many other names for this specialized field, including consultation-liaison psychiatry, medical-surgical psychiatry, psychological medicine, and psychiatric care of the complex medically ill, among others. In 2001, the Academy of Psychosomatic Medicine applied to the American Board of Psychiatry and Neurology (ABPN) for the recognition of "Psychosomatic Medicine" as a subspecialty field of psychiatry, choosing to return to the name for the field embedded in our history, our journals, and our national organizations (for a detailed account of the field, see Lyketsos et al. 2001). Subsequent formal approval was received from the American Psychiatric Association, ABPN, the Residency Review Committee (RRC) of the Accreditation Council for Graduate Medical Education (ACGME), and the American Board of Medical Specialties (ABMS). The first two certifying examinations were administered in June 2005 and 2006.

Psychosomatic Medicine has a rich history. The term *psychosomatic* was introduced by Johann Heinroth in 1818, and

Table 1: Key dates in the modern history of psychosomatic medicine

1935	Rockefeller Foundation opens first Consultation-Liaison (C/L)–Psychosomatic Units at Massachusetts General, Duke, and Colorado
1936	American Psychosomatic Society founded
1939	First issue of *Psychosomatic Medicine*
1953	First issue of *Psychosomatics*
1954	Academy of Psychosomatic Medicine (APM) founded
1975	National Institute of Mental Health (NIMH) Training Grants for C/L Psychiatry
1985	NIMH Research Development Program for C/L Psychiatry
1991	APM-recognized fellowships number 55
2001	Subspecialty application for Psychosomatic Medicine
2003	Approval as subspecialty by American Board of Medical Specialties

Table 2: Selected classic texts in psychosomatic medicine

1935	*Emotions and Body Change* (Dunbar)
1943	*Psychosomatic Medicine* (Weiss and English)
1950	*Psychosomatic Medicine* (Alexander)
1968	*Handbook of Psychiatric Consultation* (Schwab)
1978	*Organic Psychiatry* (Lishman)
1978	*Massachusetts General Hospital Handbook of General Hospital Psychiatry* (Hackett and Cassem)
1993	*Psychiatric Care of the Medical Patient* (Stoudemire and Fogel)

Table 3: Selected journals in psychosomatic medicine

Journal name	Date of initial publication
Psychosomatic Medicine	1939
Psychosomatics	1953
Psychotherapy and Psychosomatics	1953
Psychophysiology	1954
Journal of Psychosomatic Research	1956
Advances in Psychosomatic Medicine	1960
International Journal of Psychiatry in Medicine	1970
General Hospital Psychiatry	1979
Journal of Psychosomatic Obstetrics and Gynecology	1982
Journal of Psychosocial Oncology	1983
Stress Medicine	1985
Psycho-Oncology	1986

Table 4: National organizations

Academy of Psychosomatic Medicine
American Association for General Hospital Psychiatry
American Neuropsychiatric Association
American Psychosocial Oncology Society
American Psychosomatic Society
Association for Academic Psychiatry—Consultation-Liaison Section
Association for Medicine and Psychiatry
North American Society for Psychosomatic Obstetrics and Gynecology
Society for Liaison Psychiatry

Table 5: International organizations

European Association for Consultation-Liaison Psychiatry and Psychosomatics
International College of Psychosomatic Medicine
International Neuropsychiatric Association
International Organization for Consultation-Liaison Psychiatry
International Psycho-Oncology Society
World Psychiatric Association—Section of General Hospital Psychiatry

---

Felix Deutsch introduced the term *psycho-somatic medicine* around 1922 (Lipsitt 2001). Psychoanalysts and psychophysiologists pioneered the study of mind-body interactions from very different vantage points, each contributing to the growth of Psychosomatic Medicine as a clinical and scholarly field. The modern history of the field (see Table 1) perhaps starts with the Rockefeller Foundation's funding of psychosomatic medicine units in several U.S. teaching hospitals in 1935. The National Institute of Mental Health made it a priority to foster the growth of consultation-liaison psychiatry, through training grants (circa 1975) and a research development program (circa 1985).

Psychosomatic Medicine is a scholarly discipline, with classic influential texts (Table 2), many devoted journals (Table 3), and both national (Table 4) and international (Table 5) professional/scientific societies. The Academy of Psychosomatic Medicine is the only U.S. national organization primarily dedicated to Psychosomatic Medicine as a psychiatric subspecialty. The American Psychosomatic Society, an older cousin, is primarily devoted to psychosomatic research, and its members come from many disciplines (Wise 1995). While consultation-liaison psychiatry and psychosomatic medicine flourished first in the United States, exciting work now comes from around the world.

This book is a condensed and updated version of major sections of the *American Psychiatric Publishing Textbook of Psychosomatic Medicine* (Levenson 2005), and readers who wish more in-depth coverage are referred there. The first chapter of this book covers general principles in evaluation and management. The remaining chapters address issues within each of the medical specialties and subspecialties. This book has attempted to capture the diversity of our field, whose practitioners do not place equal emphasis on the syllables of "bio-psycho-social." There is not unanimity among us on some questions, and diverse opinions will be found in this book.

Psychosomatic Medicine has evolved, since its start, from a field based on clinical experience, conjecture, and theorizing into a discipline grounded in empirical research that is growing and spreading its findings into many areas of medical care (Levenson 1997).

Acknowledgments

This book has benefited from those who have gone before in creating comprehensive textbooks for our field, especially Stoudemire, Fogel, and Greenberg's *Psychiatric Care of the Medical Patient* (2000) and Wise and Rundell's *American Psychiatric Publishing Textbook of Consultation-Liaison Psychiatry* (2002).

References

Gitlin DF, Levenson JL, Lyketsos CG: Psychosomatic medicine: a new psychiatric subspecialty. Acad Psychiatry 28:4–11, 2004

Kathol RG, Stoudemire A: Strategic integration of inpatient and outpatient medical-psychiatry services, in The American Psychiatric Publishing Textbook of Consultation-Liaison Psychiatry. Edited by Wise MG, Rundell JR. Washington, DC, American Psychiatric Publishing, 2002, pp 871–888

Kornfeld DS: Consultation-liaison psychiatry and the practice of medicine. The Thomas P. Hackett Award lecture given at the 42nd annual meeting of the Academy of Psychosomatic Medicine, 1995. Psychosomatics 37:236–248, 1996

Levenson JL: Consultation-liaison psychiatry research: more like a ground cover than a hedgerow. Psychosom Med 59:563–564, 1997

Levenson JL (ed): American Psychiatric Publishing Textbook of Psychosomatic Medicine. Washington, DC, American Psychiatric Publishing, 2005

Lipowski ZJ: What does the word "psychosomatic" really mean? A historical and semantic inquiry. Psychosom Med. 46:153–71, 1984

Lipsitt DR: Consultation-liaison psychiatry and psychosomatic medicine: the company they keep. Psychosom Med 63:896–909, 2001

Lyketsos CG, Levenson JL, Academy of Psychosomatic Medicine (APM) Task Force for Subspecialization: Proposal for recognition of "PSYCHOSOMATIC MEDICINE" as a psychiatric subspecialty. Academy of Psychosomatic Medicine, July 2001

Unutzer J, Katon W, Callahan CM, et al: Collaborative care management of late-life depression in the primary care setting: a randomized controlled trial. JAMA 288: 2836–2845, 2002

Wise TN: A tale of two societies. Psychosom Med 57:303–309, 1995

1

Psychiatric Assessment and Consultation

Felicia A. Smith, M.D.

John Querques, M.D.

James L. Levenson, M.D.

Theodore A. Stern, M.D.

Psychiatric Consultation in the General Hospital

Psychiatrists who work in medical settings are charged with providing expert consultation to medical and surgical patients. Patients who are sick, preoccupied with their physical condition, and in pain are ill disposed to engage in the exploratory interviews that often typify psychiatric evaluations in other settings. The consultant must be adept at gathering the requisite diagnostic information efficiently from the data permitted by the patient's clinical condition and must be able to tolerate the sights, sounds, and smells of the sickroom. Additional visits for more history are often inevitable. In the end, the diagnosis will likely fall into one (or more) of the categories outlined in Lipowski's (1967) classification, which is still relevant today (Table 1–1).

Although the consultant is summoned by the patient's physician, in most cases the visit is unannounced and is not requested by the patient, from whom cooperation is expected. Explicitly acknowledging this reality and apologizing if the patient was not informed are often sufficient to gain the patient's cooperation. Cooperation is enhanced if the psychiatrist sits down and operates at eye level with the patient. By offering to help the patient get comfortable before and after the encounter, the consultant can increase the chances of being welcomed then and for follow-up evaluations. Starting with empathic questions about the patient's suffering establishes

TABLE 1–1.   Categories of psychiatric differential diagnoses in the general hospital

- Psychiatric presentations of medical conditions
- Psychiatric complications of medical conditions or treatments
- Psychological reactions to medical conditions or treatments
- Medical presentations of psychiatric conditions
- Medical complications of psychiatric conditions or treatments
- Comorbid medical and psychiatric conditions

Source.   Adapted from Lipowski 1967.

rapport and also guides the psychiatrist in setting the proper pace of the interview. Finally, because a psychiatric consultation will cause many patients to fear that their physician thinks they are "crazy," the psychiatrist may first need to address this fear.

The Process of the Consultation

Although rarely as straightforward as the following primer suggests, the process of psychiatric consultation should, in the end, include all the components explained below.

Speak Directly With the Referring Clinician

Requests for psychiatric consultation are notorious for being vague and imprecise. They sometimes signify only that the team recognizes that a problem exists. In speaking with a member of the team that has requested the consultation, the consultant listens to the implicit as well as the explicit messages from the other physician (Murray 2004). This brief interaction may give the consultant invaluable information about how the consultation may be useful to the team and to the patient.

Review the Current Records and Pertinent Past Records

The consultant is in a unique position to focus on details that may have been previously overlooked. For example, nurses often document salient neurobehavioral data (e.g., the level of awareness and the presence of confusion or agitation); physical and occupational therapists estimate functional abilities crucial to the diagnosis of cognitive disorders and to the choice of an appropriate level of care; and speech pathologists note alterations in articulation, swallowing, and language. All of them may have written progress notes about adherence to treatment regimens, unusual behavior, interpersonal difficulties, or family issues encountered in their care of the patient.

Review the Patient's Medications

Construction of a medication list at various time points (e.g., at home, on admission, on transfer within the hospital, and at present) is important. Special attention should be paid to medications with psychoactive effects and to those associated with withdrawal syndromes (from benzodiazepines, opiates, antidepressants, anticonvulsants, and beta-blockers). Review of order sheets or computerized order entries is not always sufficient, because patients may not always receive prescribed medications; therefore, medication administration records should also be reviewed.

Gather Collateral Data

Histories from hospitalized medically ill patients may be especially spotty and unreliable, if not nonexistent. Data from collateral sources may be of critical importance. However, psychiatric consultants must guard against prizing any single party's version of historical events over another's; family members and others may lack objectivity, be in denial, be overinvolved, or have a personal agenda to advance. Confidentiality must be valued when obtaining collateral information. Ideally, one obtains the patient's consent first; however, this may not be possible if the patient lacks capacity or if a dire emergency is in progress. Moreover, in certain situations there may be contraindications to contacting some sources of information (e.g., an employer of a patient with substance abuse or the partner of a woman who is experiencing abuse). Like any astute physician, the psychiatrist collates and synthesizes all available data and weighs each bit of information according to the reliability of its source.

Interview and Examine the Patient

Armed with information gleaned and elicited from other sources, the psychiatric consultant now makes independent observations of the patient and collects information that may be the most reliable of all because it comes from direct observations.

Mental Status Examination

A thorough mental status examination is central to the psychiatric evaluation of the medically ill patient. Because the examination is hierarchical in nature, care must be taken to complete it in a systematic fashion (Hyman and Tesar 1994).

Level of consciousness.   Level of consciousness depends on normal cerebral arousal by the reticular activating system. A patient whose level of consciousness is impaired will inevitably perform poorly on cognitive testing.

Attention.   The form of attention most relevant to the clinical mental status examination is the sustained attention that allows one to concentrate on cognitive tasks. Disruption of attention is a hallmark of delirium. Sustained attention is best tested with moderately demanding, nonauto-matic tasks, such as reciting the months backward, or, as in the Mini-Mental State Examination (Folstein et al. 1975), spelling *world* backward or subtracting 7 serially from 100. Serial subtraction is intended to be a test of attention, not arithmetic ability, so the task should be adjusted to the patient's native ability and educational level (serial 3s from 50, serial 1s from 20). An inattentive patient's performance on other parts of the mental status exam may be affected on any task requiring sustained focus.

Memory.   *Working memory* is tested by asking the patient to *register* some information (e.g., three words) and to *recall* it after an interval of at least 3 minutes, during which other testing prevents rehearsal. This task can also be considered a test of *recent memory*. *Semantic memory* is tapped by asking general-knowledge questions (e.g., "Who is the President?") and by naming and visual recognition tasks. The patient's ability to remember aspects of his or her history serves as an elegant test of *episodic memory* (as well as of *remote memory*).

Executive function.   *Executive function* refers to the abilities that allow one to plan, initiate, organize, and monitor thought and behavior. These abilities localize broadly to the frontal lobes. Frontal lobe disorders are suspected when one observes disinhibition, impulsivity, disorganization, abulia, or amotivation. Tasks that can be used to gain some insight into frontal lobe function include verbal fluency, such as listing as many animals as possible in 1 minute; motor sequencing, such as asking the patient to replicate a sequence of three hand positions; the go/no-go task, which requires the patient to tap the desk once if the examiner taps once, but not to tap if the examiner taps twice; and tests of abstraction, including questions like "What do a tree and a fly have in common?"

Language. *Language disorders* result from lesions of the dominant hemisphere. In assessing language, one should first note characteristics of the patient's speech (e.g., nonfluency or paraphasic errors) and then assess comprehension. Naming is impaired in both major varieties of aphasia, and anomia can be a clue to mild dysphasia. Reading and writing should also be assessed. Expressive (Broca's or motor) aphasia is characterized by effortful, nonfluent speech with use of phonemic paraphasias (incorrect words that approximate the correct ones in sound), reduced use of function words (e.g., prepositions and articles), and well-preserved comprehension. Receptive (Wernicke's or sensory) aphasia is characterized by fluent speech with both phonemic and semantic paraphasias (incorrect words that approximate the correct ones in meaning) and poor comprehension. The stream of incoherent speech and the lack of insight in patients with Wernicke's aphasia sometimes lead to misdiagnosis of a primary thought disorder and psychiatric referral; the clue to the diagnosis of a language disorder is the severity of the comprehension deficit. Global dysphasia combines features of Broca's and Wernicke's aphasias. Selective impairment of repetition characterizes conduction aphasia. The nondominant hemisphere plays a part in the appreciation and production of the emotional overtones of language.

Praxis. *Apraxia* refers to an inability to perform skilled actions (e.g., using a screwdriver, brushing one's teeth) despite intact basic motor and sensory abilities. These abilities can be tested by asking a patient to mime such actions or by asking the patient to copy unfamiliar hand positions. *Constructional apraxia* is usually tested with the Clock Drawing Test. *Gait apraxia* involves difficulty in initiating and maintaining gait despite intact basic motor function in

the legs. *Dressing apraxia* is difficulty in dressing caused by an inability to coordinate the spatial arrangement of clothes with the body.

Mood and affect. *Mood* and *affect* both refer to the patient's emotional state, mood being the patient's perception and affect being the interviewer's perception. Normal but intense expressions of emotion may be misperceived by nonpsychiatric physicians as evidence of psychiatric disturbance. Disturbances in mood and affect may also be the result of brain dysfunction or injury. Blunted affective expression may be a sign of Parkinson's disease. Intense affective lability (e.g., pathological crying or laughing) with relatively normal mood occurs with some diseases or injuries of the frontal lobes.

Perception. Perception in the mental status examination is primarily concerned with hallucinations and illusions. However, before beginning any part of the clinical interview and the mental status examination, the interviewer should establish whether the patient has any impairment in vision or hearing that could interfere with communication. Although hallucinations in any modality may occur in primary psychotic disorders (e.g., schizophrenia or affective psychosis), prominent visual, olfactory, gustatory, or tactile hallucinations suggest a secondary medical etiology. Olfactory and gustatory hallucinations may be manifestations of seizures, and tactile hallucinations are often seen with substance abuse.

Judgment and insight. The traditional question for the assessment of *judgment* (i.e., "What would you do if you found a letter on the sidewalk?") is much less informative than questions tailored to the problems faced by the patient being evaluated; for example, "If you couldn't stop a nosebleed, what would you do?" Similarly, questions to assess *insight* should focus on the patient's understanding of his or her illness, treatment, and life circumstances.

Further guidance on mental status examination. Particular cognitive mental status testing maneuvers are described in more detail in Table 1–2. More detailed consideration of the mental status examination can be found elsewhere (Strub and Black 2000; Trzepacz and Baker 1993).

Physical Examination

The consultation psychiatrist should be familiar with and comfortable performing neurological examinations and other selected features of the physical examination that may uncover the common comorbidities in psychiatric patients (Granacher 1981; Summers et al. 1981a, 1981b). Even with a sedated or comatose patient, simple observation and a few maneuvers that involve a laying on of hands may potentially yield a bounty of findings. Table 1–3 provides a broad outline of selected findings of the physical examination and their relevance to the psychiatric consultation.

Formulate Diagnostic and Therapeutic Strategies

By the time the consultant arrives on the scene, routine chemical and hematological tests and urinalyses are almost always available, and they should be reviewed along with any other laboratory, imaging, and electrophysiological tests. The consultant then considers what additional tests are needed to arrive at a diagnosis.

The most common screening tests in clinical practice are listed in Table 1–4. Tests should be ordered selectively, with consideration paid to sensitivity, specificity, and cost-effectiveness. Perhaps most importantly, careful thought should be given to whether the results of each test will affect the patient's management.

Neuroimaging

Neuroimaging may aid in fleshing out the differential diagnosis of neuropsychiatric conditions, although it rarely establishes the diagnosis by itself (Dougherty and Rauch 2004). In most situations, magnetic resonance imaging (MRI) is preferred over computed tomography (CT). MRI provides greater resolution of subcortical structures (e.g., basal ganglia, amygdala, and other limbic structures) of particular interest to psychiatrists. It is also superior for detection of abnormalities of the brain stem and posterior fossa. Furthermore, MRI is better able to distinguish between gray-matter and white-matter lesions. CT is most useful in cases of suspected acute intracranial hemorrhage (having occurred within the past 72 hours) and when MRI is contraindicated (in patients with metallic implants). Dougherty and Rauch (2004) suggest that the following conditions and situations merit consideration of neuroimaging: new-onset psychosis, new-onset dementia, delirium of unknown cause, prior to an initial course of electroconvulsive therapy, and an acute mental status change with an abnormal neurological examination in a patient with either a history of head trauma or an age of 50 years or older. While other physicians may tend to dismiss all but acute focal findings, psychiatrists recognize that even small abnormalities (e.g., periventricular white-matter changes) or chronic changes (e.g., cortical atrophy) have diagnostic and therapeutic implications (see Chapter 15, "Neurology and Neurosurgery").

Electrophysiological Tests

The electroencephalogram (EEG) is the most widely available test that can assess brain activity. The EEG is most often indicated in patients with paroxysmal or other symptoms suggestive of a seizure disorder, especially complex partial sei-

TABLE 1–2.   Detailed assessment of cognitive domains

Cognitive domain	Assessment
Level of consciousness and arousal	Inspect the patient
Orientation to place and time	Ask direct questions about both of these
Registration (recent memory)	Have the patient repeat three words immediately
Recall (working memory)	Have the patient recall the same three words after performing another task for at least 3 minutes
Remote memory	Ask about the patient's age, date of birth, milestones, or significant life or historical events (e.g., names of presidents, dates of wars)
Attention and concentration	Subtract serial 7s (adapt to the patient's level of education; subtract serial 3s if less educated). Spell *world* backward (this may be difficult for non-English speakers). Test digit span forward and backward. Have the patient recite the months of the year (or the days of the week) in reverse order.
Language	(Adapt the degree of difficulty to the patient's educational level)
Comprehension	Inspect the patient while he or she answers questions
	Ask the patient to point to different objects
	Ask yes or no questions
	Ask the patient to write a phrase (paragraph)
Naming	Show a watch, pen, or less familiar objects, if needed
Fluency	Assess the patient's speech
	Have the patient name as many animals as he or she can in 1 minute
Articulation	Listen to the patient's speech
	Have the patient repeat a phrase
Reading	Have the patient read a sentence (or a longer paragraph if needed)
Executive function	Determine if the patient requires constant cueing and prompting
Commands	Have the patient follow a three-step command
Construction tasks	Have the patient draw interlocked pentagons
	Have the patient draw a clock
Motor programming tasks	Have the patient perform serial hand sequences
	Have the patient perform reciprocal programs of raising fingers
Judgment and reasoning	Listen to the patient's account of his or her history and reason for hospitalization
	Assess abstraction (similarities: dog/cat; red/green)
	Ask about the patient's judgment about simple events or problems: "A construction worker fell to the ground from the seventh floor of the building and broke his two legs; he then ran to the nearby hospital to ask for medical help. Do you have any comment on this?"

TABLE 1–3.   Selected elements of the physical examination and the significance of findings

Elements	Examples of possible diagnoses
General	
General appearance healthier than expected	Somatoform disorder
Fever	Infection or NMS
Blood pressure or pulse abnormalities	Withdrawal, thyroid or cardiovascular disease
Body habitus	Eating disorders, polycystic ovaries, or Cushing's syndrome
Skin	
Diaphoresis	Fever, withdrawal, NMS
Dry, flushed skin	Anticholinergic toxicity, heat stroke
Pallor	Anemia
Changes in hair, nails, skin	Malnutrition, thyroid or adrenal disease
Jaundice	Liver disease
Characteristic stigmata	Syphilis, cirrhosis, or self-mutilation
Bruises	Physical abuse, ataxia, traumatic brain injury
Eyes	
Mydriasis	Opiate withdrawal, anticholinergic toxicity
Miosis	Opiate intoxication, cholinergic toxicity
Kayser-Fleischer pupillary rings	Wilson's disease
Neurological	
Tremors	Delirium, withdrawal syndromes, parkinsonism
Primitive reflexes present (e.g., snout, glabellar, and grasp)	Dementia, frontal lobe dysfunction
Hyperactive deep-tendon reflexes	Withdrawal, hyperthyroidism
Ophthalmoplegia	Wernicke's encephalopathy, brain stem dysfunction, dystonic reaction
Papilledema	Increased intracranial pressure
Hypertonia, rigidity, catatonia, parkinsonism	EPS, NMS
Abnormal movements	Parkinson's disease, Huntington's disease, EPS
Abnormal gait	Normal pressure hydrocephalus, Parkinson's disease, Wernicke's encephalopathy
Loss of position and vibratory sense	Vitamin B_{12} deficiency

Note.   EPS=extrapyramidal side effects; NMS=neuroleptic malignant syndrome.

zures, or pseudoseizures (see Chapter 15, "Neurology and Neurosurgery"). An EEG may also be helpful in distinguishing between neurological and psychiatric etiologies for a mute, uncommunicative patient. An EEG may be helpful in documenting the presence of generalized slowing in a delirious patient, but it rarely indicates a specific etiology of delirium and it is not indicated in every delirious patient. However, when the diagnosis of delirium is uncertain, electroencephalographic evidence of dysrhythmia may prove useful. EEGs may also facilitate the evaluation of rapidly progressive dementia or profound coma; but because findings are neither sensitive nor specific, they are not often helpful in the evaluation of space-occupying lesions, cerebral infarctions, or head injury (Bostwick and Phil-

TABLE 1–4. Common tests in psychiatric consultation

Complete blood cell count

Serum chemistry panel

Thyroid-stimulating hormone (thyrotropin) concentration

Vitamin B$_{12}$ (cyanocobalamin) concentration

Folic acid (folate) concentration

Human chorionic gonadotropin (pregnancy) test

Toxicology

   Serum

   Urine

Serological tests for syphilis

Human immunodeficiency virus tests

Urinalysis

Chest X ray

Electrocardiogram

---

brick 2002). Continuous electroencephalographic recordings with video monitoring or ambulatory electroencephalographic monitoring may be necessary in order to document abnormal electrical activity in cases of complex partial seizures or when factitious seizures are suspected. As with neuroimaging reports, the psychiatric consultant must read the electroencephalographic report, because nonpsychiatrists often misinterpret the absence of dramatic focal abnormalities (e.g., spikes) as indicative of normality, even though psychiatrically significant brain dysfunction may manifest as focal or generalized slowing or as sharp waves.

Other Tests

Other diagnostic tools may also prove useful as adjuncts. Neuropsychological testing may be helpful in diagnosis, prognosis, and treatment planning in patients with neuropsychiatric disorders. Psychological testing can help the consultant better understand a patient's emotional functioning and personality style.

Write a Note

The consultation note should be clear, concise, and free of jargon and should focus on specific diagnostic and therapeutic recommendations. Consultees fundamentally want to know what is going on with the patient and what they should and can do about it; these themes should dominate the note. Finger-pointing and criticism of the primary team or of other providers should be avoided. The consultant should also avoid rigid insistence on a preferred mode of management if there is an equally suitable alternative (Kontos et al. 2003).

The consultant should begin the note with a summary of the patient's medical and psychiatric history, the reason for the current admission, and the reason for the consultation. Next should be a brief summary of the present medical illness with pertinent findings and hospital course. Physical and neurological examinations, as well as germane laboratory results or imaging studies, should also be summarized. The consultant should then list the differential diagnosis in order of decreasing likelihood, making clear which is the working diagnosis or diagnoses. If the patient's symptoms are not likely to be due to a psychiatric disorder, this should be explicitly stated. Finally, the consultant should make recommendations or clearly describe plans in order of decreasing importance. Recommendations include ways to further elucidate the diagnosis as well as therapeutic suggestions. The consultant should include contact information in the event that the consultee has further questions.

Speak Directly With the Referring Clinician

The consultation ends in the same way that it began—with a conversation with the referring clinician. Personal contact is especially crucial if diagnostic or therapeutic suggestions are time sensitive. Some information or recommendations may be especially sensitive, whether for reasons of confidentiality or risk management, and are better conveyed verbally than fully documented in the chart. The medical chart is read by a variety of individuals, including the patient at times, and thus discretion is warranted.

Provide Periodic Follow-Up

Many consultations cannot be completed in a single visit. Rather, several encounters may be required before the problems identified by both the consultee and the consultant are resolved. Moreover, new issues commonly arise during the course of the consultative process, and a single consultation request often necessitates frequent visits, disciplined follow-up, and easy accessibility. Finally, it may be appropriate to sign off from a case when the patient stabilizes or when the consultant's opinion and recommendations are being disregarded (Kontos et al. 2003).

Conclusion

Psychiatric assessment and consultation can be crucial to seriously ill medical patients. The psychosomatic medicine psychiatrist is an expert in the diagnosis and care of psychopathology in the medically ill. The psychiatric consultant will be called on to help diagnose, understand, and manage a wide array of conditions; when effective, the consultant addresses the needs of both the patient and the medical-surgical team. In this manner, psychiatric consultation is essential to the provision of comprehensive care in the medical setting.

References

Bostwick JM, Philbrick KL: The use of electroencephalography in psychiatry of the medically ill. Psychiatr Clin North Am 25:17–25, 2002

Dougherty DD, Rauch SL: Neuroimaging in psychiatry, in Massachusetts General Hospital Psychiatry Update and Board Preparation, 2nd Edition. Edited by Stern TA, Herman JB. New York, McGraw-Hill, 2004, pp 227–232

Folstein MF, Folstein SE, McHugh PR: "Mini-Mental State": a practical method for grading the cognitive state of patients for the clinician. J Psychiatr Res 12:189–198, 1975

Granacher RP: The neurologic examination in geriatric psychiatry. Psychosomatics 22:485–499, 1981

Hyman SE, Tesar GE: The emergency psychiatric evaluation, including the mental status examination, in Manual of Psychiatric Emergencies, 3rd Edition. Edited by Hyman SE, Tesar GE. Boston, MA, Little, Brown, 1994, pp 3–11

Kontos N, Freudenreich O, Querques J, et al: The consultation psychiatrist as effective physician. Gen Hosp Psychiatry 25:20–23, 2003

Lipowski ZJ: Review of consultation psychiatry and psychosomatic medicine, II: clinical aspects. Psychosom Med 29: 201–224, 1967

Murray GB: Limbic music, in Massachusetts General Hospital Handbook of General Hospital Psychiatry, 5th Edition. Edited by Stern TA, Fricchione GF, Cassem NH, et al. Philadelphia, PA, Mosby/Elsevier, 2004, pp 21–28

Strub RL, Black FW: Mental Status Examination in Neurology, 4th Edition. Philadelphia, PA, FA Davis, 2000

Summers WK, Munoz RA, Read MR: The psychiatric physical examination, part I: methodology. J Clin Psychiatry 42:95–98, 1981a

Summers WK, Munoz RA, Read MR, et al: The psychiatric physical examination, part II: findings in 75 unselected psychiatric patients. J Clin Psychiatry 42:99–102, 1981b

Trzepacz PT, Baker RW: The Psychiatric Mental Status Examination. New York, Oxford University Press, 1993

Self-Assessment Questions

Select the single best response for each question.

1. Clinical assessment of memory and executive functions is an important component in the diagnosis and management of cognitive disorders. Regarding clinical assessment of cognitive function, all of the following are true *except*

    A. Having the patient register and then later recall specific information (e.g., three objects) is a test of episodic memory.

    B. Semantic memory is assessed by questions of general knowledge and naming of common objects.

    C. Executive function refers to the abilities that allow one to plan, initiate, organize, and monitor thought and behavior.

    D. Having the patient name as many objects in a category (e.g., names of animals) as he or she can within 1 minute assesses frontal lobe function.

    E. The go/no-go test of ability to inhibit a response assesses frontal lobe inhibitory function.

2. Language disorders involve the dominant cortical hemisphere and are important in neuropsychiatric illness encountered in psychosomatic medicine practice. Which of the following is *not* true regarding clinical presentation and assessment of the aphasias?

    A. Naming of objects is affected in Broca's (expressive) aphasia.

    B. Naming of objects is affected in Wernicke's (receptive) aphasia.

    C. Wernicke's aphasia overlaps with psychotic disorders in that both conditions feature poor insight and incoherent speech.

    D. Conduction aphasia features impaired naming with preserved repetition.

    E. Global dysphasia combines features of both Broca's and Wernicke's aphasias.

3. In the task of differentiating primary psychiatric from secondary medical etiologies of hallucinatory experiences, the affected sensory modality may guide the clinician to the more likely etiology. Which of the following types of hallucinations is often seen in substance abuse?

    A. Tactile.

    B. Auditory.

    C. Visual.

    D. Gustatory.

    E. Olfactory.

4. The adjunctive use of neuroimaging is an important part of psychosomatic medicine practice. The consultant often must determine which imaging modality is most appropriate for the clinical problem at hand. Which of the following pathological entities is better visualized by computed tomography (CT) than by magnetic resonance imaging (MRI)?

    A. Basal ganglia lesion (e.g., Parkinson's disease).

    B. Brain stem lesion with motor signs.

    C. Cerebellar tumor.

    D. Acute intracranial hemorrhage.

    E. Vascular dementia with frontal lobe signs.

5. The electroencephalogram (EEG) may be a useful diagnostic tool in psychosomatic medicine, but it is subject to some important limitations. Which of the following clinical situations is most likely to be clarified by the use of an EEG?

    A. The search for a specific etiology of an established case of delirium.

    B. An insidious onset and slowly progressive dementia.

    C. Cognitive and motor deficits suggesting cerebral infarction.

    D. Distinguishing between neurological and psychiatric etiologies for a mute, uncommunicative patient.

    E. Localization of cerebral injury in traumatic brain injury.

2 Heart Disease

Peter A. Shapiro, M.D.

Sharon L. Alspector, M.D.

THE RELATIONSHIPS BETWEEN PSYCHIATRY and cardiovascular disease are complex, including both the effects of psychosocial factors on the heart and vascular system and the effects of cardiovascular system changes on mental states. Many psychological states and traits have been identified as contributing to risk for the development or exacerbation of heart disease. Behavioral disorders such as overeating, smoking, and alcohol abuse also add to the risk of heart disease. Conversely, the experience of heart disease seems to contribute to risk for numerous psychiatric problems. Not only are the psychological effects of dealing with cardiac illness complicated and profound, but medications and other treatments for heart diseases also often have psychiatric effects. Because heart disease is so common, psychiatrists must expect to deal with the effects of cardiovascular comorbidity in the care of their patients, evaluating the role of medical factors in their mental health and recognizing the potential impact of psychiatric interventions on the cardiovascular system.

Psychiatric Disorders in Heart Disease

The development of cardiac disease in a previously well individual is associated with a variety of psychological reactions. Perhaps most fundamentally, it is difficult to maintain denial about one's mortality after a cardiac event. Viewing oneself as having heart disease has effects at every level of psychological development: increasing concerns about dependency, autonomy, control, and ability to provide for others; provoking loss of self-esteem and concern about loss of love; and inciting fears about vitality, sexuality, and mortality. The maintenance of denial has been associated with mental well-being (Levenson et al. 1989; Levine et al. 1987) and may be manifest as minimizing the severity of the event ("I just had a small attack") or attributing symptoms to a noncardiac source ("gas pains"), but excessive denial can be detrimental to health because of the failure to accept the need to maintain a treatment regimen or a delay in seeking treatment

(Cassem 1985). In contrast, inadequate denial or exaggeration of the illness can lead to invalidism or mental disorder in the cardiac patient.

Depression

Depression in Coronary Artery Disease

Depression appears to be the most common psychiatric disorder in coronary artery disease (CAD) patients (Glassman and Shapiro 1998). Numerous surveys of patients with established coronary disease, acute myocardial infarction (MI), and unstable angina indicate a point prevalence of depression consistently in the range of 15%–20% (Shapiro et al. 1997). This figure is remarkable in light of national surveys indicating a lifetime prevalence of depression of approximately 16% in the general population (Kessler et al. 2003). Three studies of patients following coronary artery bypass graft surgery also demonstrate a point prevalence of depression in the range of 20%–30% (Blumenthal et al. 2003; Connerney et al. 2001; Shapiro et al. 1998). Elevated symptom scores on depression rating scales such as the Beck Depression Inventory (BDI) are even more common and may predict subsequent major depression (Frasure-Smith et al. 1995a, 1995b).

Many studies indicate the failure to diagnose and treat depression in CAD patients (Frasure-Smith et al. 1993; Luutonen et al. 2002). In a Finnish study (Luutonen et al. 2002) of 85 consecutive post-MI patients with 18-month follow-up, the prevalence of BDI scores of 10 or greater was 21% in hospital, 30% at 6 months, and 33.9% at 18 months. Only 6 patients received mental health treatment; 2 received benzodiazepines; none received adequate antidepressant therapy (Luutonen et al. 2002). In the Montreal Heart Institute sample, none of 35 patients

identified with major depression by research interviews in the post-MI hospital stay received antidepressants (Frasure-Smith et al. 1993). In another study of patients with newly diagnosed CAD, one-sixth of the sample met the criteria for major depression; at 1-year follow-up, only one-sixth of those who were depressed had received treatment (Hance et al. 1996). The availability of good social support reduces the likelihood of persistent depression after an acute coronary event (Frasure-Smith et al. 1995b, 2000).

Depression in Congestive Heart Failure

Fewer studies have examined the prevalence of depression in patients with congestive heart failure (CHF), but as in patients with coronary disease, a point prevalence of depression approaching 20% is suggested by available data (Faris et al. 2002; Freedland et al. 1998; Jiang et al. 2001).

Anxiety

Anxiety in Coronary Artery Disease

The prevalence of anxiety disorders in CAD has not been as well studied as that of depression, but anxiety symptoms are clearly elevated in patients with acute coronary disease and in 5%–10% of patients with chronic heart disease (Sullivan et al. 2000). Many patients with coronary disease have a family history of death of the parent of the same sex as a result of the same illness. This history is often associated with the conscious fantasy that the patient's death at the age at which the parent died is inevitable, leading to considerable vigilance, avoidance, and other anxiety behaviors.

Panic and Mitral Valve Prolapse

An association of mitral valve prolapse with panic was proposed in the past on the

basis of symptoms associated with prolapse (fluttering or palpitation experiences) in patients with panic disorder and
echocardiographic findings of prolapse
(Carney et al. 1990; Gorman et al. 1988).
Depending on the echocardiographic criteria employed, 5%–20% or more of patients with panic disorder have mitral
valve prolapse (Dager et al. 1986; Liberthson et al. 1986; Margraf et al. 1988). The
nature of the link between panic and mitral valve prolapse has been questioned,
however, because panic does not occur at
higher-than-expected rates in patients
with echocardiographic mitral valve prolapse and because mitral valve prolapse occurs in many other psychiatric disorder
populations.

Anxiety and Automatic Implantable Cardioverter-Defibrillators

Malignant ventricular arrhythmias account
for a substantial fraction of fatal events in
patients with ischemic heart disease and
congestive heart failure. The use of automatic implantable cardioverter-defibrillators (AICDs) reduces mortality (DiMarco
2003), but the experience of defibrillation
is unpleasant, likened to being "kicked
in the chest." Implantable defibrillator
discharges are associated with iatrogenic
anxiety, particularly in patients who experience repetitive, frequent, or early discharges after device implantation (Heller
et al. 1998). Early experience indicated a
50% incidence of psychiatric disorders after AICD implant (adjustment disorders,
major depression, and panic disorder)
(Morris et al. 1991), but the incidence of
psychopathology has apparently diminished over time (Crow et al. 1998). Although full-fledged posttraumatic stress
disorder appears to occur in fewer than
5% of AICD patients, symptoms of the
disorder such as avoidance, hypervigi-
lance, and reexperiencing are common,

especially if patients experience multiple
sequential shocks while conscious, which
they endure with a sense of helplessness. A
variety of other reactions to implanted
defibrillators have been described, including feelings of invulnerability, dependency, and withdrawal (Fricchione et al.
1989). Nevertheless, most patients with
implanted defibrillators report satisfaction
with their experience with the device.

Delirium and Neurocognitive Dysfunction

In the cardiac surgery intensive care unit
(ICU), delirium, like beauty, is very much
in the eye of the beholder. After coronary
bypass graft surgery and open-heart procedures, it is evident that many patients
have altered mental status with impaired
level of consciousness for some days.
Whether these patients are identified as
experiencing delirium appears to depend
on the sensitivity of the observer and on
the degree to which the patient's obtunda-
tion or agitation interferes with the clinical management of the postoperative state.
Pioneering studies in the 1960s of the psychiatric aspects of heart disease included
observations of the psychiatric complications of mitral commissurotomy and mitral and aortic valve replacement (Kornfeld
et al. 1965). These studies documented a
high prevalence of delirium in early open-
heart surgery patients, a finding that led to
changes in ICU design and attention to
preservation of sleep–wake cycles and appropriate use of narcotic analgesia in
open-heart surgery. Studies demonstrating the importance of emboli from valvular structures, intracardiac thrombus, and
the cardiopulmonary bypass circuit for
subsequent cognitive impairment led to
alterations of surgical technique and bypass circuit filters (S. Newman 1989; S.
Newman et al. 1988; Willner and Rodewald 1991).

TABLE 2–1.   Selected psychiatric side effects of cardiac drugs

Drug/Class	Effects
Digoxin	Visual hallucinations (classically, yellow rings around objects); delirium; depression
Beta-blockers	Fatigue, sexual dysfunction more common than depression per se; possibly less effect with atenolol
Alpha-blockers	Depression
Lidocaine	Agitation, delirium
Carvedilol	Fatigue, insomnia
Methyldopa	Depression, confusion, insomnia
Reserpine	Depression
Clonidine	Depression
ACE inhibitors	Mood elevation or depression (rare)
Pressors (dobutamine, milrinone, dopamine)	Rarely cause psychiatric effects
Angiotensin II receptor blockers	Rarely cause psychiatric effects
Amiodarone	Mood disorders secondary to thyroid effects
Diuretics	Hypokalemia, hyponatremia can result in anorexia, weakness, apathy

Note.   ACE=angiotensin-converting enzyme.

Frequency of adverse cerebral effects after coronary artery bypass graft (CABG) was estimated at 6% at hospital discharge in a multicenter study of 2,104 patients (Roach et al. 1996). Risk factors included advanced age, history of alcohol abuse, systolic hypertension, pulmonary disease, and aortic arch atherosclerosis. A longitudinal study of 261 patients found that 53% of post-CABG patients demonstrated neurocognitive impairment 1 week after surgery; the prevalence of impairment fell to 24% at 6 months (M.F. Newman et al. 2001) Predictors of delirium after openheart surgery include older age, cerebrovascular disease, prolonged sedation, and narcotic use.

Psychiatric Side Effects of Cardiac Drugs

A few cardiac medications have psychiatric side effects (see Table 2–1). An exhaustive review is available (Brown and Stoudemire 1998).

Cardiac Neurosis

Development of cardiac neurosis can occur after a patient experiences symptoms attributed to heart disease, whether or not actual heart disease exists. In some patients, apparent clinging to symptoms of disease and the resulting disability serve as an unconscious face-saving means to escape otherwise intolerable life stress related to work, troubled intimate relationships, or other demands. Remaining in the sick role provides respite from negative affects related to one's previous psychosocial role.

Sexual Dysfunction

Sexual dysfunction after the onset of heart disease occurs as a consequence of both physical and psychological factors. Physical factors include medications, comorbid medical conditions such as peripheral vascular disease and diabetes mellitus, and low cardiac output. Psychological factors include depression, anxiety, and fear of inducing a heart attack. Coital angina makes up 5% of angina attacks, but it is rare in patients who do not have angina during strenuous physical exertion (DeBusk 2003).

Effects of Psychological Factors on the Heart and Heart Disease Risk

Depression and Risk of Coronary Heart Disease

Community prospective studies of several different populations demonstrate that a history of depressive disorder or elevated symptoms of depression as evaluated by questionnaire ratings is associated with increased risk for the subsequent development of ischemic heart disease and for coronary disease death. In studies of American, Danish, and Swedish populations, the estimated magnitude of the risk of incident disease associated with depression is 1.5- to 2.0-fold (Anda et al. 1993; Barefoot and Schroll 1996; Barefoot et al. 1996). In patients with preexisting CAD, the risk of death for patients with depression is 3- to 4-fold higher than that for nondepressed coronary patients (Carney et al. 2003; Frasure-Smith et al. 1993, 1995a; Ladwig et al. 1991).

Following CABG surgery, depression predicted recurrent cardiac events at 12 months (Connerney et al. 2001), and a recent study with 817 patients showed that moderate to severe depression symptoms on the day before surgery or even mild depression persisting from baseline to 6-month follow-up after surgery was a predictor of mortality over mean follow-up of 5.2 years, with hazard ratios of more than 2.0 (Blumenthal et al. 2003).

Depression clearly adversely affects patients' perceptions of their heart disease status and quality of life. A recent study (Ruo et al. 2003) examined 1,024 patients with stable CAD to evaluate the contributions of depressive symptoms and objective measures of cardiac function to their health status. The patients who had depressive symptoms (20%) were more likely to report coronary disease symptom burden, physical limitations, diminished quality of life, and fair to poor health.

Mechanisms Linking Depression and Coronary Artery Disease

Candidate psychophysiological mechanisms linking depression to adverse coronary disease outcomes include platelet dysfunction, autonomic dysfunction, and abnormalities of inflammation (Carney et al. 2002). Persons with depression have increased platelet reactivity to orthostatic challenge (Musselman et al. 1996) and heightened circulating levels of two markers of platelet activation (Laghrissi-Thode et al. 1997; Pollock et al. 2000), implying that depressed patients have increased likelihood of thrombus formation in response to thrombogenic stimuli.

Several measures of cardiac autonomic control, derived from time series or power spectral analyses of heart rate variability, are also deranged in depression.

Inflammation has only recently been widely recognized as another process involved in the development of atherosclerosis and acute coronary events (Libby et al. 2002). Inflammatory cytokines are elevated in coronary disease patients, and the extent of elevation of specific markers such as interleukin-6 (IL-6), tumor necrosis factor–α (TNF-α) and C reactive protein (CRP), predicts coronary and cerebrovascular disease events and progression of heart failure (Cesari et al. 2003). Depression has been shown to be associated with increases in circulating levels of IL-6 and CRP (Miller et al. 2002). In addition, when compared with nondepressed control subjects, depressed patients with CHF have increased levels of TNF-α and soluble apoptosis mediators (Parissis et al. 2004).

Depression may also exert a negative effect on cardiovascular outcomes through its negative effects on adherence to treatment recommendations.

The ENRICHD and SADHART Trials

If depression exerts a negative effect on cardiac outcomes in coronary disease, a natural and important question is whether treatment of depression improves coronary disease outcomes. Two recent trials have investigated this subject—in particular, in patients with depression after MI. In the Sertraline AntiDepressant Heart Attack Randomized Trial (SADHART) (Glassman et al. 2002), 369 patients with major depression after hospitalization for unstable angina or acute MI were randomly assigned in a double-blind study to receive treatment with sertraline, 50–200 mg/day, or placebo. The primary goal of the trial was to assess the safety of sertraline treatment, but a secondary goal was to obtain an estimate of the effect on cardiac outcomes. Although the trial was not powered to adequately test an effect on morbidity or mortality (i.e., only seven deaths occurred during the follow-up period), sertraline was superior in absolute numerical terms to placebo in the rate of recurrent MI, mortality, heart failure, and angina, suggesting that a larger study of treatment effects on mortality would be worthwhile.

Concurrent with the SADHART trial, the ENRICHD (Enhancing Recovery in Coronary Heart Disease) trial was directed primarily at addressing the effects of treatment on mortality in post-MI patients (Writing Committee for the ENRICHD Investigators 2003). In ENRICHD, patients with low social support or depression after MI were enrolled in usual care or a cognitive-behavioral therapy (CBT) intervention group. Patients in the intervention group received 6–10 sessions of treatment over 6 months following acute MI. Mortality was assessed at 30-month follow-up. A confounding element of the trial was the use of antidepressants, usually sertraline, in both arms of the trial in patients with more severe depressive symptoms. The CBT intervention was not effective in reducing mortality, and subgroup analyses did not demonstrate an effect of the intervention even in the depression subgroup. Although the use of sertraline was not randomized, it was notable that all-cause mortality in the sertraline-treated patients was only 7.4%, compared with 15.3% and 10.6% in patients who did not receive drug therapy and patients treated with tricyclic antidepressants, respectively. However, sertraline did not reduce the risk of recurrent nonfatal MI.

Suggestive convergent evidence of a possible benefit of selective serotonin reuptake inhibitor (SSRI) treatment of depression on cardiovascular disease outcomes in cardiovascular disease patients comes from a study of prophylaxis of depression after stroke (Rasmussen et al. 2003). The study demonstrated a strong prophylactic effect of sertraline on the incidence of depression, and cardiovascular adverse events during the 12-month follow-up were reduced by two-thirds in the sertraline group, compared with the patients receiving placebo.

Depression Effects on CHF Outcome

Depression also appears to carry increased mortality risk in patients with CHF. In one cohort, major depression more than doubled the risk of 3-month and 1-year mortality (Jiang et al. 2001), although the effect did not quite achieve the level of statistical significance after adjustment for other medical variables associated with mortality risk.

A multicenter study of 460 outpatients with CHF showed that, compared with nondepressed patients, patients with significant depression symptoms had both worse health status at baseline and more deterioration in health status over short-term follow-up. Depression predicted worsening of heart failure symptoms, physical and social functioning, and quality of life. Depression symptoms were the strongest predictor of decline in health status (Rumsfeld et al. 2003).

Anxiety and CAD Risk

There is little evidence in nonclinical samples that anxiety symptoms increase the risk of coronary disease or heart-disease-related mortality, with the exception of sudden cardiac death. Two prospective epidemiological studies do demonstrate an association of anxiety with sudden cardiac death. In a study involving 33,999 middle-aged male health professionals with 2-year follow-up, there were 168 new cases of coronary heart disease, including 40 fatal and 128 nonfatal events. Nonfatal events were not associated with anxiety, but the risk of fatal coronary heart disease increased with the level of phobic anxiety, and high phobic anxiety carried a three-fold increased relative risk of fatality compared with the risk in subjects with low anxiety; the excess risk was limited to cases of sudden cardiac death, with a sixfold increased risk associated with high anxiety (Kawachi et al. 1994a). The second study assessed 2,280 men free of chronic disease at baseline, with 32-year follow-up. Subjects completed an anxiety symptom rating scale at baseline. Men with anxiety scores above the ninety-eighth percentile had a 4.46-fold increased risk of sudden cardiac death and a 1.94-fold increased risk of fatal coronary heart disease, but no excess risk for angina or nonfatal MI. These hazard ratios are strongly suggestive of an association of anxiety and sudden cardiac death (Kawachi et al. 1994b).

Anger, Type A Behavior, and Hostility

Type A behavior pattern—characterized by anger, impatience, aggravation, and irritability—was linked to incident coronary disease in men in the 1970s. The Western Collaborative Group Study of more than 3,000 middle-aged men demonstrated that type A behavior was associated with a more than twofold increased risk of incident MI and of fatal coronary events (Rosenman et al. 1975). One of the few large-scale clinical trials in psychosomatic cardiology, the Recurrent Coronary Prevention Project, examined the effect of group counseling to reduce type A behavior pattern on mortality and recurrent infarction. Patients were survivors of an acute MI and were randomly assigned to usual care or added type A behavior modification groups. Follow-up in 4.5 years demonstrated a significant reduction in recurrent infarction in those assigned to type A counseling (M. Friedman et al. 1986). Subsequent studies of type A behavior pattern and CAD have been inconclusive or negative (Booth-Kewley and Friedman 1987).

Anger and hostility, considered as "toxic components" within the type A concept, have also been studied as risk factors for coronary disease but with mixed results in longitudinal observations (Barefoot et al. 1994, 1995).

Acute Mental Stress

George Engel, who championed the biopsychosocial model in medicine, provided vivid examples from the news media of acute mental stress preceding acute coronary events (Engel 1976), and epidemiological studies of disasters have helped to confirm the relationship of acute stress to risk for sudden cardiac death (Leor et al. 1996). The Northridge, California, earthquake in 1994 caused a surge in sudden cardiac deaths over the subsequent 2 days in individuals who were not physically endangered by the earthquake but resided in the immediate area (Leor et al. 1996). A preliminary, similar finding has been reported in the aftermath of the destruction of the World Trade Center in New York in 2001 (Steinberg et al. 2004). Acute stress in the laboratory, provoked by standardized tasks such as mirror-drawing, the Stroop color word test, mental arithmetic, video games, and public speaking, results in elevation in heart rate and blood pressure and alteration in indices of cardiac autonomic regulation, with diminished parasympathetic and elevated sympathetic activation, in both healthy volunteers and patients with CAD (Blumenthal et al. 1995; Jiang et al. 1996; Manuck and Krantz 1986; Rozanski et al. 1988, 1999; Sheps et al. 2002). In addition, coronary vasospasm appears to be a mechanism of mental stress–induced ischemia in at least some cases (Yeung et al. 1991). The technique of ecological momentary assessment has been used to demonstrate that emotional arousal, and especially anger during daily events, is associated with similar alterations in hemodynamic and autonomic state, and it has been estimated that acute emotional stress is a trigger for up to 20% to 30% of acute coronary events (Muller et al. 1994).

Chronic Psychosocial Stress: The INTERHEART Study

There has also been interest in looking at the effects of chronic psychosocial stressors on risk of heart disease. The INTERHEART study used a case-control design with 11,119 patients with a first myocardial infarction and 13,648 control subjects from 52 different countries to investigate the relationship of psychosocial factors to risk of myocardial infarction. The investigators discovered that people with myo-cardial infarction reported higher prevalence of the studied stress factors (work, home, financial, and major life events), suggesting that these factors are associated with increased risk of acute myocardial infarction (Rosengren et al. 2004).

Some research has been aimed at modifying these risk factors. A large meta-analysis of a variety of health education and stress reduction interventions in patients with CAD concluded that these interventions reduce the incidence of recurrent MI (29% reduction) and death (34% reduction) at 2- to 10-year follow-up. The mechanism of the effect is unclear, and more research is needed (Dusseldorp et al. 1999).

Diagnostic Issues

The most frequent problem in psychiatric diagnosis for cardiac patients is the attribution of symptoms of depression to the underlying cardiac disease or to a "normal" reaction to the illness, with the resultant underdiagnosis of depression. In an analysis of the 222 acute MI patients included in the landmark Montreal Heart Institute depression-mortality study, the investigators considered the specificity of various symptoms from the depression criteria set for a diagnosis of depression. Sleep disturbance and appetite disturbance did not help to distinguish between patients who met criteria for depressive episode and those who did not (i.e., these symptoms were common in both depressed and nondepressed patients), but fatigue and especially sadness and loss of pleasure occurred almost exclusively in patients who met criteria for a major depressive episode (Lesperance et al. 1996). This suggests that patients reporting somatic symptoms of depression should be evaluated for the presence of the cardinal mood and interest symptoms, and they should be considered depressed if these symptoms are also present. Patients with advanced heart failure often develop appetite loss and cachexia, but in the absence of loss of self-esteem, interest in ordinarily interesting events, or depressed mood, these patients should not be diagnosed with a depressive disorder.

Paroxysmal supraventricular tachycardia (PSVT) occurs in young and middle-aged adults and may manifest with symptoms of shortness of breath, chest discomfort, and apprehension. Because these features may overlap with those of generalized anxiety symptoms and panic attacks, there is a significant risk of misdiagnosis.

Atypical Chest Pain and Palpitations

Typical anginal chest pain in CAD occurs with exertion or after eating; is not exacerbated by palpation of the chest or inspiration; is described as dull, pressurelike, or burning, rather than sharp or stabbing; and is experienced across the precordium rather than in a pinpoint area of the left side of the chest. Many patients present for evaluation of atypical chest pain. While atypical features do not rule out a diagnosis of CAD, 40%–70% of patients with no history of documented CAD and few CAD risk factors have panic disorder, somatoform disorders, or depression (Alexander et al. 1994; Fleet et al. 2000). In the absence of CAD, characteristics of chest pain patients predicting panic disorder include female sex, atypical chest pain quality, younger age, lower education and income, and high self-reported anxiety (Dammen et al. 1999; Huffman and Pollack 2003).

Psychiatric disorders are also common in patients complaining of palpitations. In one study using structured diagnostic interviews and self-report questionnaires for patients undergoing ambulatory electrocardiogram (ECG) monitoring, the lifetime prevalence of any disorder was 45%, and 25% of the patients had a current disorder (Barsky et al. 1994b).

Special Issues

Heart Transplantation

Heart transplantation has been the treatment of last resort for patients with severe heart failure, and occasionally for patients with intractable recurrent myocardial ischemia or ventricular arrhythmias, for the past 2 decades. Patients eligible for heart transplantation typically have an expected survival of less than 2 years unless they receive a transplant. With transplantation, expected 5-year survival is now better than 75%. Complications can occur, and the care regimen for heart transplant patients is complicated, especially in the first few months after surgery, so transplant programs generally screen patients and exclude from candidacy those with absolute contraindications or excessive relative contraindications.

Patients awaiting transplantation often experience depression symptoms, because they perceive themselves as helpless to fundamentally affect their own chances of survival. During the waiting period, depression is often enhanced by a sense of guilt over wishes for the death of a suitable donor. Before, at the time of evaluation, and up to the time of receiving a transplant, patients may also display variable levels of denial of the seriousness of their illness and ambivalence about undergoing transplant surgery.

Following heart transplant surgery, patients receive multiple immunosuppressive antirejection medications, along with vitamins; minerals; antibacterial, antifungal, and antiviral medications; and treatments as needed for hypertension, arrhythmias, fluid retention, or other conditions. Most patients experience an initial euphoria at awakening from surgery, knowing that they have now been delivered from end-stage heart failure, but the emotional reaction depends in part on the patient's previous expectations in comparison with the state of subjective well-being in the early days after surgery. Positive feelings tend to subside as complications occur and as the patient settles into the work of rehabilitation and adjustment to the new medication regimen.

Psychiatric complications after heart transplantation are fairly common. In addition to postoperative delirium, steroid-induced mood disorders and depression not attributable to steroids occur in perhaps 20%–40% of patients in the first year after surgery (Shapiro 1990; Shapiro and Kornfeld 1989).

Hypertension

The relationship of psychological factors to the development of hypertension has been a subject of controversy, with mixed findings in large-scale observational studies.

In a cross-sectional correlation of psychological variables with mild hypertension measured in clinic visits or by ambulatory monitoring in 283 middle-aged men, there were no significant differences between normotensive and hypertensive men in any of the psychological variables assessed, including type A behavior, state and trait anger, anger expression, anxiety, psychological distress, locus of control, or attributional style (R. Friedman et al. 2001).

A 15-year prospective study of psychosocial risk factors for hypertension based on a follow-up of over 3,000 young white and black adults from four metropolitan areas of the United States used multivariate analysis and found that two components of type A behavior—namely, "time urgency–impatience" and "hostility"—were each associated with almost double the rate of incident hypertension at 15-year

follow-up. In contrast, anxiety symptoms, depression symptoms, and "achievement-striving-competitiveness" (another type A component) did not predict hypertension (Yan et al. 2003).

In another large longitudinal study, however, results differed. A population-based cohort of 3,310 normotensive persons without chronic diseases from the NHANES I Epidemiologic Follow-Up Study was followed for four waves, up to 22 years. Using combined symptoms of depression and anxiety ("negative affect") as the primary independent variable, increased negative affect was associated with increased risk for hypertension (Jonas and Lando 2000).

The main psychiatric consequence of hypertension seems to be long-term neurocognitive impairment and increased risk of dementia (Frishman 2002). Treatment that successfully controls blood pressure reduces the risk (Forette et al. 2002; Guo et al. 1999; Launer et al. 1995). The data demonstrate that dihydropyridine calcium channel blockers reduce the risk of dementia of probable Alzheimer's disease, as well as vascular or mixed dementia, and improve or maintain cognitive function in patients with impaired cognition.

Treatment Issues

Psychotherapy

Psychological reactions to the experience of heart disease include feelings of anxiety and sadness, concerns about survival and well-being, and concerns about effects on social roles and relationships and the impact on loved ones. Denial is nearly universal as an initial reaction to illness, and it can be helpful in staving off depressed and anxious mood or hurtful because of nonadherence to the treatment program. Conversely, preoccupation with disease can lead to abnormal illness behavior, unnecessary disability, and impaired quality of life. Few systematic studies of psychotherapy have been reported that specifically targeted psychological symptoms or psychiatric disorders in heart patients.

The ENRICHD trial tested the effects of a CBT intervention versus usual care in patients who had a recent MI and either low social support and/or major depression or minor depression with a history of prior major depression in a randomized trial. The trial demonstrated a modest benefit of the CBT intervention on measures of social support and depression. However, the improvement on these measures seen in the usual-care group was higher than expected, so that the effect of treatment, although statistically significant, was of small magnitude (Writing Committee for the ENRICHD Investigators 2003).

As described previously, the Recurrent Coronary Prevention Project tested the effect of group type A behavior modification on the extent of type A behavior in a cohort of post-MI patients on recurrent coronary events (M. Friedman et al. 1986). In retrospect, although the term was not used at the time, this was clearly a cognitive-behavioral psychotherapy intervention. The intervention had a strong beneficial effect on type A behavior as rated using a videotaped structured interview for the assessment of type A behavior.

Interpersonal psychotherapy (IPT) of depression focuses on present-day interpersonal problems linked to depressed mood, such as interpersonal disputes, grief after object loss, interpersonal deficits, and social role transitions. One such role transition may occur with the change in social role imposed by development of a chronic or acute medical illness (Klerman et al. 1984). Therefore IPT would seem to be readily applicable to the treatment of patients who experience depression after the onset or exacerbation of heart disease. Although a case has been reported (Stuart and Cole 1996), controlled trials of IPT in heart disease patients have not appeared.

Psychopharmacological Treatment

Common adverse cardiac effects of psychiatric drugs are shown in Table 2–2.

TABLE 2–2. Selected cardiac side effects of psychotropic drugs

Drug	Cardiac effects
Lithium	Sinus node dysfunction and arrest
SSRIs	Slowing of heart rate; occasional sinus bradycardia or sinus arrest
TCAs	Orthostatic hypotension; atrioventricular conduction disturbance; type IA antiarrhythmic effect; proarrhythmia in overdose and in setting of ischemia
MAOIs	Orthostatic hypotension
Phenothiazines	Orthostatic hypotension; QT interval prolongation; rare instances of torsades de pointes
Second-generation antipsychotics	Variable; QT interval prolongation
Carbamazepine	Type IA antiarrhythmic effects; AV block
Cholinesterase inhibitors	Decreased heart rate

Note. AV=atrioventricular; MAOI=monoamine oxidase inhibitor; SSRI=selective serotonin reuptake inhibitor; TCA=tricyclic antidepressant.

Antidepressants

Antidepressants must be used in therapeutically effective doses in cardiac patients with depression, and it is counterproductive to use inadequate doses out of fear of side effects or prolongation of metabolism. Unless the patient has severe right heart failure resulting in hepatic congestion, ascites, and jaundice, it is unlikely that metabolism of oral psychotropic medication (except for lithium) will be substantially impaired because of heart disease.

Tricyclic antidepressants (TCAs) cause orthostatic hypotension, cardiac conduction delay (bundle branch block or complete AV nodal block), and, in overdose, ventricular arrhythmias (ventricular premature depolarization, ventricular tachycardia, and ventricular fibrillation). QRS interval prolongation results from interference with phase 1 depolarization (slow Na^+ channel activity) of the action potential across the membrane of the specialized conduction tissue of the ventricle. Prolongation of the QT interval is predominantly caused by prolongation of the QRS interval, and ventricular tachycardia or fibrillation can occur if marked prolongation of the QT interval (over 500 msec) results in the R-on-T phenomenon. Nortriptyline and desipramine tend to cause less orthostatic hypotension than tertiary-amine tricyclic drugs and are better tolerated by patients with cardiac disease (Roose and Glassman 1989; Roose et al. 1986, 1987, 1989).

TCAs have quinidine-like effects on cardiac conduction and are classified as type 1A antiarrhythmic agents. Drugs of this class have been shown to increase rather than decrease mortality in post-MI patients with premature ventricular contractions (CAST Investigators 1989; CAST II Investigators 1992; Morganroth and Goin 1991), an effect believed to be mediated by episodic myocardial ischemia (Lynch et al. 1987). Consequently, TCAs should generally not be used as first-line agents for treatment of depression in ischemic heart disease patients.

SSRIs have little to no cardiac effect in healthy subjects. The most commonly observed effect is slowing of heart rate, generally by a clinically insignificant 1–2 beats/minute. The combination of beta-adrenergic blockade and serotonin reuptake inhibitors may result in additive effects on slowing of heart rate with increased risk of symptoms.

In patients with preexisting heart disease, the effects of SSRIs on cardiac function have been evaluated in several studies (Sheline et al. 1997). In the SADHART study (Glassman et al. 2002), sertraline had no effect on heart rate, blood pressure, arrhythmias, ejection fraction, or cardiac conduction, and adverse events were rare. Sertraline was effective for treatment of depression in those patients with a prior history of depression, but it did not differ from placebo in response rate for those patients with no prior history of depression.

The cardiovascular effects of other antidepressants have been less fully studied, especially in patients with cardiac disease. Bupropion appears to have few cardiovascular effects but may cause hypertension in some patients (Roose et al. 1991). Clinical experience with mirtazapine in patients with hypertension has also demonstrated instances of worsening hypertension, but the frequency of this adverse effect is unknown. Monoamine oxidase inhibitors (MAOIs) cause hypotension and orthostatic hypotension; dietary indiscretions resulting in high circulating levels of tyramine cause hypertensive crises. Consequently, there has been little interest in use of MAOIs in patients with heart disease.

Antipsychotics

Antipsychotics are used in cardiac disease patients in cases of comorbid schizophrenia or other psychotic disorders and in the management of delirium in acute cardiac care settings, such as after cardiac surgery or in ICU management of pulmonary edema, arrhythmias, or acute MI.

For chronically psychotic patients with heart disease, the choice of antipsychotic is based on side-effect profile. The principal cardiovascular effects of antipsychotic agents are orthostatic hypotension and QT interval prolongation. Orthostatic hypotension secondary to antipsychotic drugs is related to their α-adrenergic receptor– blocking effect, seen especially with the low-potency antipsychotic agents such as chlorpromazine and often accompanied by sedative effects. More attention has been paid to the less common but much more dramatic and dangerous side effect of cardiac arrest secondary to ventricular tachyarrhythmias in patients on antipsychotic drugs. A case-control study has demonstrated that current use of antipsychotics in a general population is associated with an increased risk of sudden cardiac death even at low dose and for indications other than schizophrenia (Straus et al. 2004). The characteristic tachyarrhythmia is *torsades de pointes*, a polymorphic tachycardia with the appearance of "twisting of the points" of the QRS complex (Glassman and Bigger 2001). Risk factors for torsade include QT interval prolongation of more than 500 msec, family history of sudden death, female sex, hypokalemia, hypomagnesemia, and low ejection fraction. Thioridazine is the agent most commonly associated with torsade and sudden cardiac death. Intravenous haloperidol is frequently employed in delirious open-heart surgery patients, and although it does have the potential to prolong the QT interval, its use in dosages up to 1,000 mg/24 hours has been reported without complications (Tesar et al. 1985). Clearly, electrocardiographic monitoring is important in ICU settings, and patients with a corrected QT interval (QTc) greater than 450 msec should be closely monitored. A QTc interval over 500 msec is generally considered a contraindication to use of haloperidol and other QT-prolonging agents.

Not all antipsychotic drugs have been associated with sudden cardiac death or QT prolongation, and the correlation of QT interval prolongation with risk of sudden death is not exact. For example, ziprasidone prolongs the QT interval but has not been associated with sudden death. A case-control study conducted in nursing home residents demonstrated that the conventional antipsychotics were associated with a nearly twofold increase in risk of hospitalization for ventricular arrhythmias, whereas no increased risk was associated with the use of atypical antipsychotics (Liperoti et al. 2005). In considering the use of drugs that may prolong the QT interval, factors to be reviewed in the history include familial long QT syndrome; family or personal history of sudden cardiac death, syncope, or unexplained seizure; arrhythmias; personal history of hypertension; medications that prolong the QT interval; medications that may interfere with metabolism of other QT-prolonging agents; valvular heart disease; and bradycardia (Al-Khatib et al. 2003).

Another consideration regarding these medications is the recent mandate by the U.S. Food and Drug Administration (FDA) requiring manufacturers of atypical antipsychotics to add a black box warning noting that these drugs are associated with an increased risk of death in elderly patients with dementia-related behavior problems. The reviewed studies included 5,106 patients and demonstrated a death rate of 4.5% in drug-treated patients, compared with 2.6% in those taking placebo. The causes of these deaths were either heart-related events, such as heart failure or sudden death, or infections, such as pneumonia. As a result of these findings, clinicians must consider carefully the potential risks

TABLE 2–3. Selected psychotropic drug interactions with cardiovascular drugs

Psychotropic agent	Cardiovascular agent	Effect
SSRIs	Beta-blockers	Additive bradycardic effects
SSRIs	Warfarin	Increased bleeding risk, despite little effect on INR
MAOIs	Epinephrine, dopamine	Hypertension
Lithium	Thiazide diuretics	Increased lithium level
TCAs	Guanethidine	Reduced antihypertensive efficacy of guanethidine
TCAs	Type IA antiarrhythmic agents, amiodarone	Prolonged QT interval, increased AV block
Lithium	ACE inhibitors	Increased lithium level
Phenothiazines	Beta-blockers	Hypotension

Note. ACE=angiotensin-converting enzyme; AV=atrioventricular; INR=international normalized ratio; MAOI=monoamine oxidase inhibitor; SSRI=selective serotonin reuptake inhibitor; TCA=tricyclic antidepressant.

and benefits of using these medications when treating patients with dementia and associated behavioral dyscontrol.

Anxiolytics

Benzodiazepines have no specific cardiac effects. Reduction of anxiety tends to reduce sympathetic nervous system activation and, therefore, to slow heart rate, reduce myocardial work, and reduce myocardial irritability.

Stimulants

Stimulants are often useful for treating of depressed, medically ill patients, particularly those with pronounced apathy, fatigue, or psychomotor slowing. At dosages of 5–30 mg/day, dextroamphetamine and methylphenidate are well tolerated by heart disease patients, including patients with cardiac arrhythmias and angina (Masand and Tesar 1996), and have no effects on heart rate and blood pressure.

Lithium

Lithium occasionally causes sinus node dysfunction and even sinus arrest (Mitch-ell and Mackenzie 1982). Generally, even in patients with heart disease with reduced cardiac output, lithium can be safely used by adjusting the dosage downward. Caution is necessary for patients taking diuretics, especially thiazides, and those on salt-restricted diets.

Other Mood Stabilizers

Valproic acid and lamotrigine have no cardiovascular effects. Carbamazepine resembles TCAs in having a quinidine-like type IA antiarrhythmic effect and may cause atrioventricular conduction disturbances.

Electroconvulsive Therapy (ECT)

ECT has been used safely in patients with ischemic heart disease, heart failure, and heart transplants. Acute MI or recent malignant tachyarrhythmias are relatively strong contraindications.

Cardiac–Psychiatric Drug Interactions

A few drug interactions between psychotropic and cardiovascular drugs are worth noting (see Table 2–3).

References

Alexander PJ, Prabhu SG, Krishnamoorthy ES, et al: Mental disorders in patients with noncardiac chest pain. Acta Psychiatr Scand 89:291–293, 1994

Al-Khatib SM, LaPointe NMA, Kramer JM, et al: What clinicians should know about the QT interval. JAMA 289:2120–2127, 2003

Anda R, Williamson D, Jones D, et al: Depressed affect, hopelessness, and the risk of ischemic heart disease in a cohort of U.S. adults. Epidemiology 4:285–294, 1993

Barefoot JC, Patterson JC, Haney TL, et al: Hostility in asymptomatic men with angiographically confirmed coronary artery disease. Am J Cardiol 74:439–442, 1994

Barefoot JC, Larsen S, Von der Lieth L, et al: Hostility, incidence of acute myocardial infarction, and mortality in a sample of older Danish men and women. Am J Epidemiol 142:477–484, 1995

Barefoot J, Schroll M: Symptoms of depression, acute myocardial infarction, and total mortality in a community sample. Circulation 93:1976–1980, 1996

Barefoot JC, Helms MJ, Mark DB, et al: Depression and long term mortality risk in patients with coronary artery disease. Am J Cardiol 78:613–617, 1996

Barsky AJ, Cleary PD, Coeytaux RR, et al: Psychiatric disorders in medical outpatients complaining of palpitations. J Gen Intern Med 9:306–313, 1994b

Blumenthal JA, Jiang W, Waugh RA, et al: Mental stress-induced ischemia in the laboratory and ambulatory ischemia during daily life. Association and hemodynamic features. Circulation 92:2102–2108, 1995

Blumenthal JA, Lett HS, Babyak MA, et al: Depression as a risk factor for mortality after coronary artery bypass surgery. Lancet 362:604–609, 2003

Booth-Kewley S, Friedman HS: Psychological predictors of heart disease: a quantitative review. Psychol Bull 101:343–362, 1987

Brown TM, Stoudemire A: Cardiovascular agents, in Psychiatric Side Effects of Prescription and Over the Counter Drugs. Washington, DC, American Psychiatric Press, 1998, pp 209–238

Carney RM, Freedland KE, Ludbrook PA, et al: Major depression, panic disorder, and mitral valve prolapse in patients who complain of chest pain. Am J Med 89:757–760, 1990

Carney RM, Freedland KE, Miller GE, et al: Depression as a risk factor for cardiac mortality and morbidity. A review of potential mechanisms. J Psychosom Res 53:897–902, 2002

Carney RM, Blumenthal JA, Catellier D, et al: Depression as a risk factor for mortality after acute myocardial infarction. Am J Cardiol 92:1277–1281, 2003

Cassem NH: The person confronting death, in The New Harvard Guide to Psychiatry. Edited by Nicholi AM Jr. Cambridge, MA, Harvard University Press, 1985, pp 728–758

CAST Investigators: Preliminary report: effect of encainide and flecainide on mortality in a randomized trial of arrhythmia suppression after myocardial infarction. N Engl J Med 321: 406–412, 1989

CAST II Investigators: Effect of the antiarrhythmic agent moricizine on survival after myocardial infarction. New Engl J Med 327:227–233, 1992

Cesari M, Penninx BWJH, Newman AB, et al: Inflammatory markers and onset of cardiovascular events: results from the health ABC study. Circulation 108:2317–2322, 2003

Connerney I, Shapiro PA, McLaughlin JS, et al: Relation between depression after coronary artery bypass surgery and 12-month outcome: a prospective study. Lancet 358:1766–1771, 2001

Crow SJ, Collins J, Justic M, et al: Psychopathology following cardioverter defibrillator implantation. Psychosomatics 39: 305–310, 1998

Dager SR, Comess KA, Dunner DL: Differentiation of anxious patients by two-dimensional echocardiographic evaluation of the mitral valve. Am J Psychiatry 143:533–535, 1986

Dammen T, Ekeberg O, Arnesen H, et al: The detection of panic disorder in chest pain patients. Gen Hosp Psychiatry 21:323–332, 1999

DeBusk RF: Sexual activity in patients with angina. JAMA 290: 3129–3132, 2003

DiMarco JP: Implantable cardioverter-defibrillators. N Engl J Med 349:1836–1847, 2003

Dusseldorp E, Van Elderen T, Maes S, et al: A meta-analysis of psychoeducational programs for coronary heart disease patients. Health Psychol 18:506–519, 1999

Engel GL: Psychologic factors in instantaneous cardiac death. N Engl J Med 294:664–665, 1976

Faris R, Purcell H, Henein MY, et al: Clinical depression is common and significantly associated with reduced survival in patients with non-ischaemic heart failure. Eur J Heart Fail 4:541–551, 2002

Fleet R, Lavoie K, Beitman PD: Is panic disorder associated with coronary artery disease? J Psychosom Res 48:347–356, 2000

Flockhart DA: Drug interactions. Indianapolis, IN, Indiana University School of Medicine, Division of Clinical Pharmacology, 2003. Available at: http://www.drug-interactions.com. Accessed December 2003

Forette F, Seux ML, Staessen JA, et al: Systolic Hypertension in Europe Investigators. The prevention of dementia with antihypertensive treatment: new evidence from the Systolic Hypertension in Europe (Syst-Eur) study. Arch Intern Med 162: 2046–2052, 2002

Frasure-Smith N, Lesperance F, Talajic M: Depression following myocardial infarction. Impact on 6-month survival. JAMA 270: 1819–1825, 1993

Frasure-Smith N, Lesperance F, Talajic M: Depression and 18-month prognosis following myocardial infarction. Circulation 91:999–1005, 1995a

Frasure-Smith N, Lesperance F, Talajic M: The impact of negative emotions on prognosis following myocardial infarction: is it more than depression? Health Psychol 14:388–398, 1995b

Frasure-Smith N, Lesperance F, Gravel G, et al: Social support, depression, and mortality during the first year after myocardial infarction. Circulation 101:1919–1924, 2000

Freedland KE, Carney RM, Davila-Roman VG, et al: Major depression and survival in congestive heart failure. Psychosom Med 60:118, 1998

Fricchione GL, Olson LC, Vlay SC: Psychiatric syndromes in patients with the automatic internal cardioverter defibrillator: Anxiety, psychological dependence, abuse, and withdrawal. Am Heart J 117:1411–1414, 1989

Friedman M, Thoresen CE, Gill JJ, et al: Alteration of type A behavior and its effect on cardiac recurrences in post myocardial infarction patients: summary results of the recurrent coronary prevention project. Am Heart J 112:653–665, 1986

Friedman R, Schwartz JE, Schnall PL, et al: Psychological variables in hypertension: relationship to casual or ambulatory blood pressure in men. Psychosom Med 63:19–31, 2001

Frishman WH: Are antihypertensive agents protective against dementia? A review of clinical and preclinical data. Heart Dis 4:380–386, 2002

Glassman AH, Bigger JT Jr: Antipsychotic drugs: prolonged QTc interval, Torsade de Pointes and sudden death. Am J Psychiatry 158:1774–1782, 2001

Glassman AH, Shapiro PA: Depression and the course of coronary artery disease. Am J Psychiatry 155:4–11, 1998

Glassman AH, O'Connor CM, Califf RM, et al: Sertraline treatment of major depression in patients with acute MI or unstable angina. JAMA 288:701–709, 2002

Gorman JM, Goetz RR, Fyer M, et al: The mitral valve prolapse-panic disorder connection. Psychosom Med 50:114–122, 1988

Guo Z, Fratiglioni L, Zhu L, et al: Occurrence and progression of dementia in a community population aged 75 years and older: relationship of antihypertensive medication use. Arch Neurol 56:991–996, 1999

Hance M, Carney RM, Freedland KE, et al: Depression in patients with coronary heart disease. Gen Hosp Psychiatry 18:61–65, 1996

Heller SS, Ormont MA, Lidagoster LC, et al: Psychosocial outcome after ICD implantation: a current perspective. Pacing Clin Electrophysiol 21:1207–1215, 1998

Huffman JC, Pollack MH: Predicting panic disorder among patients with chest pain: an analysis of the literature. Psychosomatics 44:222–236, 2003

Jiang W, Babyak M, Krantz DS, et al: Mental stress-induced myocardial ischemia and cardiac events. JAMA 275:1651–1656, 1996

Jiang W, Alexander J, Christopher E, et al: Relationship of depression to increased risk of mortality and rehospitalization in patients with congestive heart failure. Arch Intern Med 161:1849–1856, 2001

Jonas BS, Lando JF: Negative affect as a prospective risk factor for hypertension. Psychosom Med 62:188–196, 2000

Kawachi I, Colditz GA, Ascherio A, et al: Prospective study of phobic anxiety and risk of coronary heart disease in men. Circulation 89:1992–1997, 1994a

Kawachi I, Sparrow D, Vokonas PS, et al: Symptoms of anxiety and risk of coronary heart disease. The normative aging study. Circulation 90:2225–2229, 1994b

Kessler RC, Berglund P, Demler O, et al: The epidemiology of major depressive disorder: results from the national comorbidity survey replication (NCS-R). JAMA 289:3095–3105, 2003

Klerman GL, Weissman MM, Rounsaville BJ, et al: Interpersonal psychotherapy of depression. New York, Basic Books, 1984

Kornfeld DS, Zimberg S, Malm JR: Psychiatric complications of open heart surgery. N Engl J Med 273:287–292, 1965

Ladwig KH, Kieser M, Konig J, et al: Affective disorders and survival after acute myocardial infarction. Results from the post-infarction late potential study. Eur Heart J 12:959–964, 1991

Laghrissi-Thode F, Wagner WR, Pollack BG, et al: Elevated platelet factor 4 and beta-thromboglobulin plasma levels in depressed patients with ischemic heart disease. Biol Psychiatry 42:290–295, 1997

Launer LJ, Masaki K, Petrovitch H, et al: The association between midlife blood pressure levels and late-life cognitive function. The Honolulu-Asia Aging Study. JAMA 274:1846–1851, 1995

Leor WJ, Poole WK, Kloner RA: Sudden cardiac death triggered by an earthquake. N Engl J Med 334:413–419, 1996

Lesperance F, Frasure-Smith N, Talajic M: Major depression before and after myocardial infarction: its nature and consequences. Psychosom Med 58:99–110, 1996

Levenson JL, Mishra A, Bauernfeind RA: Denial and medical outcome in unstable angina. Psychosom Med 51:27–35, 1989

Levine J, Warrenberg S, Kerns R: The role of denial in recovery from coronary heart disease. Psychosom Med 49:109–117, 1987

Libby P, Ridker PM, Maseri A: Inflammation and atherosclerosis. Circulation 105:1135–1143, 2002

Liberthson R, Sheehan DV, King ME, et al: The prevalence of mitral valve prolapse in patients with panic disorders. Am J Psychiatry 143:511–515, 1986

Liperoti R, Gambassi G, Lapane KL, et al: Conventional and atypical antipsychotics and the risk of hospitalization for ventricular arrhythmias or cardiac arrest. Arch Intern Med 165:696–701, 2005

Luutonen S, Holm H, Salminen JK, et al: Inadequate treatment of depression after myocardial infarction. Acta Psychiatr Scand 106:434–439, 2002

Lynch JJ, Dicarlo LA, Montgomery DG, et al: Effects of flecainide acetate on ventricular tachyarrhythmia and fibrillation in dogs with recent myocardial infarction. Pharmacology 35:181–193, 1987

Manuck SB, Krantz DS: Psychophysiologic re-activity in coronary heart disease and essential hypertension, in Handbook of Stress, Reactivity, and Cardiovascular Disease. Edited by Matthews KA, Weiss SM, Detre T, et al. New York, Wiley, 1986

Margraf J, Ehlers A, Roth WT: Mitral valve prolapse and panic disorder: a review of their relationship. Psychosom Med 50:93–113, 1988

Masand PS, Tesar GE: Use of stimulants in the medically ill. Psychiatr Clin North Am 19:515–548, 1996

Miller GE, Stetler CA, Carney RM, et al: Clinical depression and inflammatory risk markers for coronary heart disease. Am J Cardiology 90:1279–1283, 2002

Mitchell JE, Mackenzie TB: Cardiac effects of lithium therapy in man: a review. J Clin Psychiatry 43:47–51, 1982

Morganroth J, Goin JE: Quinidine-related mortality in the short-to-medium-term treatment of ventricular arrhythmias. Circulation 84:1977–1983, 1991

Morris PL, Badger J, Chmielewski C, et al: Psychiatric morbidity following implantation of the automatic implantable cardioverter defibrillator. Psychosomatics 32:58–64, 1991

Muller JE, Abela GS, Nesto RW, et al: Triggers, acute risk factors and vulnerable plaques: the lexicon of a new frontier. J Am Coll Cardiol 23:809–813, 1994

Musselman DL, Tomer A, Manatunga AK, et al: Exaggerated platelet reactivity in major depression. Am J Psychiatry 153:1313–1317, 1996

Newman MF, Kirchner JL, Phillips-Bute B, et al: Longitudinal assessment of neurocognitive function after coronary-artery bypass surgery. N Engl J Med 344:395–402, 2001

Newman S: Incidence and nature of neuropsychological morbidity following cardiac surgery. Perfusion 4:93–100, 1989

Newman S, Pugsley W, Klinger L, et al: Neuropsychological consequences of circulatory arrest with hypothermia. J Clin Exp Neuropsychol 11:529–538, 1988

Parissis JT, Adamopoulos S, Rigas A, et al: Comparison of circulating proinflammatory cytokines and soluble apoptosis mediators in patients with chronic heart failure versus without symptoms of depression. Am J Cardiol 94:1326–1328, 2004

Pollock BG, Laghrissi-Thode F, Wagner WR: Evaluation of platelet activation in depressed patients with ischemic heart disease after paroxetine or nortriptyline treatment. J Clin Psychopharmacol 20:137–140, 2000

Rasmussen A, Lunde M, Poulsen DL, et al: A double-blind, placebo-controlled study of sertraline in the prevention of depression in stroke patients. Psychosomatics 44:216–221, 2003

Roach GW, Kanchuger M, Mangano CM, et al: Adverse cerebral outcomes after coronary bypass surgery. N Engl J Med 335:1857–1863, 1996

Roose SP, Glassman AH: Cardiovascular effects of tricyclic antidepressants in depressed patients with and without heart disease. J Clin Psychiatry 50:S1–S18, 1989

Roose SP, Glassman AH, Giardina EGV, et al: Nortriptyline in depressed patients with left ventricular impairment. JAMA 256:3253–3257, 1986

Roose SP, Glassman AH, Giardina EGV, et al: Tricyclic antidepressants in depressed patients with cardiac conduction disease. Arch Gen Psychiatry 44:273–275, 1987

Roose SP, Glassman AH, Dalack GW: Depression, heart disease, and tricyclic antidepressants. J Clin Psychiatry 50:12–16, 1989

Roose SP, Dalack GW, Glassman AH, et al: Cardiovascular effects of bupropion in depressed patients with heart disease. Am J Psychiatry 148:512–516, 1991

Rosengren A, Hawken S, Ounpuu S, et al: Association of psychosocial risk factors with risk of acute myocardial infarction in 11,119 cases and 13,648 controls from 52 countries (the INTERHEART study): case-control study. Lancet 2004. Available at: http://www.thelancet.com. Published online September 3, 2004.

Rosenman RH, Brand RJ, Jenkins CD, et al: Coronary heart disease in the Western Collaborative Group Study. Final follow-up experience of 8½ years. JAMA 233:872–877, 1975

Rozanski A, Bairey CN, Krantz DS, et al: Mental stress and the induction of silent myocardial ischemia in patients with coronary artery disease. N Engl J Med 318:1005–1012, 1988

Rozanski A, Blumenthal JA, Kaplan J: Impact of psychological factors on the pathogenesis of cardiovascular disease and implications for therapy. Circulation 99:2192–2217, 1999

Rumsfeld JS, Havranek E, Masoudi FA, et al: Depressive symptoms are the strongest predictors of short-term declines in health status in patients with heart failure. J Am Coll Cardiol 42:1811–1817, 2003

Ruo B, Rumsfeld JS, Hlatky MA, et al: Depressive symptoms and health-related quality of life. The Heart and Soul Study. JAMA 290:215–221, 2003

Shapiro PA: Life after heart transplantation. Prog Cardiovasc Dis 32:405–418, 1990

Shapiro PA, Kornfeld DS: Psychiatric outcome of heart transplantation. Gen Hosp Psychiatry 11:352–357, 1989

Shapiro PA, Lidagoster L, Glassman AH: Depression and heart disease. Psychiatr Ann 27:347–352, 1997

Shapiro PA, DePena M, Lidagoster L, et al: Depression after coronary artery bypass graft surgery (abstract). Psychosom Med 60:108, 1998

Sheline YI, Freedland KE, Carney RM: How safe are serotonin reuptake inhibitors for depression in patients with coronary heart disease? Am J Med 102:54–59, 1997

Sheps DS, McMahon RP, Becker L, et al: Mental stress-induced ischemia and all-cause mortality in patients with coronary artery disease: results from the Psychophysiological Investigations of Myocardial Ischemia study. Circulation 105: 1780–1784, 2002

Steinberg JS, Arshad A, Kowalski M, et al: Increased incidence of life-threatening ventricular arrhythmias in implantable defibrillator patients after the World Trade Center attack. J Am Coll Cardiol 44:1261–1264, 2004

Straus SMJM, Bleumink GS, Dieleman JP, et al: Antipsychotics and the risk of sudden cardiac death. Arch Intern Med 164:1293–1297, 2004

Stuart S, Cole V: Treatment of depression following myocardial infarction with interpersonal psychotherapy. Ann Clin Psychiatry 8:203–206, 1996

Sullivan M, LaCroix AX, Spertus JS, et al.: Effects of anxiety and depression on symptoms and function in patients with coronary heart disease: A five-year prospective study. Psychosomatics 41:187, 2000

Tesar GE, Murray GB, Cassem NH: Use of high dose intravenous haloperidol in the treatment of agitated cardiac patients. J Clin Psychopharmacol 5:344–347, 1985

Willner A, Rodewald G: The Impact of Cardiac Surgery on the Quality of Life: Neurological and Psychological Aspects. New York, Plenum, 1991

Writing Committee for the ENRICHD Investigators: Effects of treating depression and low perceived social support on clinical events after myocardial infarction: the enhancing recovery in coronary heart disease patients (ENRICHD) randomized trial. JAMA 289:3106–3116, 2003

Yan LL, Liu K, Matthews KA, et al: Psychosocial factors and risk of hypertension: the coronary artery risk development in young adults (CARDIA) study. JAMA 290:2138–2148, 2003

Yeung AC, Vekshstein VI, Krantz DS, et al: The effect of atherosclerosis on the vasomotor response of coronary arteries to mental stress. N Engl J Med 325:1551–1556, 1991

Self-Assessment Questions

Select the single best response for each question.

1. Depression and anxiety in heart disease patients may significantly affect quality of life and may complicate medical management. All of the following statements are true *except*

    A. Depression is the most common comorbid psychiatric illness in coronary artery disease patients.

    B. The prevalence of major depression following coronary artery bypass graft (CABG) is 20%–30%.

    C. The point prevalence of major depression in congestive heart failure (CHF) approaches 20%.

    D. Panic disorder occurs at a much higher rate in patients with mitral valve prolapse confirmed by echocardiography than in healthy control subjects.

    E. Subsyndromal posttraumatic stress disorder (PTSD) is common in patients with automatic implantable cardioverter-defibrillators (AICDs).

2. A cardiac patient presents to a psychiatrist with a complaint of mood symptoms and of seeing yellow rings around objects in the visual field. The medication most likely responsible for these symptoms is

    A. Reserpine.

    B. Digoxin.

    C. Clonidine.

    D. Beta-blocker.

    E. Alpha-blocker.

3. Regarding cardiac transplantation surgery for end-stage cardiac disease and its psychiatric implications, all of the following are true *except*

    A. Patients awaiting transplantation commonly experience depression secondary to their helplessness to influence their own chances of survival.

    B. Patients on transplant waiting lists often experience guilt about the need for another patient to die to give them a heart.

    C. Patients on transplant waiting lists tend to minimize and/or deny their illness and to display ambivalence about the surgery.

    D. Most patients experience an initial depression at awakening from transplant surgery.

    E. Steroid-induced mood disorder and other types of depression are seen in 20%–40% of patients during the first postoperative year.

4. Regarding cardiac implications of antidepressants and antipsychotics, all of the following are true *except*

    A. Tricyclic antidepressants (TCAs) can increase mortality in post–myocardial infarction (MI) patients with premature ventricular contractions (PVCs).

    B. Selective serotonin reuptake inhibitors (SSRIs) plus concurrent use of beta-blockers have been shown to lead to symptomatic bradycardia.

    C. Ziprasidone increases the QTc interval and has been associated with an increased risk of sudden death.

D. A QTc interval greater than 500 msec contraindicates the use of haloperidol and thioridazine.

E. Among the antipsychotics, thioridazine carries the highest risk of torsades de pointes.

5. Which of the following psychotropic medications is associated with a quinidine-like type IA antiarrhythmic effect?

A. Carbamazepine.

B. Valproate.

C. Lithium carbonate.

D. Lamotrigine.

E. Buspirone.

3 Lung Disease

Kathy Coffman, M.D.

James L. Levenson, M.D.

IN THIS CHAPTER, we review psychiatric aspects of the major pulmonary disorders, as well as lung transplantation and the use of psychiatric drugs in pulmonary patients.

Common Pulmonary Disorders

Asthma

Asthma is the most common chronic disease in the United States, affecting 5%–7% of the population, or roughly 17 million people (American Lung Association 2000; Barnes and Woolcock 1998). This chapter focuses on asthma in adults (see Chapter 17, "Pediatrics," for discussion of asthma in children). Mortality has risen steadily since the early 1980s and is highest among Puerto Ricans (40.9 per million) and non-Hispanic blacks (38.1 per million) (National Center for Health Statistics 2000).

Comorbidity With Psychiatric Disorders

Asthma may be misdiagnosed as an anxiety disorder, and some anxiety disorders (panic, social anxiety) may be mislabeled as asthma. In one study, 31% of patients who had been given an asthma diagnosis had a negative methacholine inhalation challenge test, indicating no airway hyperresponsiveness. Among patients without bronchial reactivity, social phobia was 10 times more common than in patients who actually had asthma (Schmaling et al. 1999).

Of course, patients may frequently have both asthma and anxiety. Anxiety is increased by attacks of asthma, anticipation of attacks in response to certain triggers, and side effects of medications for asthma (ten Thoren and Petermann 2000).

Some have reported a high comorbidity between asthma and panic disorder and other anxiety disorders (Schmaling et al. 1999). A study of 230 outpatients with asthma revealed that almost half had a positive screen for depressive symptoms (Mancuso et al. 2000).

Psychological Factors in Asthma

Psychosomatic theories about asthma were proposed by French and Alexander in 1939–1941, based on the hypothesis that a central conflict revolved around unconscious dependency issues with the mother and fear of separation. However, these theories have little empirical support (Greenberg et al. 1996).

Few prospective studies of the relationship of psychosocial variables to pulmonary function in patients with asthma have been reported.

No particular personality type is more susceptible to development of asthma (Garden and Ayres 1993). Similar to panic disorder patients, those with asthma have a tendency to hold catastrophic beliefs (Giardino et al. 2002).

Asthma attacks have long been thought to be provoked by psychological distress. There was a 27% increase in severity of asthma symptoms in patients surveyed in New York City 5–9 weeks after the September 11, 2001, terrorist attacks (Centers for Disease Control and Prevention 2002), and posttraumatic stress disorder (PTSD) was a significant predictor of asthma symptom severity (Fagan et al. 2003).

Psychological factors and psychosocial problems in hospitalized asthma patients were a more powerful predictor of which patients required intubation than any other examined variable (e.g., smoking, infection, prior hospitalization) (LeSon and Gershwin 1996). Several psychological factors in asthma patients may be associated with asthma deaths, such as poor adherence with follow-up visits and poor inhaler technique, psychosis, financial problems, and learning difficulties (Sturdy et al. 2002).

From a physiological perspective, the vagus nerve is thought to mediate airway reactivity to emotion (Isenberg et al. 1992). The upper airways innervated by cholinergic neurons may be affected more by suggestion and emotion than smaller airways (Lehrer et al. 1986).

Psychological factors may also influence asthma through behavioral mechanisms. Psychological morbidity is associated with high levels of denial and delays in seeking medical care (D.A. Campbell et al. 1995; Miles et al. 1997), as well as less medication adherence (Cluley and Cochrane 2001). Emotional distress associated with disease and treatment was related to noncompliance (Put et al. 2000).

Interventions With Asthma Patients

Adjuvant forms of treatment for asthma may involve psychological interventions such as biofeedback, education programs, hypnosis, stress management, symptom perception, and yoga (Lehrer et al. 2002).

Biofeedback-assisted relaxation produced improvement in FEV1/FVC (ratio of forced expiratory volume after 1 second to forced vital capacity) at posttest and decreased severity of asthma and bronchodilator usage with changes in white blood cell populations over time, suggesting decreased inflammation (Kern-Buell et al. 2000).

Cystic Fibrosis

In the United States, cystic fibrosis (CF) affects over 18,000 children under the age of 18 (1 in 2,500 births). CF is the most common hereditary disease in white children, and it is also seen in other races. Survival improved from a median age of 12 years in 1966 to 40 years by 2001 (Jaffe and Bush 2001), so adults living with CF are a relatively recent and growing population. (See Chapter 17, "Pediatrics," for information on CF in children.)

Psychological Factors in Cystic Fibrosis

Several authors have described growing up with CF from a child's perspective. Knowing the key issues involved can enhance effectiveness of therapeutic interventions (Christian and D'Auria 1997; Hains et al. 1997; Llewellyn 1998).

There are few studies of psychological functioning in adults with CF. One study showed that adults with CF did not display significant levels of depression, anxiety, or any other psychopathology (D.L. Anderson et al. 2001).

Coping responses and reasons for non-adherence to medical regimens were systematically explored in 60 adult CF patients, showing that adherent patients more often used optimistic acceptance and hopefulness, whereas nonadherent patients used avoidant strategies (Abbott et al. 2001).

A comparison of pre–lung transplant quality of life in 58 patients with CF versus 52 patients with other types of end-stage lung disease revealed that the CF patients had lower levels of anxiety, were more likely to be working, and used more functional coping methods (Burker et al. 2000).

However, anxiety has been seen in 50%–60% of CF patients (Hains et al. 1997), with increases in depressive symptoms in older teenagers and young adults (Benner 1993). Noncompliance with the medical regimen has been estimated to be at least 35% (Czajkowski and Koocher 1987).

Chronic Obstructive Pulmonary Disease

Almost 16 million Americans have chronic obstructive pulmonary disease (COPD): 14 million with chronic bronchitis and 2 million with emphysema. COPD ranks fourth as a cause of death in the United States after heart disease, cancer, and stroke. Cigarette smokers are 10 times as likely to die of COPD as nonsmokers.

COPD results in progressive declines in arterial oxygen, with carbon dioxide increasing late in the course of the disease. Hypoxia causes confusion, disorientation, altered consciousness, muscle twitching, tremor, and seizures. Mild hypoxia can be accompanied by irritability, mental slowing, and impairment of memory with poor reasoning and perseveration. Prolonged hypoxia can result in permanent memory deficits or dementia (Lishman 1987). Patients with hypercapnea may be lethargic and have auditory and visual hallucinations (Lishman 1987).

Comorbidity With Psychiatric Disorders

Nicotine dependence is the most commonly associated psychiatric condition in patients with COPD. More than 80% of COPD cases are associated with tobacco smoking (Tashkin et al. 2001). Alcohol abuse aggravates COPD because of a higher rate of severe community-acquired pneumonia, particularly aspiration pneumonia (Ewig and Torres 1999). Sexual dysfunction is common in COPD (Ibanez et al. 2001).

Major depression is also very common in patients with COPD, partly due to an increased prevalence of depression in smokers (Aydin and Ulusahin 2001; Withers et al. 1999; Yohannes et al. 2000). In one study, clinical depression was found in 42% of the patients (Yohannes et al. 2000), yet only about one-fifth of COPD patients with major depression are treated with antidepressants. Depression may adversely impact rehabilitation and contribute to difficulty ceasing tobacco use (Borson et al. 1998).

Anxiety is also common in COPD (Aydin and Ulusahin 2001; Withers et al. 1999; Yohannes et al. 2000). The prevalence of panic disorder in COPD patients remains controversial. In one study, 37% of COPD patients reported having had a panic attack (Porzelius et al. 1992). Another study found that COPD patients had symptoms similar to those of agoraphobic patients (Klonoff and Kleinhenz 1993).

Cognitive dysfunction is also very common in COPD and is improved by supplemental oxygen. Those receiving continuous oxygen treatment had better neuropsychological performance and survival at 12 months than did those receiving nocturnal oxygen treatment only (Heaton et al. 1983). Rates of neuropsychological impairment rose from 27% in those with mild hypoxemia to 61% in those with severe hypoxemia (Grant et al. 1987). About 30% of COPD patients showed immediate memory impairment (Fioravanti et al. 1995). Of the COPD patients tested at discharge after a first episode of acute respiratory failure requiring mechanical ventilation, 47% showed Mini-Mental State Examination scores below 24, compared with 3% of stable COPD control subjects receiving continuous oxygen treatment (Ambrosino et al. 2002). Anterior cerebral hypoperfusion has been demonstrated on single-photon emission computed tomography in hypoxemic COPD patients (Antonelli Incalzi et al. 2003).

Psychological Factors in COPD

As with other medical illnesses, measurement of physical symptoms in COPD may be confounded by psychological symptoms, and vice versa. One study of COPD patients showed that patients with more severe physical symptoms had more negative mood symptoms (Small and Graydon 1992).

Results have not been consistent in correlating quality of life and various measures of pulmonary function. Those with higher levels of positive social support had better quality of life with less depression and anxiety. Lower quality of life was seen when catastrophic withdrawal coping strategies were employed by the patients (McCathie et al. 2002).

Depression and anxiety in COPD patients have led to lower exercise tolerance (Withers et al. 1999), noncompliance with treatment (Bosley et al. 1996), and increased disability (Aydin and Ulusahin 2001). In one study, those with anxiety or depression had a higher rate of relapse within 1 month after emergency treatment (53%) compared with those in the group without anxiety or depression (19%) (Dahlen and Janson 2002).

On the basis of clinical experience, Dudley et al. (1985) observed that when

patients and physicians face COPD, they may feel helpless. The patient may avoid emotional expression because it exacerbates his or her sense of dyspnea. Denial, suppression of affect, repression, and isolation are frequently used as coping strategies in COPD patients (Dudley et al. 1985). Chronic steroid use may also exacerbate depression, emotional lability, or irritability, which in turn further strains interpersonal relationships.

Dependence on supplemental oxygen can be socially stigmatizing. Some cannot accept the need for oxygen, whereas others exceed the amount prescribed, posing a risk of carbon dioxide retention and lethargy.

The Veterans Administration Normative Aging Study found that optimism in older men with COPD predicted higher levels of pulmonary function and a slower rate of pulmonary function decline (independent of smoking status) (Kubzansky et al. 2002).

Interventions With COPD Patients

Psychotherapeutic, psychopharmacological, and rehabilitation intervention trials in COPD have been recently reviewed in detail elsewhere (Brenes 2003). The first priority in the rehabilitation of patients with COPD is smoking cessation. A small fraction of patients may benefit from bilateral lung volume reduction surgery (Wurtemberger and Hutter 2001).

The goals of treatment are to relieve symptoms, improve physical functioning via rehabilitation, and improve patients' coping skills (Small and Graydon 1992). Patients with dyspnea may avoid all activity and become homebound. Exercise may help build endurance and help patients learn to pace themselves. A treatment plan with realistic goals can counteract helplessness (Dudley et al. 1985).

A study of the impact of inpatient pulmonary rehabilitation found 29.2% of patients with significant anxiety on admission and 15% with significant depression (Withers et al. 1999). Pulmonary rehabilitation can increase patients' sense of control over COPD (Lacasse et al. 2002).

Predictors of nonadherence with an outpatient pulmonary rehabilitation program were investigated by Young et al. (1999). Noncompleters were more likely to be currently smoking, divorced, and living alone in rented accommodations and were less likely to use inhaled corticosteroids (Young et al. 1999).

Rose et al. (2002) reviewed 25 published studies of psychological treatments for reduction of anxiety in patients with COPD. There is insufficient evidence to recommend a specific psychological treatment for anxiety in COPD, though relaxation techniques are useful in motivated patients (Rose et al. 2002).

Sarcoidosis

Sarcoidosis is characterized by noncaseating granulomatous involvement of lymph nodes and other tissues. Sarcoidosis affects black patients more than whites in the United States (40 per 100,000 vs. 5 per 100,000). In Europe, Swedes and Danes have high prevalence rates (American Lung Association 2000). Onset of the illness is usually between ages 20 and 40. The disease often follows a relapsing and remitting course, with recovery in 80% of patients, but about 5% die from sarcoidosis. Patients often have a dry cough, shortness of breath, fatigue, and weight loss. Fatal complications include progressive respiratory impairment, infection, cardiac disease, and renal failure.

Central Nervous System Sarcoidosis

Sarcoidosis may affect the central nervous system (CNS) in 5% of patients. Neurosarcoidosis may involve cranial nerves and cause peripheral neuropathies (and rarely choreoathetosis). In 30% of cases, the cerebrospinal fluid may be normal (Stoudemire et al. 1983). Pituitary involvement may result in diabetes insipidus or the syndrome of inappropriate antidiuretic hormone secretion (SIADH) with hyponatremia, hypercalcemia, hyperprolactinemia, menstrual cycle changes, or hypogonadism (see Bullman et al. 2000; Delaney 1977; Mino et al. 2000; Sharma 1975).

CNS disease may alter cognition (Mathews 1965; Silverstein et al. 1965). CNS sarcoidosis can mimic depressive stupor, Wernicke-Korsakoff psychosis, classic paranoid psychosis, and schizophreniform disorder (Hook 1954; Sabaawi et al. 1992; Suchenwirth and Dold 1969; Zerman 1952). Psychotic symptoms rapidly remit with steroids. Patients with CNS sarcoidosis may present with seizures (Thompson and Checkley 1981).

Psychological Factors in Sarcoidosis

Sarcoidosis has been rarely investigated from the psychological standpoint. One study found that increased life stress predicted impairment of lung function, suggesting the potential benefit of relaxation exercises and stress management (Klonoff and Kleinhenz 1993). Some patients with sarcoidosis have been mistakenly labeled as having somatization disorder (deGruy et al. 1987).

Hoitsma et al. (2003) found that 72% of sarcoidosis patients had pain, including arthralgia (53.8%), muscle pain (40.2%), headache (28%), and chest pain (26.9%), suggesting that pain management may be beneficial.

Pulmonary Fibrosis

The etiology of idiopathic pulmonary fibrosis (IPF) is unknown, but the prevalence is roughly 3–5 per 100,000. Pulmonary fibrosis also may be caused by inhalation of a variety of agents, radiation, and rheumatological disorders, especially systemic sclerosis.

Psychological factors have received little attention in IPF. Dyspnea is the most important factor in determining quality of life in IPF (DeVries et al. 2001; Martinez et al. 2000).

Tuberculosis

The incidence of tuberculosis (TB) had been declining for more than 70 years but began to rise again over the last decade in the United States, Western Europe, Asia, and Africa due to AIDS, homelessness, and the failure to fund public health systems. There are about 2.9 million deaths per year and nearly 8 million new cases per year in the world (Bloom et al. 1996). See Chapter 10, "Infectious Diseases," for a discussion of CNS tuberculosis.

Psychiatrists may be asked to make capacity determinations in patients who are nonadherent with TB treatment (O'Dowd et al. 1998). One survey of TB detainees showed that 81% had drug or alcohol abuse, 46% were homeless, and 28% had mental illness (Oscherwitz et al. 1997).

Since alcoholic patients are more susceptible to TB (Sternbach 1990), and drug dependence is also a risk factor (Reichman et al. 1979), access to adequate substance abuse treatment may be essential for recovery from TB and for preventing relapse.

Psychiatrists must be attuned to neuropsychiatric symptoms such as mania and psychosis during treatment with isoniazid (Alao and Yolles 1998), probably related to its being a weak inhibitor of monoamine oxidase. Pyridoxine deficiency may play a role in the etiology of isoniazid-related psychosis. Acute overdosage with isoniazid, causing convulsions (controlled by giving pyridoxine), has been reported (Ebadi et al. 1982). Pellagra encephalopathy has been seen because isoniazid inhibits conversion of tryptophan to niacin (Ishii and Nishihara 1985).

Hyperventilation

Hyperventilation is a common presenting complaint in emergency rooms, leading to psychiatric consultation (Nguyen et al. 1992). These patients briefly experience an increase in the rate and depth of breathing and may have dizziness or syncope from the respiratory alkalosis and cerebral vasoconstriction that result. Symptoms of carpopedal spasm, myoclonic jerks, or paresthesias may frighten the patient or relatives and result in an emergency room visit.

The incidence of hyperventilation syndrome (HVS) may be as high as 6%–11% of the general population (Lachman et al. 1992), and HVS may recur.

Differential diagnosis for hyperventilation includes medical and psychiatric disorders. Medical illnesses confused with HVS include angina, arrhythmia, asthma (Demeter and Cordasco 1986), carbon monoxide poisoning (Skorodin et al. 1986), diabetic ketoacidosis (Treasure et al. 1987), pulmonary emboli (Hoegholm et al. 1987), epilepsy, hypoglycemia, ingestion of salicylates (Rognum et al. 1987), Meniere disease, tetany (Hehrmann 1996), and vasovagal syncope. There have also been reports of neurological causes of hyperventilation, including thalamic infarct (Scialdone 1990), Cheyne-Stokes breathing (Liippo et al. 1992), and traumatic vestibular hyperreactivity after whiplash injury (Fischer et al. 1995).

Medications reported to cause central hyperventilation include carbamazepine, salicylates, and topiramate. Central hyperventilation resolves promptly within a day or two after discontinuation of these drugs (Lasky and Brody 2000; Mizukami et al. 1990).

Psychiatric disorders to consider in HVS include conversion disorder, histrionic personality disorder, panic disorder, phobic disorders, hypochondriasis, substance abuse, and mass psychogenic illness

(Araki and Honma 1986). Estimates of the overlap between HVS and panic disorder are between 35% and 83% (Cowley and Roy-Byrne 1987; deRuiter et al. 1989; Hoes et al. 1987). The relationship between HVS and panic disorder is controversial.

Various treatments for HVS have been employed over the years, such as the use of antidepressants (Saarijarvi and Lehtinen 1987), intravenous sedatives (Hirokawa et al. 1995), beta-blockers (Van De Ven et al. 1995), breathing retraining (DeGuire et al. 1992, 1996; Pinney et al. 1987), and hypnosis (Conway et al. 1988).

Although having patients with acute hyperventilation rebreathe into a brown paper bag is a traditional technique used in the emergency department, death resulted in three cases where this treatment was mistakenly applied to patients with hypoxia or myocardial ischemia (Callaham 1989).

Vocal Cord Dysfunction

Vocal cord dysfunction (VCD) is a respiratory syndrome often confused with asthma, although they frequently occur together (Newman et al. 1995). VCD may also co-occur with HVS (Brugman 2003). The disorder may present in childhood, adolescence, or adulthood. Patients may appear in severe respiratory distress yet rarely present with hypoxemia. In contrast to asthma, in VCD wheezing will be loudest over the larynx and more pronounced in the inspiratory phase, but the chest is otherwise clear. Also unlike asthma, VCD attacks typically have rapid onset and equally rapid resolution. VCD may lead to frequent emergency department visits and hospitalizations, high doses of (ineffective) asthma medications, and unnecessary intubation (Bahrainwala and Simon 2001). The differential diagnosis of VCD includes asthma, HVS, neurological disorders (e.g., spasmodic dysphonia and laryngeal nerve injury), and angioedema (Brugman 2003).

In most patients, VCD appears not to be a primary psychiatric disorder but rather a conditioned response, which may result in secondary anxiety. The onset of VCD is typically preceded by allergy, asthma, reflux, irritant exposure (Perkner et al. 1998), or a dyspneic episode in athletes (Newsham et al. 2002). Case reports and retrospective case series noted strong dependency needs and fears of separation in patients with VCD and its acute precipitation following psychosocial stress. Other referred cases of VCD may represent conversion disorder, posttraumatic stress disorder, somatization disorder, or factitious illness.

There is no empirically proven treatment for VCD, although speech therapy alone (Brugman 2003), psychotherapy or antipanic pharmacotherapy, and biofeedback have been reported as helpful (Earles et al. 2003).

Lung Cancer

Lung cancer is the most common cause of cancer death in the United States and the world. Smoking tobacco is the primary cause of most lung cancers (Strauss 1998).

A review of quality of life in lung cancer patients from 1970 to 1995 noted that over 80% of lung cancer patients died within a year of diagnosis, because many were diagnosed late (Montazeri et al. 1998). More than 50 instruments have been used to measure quality of life in patients with lung cancer. Psychological distress and lower quality of life have been correlated with even moderate weight loss (Ovesen et al. 1993). Symptoms of psychological distress are common in lung cancer. One study showed that newly diagnosed lung cancer patients had frequent insomnia (52%), loss of libido (48%), loss of interest in or ability to work (33%), concerns about their families (29%), and poor concentration (19%) (Ginsburg et al. 1995). Another study found predictors of psychological distress in ambulatory lung cancer patients included having a helpless or hopeless coping style (Akechi et al. 1998).

A study of newly diagnosed patients with unresectable non–small cell cancer of the lung described the most common psychiatric diagnosis as nicotine dependence (67%). Depression did not increase over the course of the illness. Pain management was key in relieving depression (Akechi et al. 2001). Type of lung cancer may influence the rate of depression. In one study, the rate of depression was nearly three times higher in those with small cell cancer (25%) than in those with non–small cell cancer (9%). The most important risk factor for depression was functional impairment (Hopwood and Stephens 2000).

Fatigue is more common at diagnosis with lung cancer than most other cancers: 50% of those with inoperable non–small cell cancer reported severe fatigue (Stone et al. 2000). Adaptive behaviors can reduce fatigue even with low hemoglobin levels (Olson et al. 2002).

Given the high rate of dyspnea in lung cancer patients, one might expect that many patients would cease tobacco use. This is not the case, despite evidence that continued smoking after lung cancer diagnosis decreases treatment efficacy, increases complications, increases risk of recurrence and occurrence of another primary tumor, and decreases survival time (Schnoll et al. 2002).

Do psychological factors alter the course of lung cancer? One study of lung cancer patients found that self-report of depressive coping was an independent predictor of decreased survival time at 8- and 10-year follow-up (Faller and Bulzebruck 2002; Faller et al. 1997). Psychological factors may also influence response to treatment. For example, anxiety or depression may predict increased nausea scores after chemotherapy (Takatsuki et al. 1998).

Little has been written on coping in lung cancer. One study noted four common coping strategies among 50 patients with stages III and IV adenocarcinoma of the lung: seeking of social support, problem solving, self-control, and positive reappraisal (Chernecky 1999).

Procedures

Lung Transplantation

Indications and Contraindications

The first lung transplant was performed in 1963, but it was 20 years before the first successful operation in 1983 (Ochoa and Richardson 1999) (see also Chapter 14, "Organ Transplantation"). The most common indication is COPD, which accounts for about 45% of lung transplants (Hosenpud et al. 1998). Transplants are also performed for those with CF, IPF, Eisenmenger syndrome, primary pulmonary hypertension, and a number of other pulmonary diseases (Etienne et al. 1997). Patients are generally listed when their quality of life has declined and transplant would confer a survival benefit, given the waiting time of up to 2 years once the patient is listed for transplant (Maurer et al. 1998).

Exclusion criteria vary from one transplant center to another. Psychiatric factors that are considered to be absolute contraindications to lung transplantation include active alcoholism, drug abuse or cigarette use, severe psychiatric illness, and noncompliance with treatment (Aris et al. 1997; Paradowski 1997; Snell et al. 1993).

There are four main approaches to lung transplantation: single-lung transplantation, bilateral sequential transplantation, heart–lung transplantation, and single-lobe donation from living donors

(Arcasoy and Kotloff 1999). Living donor donation has been controversial because of the uncertainty regarding risks to the donor (Barr et al. 1998).

Medical and Surgical Outcomes

Patient survival in the United States at 1 year and 3 years after lung transplant is currently 77% and 58%, respectively. For comparison, the corresponding survival figures after heart transplant are 85% and 77% (Trulock 2003). Exercise capacity improves, with about 80% of recipients reporting no limitations in activity within 1 year of transplant. Quality of life remains stable for the first few years if the course is uncomplicated, but those who develop bronchiolitis obliterans show a sharp decline in quality of life (Paris et al. 1998).

Early complications after lung transplantation include primary graft failure, stenosis of the anastomosis, and a higher rate of infectious complications than in other solid organ transplantation (Christie et al. 1998; Kramer et al. 1993).

Psychological Factors and Quality of Life

Until recently, there were few studies in this area. All available studies are limited by small size. Cohen et al. (1998) described 32 recipients reporting better quality of life posttransplant. No pretransplant psychological variables were found to be associated with the length of survival posttransplant (Cohen et al. 1998).

Stilley et al. (1999) studied 36 lung recipients and 14 heart–lung recipients, noting no differences in psychological data between the two transplant types. Recipients showed lower hostility than a normative sample. On the Hopkins Symptom Checklist–90 (SCL-90), recipients had about double the rates of depression and anxiety compared with the control group, with lung recipients having higher rates than heart–lung recipients (Stilley et al. 1999).

Limbos et al. (2000) observed that most lung transplant recipients reported significant improvement in general health, self-esteem, social functioning, quality of life, anxiety, and depression.

Psychological Interventions

Napolitano et al. (2002) found that inexpensive telephone-based supportive and cognitive-behavioral therapy for lung transplant candidates were efficacious.

Teichman et al. (2000) studied adherence to treatment regimens after lung transplant and found that patients became less compliant the further from the time of transplant, suggesting that periodic reeducation after transplantation may improve adherence.

Terminal Weaning

Patients with end-stage pulmonary disease caused by amyotrophic lateral sclerosis, COPD, CF, IPF, lung cancer, or other diseases may request terminal weaning. Although *terminal* implies that the withdrawal of ventilator support will inevitably end in death, patients do not always die shortly after discontinuation of ventilatory support. In one study, 8% of patients survived and were discharged (M.L. Campbell 1994). The phrase "discontinuation of ventilator support" or "withdrawal of mechanical ventilation" may be used as an alternative (Apelgren 2000; Daly et al. 1993).

The patient must be aware that death is the most likely outcome when ventilator support is discontinued and make the decision after due deliberation (Daly et al. 1993).

The patient's goals should guide the process of withdrawing ventilator support (J. Anderson and O'Brien 1995). If the patient shows ambivalence about terminal weaning or it is unclear whether the patient has sufficient mental capacity to make a well-thought-out decision, consultation from a psychiatrist should be obtained. The first step in evaluation is to explore why the patient has requested discontinuation of ventilator support. Depression, delirium, and concerns about burdening the family require different interventions. In difficult cases, in addition to the psychiatrist, involvement of the hospital's ethics committee, chaplain, social worker, and legal counsel may be helpful.

Patients should be told that the weaning process may be stopped at any time if they wish. Withdrawal of the ventilator may follow the withdrawal of pressors, antibiotics, and enteral feeding (Brody et al. 1997). In a conscious patient, a gradual decrease in FIO_2, with decreased positive end-expiratory pressure (PEEP) and decrease in respiratory rate over several hours, has been advocated (Grenvik 1983).

Adjunctive medication may alleviate distress. Opiates have been used for pain relief and to decrease gasping, coughing, or the sensation of shortness of breath; to provide sedation; and to decrease anxiety in the patient. Documentation of the physician's intent in administering opiates is important to show that the medication is being used as a comfort measure and not to hasten death. Benzodiazepines may decrease anxiety and prevent myoclonus or twitching that may be unsettling to the family (Faber-Langendoen 1994). Phenobarbital may control twitching not relieved by benzodiazepines. Low-dose haloperidol may be used intravenously for anxiety that is not relieved by benzodiazepines or if the patient is delirious.

The family should be educated prior to the procedure that the medications used will prevent the patient from having awareness of bodily events and may induce euphoria.

Use of paralytic agents is discouraged because they may prevent the patient from signaling if there is any distress. Staff members should remain at the bedside to attend to the patient and provide comfort to the family (Benner 1993; Daly et al. 1993).

Psychopharmacology in Pulmonary Disease

Anxiety

Anxiety in pulmonary patients may be caused by breathlessness, bronchospasm, excessive secretions, or hypoxia, so the first step in treatment of anxiety is optimization of management of the patient's respiratory illness. Many drugs used to treat pulmonary disease may cause anxiety. Theophylline can cause anxiety, nausea, tremor, and restlessness, especially at higher doses. Beta-adrenergic bronchodilators can cause marked anxiety, tachycardia, and tremor, particularly in patients who overuse their inhalers. Nonprescription asthma preparations contain nonselective sympathomimetics, which cause anxiety and, at high doses, may cause psychosis and seizures.

Buspirone may be used in anxious pulmonary patients with hypercapnia or sleep apnea (Craven and Sutherland 1991; Mendelson et al. 1991). Buspirone can be combined with theophylline and terbutaline (Kiev and Domantay 1988).

In COPD patients who do not retain carbon dioxide, prudent doses of benzodiazepines may decrease breathlessness. In elderly patients, shorter-acting benzodiazepines with no active metabolites, such as alprazolam, lorazepam, and oxazepam, are preferred. Zolpidem does not alter respiratory drive in COPD patients but may cause rebound insomnia. Diazepam has no effect on breathlessness and may decrease exercise tolerance. Selective serotonin reuptake inhibitors (SRRIs) may also be helpful in treating panic symptoms and do not have pulmonary side effects. Beta-blockers should not be used for anxiety in asthma patients, because of resulting bronchoconstriction.

Depression

When choosing an antidepressant, the side-effect profile and cytochrome P450 interactions with pulmonary drugs should be considered. Generally, SSRIs other than fluvoxamine are effective and have few drug interactions that are problematic in pulmonary patients (Ciraulo and Shader 1990; Smoller et al. 1998).

Many pulmonary patients may be on medications that can prolong the QT interval, so reviewing the electrocardiogram (ECG) is prudent when considering treatment with a tricyclic antidepressant. In elderly patients or in patients with COPD or sleep apnea, the sedating tricyclic antidepressants are best avoided (DeVane 1998).

Psychosis

Pulmonary patients may have primary psychotic disorders, such as bipolar disorder or schizophrenia, or may become psychotic because of medications such as beta-agonists, cycloserine, isoniazid, or corticosteroids. The incidence of steroid psychosis is dose-related, seen in less than 1% of patients taking 40 mg or less of prednisone per day versus 28% taking 80 mg daily (Boston Collaborative Drug Surveillance Program 1972).

Typical neuroleptics such as haloperidol at high doses may cause laryngospasm, akathisia, and paradoxical intercostal muscle movements that, in turn, may cause restlessness and interfere with breathing. Tardive dyskinesia sometimes affects the diaphragm and other muscles used in breathing, so for chronic treatment, newer drugs with lower incidence of extrapyramidal side effects may be preferred.

Drug Interactions Between Psychotropic and Pulmonary Drugs

The psychiatrist should consider potential interactions when prescribing psychotropic medications to patients with pulmonary disease. Theophylline levels may be reduced 50%–80% by tobacco smoking. Nicotine gum does not have this effect. Al-

cohol can reduce clearance of theophylline by as much as 30% for up to 24 hours. Most pulmonary medications do not affect lithium levels, but theophylline can lower lithium levels by 20%–30%. Theophylline preparations administered concurrently with electroconvulsive therapy can prolong seizure duration (Peters et al. 1984).

Rifampin is a cytochrome P450 3A4 substrate and so may compete with many psychotropic drugs, including the antidepressants amitriptyline, imipramine, fluoxetine, sertraline, bupropion, venlafaxine, and trazodone. Rifampin may compete through the same site with anticonvulsants (e.g., carbamazepine, tiagabine, and valproate) and with benzodiazepines, zolpidem, and haloperidol. Montelukast sodium may have similar interactions to those of rifampin, because of metabolism via 3A4 and 2C9.

References

Abbott J, Dodd M, Gee L, Webb K: Ways of coping with cystic fibrosis: implications for treatment adherence. Disabil Rehabil 23:315–24, 2001

Akechi T, Kugaya A, Okamura H, et al: Predictive factors for psychological distress in ambulatory lung cancer patients. Support Care Cancer 6:281–286, 1998

Akechi T, Okamura H, Nishiwaki Y, et al: Psychiatric disorders and associated and predictive factors in patients with unresectable nonsmall cell lung carcinoma: a longitudinal study. Cancer 92:2609–2622, 2001

Alao AO, Yolles JC: Isoniazid-induced psychosis. Ann Pharmacother 32:889–891, 1998

Ambrosino N, Bruletti G, Scala V, et al: Cognitive and perceived health status in patients with chronic obstructive pulmonary disease surviving acute or chronic respiratory failure: a controlled study. Intensive Care Med 28:170–177, 2002

American Lung Association: Minority Lung Disease Data 2000. Available at: http://www.lungusa.org. Accessed January 2000.

Anderson DL, Flume PA, Hardy KK: Psychological functioning of adults with cystic fibrosis. Chest 119:1079–1084, 2001

Anderson J, O'Brien M: Challenges for the future: the nurse's role in weaning patients from mechanical ventilation. Intensive Crit Care Nurs 11:2–5, 1995

Antonelli Incalzi R, Marra C, Giordano A, et al: Cognitive impairment in chronic obstructive pulmonary disease—a neuropsychological and SPECT study. J Neurol 250:325–332, 2003

Apelgren KN: "Terminal" wean is the wrong term. Crit Care Med 28:3576–3577, 2000

Araki S, Honma T: Mass psychogenic systemic illness in school children in relation to the Tokyo photochemical smog. Arch Environ Health 41:159–162, 1986

Arcasoy SM, Kotloff RM: Lung transplantation. N Engl J Med 340:1081–1091, 1999

Aris RM, Gilligan PH, Neuring IP, et al: The effect of panresistant bacteria in cystic fibrosis patients on lung transplant outcome. Am J Respir Crit Care Med 155:1699–1704, 1997

Aydin IO, Ulusahin A: Depression, anxiety comorbidity, and disability in tuberculosis and chronic obstructive pulmonary disease patients: applicability of GHQ-12. Gen Hosp Psychiatry 23:77–83, 2001

Bahrainwala AH, Simon MR: Wheezing and vocal cord dysfunction mimicking asthma. Curr Opin Pulm Med 7:8–13, 2001

Barnes PJ, Woolcock AJ: Difficult asthma. Eur Respir J 12: 1209–1218, 1998

Barr ML, Schenkel FA, Cohen RG, et al: Recipient and donor outcomes in living related and unrelated lobar transplantation. Transplant Proc 30:2261–2263, 1998

Benner KL: Terminal weaning: a loved one's vigil. Am J Nurs 93:22–25, 1993

Bloom BB, Humphries DE, Kuang PP, et al: Structure and expression of the promoter for the R4/ALK5 hu type I transforming growth factor-beta receptor: regulation by TGF-beta. Biochim Biophys Acta 1312:243–248, 1996

Borson S, Claypoole K, McDonald GJ: Depression and chronic obstructive pulmonary disease: treatment trials. Semin Clin Neuropsychiatry 3:115–130, 1998

Bosley CM, Corden ZM, Rees PJ, et al: Psychological factors associated with use of home nebulized therapy for COPD. Eur Respir J 9:2346–2350, 1996

Boston Collaborative Drug Surveillance Program: Acute adverse reaction to prednisone in relation to dosage. Clin Pharmacol Ther 13:694–697, 1972

Brenes GA: Anxiety and chronic obstructive pulmonary disease: prevalence, impact, and treatment. Psychosom Med 65: 963–970, 2003

Brody H, Campbell ML, Faber-Langendoen, et al: Withdrawing intensive life-sustaining treatment—recommendations for compassionate clinical management. N Engl J Med 336: 652–657, 1997

Brugman SM: The many faces of vocal cord dysfunction: what 36 years of literature tell us. Am J Respir Crit Care Med 167: A588, 2003

Bullman C, Faust M, Hoffmann A, et al: Five cases with central diabetes insipidus and hypogonadism as first presentation of neurosarcoidosis. Eur J Endocrinol 142:365–372, 2000

Burker EJ, Carels RA, Thompson LF, et al: Quality of life in patients awaiting lung transplant: cystic fibrosis versus other end-stage lung diseases. Pediatr Pulmonol 30:453–460, 2000

Callaham M: Hypoxic hazards of traditional paper bag rebreathing in hyperventilating patients. Ann Emerg Med 18:622–628, 1989

Campbell DA, Yellowlees PM, McLennan G, et al: Psychiatric and medical features of near fatal asthma. Thorax 50:254–259, 1995

Campbell ML: Terminal weaning: it's not simply "pulling the plug." Nursing 24:34–39, 1994

Centers for Disease Control and Prevention: Self-reported increase in asthma severity after the September 11 attacks on the World Trade Center—Manhattaan, New York, 2001. MMWR Morb Mortal Wkly Rep 51:781–784, 2002

Chernecky C: Temporal differences in coping, mood, and stress with chemotherapy. Cancer Nurs 22:266–276, 1999

Christian BJ, D'Auria JP: The child's eye: memories of growing up with cystic fibrosis. J Pediatr Nurs 12:3–12, 1997

Christie JD, Bavaria JE, Palevsky HI, et al: Primary graft failure following lung transplantation. Chest 114:51–60, 1998

Ciraulo DA, Shader RI: Fluoxetine drug-drug interactions II. J Clin Psychopharmacol 10:213–217, 1990

Cluley S, Cochrane GM: Psychological disorder in asthma is associated with poor control and poor adherence to inhaled steroids. Respir Med 95:37–39, 2001

Cohen L, Littlefield C, Kelly P, et al: Predictors of quality of life and adjustment after lung transplantation. Chest 113:633–644, 1998

Conway AV, Freeman LJ, Nixon PG: Hypnotic examination of trigger factors in the hyperventilation syndrome. Am J Clin Hypn 30:286–304, 1988

Cowley DS, Roy-Byrne PP: Hyperventilation and panic disorder. Am J Med 83:929–937, 1987

Craven J, Sutherland A: Buspirone for anxiety disorders in patients with severe lung disease (letter). Lancet 338:249, 1991

Czajkowski DR, Koocher GP: Medical compliance and coping with cystic fibrosis. J Child Psychol Psychiatry 28:311–319, 1987

Dahlen I, Janson C: Anxiety and depression are related to the outcome of emergency treatment in patients with obstructive pulmonary disease. Chest 122:1633–1637, 2002

Daly BJ, Newlon B, Montenegro HD, et al: Withdrawal of mechanical ventilation: ethical principles and guidelines for terminal weaning. Am J Crit Care 2:217–223, 1993

deGruy F, Crider J, Hashimi DK, et al: Somatization disorder in a university hospital. J Fam Pract 25:579–584, 1987

DeGuire S, Gevirtz R, Kawahara Y, et al: Hyperventilation syndrome and the assessment of treatment for functional cardiac symptoms. Am J Cardiol 70:673–677, 1992

DeGuire S, Gevirtz R, Hawkinson D, et al: Breathing retraining: a 3-year follow-up study of treatment for hyperventilation syndrome and associated functional cardiac symptoms. Biofeedback Self Regul 21:191–198, 1996

Delaney P: Neurologic manifestations in sarcoidosis: review of the literature, with a report of 23 cases. Ann Intern Med 87: 336–345, 1977

Demeter SL, Cordasco EM: Hyperventilation syndrome and asthma. Am J Med 81:989–994, 1986

deRuiter C, Garssen B, Rijken H, et al: The hyperventilation syndrome in panic disorder, agoraphobia and generalized anxiety disorder. Behav Res Ther 27:447–452, 1989

DeVane CL: Principles of pharmacokinetics and pharmacodynamics, in Textbook of Psychopharmacology, 2nd Edition. Edited by Schatzberg AF, Nemeroff CB. American Psychiatric Press, Washington, DC, London, pp 155–169, 1998

DeVries J, Kessels BL, Drent M: Quality of life of idiopathic pulmonary fibrosis patients. Eur Respir J 17:954–961, 2001

Dudley DL, Sitzman J, Rugg M: Psychiatric aspects of patients with chronic obstructive pulmonary disease. Adv Psychosom Med 14:64–77, 1985

Earles J, Kerr B, Kellar M: Psychophysiologic treatment of vocal cord dysfunction. Ann Allergy Asthma Immunol 90:669–671, 2003

Ebadi M, Gessert CF, Al-Sayegh A: Drug-pyridoxal phosphate interactions. Q Rev Drug Metab Drug Interact 4:289–331, 1982

Etienne B, Bertocchi M, Gamondes JP, et al: Successful double-lung transplantation for bronchioalveolar carcinoma. Chest 112:1423–1424, 1997

Ewig S, Torres A: Severe community-acquired pneumonia. Clin Chest Med 20:575–587, 1999

Faber-Langendoen K: The clinical management of dying patients receiving mechanical ventilation: a survey of physician practice. Chest 106:880–888, 1994

Fagan J, Galea S, Ahern J, et al: Relationship of self-reported asthma severity and urgent health care utilization to psychological sequelae of the September 11, 2001 terrorist attacks on the World Trade Center among New York City area residents. Psychosom Med 65:993–996, 2003

Faller H, Bulzebruck H: Coping and survival in lung cancer: a 10-year follow-up. Am J Psychiatry 159:2105–2107, 2002

Faller H, Bulzebruck H, Schilling S, et al: Do psychological factors modify survival of cancer patients? II: results of an empirical study with bronchial carcinoma patients. Psychother Psychosom Med Psychol 47:206–218, 1997

Fioravanti M, Nacca D, Amati S, et al: Chronic obstructive pulmonary disease and associated patterns of memory decline. Dementia 6:39–48, 1995

Fischer AJ, Huygen PL, Folgering HT, et al: Vestibular hyperreactivity and hyperventilation after whiplash injury. J Neurol Sci 132:35–43, 1995

Garden GM, Ayres JG: Psychiatric and social aspects of brittle asthma. Thorax 48:501–505, 1993

Giardino ND, Schmaling KB, Afari N: Relationship satisfaction moderates the association between catastrophic cognitions and asthma symptoms. J Asthma 39:749–756, 2002

Ginsburg ML, Quirt C, Ginsburg AD, et al: Psychiatric illness and psychosocial concerns of patients with newly diagnosed lung cancer. CMAJ 152:1961–1963, 1995

Grant I, Prigatoano GP, Heaton RK, et al: Progressive neuropsychological impairment and hypoxemia. Relationship in chronic obstructive pulmonary disease. Arch Gen Psychiatry 44:999–1006, 1987

Greenberg, DB, Halperin P, Kradin RL, et al: Internal medicine and medical subspecialties, in Textbook of Consultation-Liaison Psychiatry. Washington, DC, American Psychiatric Press, 1996, pp 565–566

Grenvik A: "Terminal weaning": discontinuance of life-support therapy in the terminally ill patient. Crit Care Med 11:394–395, 1983

Hains AA, Davies WH, Behrens D, et al: Cognitive behavioral interventions for adolescents with cystic fibrosis. J Pediatr Psychol 22:669–687, 1997

Heaton RK, Grant I, McSweeney AJ, et al: Psychologic effects of continuous and nocturnal oxygen therapy in hypoxemic chronic obstructive pulmonary disease. Arch Intern Med 143:1941–1947, 1983

Hehrmann R: Hypocalcemic crisis. Hypoparathyroidism—non-parathyroid origin—the most frequent form: hyperventilation syndrome [in German]. Fortschr Med 114:223–226, 1996

Hirokawa Y, Kondo T, Ohta Y, et al: Clinical characteristics and outcome of 508 patients with hyperventilation syndrome. Nihon Kyobu Shikkan Gakkai Zasshi 33:940–946, 1995

Hoegholm A, Clementsen P, Mortensen SA: Syncope due to right atrial thromboembolism: diagnostic importance of two-dimensional echocardiography. Acta Cardiol 42:469–473, 1987

Hoes MJ, Colla P, Van Doorn P et al: Hyperventilation and panic attacks. J Clin Psychiatry 48:435–437, 1987

Hoitsma E, DeVries J, van Santen-Hoeufft M, et al: Impact of pain in a Dutch sarcoidosis patient population. Sarcoidosis Vasc Diffuse Lung Dis 20:33–39, 2003

Hook O: Sarcoidosis with involvement of the nervous system. Report of nine cases. Arch Neurol Psychiatry 71:554–575, 1954

Hopwood P, Stephens RJ: Depression in patients with lung cancer: prevalence and risk factors derived from quality-of-life data. J Clin Oncol 18:893–903, 2000

Hosenpud JD, Bennett LE, Keck BM, et al: The registry of the international society for heart and lung transplantation: fifteenth official report—1998. J Heart Lung Transplant 17: 656–668, 1998

Ibanez M, Aguilar JJ, Maderal MA, et al: Sexuality in chronic respiratory failure: coincidences and divergences between patients and primary caregiver. Respir Med 95:975–979, 2001

Isenberg SA, Lehrer PM, Hochron S: The effects of suggestion and emotional arousal on pulmonary function in asthma: a review and a hypothesis regarding vagal mediation. Psychosom Med 54:192–216, 1992

Ishii N, Nishihara Y: Pellagra encephalopathy among tuberculous patients: its relation to isoniazid therapy. J Neurol Neurosurg Psychiatry 48:628–634, 1985

Jaffe A, Bush A: Cystic fibrosis: a review of the decade. Monaldi Arch Chest Dis 56:240–247, 2001

Kern-Buell CL, McGrady AV, Conran PB, et al: Asthma severity, psychophysiological indicators of arousal, and immune function in asthma patients undergoing biofeedback-assisted relaxation. Appl Psychophysiol Biofeedback 25:79–91, 2000

Kiev A, Domantay AG: A study of buspirone coprescribed with bronchodilators in 82 anxious ambulatory patients. J Asthma 25:281–284, 1988

Klonoff EA, Kleinhenz ME: Psychological factors in sarcoidosis: the relationship between life stress and pulmonary function. Sarcoidosis Vasc Diffuse Lung Dis 10:118–124, 1993

Kramer MR, Marshall SE, Starnes VA, et al: Infectious complications in heart-lung transplantation: analysis in 200 episodes. Arch Intern Med 153:2010–2016, 1993

Kubzansky LD, Wright RJ, Cohen S, et al: Breathing easy: a prospective study of optimism and pulmonary function in the normative aging study. Ann Behav Med 24:345–353, 2002

Lacasse Y, Brosseau L, Milne S, et al: Pulmonary rehabilitation for chronic obstructive pulmonary disease. Cochrane Database Syst Rev 3:CD003793, 2002

Lachman A, Gielis O, Thys P, et al: Hyperventilation syndrome: current advances. Rev Mal Respir 9:277–285, 1992

Lasky JA, Brody AR: Interstitial fibrosis and growth factors. Environ Health Perspect 108 (suppl 4):751–762, 2000

Lehrer PM, Hochron SM, McCann B, et al: Relaxation decreases large-airway but not small-airway asthma. J Psychosom Res 30:13–25, 1986

Lehrer P, Feldman J, Giardino N, et al: Psychological aspects of asthma. J Consult Clin Psychol 70:691–711, 2002

LeSon S, Gershwin ME: Risk factors for asthmatic patients requiring intubation. J Asthma 33:27–35, 1996

Liippo K, Puolijoki H, Tala E: Periodic breathing imitating hyperventilation syndrome. Chest 102:638–639, 1992

Limbos MM, Joyce DP, Chan CK, et al: Psychological functioning and quality of life in lung transplant candidates and recipients. Chest 118:408–416, 2000

Lishman WA: Endocrine diseases and metabolic disorders, in Organic Psychiatry. London, Blackwell, 1987, pp 466–467, 651

Llewellyn K: CF and me. Interview by Anna Sidey. Paediatr Nurs 10:21–22, 1998

Mancuso CA, Peterson MG, Charlson ME: Effects of depressive symptoms on health-related quality of life in asthma patients. J Gen Intern Med 15:301–310, 2000

Martinez TY, Pereira CA, Dos Santos ML, et al: Evaluation of the short-form 36-item questionnaire to measure health-related quality of life in patients with idiopathic pulmonary fibrosis. Chest 117:1627–1632, 2000

Mathews WB: Sarcoidosis of the nervous system. J Neurol Neurosurg Psychiatry 28:23–29, 1965

Maurer JR, Frost AE, Estenne M et al: International guidelines for the selection of lung transplant candidates. J Heart Lung Transplant 17:703–709, 1998

McCathie HC, Spence SH, Tate RL: Adjustment to chronic obstructive pulmonary disease: the importance of psychological factors. Eur Respir J 19:47–53, 2002

Mendelson WB, Maczaj M, and Holt J: Buspirone administration to sleep apnea patients. J Clin Psychopharmacol 11:71–72, 1991

Miles JF, Garden GM, Tunnicliffe WS, et al: Psychological morbidity and coping skills in patients with brittle and non-brittle asthma: a case-control study. Clin Exp Allergy 27:1151–1159, 1997

Mino M, Narita N, Ikeda H: A case of a pituitary mass in association with sarcoidosis. No To Shinkei 52:253–257, 2000

Mizukami K, Naito Y, Yoshida M, et al: Mental disorders induced by carbamazepine. Jpn J Psychiatry Neurol 44:59–63, 1990

Montazeri A, Gillis CR, McEwen J: Quality of life in patients with lung cancer: a review of literature from 1970 to 1995. Chest 113:467–481, 1998

Napolitano MA, Babyak MA, Palmer S, et al: Effects of a telephone-based psychosocial intervention for patients awaiting lung transplantation. Chest 122:1176–1184, 2002

National Center for Health Statistics: Vital And Health Statistics: Current Estimates from the National Health Interview Survey. U.S. Department of Health and Human Services, 1990–1993. National Vital Statistics Reports 48:26, 2000

Newman KB, Mason UG 3rd, Schmaling KB: Clinical features of vocal cord dysfunction. Am J Respir Crit Care Med 152 (4 pt 1):1382–1386, 1995

Newsham KR, Klaben BK, Miller VJ, et al: Paradoxical vocal-cord dysfunction: management in athletes. J Athl Train 37:325–328, 2002

Nguyen VQ, Byrd RP, Fields CL, et al: DaCosta's syndrome: chronic symptomatic hyperventilation. J Ky Med Assoc 90:221–334, 1992

Ochoa LL, Richardson GW: The current status of lung transplantation: a nursing perspective. AACN Clin Issues 10:229–239, 1999

O'Dowd MA, Jaramillo J, Dubler N, et al: A noncompliant patient with fluctuating capacity. Gen Hosp Psychiatry 20:317–324, 1998

Olson K, Tom B, Hewitt J, et al: Evolving routines: preventing fatigue associated with lung and colorectal cancer. Qual Health Res 12:655–670, 2002

Oscherwitz T, Tulsky JP, Roger S, et al: Detention of persistently nonadherent patients with tuberculosis. JAMA 278:843–846, 1997

Ovesen L, Hannibal J, Mortensen EL: The interrelationship of weight loss, dietary intake, and quality of life in ambulatory patients with cancer of the lung, breast, and ovary. Nutr Cancer 19:159–167, 1993

Paradowski LJ: Saprophytic fungal infections and lung transplantation revisited. J Heart Lung Transplant 16:524–531, 1997

Paris WP, Diercks M, Bright J, et al: Return to work after lung transplantation. J Heart Lung Transplant 17:430–436, 1998

Perkner JJ, Fennelly KP, Balkissoon R, et al: Irritant-associated vocal cord dysfunction. J Occup Environ Med 40:136–143, 1998

Peters SG, Wochos DN, Peterson GC: Status epilepticus as a complication of concurrent electroconvulsive and theophylline therapy. Mayo Clin Proc 59:568–570, 1984

Pinney S, Freeman LJ, Nixon PG: Role of the nurse counselor in managing patients with the hyperventilation syndrome. J R Soc Med 80:216–218, 1987

Porzelius J, Vest M, Nochomovitz M: Respiratory function, cognitions, and panic in chronic obstructive pulmonary patients. Behav Res Ther 30:75–77, 1992

Put C, Van den Bergh O, Demedts M, et al: A study of the relationship among self-reported noncompliance, symptomatology, and psychological variables in patients with asthma. J Asthma 37:503–510, 2000

Reichman LB, Felton CP, Edsall JR: Drug dependence, a possible new risk factor for tuberculosis disease. Arch Intern Med 139:337–339, 1979

Rognum TO, Olaisen B, Teige B: Hyperventilation syndrome. Could acute salicylic acid poisoning be the cause? [in Norwegian]. Tidsskr Nor Laegforen 107:1043, 1050, 1987

Rose C, Wallace L, Dickson R, Ayres J, Lehman R, Searle Y, Burge PS: The most effective psychologically-based treatments to reduce anxiety and panic in patients with chronic obstructive pulmonary disease (COPD): a systematic review. Patient Educ Couns 47:311–318, 2002

Saarijarvi S, Lehtinen P: The hyperventilation syndrome treated with antidepressive agents. Duodecim 103:417–420, 1987

Sabaawi M, Gutierrez-Nunez J, Fragala MR: Neurosarcoidosis presenting as schizophreniform disorder. Int J Psychiatry Med 22:269–274, 1992

Schmaling KB, Niloofar A, Barnhart S, et al: Medical and psychiatric predictors of airway reactivity. Respir Care 44:1452–1457, 1999

Schnoll RA, Malstrom M, James C, et al: Correlates of tobacco use among smokers and recent quitters diagnosed with cancer. Patient Educ Couns 46:137–145, 2002

Scialdone AM: Thalamic hemorrhage imitating hyperventilation. Ann Emerg Med 19:817–819, 1990

Sharma, OP: Sarcoidosis: A Clinical Approach. Springfield, IL, Charles C Thomas, 1975

Silverstein A, Feuer M, Siltzback L: Neurologic sarcoidosis. Arch Neurol 12:1–11, 1965

Skorodin MS, King F, Sharp JT: Carbon monoxide poisoning presenting as hyperventilation syndrome. Ann Intern Med 105:631–632, 1986

Small SP, Graydon JE: Perceived uncertainty, physical symptoms, and negative mood in hospitalized patients with chronic obstructive pulmonary disease. Heart Lung 21: 568–574, 1992

Smoller JW, Pollack MH, Systrom D, et al: Sertraline effects on dyspnea in patients with obstructive airways disease. Psychosomatics 39:24–29, 1998

Snell G, deHoyos A, Krajden M, et al: *Pseudomonas capacia* in lung transplantation recipients with cystic fibrosis. Chest 103:466–471, 1993

Sternbach GL: Infections in alcoholic patients. Emerg Med Clin North Am 8:793–803, 1990

Stilley C, Dew MA, Stukas AA, et al: Psychological symptom levels and their correlates in lung and heart-lung transplant recipients. Psychosomatics 40:503–509, 1999

Stone P, Richards M, A'Hern R, et al: A study to investigate the prevalence, severity and correlates of fatigue among patients with cancer in comparison with a control group of volunteers without cancer. Ann Oncol 11:561–567, 2000

Stoudemire A, Linfors E, Houpt JL, et al: Central nervous system sarcoidosis. Gen Hosp Psychiatry 5:129–132, 1983

Strauss GM: Bronchogenic carcinoma, in Textbook of Pulmonary Disease, 6th Edition. Edited by Baum GL, Grapo JD, Celli BR. Philadelphia, PA, Lippincott-Raven, 1998, p 1329

Sturdy PM, Victor CR, Anderson HR, et al: Mortality and severe morbidity working group of the national asthma task force. Psychological, social and health behavior risk factors for deaths certified as asthma: a national case-control study. Thorax 57:1034–1039, 2002

Suchenwirth R, Dold V: Functional psychoses in sarcoidosis. Verh Dtsch Ges Inn Med 75:757–759, 1969

Takatsuki K, Kado T, Satouchi M, et al: Psychiatric studies of chemotherapy and chemotherapy-induced nausea and vomiting of patients with lung or thymic cancer. Gan To Kagaku Ryoho 25:403–408, 1998

Tashkin D, Kanner R, Bailey W, et al: Smoking cessation in patients with chronic obstructive pulmonary disease: a double-blind, placebo-controlled, randomised trial. Lancet 357: 1571–1575, 2001

Teichman BJ, Burker EJ, Weiner M, et al: Factors associated with adherence to treatment regimens after lung transplantation. Prog Transplant 10:113–121, 2000

ten Thoren C, Petermann F: Reviewing asthma and anxiety. Respir Med 94:409–415, 2000

Thompson C, Checkley S: Short term memory deficit in a patient with cerebral sarcoidosis. Br J Psychiatry 139:160–161, 1981

Treasure RA, Fowler PB, Millington HT, et al: Misdiagnosis of diabetic ketoacidosis as hyperventilation syndrome. BMJ (Clin Res Ed) 294:630, 1987

Trulock EP, Edwards LB, Taylor DO, et al: The Registry of the International Society for Heart and Lung Transplantation: Twentieth official adult lung and heart-lung transplant report—2003. J Heart Lung Transplant 22:625–635, 2003. Available at: http://www.ustransplant.org/annual_reports/archives/2003/Preface_Contributors.htm#citataion

Van De Ven LL, Mouthan BJ, Hoes MJ: Treatment of the hyperventilation syndrome with bisoprodol: a placebo-controlled clinical trial. J Psychosom Res 39:1007–1013, 1995

Withers NJ, Rudkin ST, White RJ: Anxiety and depression in severe chronic obstructive pulmonary disease: the effects of pulmonary rehabilitation. J Cardiopulm Rehabil 19:362–365, 1999

Wurtemberger G, Hutter BO: The significance of health related quality of life for the evaluation of interventional measures in patients with COPD. Pneumologie 55:91–99, 2001

Yohannes AM, Baldwin RC, Connolly MJ: Depression and anxiety in elderly outpatients with chronic obstructive pulmonary disease: prevalence, and validation of the BASDEC screening questionnaire. Int J Geriatr Psychiatry 15:1090–1096, 2000

Young P, Dewse M, Fergusson W, Kolbe J: Respiratory rehabilitation in chronic obstructive pulmonary disease: predictors of nonadherence. Eur Respir J 13:855–859, 1999

Zerman W: Die Meningoencephalitis. Nervenarzt 23:43–52, 1952

Self-Assessment Questions

Select the single best response for each question.

1. Which of the following statements concerning psychological factors in asthma is *false?*
   A. People with Cluster B personality disorders are more likely to have asthma.
   B. Psychological factors may influence asthma through behavioral mechanisms.
   C. Poor adherence with follow-up visits and poor inhaler technique may be associated with asthma deaths.
   D. Patients with asthma are more likely to hold catastrophic beliefs or cognitions.
   E. Asthma attacks may be provoked by psychological distress.

2. In patients with chronic obstructive pulmonary disease (COPD), anxiety and depression have been found to be associated with
   A. Higher relapse after emergency treatment.
   B. Increased disability.
   C. Lower exercise tolerance.
   D. Noncompliance with treatment.
   E. All of the above.

3. Regarding sarcoidosis, which of the following statements is *true?*
   A. Sarcoidosis affects white patients more than African American patients.
   B. In Europe, Italians have high prevalence rates.
   C. Onset of the illness usually occurs between the ages of 20 and 40 years.
   D. The disease follows a progressive, downhill course, with nearly 25% of patients dying from it.
   E. All of the above.

4. Psychiatric factors that are considered to be absolute contraindications to lung transplantation include all of the following *except*
   A. Active alcoholism.
   B. Anxiety disorders.
   C. Noncompliance with treatment.
   D. Drug abuse.
   E. Cigarette use.

5. In the treatment of anxiety disorders in pulmonary disease, which of the following classes of psychotropic medications are contraindicated due to the risk of inducing vasospasm?
   A. Buspirone.
   B. Short-acting benzodiazepines.
   C. Long-acting benzodiazepines.
   D. SSRIs.
   E. Beta-blockers.

4 Gastrointestinal Disorders

Francis Creed, M.D., F.R.C.P., F.R.C.Psych., F.Med.Sci.
Kevin W. Olden, M.D.

THE CLOSE RELATIONSHIP between the gut and the psyche means that there are many examples of biopsychosocial relationships in the patient population seen by gastroenterologists. The consulting psychiatrist can expect to see a large number of patients with functional gastroenterological disorders, which comprise approximately half of all patients seen by gastroenterologists (Thompson et al. 2000). Psychiatrists in medical settings can also expect to see patients with organic diseases, such as liver disease and inflammatory bowel disease, where psychiatric disorders can influence management and outcome. Some patients are seen routinely by psychiatrists prior to liver transplant (see Chapter 14, "Organ Transplantation") or before the start of interferon treatment for chronic hepatitis C.

Functional Gastrointestinal Disorders

The broad categorization of disorders into *functional* and *organic* (or *structural*) has helped to facilitate research into the psychological factors that are important in the functional disorders. It has also helped with the adaptation of the biopsychosocial model in gastroenterology (Drossman 1998; Drossman et al. 1999).

The functional and organic terminology may, however, reinforce dualistic thinking—the separation of mind and body. Furthermore, some gastroenterologists falsely equate *functional* with *psychiatric*, which leads them to ignore psychiatric disorders in patients with organic disease.

In clinical practice, the identification and treatment of psychiatric disorders in patients with gastrointestinal (GI) disorders can be very rewarding. Many patients with functional GI disorders may experience considerable improvement in their symptoms when a concurrent psychiatric disorder is successfully identified and treated. In structural (organic) disorders, the GI symptoms may not change as dramatically when coexisting depression or anxiety is treated, but patients may experience substantial improvement in their health-related quality of life—that is, they can cope with their symptoms, treatment, and lifestyle changes much more successfully.

The Relationship Between Psychiatric Disorders and Gastrointestinal Diseases

Our understanding of the relationship between psychiatric and GI disorders has developed considerably over the last two decades. The *Diagnostic and Statistical Manual of Mental Disorders* (DSM; American Psychiatric Association 2000) has been mirrored by a similar symptom-based classification of the functional GI disorders, the so-called Rome criteria (Drossman et al. 2000a). Such a classification has caused much discussion among gastroenterologists, who are used to making diagnoses on the basis of observable structural abnormalities. This has implications for clinical practice because some gastroenterologists may give the impression to patients that complaints based on structural abnormalities of the gut are "real," whereas complaints without any abnormalities seen on endoscopy or imaging studies may be dismissed as they turn out to be "only" functional. When this occurs, the psychiatrist must first deal with patients feeling angry or devalued before a full clinical appraisal of symptoms is commenced (Creed and Guthrie 1993; Guthrie and Creed 1996).

Peptic Ulcer

It has been estimated that approximately 10% of individuals in Western countries will develop a peptic ulcer sometime during their lifetime (Rosenstock and Jorgensen 1995). The two major risk factors associated with the development of both gastric and duodenal ulcers are the use of nonsteroidal anti-inflammatory drugs (NSAIDs) and the presence of infection with *Heliobacter pylori* (Kurata et al. 1997).

However, despite the importance of *H. pylori* in the etiology of peptic ulcer, significant psychosocial dimensions remain to be considered with this disorder.

Prevalence of Psychiatric Disorders

Although the prevalence of anxiety and depressive disorders appears increased in patients with peptic ulcer disease (Table 4–1), this is not a firm conclusion because of methodological weaknesses with many studies (Lewin and Lewis 1995). One of the most comprehensive studies included patients with peptic ulcer and inflammatory bowel diseases of recent onset (Craig 1989); 16% of patients had definite psychiatric disorders, and a further 32% had borderline ("subthreshold") psychiatric disorders. Subthreshold disorders may impair health-related quality of life and lead to a worse prognosis, so psychiatric or psychological treatments should not be confined to people who meet the DSM criteria for a psychiatric disorder (Creed et al. 2002).

The onset, perpetuation, and recurrence of peptic ulcers are associated with stressful life events. This has been demonstrated after earthquakes, where stress and the presence of *H. pylori* interacted (Matsushima et al. 1999). Onset or relapse of peptic ulcer disease is associated with chronic stressors involving goal frustration, in which the individual is repeatedly prevented from reaching a much-treasured goal (Craig 1989; Ellard et al. 1990). Such frustration may reflect a personality type associated with continuing to strive toward a goal even when success is unlikely.

The personality traits of social withdrawal, suspiciousness, hostility, and dependency may be associated with increased cigarette and alcohol consumption, which contributes to development of peptic ulcers (Levenstein 2000).

Psychosomatic medicine specialists should be prepared to discuss these finding with patients as part of a strategy to prevent

TABLE 4–1. Prevalence of psychiatric disorder in peptic ulcer disease

Study	Psychiatric disorder measure	Peptic ulcer disease, no.	Control subjects, no.	Statistical significance
Langeluddecke et al. 1987	STAI, ZDS	63	50 (medically ill patients)	No significant difference from MI patients
Langeluddecke et al. 1987	STAI, ZDS	83	59 (dyspepsia patients)	Less anxious than dyspepsia patients
Tennant et al. 1986	STAI, ZDS	87	Population normative data	Higher anxiety and depression scores than norms
Craig 1989	PSE	56[a]	79 (functional bowel disorders)[b] 135 (healthy control subjects)[b]	Prevalence of psychiatric disorder less than in patients with functional GI disorder and more than in healthy control subjects
Magni et al. 1982	KSSRT	25 (duodenal ulcer) 36 (acute gastroduodenitis)	61 (matched control subjects)	Both groups more anxious than control subjects Higher depression and somatization scores only in acute gastroduodenitis group

Note. GI=gastrointestinal; KSSRT=Kellner-Sheffield Symptom Rating Test; MI=myocardial infarction; PSE=Present State Examination; STAI=State-Trait Anxiety Inventory; ZDS=Zung Depression Scale.
[a]16% had psychiatric disorders.
[b]34% of patients with functional GI disorder and 8% of control subjects had psychiatric disorders.

recurrent ulcers. Some patients understand the association between *H. pylori* and peptic ulcer as a one-to-one relationship, excluding the possibility that outcome might be influenced by their own behavior.

Health-Related Quality of Life

Health-related quality of life is impaired most severely in people with gastric or duodenal ulcers, which are accompanied by anxiety or depression (Dimenas et al. 1995). Depression also adversely affects the outcome of standard treatment for peptic ulcer (Xuan et al. 1999).

Inflammatory Bowel Disease

Idiopathic inflammatory bowel disease (IBD) represents a spectrum of illnesses from ulcerative colitis and Crohn's disease to the less common but emerging disorders of microscopic colitis, collagenous colitis, and lymphocytic colitis.

Prevalence of Psychiatric Disorders

Patients with IBD show a higher prevalence of psychological disorder than the general population, but a lower prevalence of psychological disorder than patients with functional bowel disorder (Walker et al. 1995). The rate, mostly in the range of 21% to 35%, is similar to that found in other chronic physical illnesses (Creed et al. 2002). Mood disorder appears to be more common in older patients and in those with a previous history of psychiatric disorder (Acosta-Ramirez et al. 2001).

Stress, Psychiatric Disorder, and Gastrointestinal Function

The relationship between psychiatric disorder and IBD is unclear (Table 4–2). Some patients with IBD may be particularly vulnerable to developing psychiatric disorder because of experiences that are independent of the disease process (e.g., childhood victimization and abuse) (Walker et al. 1996). Most studies have failed to find an association with stress (North et al. 1991), but two studies suggest that relapse is predicted by depression (Kurina et al. 2001; Mittermaier et al. 2004). Many authors report psychiatric disorder only in close relationship with increased disease activity, suggesting that the former is a consequence of an IBD flare (North et al. 1991).

Some patients with IBD may avidly attribute their symptoms to stress. This can be maladaptive if patients conclude the disease is somehow their (or someone else's) fault or if patients use it to rationalize the avoidance of chronic drug therapy. It should be pointed out that general stress reduction measures may be helpful, but they are not an alternative to close adherence to the prescribed medications (Maunder and Esplen 2001; Maunder et al. 1997).

Health-Related Quality of Life

There is clear evidence that anxiety and depression impair health-related quality of life in IBD (Guthrie et al. 2002; Nordin et al. 2002; Turnbull and Vallis 1995; Walker et al. 1996). Even after adjustment for severity of IBD, anxiety and depressive disorders, including subthreshold disorders, are associated with worse physical function, role limitation, health perception, and pain. There is preliminary evidence that health-related quality of life improves if psychiatric morbidity is treated (Walker et al. 1996), and this should be the main aim of psychiatric treatment in people with concurrent psychiatric disorders and IBD.

The presence of psychiatric disorder in patients with IBD is also associated with many GI symptoms that are typical of irritable bowel syndrome (IBS)—abdominal pain that is relieved by defecation; bloating; and altered bowel habits. People with IBD who also have these comorbid IBS symptoms have the greatest impairment of health-related quality of life of all patients with IBD (Simren et al. 2002). Clinicians should therefore ask about IBS-type symptoms even in patients with IBD and anticipate that these symptoms may improve with psychiatric treatment.

Relationship Between Health Care Utilization and Psychological and Disease-Related Variables

Although severity of IBD is the main predictor of health care service use, especially hospitalization, a number of psychological and social variables are also important independent predictors. These include depression (Guthrie et al. 2002), emotional and social functioning, and patients' concerns (Drossman et al. 1991). Because many patients with IBD are young and striving to lead a normal life, any intervention that reduces the time spent visiting doctors is beneficial—another reason for energetically treating any concurrent psychiatric disorder.

Functional Gastrointestinal Disorders: Irritable Bowel Syndrome and Functional Dyspepsia

Functional GI disorders represent a spectrum of disorders of function, which en-

TABLE 4–2. Prevalence of psychiatric disorder in patients with inflammatory bowel disease

Study	Psychiatric disorder measure	Total no.	Ulcerative colitis and Crohn's disease patients		Comment
			Percent with psychiatric disorder		
Helzer et al. 1982	Standardized psychiatric interview/ Feighner criteria	50	26		Prevalence similar to that in other medically ill patients (30%)
Andrews et al. 1987	DSM-III	162	33		No difference between Crohn's disease and ulcerative colitis groups
Tarter et al. 1987	DIS/DSM-III	53	26 (anxiety) 15 (panic) 10 (depression)		Greater prevalence than in control subjects
Magni et al. 1991		50	22 (lifetime) 62 (current)		More than in control subjects
Walker et al. 1996	DIS	40	35		No difference between IBD groups
de Boer et al. 1998	CES-D	224	32		No difference between IBD groups
Guthrie et al. 2002	HADS	112	26		No difference between IBD groups
Rose et al. 2002	CES-D	66	21		No control group

Note. CES-D=Center for Epidemiologic Studies Depression Scale; DIS=Diagnostic Interview Schedule; HADS=Hospital Anxiety and Depression Scale; IBD=inflammatory bowel disease.

TABLE 4–3. Rome II criteria for irritable bowel syndrome

At least 12 weeks or more, which need not be consecutive, in the preceding 12 months of abdominal discomfort or pain that has two out of the following three features:

- Relieved with defecation
- Onset associated with a change in frequency of stool
- Onset associated with a change in form (appearance) of stool

Symptoms that cumulatively support the diagnosis of irritable bowel syndrome:

- Abnormal stool frequency (for research purposes, "abnormal" may be defined as more than three bowel movements per day or less than three bowel movements per week)
- Abnormal stool form (lumpy/hard or loose/watery stool)
- Abnormal stool passage (straining, urgency, or feeling of incomplete evacuation)
- Passage of mucus
- Bloating or feeling of abdominal distension

---

compasses the functional esophageal disorders, such as noncardiac chest pain and functional dysphagia; functional dyspepsia (previously called nonulcer dyspepsia); IBS; and functional constipation, functional diarrhea, and functional abdominal pain. The sine qua non of a functional GI disorder is the lack of structural or biochemical abnormalities that could explain the patient's symptoms, which requires that the diagnosis of functional GI disorders be symptom based.

The most common functional GI disorder is IBS, which comes in three general clinical forms: with constipation, with diarrhea, and with an alternating pattern of diarrhea and constipation. The diagnostic criteria for IBS are outlined in Table 4–3.

Prevalence of Psychiatric Disorders

The prevalence of anxiety, panic, and mood disorders in patients attending gastroenterology clinics with functional bowel disorders (50%–60%) is approximately twice that of IBD (Drossman et al. 2000a, 2002). The prevalence is similar across diagnostic groups such as patients with IBS, functional dyspepsia, functional abdominal pain, and noncardiac chest pain (Biggs 2004; Dimenas et al. 1995). Anxiety is more prominent in first-time attenders, but depression seems more prominent in those who have chronic symptoms and who have been attending the clinic over a long period without remission (Guthrie et al. 1992). Panic disorder is frequent in some specialist settings (Lydiard et al. 1993). High levels of psychological distress are found in people who have numerous bodily symptoms outside of the GI tract (so-called extraintestinal symptoms), including fibromyalgia (Sperber et al. 2000; Whitehead et al. 2002).

The onset of anxiety or mood disorder precedes or coincides with the onset of the bowel disorder in approximately two-thirds of IBS patients (Craig 1989; Ford et al. 1987). This suggests a close link between the psychiatric disorder and gut symptoms. The presence of (untreated) psychiatric disorder predicts a poor outcome, and conversely, reduction of psychiatric symptoms is associated with reduction of bowel symptoms (Creed 1999).

Stress precedes the onset of functional bowel disorders, whether there is concurrent psychiatric disorder or not (Creed et al. 1988; Drossman et al. 1988). The most common stresses relate to difficult personal relationships—marital separations, divorce, and other relationship breakups. Many patients tend to deny the importance of such events and claim that any psychological or social difficulties are the result of the bowel disorder rather than stress. Careful history taking with sufficient attention paid to time course of events will usually demonstrate the correct sequence.

Social stress is also the single most important predictor of outcome in patients with IBS who attend a gastroenterology clinic (Bennett et al. 1998). Failure to address the stressor(s) may therefore lead to persistent symptoms. Some patients are reluctant to discuss social stress, protesting that it is unrelated to the bowel disorder (Creed and Guthrie 1993). For most patients, however, a clear explanation of the purpose of doing so leads to a fruitful discussion. For example, a series of patients with dyspepsia were asked to list their main complaints, and about two-thirds spontaneously mentioned "anxiety" before "dyspepsia"; therefore, an open question may enable the psychiatrist to rapidly elicit a person's concerns (Haug et al. 1995).

Health-Related Quality of Life

Anxiety and mood disorders play a large part in the impairment of health-related quality of life observed in IBS (Creed et al. 2001; Walker et al. 1995; Whitehead et al. 1996). As in other medical conditions, the effects of physical and psychological symptoms are approximately additive in terms of their effect on quality of life (Creed et al. 2001, 2002). In dyspepsia, psychological distress is a better predictor of health-related quality of life than the severity of the dyspepsia (Quartero et al. 1999), and the considerable impairment of health-related quality of life attributed to IBS may be the result of concurrent psychiatric disorders (Creed et al. 2005; Drossman et al. 2000b). In other words, there is a good prospect of improvement of health-related quality of life when the anxiety or mood disorder is satisfactorily

treated, as has been demonstrated with both antidepressants and psychotherapy (Creed et al. 2003; Drossman et al. 2003; Guthrie et al. 1991; Hamilton et al. 2000).

Relationship Between Health Care Utilization and Psychological and Disease-Related Variables

Many people with functional dyspepsia or IBS do not consult a doctor (Drossman et al. 1988). Those who do so have more severe abdominal pain than nonconsulters, but they also have more anxiety and depression and, in particular, more worries about their health—especially fears of cancer (Creed 1999; Gomborone et al. 1995; Kettell et al. 1992; Koloski et al. 2003; Lydiard and Jones 1989). Adequately addressing these worries in the gastroenterology clinic may lead to fewer subsequent visits (van Dulmen et al. 1995). Psychiatrists should routinely ask about such fears and be prepared to deal with them directly, because they often persist even after diagnostic investigations have been normal (Lucock et al. 1997).

The sources of persistent health anxiety are not fully understood, but lack of social support and early life experience, including illness in the family, abuse, or neglect, both may play a part (Biggs et al. 2003; Whitehead et al. 1982). It is crucial for the psychiatrist to fully explore concerns about serious illness with the patient; such concerns are often related to illness in family members or remarks made to the individual by a physician that play on the patient's mind.

Sexual Abuse and Functional Gastrointestinal Disorders

There is an established literature demonstrating an association between IBS and a history of childhood sexual abuse (Delvaux et al. 1997; Drossman et al. 1990, 1995; Leserman et al. 1996, 1998; Walker et al.

1995), although there are some inconsistencies (Biggs 2004; Talley et al. 1995), including in population-based studies (Talley et al. 1998). It appears that a history of sexual abuse might be a predictor of chronicity and severity of a disorder (Longstreth et al. 1993) and may not be specific to IBS (Katon et al. 2001).

Reported childhood sexual abuse or related trauma is associated with increased health care utilization in functional bowel disorders (Biggs et al. 2003; Guthrie and Creed 2003; Leserman et al. 1998). Self-reported abuse is associated with complaints in adulthood of a greater number of bodily symptoms; this may be associated with a lower pain threshold and a tendency to be hypervigilant about bodily symptoms (Salmon et al. 2003). Perhaps the mechanism most commonly involves mood, panic, and other anxiety disorders, which occur in those subjected to abuse during childhood (Blanchard et al. 2002). As we have seen, these psychiatric disorders are more common in functional bowel disorders than organic GI diseases, and they are independently associated with higher health care utilization in IBS (Budavari and Olden 2003).

In clinical practice, it is important for psychiatrists to routinely assess possible childhood abuse in patients with functional GI disorders, especially those who have not responded to treatment. Whatever the type of disorder, patients will usually not have had the opportunity to speak to their gastroenterologist about such intimate aspects of their life (Drossman et al. 1990).

Other Functional Gastrointestinal Disorders

The other functional GI disorders, for example, gastroesophageal reflux, globus, functional abdominal pain, and cyclic vomiting, are described in the Rome book (Drossman et al. 2000a). They often co-exist with other functional GI disorders, and their features are very similar to the two disorders described here; anxiety and depression are common. Clinical assessment and treatment follow the general pattern described in this chapter, with the exception that speech therapy may be helpful for globus (Khalil et al. 2003).

Liver Disease

A variety of liver diseases are important in psychosomatic medicine. We focus here primarily on hepatitis C virus (HCV) infection. Viral hepatitides are also discussed in Chapter 10, "Infectious Diseases." In the developed nations, alcohol is the most common cause of liver disease. Most forms of chronic liver disease can result in cirrhosis, leading to hepatic encephalopathy, which may manifest with symptoms of psychosis, mania, depression, apathy, or confusion before becoming a frank delirium (Dieperink et al. 2000) (see Chapter 14, "Organ Transplantation"). Wilson's disease (Chapter 15, "Neurology and Neurosurgery") and the porphyrias (Chapter 6, "Endocrine Disorders") are rare diseases affecting the liver whose first symptoms may be psychiatric.

Fatigue is a common symptom in liver disease and may be caused by the disease, its treatment, or a comorbid depression. In one study of patients with primary biliary cirrhosis, fatigue was more closely associated with depression than with liver disease (Cauch-Dudek et al. 1998). Depression is also common in people undergoing liver transplantation, and there is some evidence that the depression may improve following transplantation (see Chapter 14, "Organ Transplantation").

Chronic liver disease leads to significantly impaired health-related quality of life; successful treatment, either by transplant or by antiviral treatment, may lead to improvement (De Bona et al. 2000; Dieperink et al. 2000). Depression also predicts impaired health-related quality of life (Fontana et al. 2001). Thus, treatment of depression in patients with chronic liver disease is important for three reasons: in its own right, to improve health-related quality of life, and to facilitate treatment of liver disease.

Chronic Hepatitis C Virus Infection

Chronic HCV (previously known as non-A, non-B hepatitis) has become the major cause of chronic liver disease in the United States, with a prevalence of 1.8% of the population. It is estimated that 4 million Americans are infected with HCV (Alter 1997).

HCV infection is acquired through intravenous drug abuse, a strong risk factor for other psychiatric disorders (Dwight et al. 2000). Individuals with HCV infection are more likely to have major depressive disorder, posttraumatic stress disorder (PTSD), and anxiety disorders as well as alcohol- and drug-use disorders (El-Serag et al. 2002). Studies of war veterans with HCV have recorded a very high prevalence of alcohol and drug abuse (80%) combined with current depression and PTSD, which occurred in 60% of the sample (Nguyen et al. 2002).

In contrast to HCV, hepatitis B virus (HBV) is acquired mainly through sexual contact and through maternal–fetal transmission. It is much less likely to induce depression or other psychiatric symptoms as compared with HCV, and thus HBV is less of an issue for the consultation psychiatrist.

A major concern now lies in the increased chance of developing significant depression with interferon (antiviral) treatment of hepatitis C. Interferon treatment has significant side effects, including fatigue, neurological and cognitive symptoms, and depression (fulfilling the criteria for major depression in approximately one-third of people) (Bonaccorso et al. 2002;

Horikawa et al. 2003; Kraus et al. 2003). Suicidal ideation occurs frequently and has led to cessation of treatment. In one study, 58% of individuals receiving interferon had a diagnosable psychiatric illness after initiation of therapy (Kraus et al. 2003).

In patients with chronic HCV infection, severity of depressive symptoms is highly correlated with fatigue severity, but measures of hepatic disease severity, interferon dosage, and severity of comorbid medical illnesses are not (Dwight et al. 2000). Patients' symptoms of listlessness, anhedonia, fatigue, and physical pain may be mistaken as manifestations of their liver disease; however, it is much more likely that these symptoms are the result of a comorbid psychiatric disorder, most likely major depressive disorder (Porcelli et al. 1996; Wessely and Pariante 2002).

Antidepressants, most often selective serotonin reuptake inhibitors (SSRIs), are useful in the treatment of depressive disorder during interferon-alfa treatment. Paroxetine (Kraus et al. 2001, 2002), sertraline (Schramm et al. 2000), and citalopram (Gleason et al. 2002) have all been effective in clinical trials for the treatment of interferon-induced depression in patients infected with HCV.

Diagnostic Issues

The diagnosis of psychiatric disorders in gastroenterology patients does not usually present great difficulties. Some GI symptoms, such as pain, anorexia, or constipation, may be ambiguous (i.e., resulting from either psychiatric or GI disorders), but there are usually a host of other somatic and psychological symptoms that enable the psychiatrist to diagnose anxiety or depressive disorders. Somatization and somatoform pain disorders may be more difficult to distinguish from GI disorders, because both present with physical symptoms; but the diagnosis will usually become apparent after a careful history and physical and psychiatric examinations.

A common problem lies in persuading gastroenterologists and primary care doctors to recognize anxiety or depressive disorders early in their management of GI diseases. The search for possible organic causes of symptoms such as abdominal pain and diarrhea can become very extensive, increasing health anxiety. The doctor's attention can be drawn to the possibility of a psychiatric disorder by the use of a simple screening questionnaire such as the Beck Depression Inventory (BDI) (Beck et al. 1961) or the Hospital Anxiety and Depression Scale (HADS) (Drossman et al. 2000a; Zigmond and Snaith 1983).

Rarely, but especially in older people, an undiagnosed depressive illness can lead to marked diarrhea (as a manifestation of accompanying anxiety), abdominal pain, and weight loss. These symptoms may lead to the suspicion of an underlying GI malignancy and numerous investigations. Psychiatrists should be prepared to treat such a person energetically with antidepressants and monitor closely both the depressive and GI symptoms. If two disorders are present—a malignancy and depression—sleep, pain, mood, and hopelessness might improve, but weight and diarrhea might not.

Patients with carcinoma of the pancreas have a reputation for presenting first with depression (Passik and Breitbart 1996) (see Chapter 7, "Oncology"). Gastroenterologists may encounter patients with unsuspected anorexia nervosa with chronic diarrhea, generalized weakness, and hypokalemia from laxative abuse, or chronic vomiting either self-induced or from ipecac abuse. Psychiatric symptoms in patients with ostomies are discussed in Chapter 13, "Surgery."

Treatment

Clinical Assessment

The clinical psychiatric assessment of patients with GI disorders is similar to that in other medical disorders (see Chapter 1, "Psychiatric Assessment and Consultation"). In this section, we emphasize points relevant to patients seen by psychiatrists referred from gastroenterologists.

Accurate Dating of Symptom Onset

Careful history taking should establish several dates: the date of onset and exacerbation of the GI symptoms and the date of onset of depressive or anxiety symptoms. These dates may be compared to the dates of any important life events to establish an accurate time course. Thus, for instance, discovery of a spouse's extramarital affair may be followed by onset of anxiety symptoms, later marital separation, and subsequent simultaneous onset of depressive symptoms, abdominal pain, and diarrhea. This sequence suggests that the bowel symptoms are related to stress. It does *not*, however, prove that the symptoms are caused by a functional, as opposed to an organic, disorder, because symptoms of IBD may also get worse with stress and precipitate anxiety or depression. The time sequence allows the psychiatrist to evaluate any suggestion from the patient that the depression is unrelated or is simply a reaction to the bowel disturbance. It also allows a full exploration of the patient's feelings about the life events.

Systems Review

It is also important to perform a thorough review of symptoms in other bodily systems. By eliciting all of the patient's bodily symptoms, the psychiatrist makes the patient *feel understood*, which is the first stage of management of a patient with medically unexplained symptoms (Morriss et al. 1999).

Health Anxiety, Early Experiences, and Attitudes

It is important to elicit fears of cancer or other serious illness. Satisfactory consultation with a gastroenterologist leads to reduction in fears of cancer and to decreased preoccupation and helplessness in relation to the pain (van Dulmen et al. 1995). However, if these issues have not been addressed previously, the psychiatrist should address them and explore possible reasons, such as serious illness in the family; depressive, panic, and other anxiety disorders; and hypochondriacal personality traits (Colgan et al. 1988a).

As noted earlier in this chapter, sexual abuse in childhood and related traumatic experiences may be important in patients with functional GI disorders, especially those with high health care utilization.

In their extreme forms, the illness attitudes and behaviors seen in patients with functional GI disorders may amount to a psychiatric diagnosis of a somatoform disorder or a factitious disorder or malingering.

Measurement and Monitoring

Nowadays, psychiatrists often use standardized instruments to measure the severity of depressive or anxiety disorders, particularly for screening and in research. Many common psychiatric instruments include GI symptoms, so it may be wise to consider the total score with and without these symptoms included, especially in borderline cases. For example, the BDI has items concerning aches and pains, upset stomach, constipation, and changes in appetite (Beck et al. 1961). The HADS (Zigmond and Snaith 1983) was designed for use in medical populations and may be particularly useful in GI patients because it specifically excludes items concerning bodily symptoms. The Rome committee has reviewed the instruments commonly used (Drossman et al. 1999, 2000a).

Pharmacological Treatment

Functional Gastrointestinal Syndromes

Pharmacological treatment of IBS has been recently reviewed (Talley 2003). There is clear evidence of the effectiveness of tricyclic antidepressants (TCAs) in IBS (Clouse 2003; Jackson et al. 2000). Systematic reviews of the existing literature show an odds ratio of 4.2 (95% CI: 2.3 to 7.9) for the efficacy of TCAs over placebo, mostly measured in terms of pain relief (Jackson et al. 2000). The mechanism of the benefit derived from TCAs in functional bowel disorders is not entirely clear. They are effective in low doses with rapid onset, suggesting the benefits may be the result of analgesic and anticholinergic effects. Imipramine was helpful in chest pain in one study (Cannon et al. 1994), but the mechanisms of action are also not clear.

Too few studies have examined the effect of SSRI antidepressants to be clear about their efficacy, but they are active in doses that are effective in clinical depression, and the onset of action is slower, suggesting that they act through a different mechanism from TCAs (Creed et al. 2003; Kirsch and Louie 2000; Masand et al. 2002).

In larger studies, effectiveness of TCAs and SSRIs in improving abdominal pain is related to medication adherence (Creed et al. 2003; Drossman et al. 2003). Some patients with constipation-predominant IBS cannot tolerate TCAs, and some with diarrhea may experience an increase in diarrhea with SSRIs. Dropout rates are high for either class of drug unless special effort is made to promote adherence (Clouse 2003; Creed et al. 2003). Newer drugs developed for IBS have been agonists and antagonists of enteric serotonin receptors (e.g., alosetron, tegaserod), but they do not seem to interact adversely with SSRIs.

In clinical practice, it is important to decide why antidepressants are being used—for their analgesic properties in people who have severe pain or to treat a concurrent depressive illness—and to carefully explain this to the patient. On many occasions, doctors have prescribed low-dose antidepressants for patients' pain, only to be told later that these patients did not take (or stopped taking) the medication because they learned that the drug is an antidepressant and they did not consider themselves depressed.

The Rome committee has reviewed in detail the use of psychotropic drugs in treating functional GI disorders (Drossman et al. 2000a). Antidepressants have also been used with some degree of success for functional dyspepsia (Mertz et al. 1998). A number of other agents may also provide symptom relief (see Stanghellini et al. 2003).

Depression in People With Organic Gastrointestinal Disorders

Antidepressant treatment for interferon-induced depression was discussed earlier in this chapter (see subsection "Chronic Hepatitis C Virus Infection").

Psychological Treatment

Functional Gastrointestinal Disorders

There have been many studies of psychological treatments of functional bowel disorders, but the sample sizes have been small in some studies, and different therapies and different measures have been used (Spanier et al. 2003). However, the overall evidence suggests that these treatments are helpful (Lackner et al. 2004). There seems to be no difference according to specific treatment—dynamic interpersonal therapy, cognitive-behavioral therapy, hypnosis, and relaxation training all appeared to be successful. It is not clear whether these therapies have a specific effect on gut function or whether they act in a general way by reducing tension or improving interpersonal relationships and assertiveness. Because of their time-consuming nature

and associated expense, psychological treatments tend to be reserved for the more severe cases.

In clinical practice, the choice between an antidepressant and psychotherapy may be made by patient preference. Often the latter is preferred. Because psychotherapy and pharmacotherapy probably have different modes of action, it is reasonable to assume that they may have synergistic effects, so it is responsible to try a combination (Olden and Drossman 2000). A patient with depressive disorder and excessive concern about serious illness might benefit from antidepressant treatment combined with cognitive-behavioral therapy.

Peptic Ulcer and Inflammatory Bowel Disease

There is nearly always a need to provide proper education and support to patients with organic GI diseases (peptic ulcer and IBD). The provision of information can lead to decreasing patient anxiety, empowering patients to participate more fully in their care and to obviate unnecessary worries such as an undue fear of cancer and the like.

Both dynamic interpersonal therapy and hypnosis have been studied in patients with peptic ulcer. These studies are interesting because they employed the same treatment method for patients with peptic ulcer as they did for patients with IBS. One used dynamic psychotherapy (Sjodin et al. 1985), and the other used hypnotherapy (Colgan et al. 1988b). Both found a more pronounced positive result in IBS, but the psychological treatments had a clear beneficial effect on ulcer symptoms compared to the control condition. This is a reminder that psychological factors may play a part in the etiology or perpetuation of the symptoms of peptic ulcer disease.

Psychotherapy trials, both controlled and uncontrolled, have not shown a benefit in improving outcome in IBD (Jantschek et al. 1998; Maunder and Esplen 2001).

Conclusion

The detection and treatment of psychiatric disorders in patients presenting to gastroenterologists is an important aspect of clinical practice. Whereas anxiety and depression have a more prominent role in functional gastrointestinal disorders, they have important effects on treatment, outcome, and quality of life in patients with "organic" gastrointestinal disorders as well. Chronic hepatitis C infection is of particular concern, both because of its frequency in patients with serious mental illness and substance abuse and because of the psychiatric side effects associated with its treatment.

References

Acosta-Ramirez D, Pagan-Ocasio V, Torres EA: Profile of the inflammatory bowel disease patient with depressive disorders. P R Health Sci J 20:215–220, 2001

Alter MJ: Epidemiology of hepatitis C. Hepatology 26 (suppl): 62S–65S, 1997

American Psychiatric Association: Diagnostic and Statistical Manual of Mental Disorders, 4th Edition, Text Revision. Washington, DC, American Psychiatric Association, 2000

Andrews H, Barczak P, Allan RN: Psychiatric illness in patients with inflammatory bowel disease. Gut 28:1600–1604, 1987

Beck AT, Ward CH, Mendelson M, et al: An inventory for measuring depression. Arch Gen Psychiatry 14:561–571, 1961

Bennett EJ, Tennant CC, Piesse C, et al: Level of chronic life stress predicts clinical outcome in irritable bowel syndrome. Gut 43:256–262, 1998

Biggs AMA: Effect of childhood adversity on health related quality of life in patients with upper abdominal or chest pain. Gut 53:180–186, 2004

Biggs AM, Aziz Q, Tomenson B, et al: Do childhood adversity and recent social stress predict health care use in patients presenting with upper abdominal or chest pain? Psychosom Med 65:1020–1028, 2003

Blanchard EB, Keefer L, Payne A, et al: Early abuse, psychiatric diagnoses and irritable bowel syndrome. Behav Res Ther 40:289–298, 2002

Bonaccorso S, Marino V, Biondi M, et al: Depression induced by treatment with interferon-alpha in patients affected by hepatitis C virus. J Affect Disord 72:237–241, 2002

Budavari AI, Olden KW: Psychosocial aspects of functional gastrointestinal disorders. Gastroenterol Clin North Am 32: 477–506, 2003

Cannon RO, Quyyumi AA, Mincemoyer R, et al: Imipramine in patients with chest pain despite normal coronary angiograms. N Engl J Med 20:1411–1417, 1994

Cauch-Dudek K, Abbey S, Stewart DE, et al: Fatigue in primary biliary cirrhosis. Gut 43:705–710, 1998

Clouse RE: Antidepressants for irritable bowel syndrome (therapy update). Gut 52:598–599, 2003

Colgan S, Creed F, Klass H: Symptom complaints, psychiatric disorder and abnormal illness behaviour in patients with upper abdominal pain. Psychol Med 18:887–892, 1988a

Colgan SM, Faragher EB, Whorwell PJ: Controlled trial of hypnotherapy in relapse prevention of duodenal ulceration. Lancet 1(8598):1299–1300, 1988b

Craig TKJ: Abdominal pain, in Life Events and Illness. Edited by Brown GW, Harris TO. New York, Guilford, 1989, pp 233–259

Creed F: The relationship between psychosocial parameters and outcome in irritable bowel syndrome. Am J Med 107:74S–80S, 1999

Creed F, Guthrie E: Techniques for interviewing the somatising patient. Br J Psychiatry 162:467–471, 1993

Creed F, Craig T, Farmer R: Functional abdominal pain, psychiatric illness, and life events. Gut 29:235–242, 1988

Creed F, Ratcliffe J, Fernandez L, et al: Health-related quality of life and health care costs in severe, refractory irritable bowel syndrome. Ann Intern Med 134:860–868, 2001

Creed F, Morgan R, Fiddler M, et al: Depression and anxiety impair health-related quality of life and are associated with increased costs in general medical inpatients. Psychosomatics 43:302–309, 2002

Creed F, Fernandes L, Guthrie E, et al: The cost-effectiveness of psychotherapy and paroxetine for severe irritable bowel syndrome. Gastroenterology 124:303–317, 2003

Creed F, Ratcliffe J, Fernandes L, et al: Outcome in severe irritable bowel syndrome with and without accompanying depressive, panic and neurasthenic disorders. Br J Psychiatry 186:507–515, 2005

de Boer AG, Sprangers MA, Bartelsman JF, et al: Predictors of health care utilization in patients with inflammatory bowel disease: a longitudinal study. Eur J Gastroenterol Hepatol 10:783–789, 1998

De Bona M, Ponton P, Ermani M, et al: The impact of liver disease and medical complications on quality of life and psychological distress before and after liver transplantation. J Hepatol 33: 609–615, 2000

Delvaux M, Denis P, Allemand H: Sexual abuse is more frequently reported by IBS patients than by patients with organic digestive diseases or controls. Results of a multicentre inquiry. French Club of Digestive Motility. Eur J Gastroenterol Hepatol 9: 345–352, 1997

Dieperink E, Willenbring M, Ho SB: Neuropsychiatric symptoms associated with hepatitis C and interferon alpha: a review. Am J Psychiatry 157:867–876, 2000

Dimenas E, Glise H, Hallerback B, et al: Well-being and gastrointestinal symptoms among patients referred to endoscopy owing to suspected duodenal ulcer. Scand J Gastroenterol 30:1046–1052, 1995

Drossman DA: Presidential address: gastrointestinal illness and the biopsychosocial model. Psychosom Med 60:258–267, 1998

Drossman DA, McKee DC, Sandler RS, et al: Psychosocial factors in the irritable bowel syndrome. A multivariate study of patients and nonpatients with irritable bowel syndrome. Gastroenterology 95:701–708, 1988

Drossman DA, Leserman J, Nachman G, et al: Sexual and physical abuse in women with functional or organic gastrointestinal disorders. Ann Intern Med 113:828–833, 1990

Drossman DA, Leserman J, Mitchell CM, et al: Health status and health care use in persons with inflammatory bowel disease. A national sample. Dig Dis Sci 36:1746–1755, 1991

Drossman DA, Talley NJ, Leserman J, et al: Sexual and physical abuse and gastrointestinal illness: review and recommendations. Ann Intern Med 123:782–794, 1995

Drossman DA, Creed FH, Olden KW, et al: Psychosocial aspects of the functional gastrointestinal disorders. Gut 45 (suppl 2):II25–II30, 1999

Drossman DA, Creed FH, Olden KW, et al: Psychosocial aspects of the functional gastrointestinal disorders, in Rome II: The Functional Gastrointestinal Disorders. Edited by Drossman DA, Corazziari E, Talley NJ, et al. McLean, VA, Degnon Associates, 2000a, pp 157–245

Drossman DA, Whitehead WE, Toner BB, et al: What determines severity among patients with painful functional bowel disorders? Am J Gastroenterol 95:974–980, 2000b

Drossman DA, Camilleri M, Mayer EA, et al: AGA technical review on irritable bowel syndrome. Gastroenterology 123: 2108–2131, 2002

Drossman DA, Toner BB, Whitehead WE, et al: Cognitive-behavioral therapy versus education and desipramine versus placebo for moderate to severe functional bowel disorders. Gastroenterology 125:19–31, 2003

Dwight MM, Kowdley KV, Russo JE, et al: Depression, fatigue, and functional disability in patients with chronic hepatitis C. J Psychosom Res 49:311–317, 2000

Ellard K, Beaurepaire J, Jones M, et al: Acute chronic stress in duodenal ulcer disease. Gastroenterology 99:1628–1632, 1990

El-Serag HB, Kunik M, Richardson P, et al: Psychiatric disorders among veterans with hepatitis C infection. Gastroenterology 123:476–482, 2002

Fontana RJ, Moyer CA, Sonnad S, et al: Comorbidities and quality of life in patients with interferon-refractory chronic hepatitis C. Am J Gastroenterol 96:170–178, 2001

Ford MJ, Miller PM, Eastwood J, et al: Life events, psychiatric illness and the irritable bowel syndrome. Gut 28:160–165, 1987

Gleason OC, Yates WR, Isbell MD, et al: An open-label trial of citalopram for major depression in patients with hepatitis C. J Clin Psychiatry 63:194–198, 2002

Gomborone J, Dewsnap P, Libby G, et al: Abnormal illness attitudes in patients with irritable bowel syndrome. J Psychosom Res 39:227–230, 1995

Guthrie E, Creed FH: Basic skills, in Seminars in Liaison Psychiatry. Edited by Guthrie E, Creed FH. London, Gaskell Press, 1996, pp 21–52

Guthrie E, Creed F: Cluster analysis of symptoms and health seeking behaviour differentiates subgroups of patients with severe irritable bowel syndrome. Gut 52:1616–1622, 2003

Guthrie E, Creed F, Dawson D, et al: A controlled trial of psychological treatment for the irritable bowel syndrome. Gastroenterology 100:450–457, 1991

Guthrie EA, Creed FH, Whorwell PJ, et al: Outpatients with irritable bowel syndrome: a comparison of first time and chronic attenders. Gut 33:361–363, 1992

Guthrie E, Jackson J, Shaffer J, et al: Psychological disorder and severity of inflammatory bowel disease predict health-related quality of life in ulcerative colitis and Crohn's disease. Am J Gastroenterol 97:1994–1999, 2002

Hamilton J, Guthrie E, Creed F, et al: A randomized controlled trial of psychotherapy in patients with chronic functional dyspepsia. Gastroenterology 119:661–669, 2000

Haug TT, Wilhelmsen I, Ursin H, et al: What are the real problems for patients with functional dyspepsia? Scand J Gastroenterol 30:97–100, 1995

Helzer JE, Stillings WA, Chammas S, et al: A controlled study of the association between ulcerative colitis and psychiatric diagnoses. Dig Dis Sci 27:513–518, 1982

Horikawa N, Yamazaki T, Izumi N, et al: Incidence and clinical course of major depression in patients with chronic hepatitis type C undergoing interferon-alpha therapy: a prospective study. Gen Hosp Psychiatry 25:34–38, 2003

Jackson JL, O'Malley PG, Tomkins G, et al: Treatment of functional gastrointestinal disorders with antidepressant medications: a meta-analysis. Am J Med 108:65–72, 2000

Jantschek G, Zeitz M, Pritsch M, et al: Effect of psychotherapy on the course of Crohn's disease. Results of the German prospective multicenter psychotherapy treatment study on Crohn's disease. German Study Group on Psychosocial Intervention in Crohn's Disease. Scand J Gastroenterol 33: 1289–1296, 1998

Katon W, Sullivan M, Walker E: Medical symptoms without identified pathology: relationship to psychiatric disorders, childhood and adult trauma, and personality traits. Ann Intern Med 134:917–925, 2001

Kettell J, Jones R, Lydiard S: Reasons for consultation in irritable bowel syndrome: symptoms and patient characteristics. Br J Gen Pract 42:459–461, 1992

Khalil HS, Bridger MW, Hilton-Pierce M, et al: The use of speech therapy in the treatment of globus pharyngeus patients. A randomised controlled trial. Rev Laryngol Otol Rhinol (Bord) 124:187–190, 2003

Kirsch MA, Louie AK: Paroxetine and irritable bowel syndrome. Am J Psychiatry 157: 1523–1524, 2000

Koloski NA, Talley NJ, Boyce PM: Does psychological distress modulate functional gastrointestinal symptoms and health care seeking? A prospective, community Cohort study. Am J Gastroenterol 98:789–797, 2003

Kraus MR, Schafer A, Scheurlen M: Paroxetine for the prevention of depression induced by interferon alfa. N Engl J Med 345:375–376, 2001

Kraus MR, Schafer A, Faller H, et al: Paroxetine for the treatment interferon–induced depression in chronic hepatitis C. Aliment Pharmacol Ther 16:1091–1099, 2002

Kraus MR, Schafer A, Faller H, et al: Psychiatric symptoms in patients with chronic hepatitis C receiving interferon alfa-2b therapy. J Clin Psychiatry 64:708–714, 2003

Kurata JH, Nogawa AN, Noritake D: NSAIDs increase risk of gastrointestinal bleeding in primary care patients with dyspepsia. J Fam Pract 45:227–235, 1997

Kurina LM, Goldacre MJ, Yeates D, et al: Depression and anxiety in people with inflammatory bowel disease. J Epidemiol Community Health 55:716–720, 2001

Lackner JM, Mesmer C, Morley S, et al: Psychological treatments for irritable bowel syndrome: a systematic review and meta-analysis. J Consult Clin Psychol 72:1100–1113, 2004

Langeluddecke P, Goulston K, Tennant C: Type A behaviour and other psychological factors in peptic ulcer disease. J Psychosom Res 31:335–340, 1987

Leserman J, Drossman DA, Li Z, et al: Sexual and physical abuse history in gastroenterology practice: how types of abuse impact health status. Psychosom Med 58:4–15, 1996

Leserman J, Li Z, Drossman DA, et al: Selected symptoms associated with sexual and physical abuse history among female patients with gastrointestinal disorders: the impact on subsequent health care visits. Psychol Med 28:417–425, 1998

Levenstein S: The very model of a modern etiology: a biopsychosocial view of peptic ulcer. Psychosom Med 62:176–185, 2000

Lewin J, Lewis S: Organic and psychosocial risk factors for duodenal ulcer. Psychosom Res 39:531–548, 1995

Longstreth GF, Wolde-Tsadik G: Irritable-bowel symptoms in HMO examinees. Prevalence, demographics and clinical correlates. Dig Dis Sci 38:1581–1589, 1993

Lucock MP, Morley S, White C, et al: Responses of consecutive patients to reassurance after gastroscopy: results of self-administered questionnaire survey. BMJ 315:572–575, 1997

Lydiard S, Jones R: Factors affecting the decision to consult with dyspepsia: comparison of consulters and nonconsulters. Br J Gen Pract 39:495–498, 1989

Lydiard RB, Fossey MD, Marsh W, et al: Prevalence of psychiatric disorders in patients with irritable bowel syndrome. Psychosomatics 34:229–234, 1993

Magni G, Salmi A, Paterlini A, et al: Psychological distress in duodenal ulcer and acute gastroduodenitis. A controlled study. Dig Dis Sci 27:1081–1084, 1982

Magni G, Bernasconi G, Mauro P, et al: Psychiatric diagnoses in ulcerative colitis. A controlled study. Br J Psychiatry 158: 413–415, 1991

Masand PS, Gupta S, Schwartz TL, et al: Does a preexisting anxiety disorder predict response to paroxetine in irritable bowel syndrome? Psychosomatics 43:451–455, 2002

Matsushima Y, Aoyama N, Fukuda H, et al: Gastric ulcer formation after the Hanshin-Awaji earthquake: a case study of *Helicobacter pylori* infection and stress-induced gastric ulcers. Helicobacter 4:94–99, 1999

Maunder RG, Esplen MJ: Supportive-expressive group psychotherapy for persons with inflammatory bowel disease. Can J Psychiatry 46:622–626, 2001

Maunder RG, de Rooy EC, Toner BB, et al: Health-related concerns of people who receive psychological support for inflammatory bowel disease. Can J Gastroenterol 11:681–685, 1997

Mertz H, Fass R, Kodner A, et al: Effect of amitriptyline on symptoms, sleep, and visceral perception in patients with functional dyspepsia. Am J Gastroenterol 93:160–165, 1998

Mittermaier C, Dejaco C, Waldhoer T, et al: Impact of depressive mood on relapse in patients with inflammatory bowel disease: a prospective 18-month follow-up study. Psychosom Med 66:79–84, 2004

Morriss RK, Gask L, Ronalds C, et al: Clinical and patient satisfaction outcomes of a new treatment for somatized mental disorder taught to general practitioners. Br J Gen Pract 49:263–267, 1999

Nguyen HA, Miller AI, Dieperink E, et al: Spectrum of disease in U.S. veteran patients with hepatitis C. Am J Gastroenterol 97:1813–1820, 2002

Nordin K, Pahlman L, Larsson K, et al: Health-related quality of life and psychological distress in a population-based sample of Swedish patients with inflammatory bowel disease. Scand J Gastroenterol 37:450–457, 2002

North CS, Alpers DH, Helzer JE, et al: Do life events or depression exacerbate inflammatory bowel disease? Ann Intern Med 114:381–386, 1991

Olden KW, Drossman DA: Psychologic and psychiatric aspects of gastrointestinal disease. Med Clin North Am 84:1313–1327, 2000

Passik SD, Breitbart WS: Depression in patients with pancreatic carcinoma. Diagnostic and treatment issues. Cancer 78:615–626, 1996

Porcelli P, Leoci C, Guerra V: A prospective study of the relationship between disease activity and psychologic distress in patients with inflammatory bowel disease. Scand J Gastroenterol 31:792–796, 1996

Quartero AO, Post MW, Numans ME, et al: What makes the dyspectic patient feel ill? A cross sectional survey of functional health status, *Helicobacter pylori* infection, and psychological distress in dyspeptic patients in general practice. Gut 45:15–19, 1999

Rose M, Hildebrandt M, Fliege H, et al: T-cell immune parameters and depression in patients with Crohn's disease. J Clin Gastroenterol 34:40–48, 2002

Rosenstock SJ, Jorgensen T: Prevalence and incidence of peptic ulcer disease in a Danish County—a prospective cohort study. Gut 36:819–824, 1995

Salmon P, Skaife K, Rhodes J: Abuse, dissociation, and somatization in irritable bowel syndrome: towards an explanatory model. J Behav Med 26:1–18, 2003

Schramm TM, Lawford BR, Macdonald GA, et al: Sertraline treatment of interferon-alfa-induced depressive disorder. Med J Aust 173:359–361, 2000

Simren M, Axelsson J, Gillberg R, et al: Quality of life in inflammatory bowel disease in remission: the impact of IBS-like symptoms and associated psychological factors. Am J Gastroenterol 97:389–396, 2002

Sjodin I, Svedlund J, Ottosson JO, et al: Controlled study of psychotherapy in chronic peptic ulcer disease. Psychosomatics 27:187–191, 1985

Spanier JA, Howden CW, Jones MP: A systematic review of alternative therapies in the irritable bowel syndrome. Arch Intern Med 163:265–274, 2003

Sperber AD, Carmel S, Atzmon Y, et al: Use of the Functional Bowel Disorder Severity Index (FBDSI) in a study of patients with the irritable bowel syndrome and fibromyalgia. Am J Gastroenterol 95:995–998, 2000

Stanghellini V, De Ponti F, De Giorgio R, et al: New developments in the treatment of functional dyspepsia. Drugs 63:869–892, 2003

Talley NJ: Evaluation of drug treatment in irritable bowel syndrome. Br J Clin Pharmacol 56:362–369, 2003

Talley NJ, Fett SL, Zinsmeister AR: Self-reported abuse and gastrointestinal disease in outpatients: association with irritable bowel-type symptoms. Am J Gastroenterol 90:366–371, 1995

Talley NJ, Boyce PM, Jones M: Is the association between irritable bowel syndrome and abuse explained by neuroticism? A population-based study. Gut 42: 47–53, 1998

Tarter RE, Switala J, Carra J, et al: Inflammatory bowel disease: psychiatric status of patients before and after disease onset. Int J Psychiatry Med 17:173–181, 1987

Tennant C, Goulston K, Langeluddecke P: Psychological correlates of gastric and duodenal ulcer disease. Psychol Med 16:365–371, 1986

Thompson WG, Longstreth G, Drossman DA, et al: Functional bowel disorders, in Rome II: The Functional Gastrointestinal Disorders. Edited by Drossman DA, Corazziari E, Talley NJ, et al. McLean, VA, Degnon Associates, 2000, p 355

Turnbull GK, Vallis TM: Quality of life in inflammatory bowel disease: the interaction of disease activity with psychosocial function. Am J Gastroenterol 90:1450–1454, 1995

van Dulmen AM, Fennis JFM, Mokkink HGA, et al: Doctor-dependent changes in complaint-related cognitions and anxiety during medical consultations in functional abdominal complaints. Psychol Med 25:1011–1018, 1995

Walker EA, Gelfand AN, Gelfand MD, et al: Psychiatric diagnoses, sexual and physical victimization and disability in patients with irritable bowel syndrome or inflammatory bowel disease. Psychol Med 25:1259–1267, 1995

Walker EA, Gelfand MD, Gelfand AN, et al: The relationship of current psychiatric disorder to functional disability and distress in patients with inflammatory bowel disease. Gen Hosp Psychiatry 18:220–229, 1996

Wessely S, Pariante C: Fatigue, depression and chronic hepatitis C infection. Psychol Med 32:1–10, 2002

Whitehead WE, Winget C, Fedoravicius AS, et al: Learned illness behavior in patients with irritable bowel syndrome and peptic ulcer. Dig Dis Sci 27:202–208, 1982

Whitehead WE, Burnett C, Cook E, et al: Impact of irritable bowel syndrome on quality of life. Dig Dis Sci 41:2248–2253, 1996

Whitehead WE, Palsson O, Jones KR: Systematic review of the comorbidity of irritable bowel syndrome with other disorders: what are the causes and implications? Gastroenterology 122:1140–1156, 2002

Xuan J, Kirchdoerfer LJ, Boyer JG, et al: Effects of comorbidity on health-related quality of life scores: an analysis of clinical trials data. Clin Ther 21: 383–403, 1999

Zigmond AS, Snaith RP: The Hospital Anxiety and Depression Scale. Acta Psychiatr Scand 67:361–370, 1983

Self-Assessment Questions

Select the single best response for each question.

1. Peptic ulcer disease is a common gastrointestinal illness, with a substantial psychiatric component in many cases. All of the following statements are true *except*
    A. The clinical use of nonsteroidal anti-inflammatory drugs (NSAIDs) has been identified as a major risk factor for the development of peptic ulcer disease.
    B. The presence of gut infection with *Helicobacter pylori* is associated with the development of peptic ulcer disease.
    C. It has been estimated that approximately 25% of individuals in Western countries will develop peptic ulcer disease.
    D. The prevalence of anxiety and depressive disorders appears increased in patients with peptic ulcer disease.
    E. Stressful life events have been associated with the onset, perpetuation, and recurrence of peptic ulcers.

2. Inflammatory bowel disease (IBD), which includes Crohn's disease and ulcerative colitis, is commonly associated with behavioral and emotional factors, which may lead to involvement of the psychosomatic medicine physician. Which of the following statements is *true?*
    A. The prevalence rate of psychiatric disorders is much higher in IBD (40%–50%) than in other chronic physical illnesses.
    B. The relationship between psychiatric disorders and stress and IBD has been clearly delineated.
    C. There is no clear evidence to suggest that anxiety and depression impair health-related quality of life in patients with IBD.
    D. Because of the seriousness of medical complications, IBD patients have a higher risk of comorbid psychiatric illness compared with patients with functional bowel disorder.
    E. Among IBD patients, mood disorders are more common in older patients and in those with a history of previously diagnosed psychiatric illness.

3. Irritable bowel syndrome (IBS) and functional dyspepsia are considered to be functional gastrointestinal disorders. Which of the following statements is *true?*
    A. The most common functional gastrointestinal disorder is functional dyspepsia.
    B. The prevalence of anxiety and mood disorders in patients with functional gastrointestinal illness is between 30% and 40%.
    C. Patients with chronic functional gastrointestinal disorders are more likely to present with anxiety, whereas first-time clinic patients usually present with depression.
    D. Psychiatric treatment of anxiety and mood disorders in these patients is associated with improved health-related quality of life.
    E. Patients with functional dyspepsia or IBS who consult physicians are less likely to have depression than equivalent patients who do not seek medical care.

4. Speech therapy has been found to be useful for symptomatic relief of which of the following functional gastrointestinal illnesses?

   A. Globus.
   B. Gastroesophageal reflux.
   C. Functional abdominal pain.
   D. Cyclic vomiting.
   E. IBS.

5. Antidepressant therapy may be helpful in managing IBS patients. Among the following classes, which has been clearly shown to be of benefit in IBS?

   A. Tricyclic antidepressants (TCAs).
   B. Monoamine oxidase inhibitors (MAOIs).
   C. Selective serotonin reuptake inhibitors (SSRIs).
   D. Selective norepinephrine reuptake inhibitors (SNRIs).
   E. Trazodone and nefazodone.

5 Renal Disease

Lewis M. Cohen, M.D.

Norman B. Levy, M.D.

Edward G. Tessier, Pharm.D., M.P.H.

Michael J. Germain, M.D.

NEPHROLOGY HAS RECOGNIZED the need for psychiatric consultation since the initial development of kidney dialysis in the late 1960s. Nearly universal access to treatment followed passage of the 1972 End-Stage Renal Disease amendment to the Social Security Act, which provided government subsidy for dialysis. Subsequently, the population has steadily grown, aged, and become more severely ill (McBride 1990). Psychiatry's potential role in the collaborative care of patients with renal disease is increasing.

Each year, approximately 80,000 Americans develop end-stage renal disease (ESRD). More than 340,000 individuals are treated for kidney failure (U.S. Renal Data System 2002); 240,000 people are receiving maintenance dialysis, and 100,000 have a functioning kidney transplant. Every year data have been collected, the average age of the ESRD incident population has increased. In 1986, the mean age was 56 years, and by 1995, it was 60 years

(National Institutes of Health 2000). The fastest growth has occurred among the oldest age groups.

The causes of renal failure include diabetes; hypertension; generalized arteriosclerosis; lupus; AIDS; and primary renal diseases, such as chronic glomerulonephritis, chronic interstitial nephritis, polycystic kidney disease, and other hereditary and congenital disorders. In 1999, only 9% of dialysis patients were free of significant comorbid conditions. Diabetes is now found in almost half of ESRD incident cases, and because of its plethora of microvascular and macrovascular complications, diabetes patients are especially likely to have increased morbidity (Lea and Nicholas 2002).

In some surveys, almost two-thirds of ESRD patients rate quality of life as being less than "good" (Levy and Wynbrandt 1975; Roberts and Kjellstrand 1988). In a recent survey at nine New England dialysis clinics involving 619 patients, 57% of the sample reported that physical health problems during the previous 4 weeks forced them to cut down on the amount of time spent on work or other activities, 69% accomplished less than they would prefer, and 71% were limited in the kind of work or activities that they could pursue (Poppel et al. 2003). A study of 14,815 dialysis patients demonstrated a significant correlation between mortality and mental health and physical function scores on the SF-36 Health Survey (Knight et al. 2003).

While there have been advances in the technology and treatments of renal transplantation and dialysis, clinical challenges presented by the patient population steadily mount.

Renal transplantation (see also Chapter 14, "Organ Transplantation," and Chapter 17, "Pediatrics") is the treatment of choice for many patients, and if a transplant is successful, the patient's survival (U.S. Renal Data System 2002; Wolfe et al. 1999) and quality of life (Franke et al. 2003; Laupacis et al. 1996) are almost always better than they would be with dialysis. The major issue in transplantation is the shortage of donor organs.

Peritoneal dialysis and *hemodialysis* are the two forms of dialysis. In peritoneal dialysis, dialysate fluid is introduced and then removed from the peritoneal space through an indwelling catheter. Peritoneal dialysis may be performed by a machine in the home at night (continuous cycling peritoneal dialysis, or CCPD) or manually at home four to six times per day (continuous ambulatory peritoneal dialysis, or CAPD). Only 11% of ESRD patients use peritoneal dialysis as the initial mode of renal replacement therapy (U.S. Renal Data System 1997a). Hemodialysis may be conducted at the patient's home, but it usually takes place at dialysis units for 4-hour sessions held three times per week. Home dialysis requires the participation of another person, who must be available

to assist with treatment. There has been a great deal of recent interest in daily and nocturnal dialysis done at home or in a dialysis facility (Lockridge et al. 2001). Data suggest that this new approach may result in improved quality of life and health. Although patients have not been randomized to dialysis modalities, most studies continue to show that patients receiving peritoneal dialysis rate their care higher than do those receiving hemodialysis (Rubin et al. 2004).

Psychiatric Disorders in Renal Disease

In a review of psychiatric illness involving 200,000 U.S. dialysis patients, almost 10% had been hospitalized with a psychiatric diagnosis, and this was the primary reason for hospitalization of 25% of the subgroup (Kimmel et al. 1993). Depression and other affective disorders were the most common diagnoses, followed by delirium and dementia. Compared with other medical illnesses, depression as the primary diagnosis was higher in renal failure patients than in those with ischemic heart disease and cerebrovascular disease (Kimmel et al. 1993).

Studies of depression and ESRD have reported prevalence rates ranging from 0% to 100% (Cohen-Cole and Stoudemire 1987; Kimmel 2000, 2002), reflecting widely variable definitions, criteria, and measurement methods.

Because depression frequently follows loss, its occurrence is understandable in the context of dialysis, where patients commonly lose strength, energy, sexual ability, employment, physical freedom, and independence. Another potential contributing factor to depression is survival guilt, when a fellow dialysis patient dies (Vamos 1997). A recent study highlighted the significance of comorbid disorders (e.g., diabetes) and job status in the etiology of clinical depression (Chen et al. 2003). Examination of the ESRD literature suggests that subsyndromal depressive syndromes are likely in about 25% of patients; and major depression is likely in 5%–22% of patients (O'Donnell and Chung 1997).

Our own diagnostic approach entails describing the criteria for major depression, asking whether the patient believes he or she is depressed, and then documenting the existence of associated factors, such as depressive episodes prior to the onset of renal failure, a family history of depression, and previous suicide attempts (Cohen 1998; Cohen et al. 2000). The presence of depressive affect and cognition, such as poor self-esteem, worthlessness, hopelessness, and helplessness, is valuable in arriving at the correct diagnosis.

Major depression appears to be frequently unrecognized and untreated (Finkelstein and Finkelstein 2000). In a recent study of Connecticut dialysis patients (N=123) initiating dialysis treatment, almost half (44%) of the sample scored above the depressed range on the Beck Depression Inventory (score=15), but only 16% of these patients were receiving antidepressant medications (Watnick et al. 2003).

Suicide, the ultimate complication of depression, is reportedly more common among dialysis patients than in the general population (Abram et al. 1971; Haenel et al. 1980; Kimmel 2001). ESRD suicide rates were originally calculated by combining ordinary clinical suicides with deaths following dialysis discontinuation and deaths caused by noncompliance (Abram et al. 1971). Kishi and Kathol (2002) observed that suicide in the context of terminal illness is increasing, and although suicide usually is a consequence of comorbid major depression or alcohol abuse, it also may occur in the absence of demonstrable psychiatric illness.

Anxiety and depression are the most common psychological symptoms seen in the physically ill (Lefebvre et al. 1972); this is also true in ESRD. Anxiety may be especially present during dialysis treatments.

Substance use disorders, such as cocaine or heroin dependence, can directly lead to ESRD (Norris et al. 2001). They may also result in HIV infection and, later, AIDS, which can secondarily cause renal failure.

Cognitive disorders are common in the ESRD patient population and may be related to uremia, a variety of medical comorbidities (e.g., electrolyte disturbances, severe malnutrition, impaired metabolism, cerebrovascular disease), or adverse effects of treatment. *Uremia* refers to the clinical syndrome resulting from profound loss of renal function. Central nervous system symptoms may begin with mild cognitive dysfunction, fatigue, and headache, progressing to a usually hypoactive delirium and, if untreated, coma. Restless legs syndrome, muscle cramps, and sleep disorders are also common. Other common symptoms include pruritus, anorexia, nausea, vomiting, and metabolic abnormalities.

Many patients will tend to note progressive impairment as their day for dialysis approaches (Levy and Cohen 2000). After dialysis, they may experience a short period of delirium lasting from minutes to hours that is termed "dysequilibrium syndrome," likely caused by the rapid changes in fluid and electrolytes during the dialysis session. Acute changes in mental status are not commonly seen in CAPD, because this procedure is slow, continuous, and without sudden fluxes of fluid and electrolytes. The presence of a transient metabolic encephalopathy can be confirmed by an electroencephalogram, demonstrating diffuse slowing.

The usual types of dementia, such as vascular and Alzheimer's, are increasingly encountered as the ESRD population continues to age. Vascular dementia is especially common because of the high prevalence of diabetes, hypertension, and atherosclerosis in ESRD patients.

Effects of Psychological Factors on Choice of Modality and Compliance

In renal failure, the choice of treatment involves center hemodialysis versus various methods of self-care, such as home hemodialysis, CAPD, and CCPD. The physician's orientation and preferences are often the main factors that influence treatment choice; ideally, the patient's preferences should be paramount. In contrast with European nephrologists, most American nephrologists treat patients with hemodialysis. Nephrologists who work in medical centers where renal transplantation is the centerpiece of treatment and hemodialysis space is limited will tend, when feasible, to favor transplantation.

Psychosocial factors have a significant impact on the choice of treatment modality (Maher et al. 1983). A medical history marked by noncompliance argues against modalities of self-care. This is especially true for transplantation, where nonadherence to immunosuppressant treatment will generally result in organ rejection (Surman 1989). Modality decisions must take into account the social support system of the individual patient. In order for home dialysis to take place, it is essential not only that the patient have a home but also that another individual be available to provide care. The very independent patient will tend to favor modalities of self-care, whereas the dependent person will tend to prefer being cared for.

Compliance is a common problem and is often a central issue in the management of patients. Compliance is a complex, multidimensional array of behaviors, and its relationship with health outcomes in dialysis patients is difficult to study. However, the widespread belief among physicians and nurses that noncompliance results in worse outcomes, including higher mortality in ESRD, is supported by a large multicenter study (Leggat et al. 1997). It is difficult enough for the dialysis patient to engage in a lifelong procedure that occurs daily in the case of CAPD, and three times weekly in the case of hemodialysis, but the burdens of dietary restrictions and required medications add major compliance chores. Hemodialysis patients in particular, and peritoneal patients to a lesser degree, need to restrict their intake of protein, sodium, potassium (fruit), phosphates (dairy), and, most difficult of all, fluids.

There is no validated method to measure compliance, but clinical indices include dialysis attendance, interdialytic weight gain, serum potassium, and medication adherence. Lack of adherence to treatment regimens is believed to be a common cause for inadequate dialysis and poor outcome (Kaveh and Kimmel 2001). Common noncompliant behaviors include skipping or missing dialysis sessions, and dietary and medication indiscretions. According to self-report, one peritoneal dialysis exchange per week is missed by 12% of patients, and two to three exchanges per week are skipped by 5% of patients (U.S. Renal Data System 1997b). Noncompliance is more common in younger patients, those without diabetes, and black and Hispanic patients, as compared with white and Asian patients (Blake et al. 2000). Among the factors associated with noncompliance are depression, hostility toward authority, memory impairment, ethnic barriers, and financial problems (Anderson and Kirk 1982). The field of nephrology appreciates that appropriate patient and modality selection needs to be combined with a multidisciplinary approach to improve adherence (Raj 2002), with particular attention accorded to patient education (Golper 2001).

Diagnostic Issues

Progressive uremia and its treatment modalities are associated with both physical and psychological symptoms, and it is often difficult to delineate the etiology, particularly when patients have comorbid systemic disorders, such as diabetes. It is important to understand that dialysis only partially corrects the uremic state equivalent to less than 10 cc/min glomerular filtration rate, and in three-times-per-week hemodialysis, this clearance is provided only intermittently. This limited amount of clearance of uremic toxins is enough to prevent death; however, patients may remain symptomatic. There has been relatively little research focused on identifying common symptoms and examining different treatment approaches (Weisbord et al. 2003).

In the nephrology literature, there is a lack of clarity around the term *depression* and whether it refers to the affective symptom or the psychiatric disorder (Cohen 1996). Most ESRD research studies have relied on instruments that determine the severity of the symptom (Craven et al. 1988; Kimmel et al. 1998; Smith et al. 1985). In contrast, psychiatric studies in the medically ill now more often rely on the combination of such measures with a structured diagnostic interview based on DSM-IV criteria (American Psychiatric Association 2000) (e.g., Chochinov et al. 1994; Sullivan et al. 1999). In addition, the evaluation of depression is complicated by the fact that the somatic signs and symptoms of ESRD may fulfill the criteria for major depressive disorder. Many patients have diminished appetite, loss of energy, dryness of the mouth, constipation, and diminished sexual interest. However, during interviews some individuals will adamantly maintain that they are not depressed, and it is likely that the vegetative symptoms are being produced by the kidney failure and renal replacement therapy.

Withholding or Withdrawing Dialysis: Renal Palliative Care

Psychiatrists have an opportunity to participate in the ongoing integration of palliative medicine and nephrology (Cohen and Germain 2003). Recent ESRD patient demographics reveal a robust increase in numbers, severity of comorbid illnesses, and age (Weisbord et al. 2003). Consequently, it should be no surprise that despite continuing improvements in technology, more than 65,000 Americans with ESRD will die this year, and the annual mortality rate is around 23% (U.S. Renal Data System 2002). This mortality rate is comparable to that of non-Hodgkin's lymphoma and higher than that of prostate (0.2%), breast (2.4%), colorectal (17.4%), and ovarian (20.8%) cancer (Ries et al. 2002). The expected remaining lifetime of dialysis patients is one-quarter to one-fifth that of the age- and sex-matched general population (U.S. Renal Data System 2003). Although the figures are better for transplant patients, their expected remaining lifetime is still only 70%–80% that of the general population. Multidisciplinary involvement is needed to lift the denial of death and improve the provision of end-of-life care and symptom management (Cohen et al. 1997).

Psychiatrists can play a crucial role in the complex determinations to withhold or withdraw renal replacement treatment. Treatment guidelines have been developed by a task force from the Renal Physician's Association, American Society of Nephrology, National Kidney Foundation, and other renal organizations (Moss et al. 2000). Guidelines also exist or are under development in other nations—for example, Japan (Sakaguchi and Akizawa 2002) and Italy (Buzzi et al. 2001). The U.S. guidelines, which directed attention to the ethical and psychological issues in decisions to withhold or withdraw renal replacement treatment, were prompted by the finding that the percentage of patient deaths preceded by decisions to stop dialysis steadily increased during the 1990s. In the United States, between 1990 and 1995, more than 20,000 deaths were preceded by dialysis discontinuation (Leggat et al. 1997). During the same period of time, beginning in 1995, there were 36,000 withdrawal deaths in the incident sample of patients (U.S. Renal Data System 2002). Furthermore, an unknown number of patients die after they or their families decide to withhold or not initiate dialysis. All of these decisions are emotionally complex and stressful for patients, caregivers, and staff. Psychiatrists can assist with determinations of patient capacity and also the potential influence of depression or other psychosocial factors.

In providing better end-of-life care for this very ill population, attention should focus on the following issues:

- Early frank discussions concerning prognosis and goals of care
- Attention to symptoms at all stages of the disease process
- Early hospice referrals
- Maximal palliative care at the end of life

The decision not to start dialysis is probably more common than withdrawal from dialysis. Patients who are already uremic at the time of decision to initiate dialysis may be encephalopathic and lack sufficient decision-making capacity. If dialysis is otherwise indicated and the patient is refusing dialysis, it is appropriate to seek legal authorization to provide involuntary dialysis until the patient's mental status has improved enough to enable an informed decision. Utmost sensitivity is needed in making withholding or discontinuation decisions, and one needs to be alert to cultural biases, countertransference, and other complicating factors. There are significant differences, even among the English-speaking nations, between countries in how

often dialysis is offered and the relative factors affecting the decision. American nephrologists offer dialysis more often and give more weight to patient or family wishes and fear of lawsuit than do British or Canadian nephrologists. British nephrologists more often consider their perception of patients' quality of life as a reason to provide or not provide dialysis than do their American counterparts (McKenzie et al. 1998). Primary care physicians can also withhold dialysis by not referring the patients to nephrologists for evaluation of their progressive renal failure. One study among physicians in West Virginia, for example, found that 20 of 76 primary care providers (26%) had effectively withheld dialysis for at least one patient through nonreferral to a nephrologist (Sekkarie and Moss 1998).

The following conditions are considered appropriate reasons to withhold dialysis based on recently published U.S. guidelines (Moss et al. 2000):

- Severe and irreversible dementia
- Permanent unconsciousness (as in a persistent vegetative state)
- End-stage cancer or end-stage lung, liver, or heart disease in patients who need considerable assistance with activities of daily living and may be confined to bed or chair or involved in a hospice program
- Severe mental disability in patients who are uncooperative with the procedure of dialysis itself, are unable to interact with the environment or other people, or are persistently combative with family or staff
- Severe, continued, and unrelenting pain, when dialysis may prolong life for a short period of time but will also prolong suffering
- Hospitalization (especially among the elderly) with multiple organ system failure that persists after 3 days of intensive therapy

Withdrawal from dialysis is often appropriate for the dying dialysis patient. It provides the patient and family with the blessing of a quick death (Cohen et al. 2003). The mean time to death after stopping dialysis is 8 days, and dialysis termination does not cause pain or discomfort (Cohen et al. 2001). It typically results in lethargy progressing to coma. Psychiatrists have an important opportunity to assist in the effort to integrate palliative care in the treatment of this population.

Treatment Issues

Psychotherapy

A wide variety of forms of psychotherapy may be helpful. In a study of five Boston patients (Surman and Tolkoff-Rubin 1984), hypnosis was successful in curtailing psychiatric symptoms. In a study of 116 patients, Cummings et al. (1981) demonstrated that behavioral contracting and weekly telephone contacts were effective in the short term in improving compliance with medical regimens. More recently, behavioral interventions were shown to improve compliance with fluid restriction in both a small quasi-experimental study (Sagawa et al. 2003) and a controlled trial (Christensen et al. 2002). A controlled trial of group therapy in Israeli dialysis patients showed a significant decrease in psychological distress and interdialytic weight gain in those who received group therapy (Auslander and Buchs 2002).

Any form of psychotherapy stands the best chance of success if conducted during dialysis treatment sessions (Levy 1999). Patients with ESRD feel overdoctored and overburdened by the time requirements of treatment. Groups that have been most successful are those that have a strong educational component. This component may comprise lectures from social workers, nutritionists, transplant surgeons, and nephrologists. Such sessions are especially valuable in the earliest phases of groups, when patients may be most hesitant to talk about themselves. As time progresses, personal stories and problems usually emerge. Individual psychotherapy is mainly limited to those few patients who see themselves as having psychological problems and who are willing and able to engage in this form of treatment.

Miscellaneous Treatment Issues

Aggression, irritability, drug abuse, persistent insomnia, and noncompliance are frequent reasons for referral. During the past several years, the authors have also received increasing requests from nephrologists to assist in determinations of capacity, as well as issues related to dialysis discontinuation decisions.

When it comes to delirium and dementia, the basic treatment involves recognition and correction of the underlying pathology. Intensified dialysis, parathyroidectomy, and improved control of diabetes mellitus can each prove to be ameliorative. Neuroleptics or benzodiazepines may provide symptomatic treatment of agitation and delusions, and antidepressant medications can likewise be highly effective (Levy and Cohen 2001).

Sexual disorders and erectile dysfunction are common in the ESRD population, and these may sometimes result in consultations or requests for counseling. Many different behavioral and physical therapies offer the hope of some improvement. The latter include vacuum tumescence therapy, renal transplantation, use of recombinant human erythropoietin, and sildenafil (Rosas et al. 2001).

Psychopharmacology

Most psychotropic medications are fat soluble with large volumes of distribution.

With the exception of lithium, they are metabolized in the liver, and metabolites are eliminated in urine and bile. The majority of these drugs can be safely used in ESRD patients, but attention must be paid to medications with active metabolites, those that may be highly plasma-protein bound, and those with altered pharmacokinetics or pharmacodynamics.

When dose adjustments of psychiatric drugs in ESRD are required, it is usually because of comorbidities (e.g., diabetic autonomic neuropathy) and concurrent drug therapy (e.g., other agents metabolized by cytochrome P450 enzyme systems, and those with pharmacodynamic interactions) rather than the ESRD per se. Psychopharmacological management of transplant patients requires an appreciation of potential interactions with immunosuppressant medications (Robinson and Levenson 2001). Given the size of the population, there has been a dearth of systematic investigations; for example, although antidepressants are frequently prescribed for patients with ESRD, there is only one very small controlled clinical trial (Blumenfield et al. 1997).

Conclusion

As the techniques of dialysis and transplantation have advanced, patients are living longer. Because comorbid psychiatric disorders are widely prevalent among the dialysis and renal transplant populations, psychiatrists can play a vital role in management, including choice of treatment modality and promotion of compliance, as well as in palliative care for patients who wish to decline or discontinue dialysis. Finally, specific psychotherapeutic techniques and psychopharmacological interventions must be tailored to meet the special needs of patients with compromised renal function.

References

Abram HS, Moore GL, Westervelt BS Jr: Suicidal behavior in chronic dialysis patients. Am J Psychiatry 127:1199–1204, 1971

American Psychiatric Association: Diagnostic and Statistical Manual of Mental Disorders, 4th Edition, Text Revision. Washington, DC, American Psychiatric Association, 2000

Anderson RJ, Kirk LM: Methods of improving compliance in chronic disease states. Arch Intern Med 142:1673–1675, 1982

Auslander GK, Buchs A: Evaluating an activity intervention with hemodialysis patients in Israel. Soc Work Health Care 35:407–423, 2002

Blake PG, Korbert SM, Blake R, et al: A multicenter study of noncompliance with continuous ambulatory peritoneal dialysis exchanges in U.S. and Canadian patients. Am J Kidney Dis 35:506–514, 2000

Blumenfield M, Levy NB, Spinowitz B, et al: Fluoxetine in depressed patients on dialysis. Int J Psychiatry Med 27:71–80, 1997

Buzzi F, Cecioni R, Di Paolo M, et al: Bioethics in nephrology: guidelines for decision-making in Italy. J Nephrol 14:93–97, 2001

Chen YS, Wu SC, Wang SY, et al: Depression in chronic haemodialysed patients. Nephrology (Carlton) 8:121–126, 2003

Chochinov HM, Wilson KG, Enns M, et al: Prevalence of depression in the terminally ill: Effects of diagnostic criteria and symptom threshold judgments. Am J Psychiatry 51: 537–540, 1994

Christensen AJ, Moran PJ, Wiebe JS, et al: Effect of a behavioral self-regulation intervention on patient adherence in hemodialysis. Health Psychol 21:393–397, 2002

Cohen LM: Renal disease, in American Psychiatric Press Textbook of Consultation-Liaison Psychiatry. Edited by Rundell JR, Wise M. Washington, DC, American Psychiatric Press, 1996, pp 573–578

Cohen LM: Suicide, hastening death, and psychiatry. Arch Intern Med 158:1973–1976, 1998

Cohen LM, Germain MJ: Palliative and supportive care, in Therapy of Nephrology and Hypertension: A Companion to Brenner's The Kidney, 2nd Edition. Edited by Brady HR, Wilcox CS. Philadelphia, PA, Elsevier, 2003, pp 753–756

Cohen LM, McCue J, Germain M, et al: Denying the dying: advance directives and dialysis discontinuation. Psychosomatics 38:27–34, 1997

Cohen LM, Steinberg MD, Hails KC, et al: The psychiatric evaluation of death-hastening requests: lessons from dialysis discontinuation. Psychosomatics 41:195–203, 2000

Cohen LM, Reiter G, Poppel D, et al: Renal palliative care, in Palliative Care for Non-Cancer Patients. Edited by Addington-Hall J, Higginson I. London, Oxford University Press, 2001, pp 103–113

Cohen LM, Germain MJ, Poppel DM: Practical considerations in dialysis withdrawal: "to have the option is a blessing." JAMA 289:2113–2119, 2003

Cohen-Cole SA, Stoudemire A: Major depression and physical illness: special considerations in diagnosis and biologic treatment. Psychiatr Clin North Am 10:1–17, 1987

Craven JL, Rodin GM, Littlefield C: The Beck Depression Inventory as a screening device for major depression in renal dialysis patients. Int J Psychiatry Med 18:365–374, 1988

Cummings KB, Becker M, Kirscht JP, et al: Intervention strategies to improve compliance with medical regimens by ambulatory hemodialysis patients. J Behav Med 4:111–127, 1981

Finkelstein FO, Finkelstein SH: Depression in chronic dialysis patients: assessment and treatment. Nephrol Dial Transplant 15:191–192, 2000

Franke GH, Reimer J, Philipp T, et al: Aspects of quality of life through end-stage renal disease. Qual Life Res 12:103–115, 2003

Golper T: Patient education: can it maximize the success of therapy? Nephrol Dial Transplant 16 (suppl 7):20–24, 2001

Haenel T, Brunner F, Battegay R: Renal dialysis and suicide: occurrence in Switzerland and Europe. Compr Psychiatry 21:140–145, 1980

Kaveh K, Kimmel PL: Compliance in hemodialysis patients: multidimensional measures in search of a gold measure. Am J Kidney Dis 37:244–266, 2001

Kimmel PL: Just whose quality of life is it anyway? Kidney Int 57:S74, S113–S120, 2000

Kimmel PL: Nephrology forum. Psychosocial factors in dialysis patients. Kidney Int 59:1599–1613, 2001

Kimmel PL: Depression in patients with chronic renal disease: What we know and what we need to know. J Psychosom Res 53:951–956, 2002

Kimmel PL, Weihs K, Peterson RA: Survival in hemodialysis patients: the role of depression. J Am Soc Nephrol 3:12–27, 1993

Kimmel PL, Thamer M, Richard CM, et al: Psychiatric illness in patients with end-stage renal disease. Am J Med 105:214–221, 1998

Kishi Y, Kathol RG: Assessment of patients who attempt suicide. Prim Care Companion J Clin Psychiatry 4:132–136, 2002

Knight EL, Ofsthun N, Teng M, et al: The association between mental health, physical function, and hemodialysis mortality. Kidney Int 63:1843–1851, 2003

Laupacis A, Keown P, Pus N, et al: A study of the quality of life and cost-utility of renal transplantation. Kidney Int 50:235–42, 1996

Lea JP, Nicholas SB: Diabetes mellitus and hypertension: Key risk factors for kidney disease. J Natl Med Assoc 94:7S–15S, 2002

Lefebvre P, Nobert A, Crombez JC: Psychological and psychopathological reactions in relation to chronic hemodialysis. Can Psychiatr Assoc J 17:9–13, 1972

Leggat JE Jr, Bloembergen WE, Levine G, et al: An analysis of risk factors for withdrawal from dialysis before death. J Am Soc Nephrol 8:1755–1763, 1997

Levy NB: Renal failure, dialysis and transplantation, in Psychiatric Treatment of the Medically Ill. Edited by Robinson RG. New York, Marcel Dekker, 1999, pp 141–153

Levy NB, Cohen LM: End-stage renal disease and its treatment: dialysis and transplantation, in Psychiatric Care of the Medical Patient, 2nd Edition. Edited by Stoudemire A, Fogel BS, Greenberg D. London, Oxford University Press, 2000, pp 791–800

Levy NB, Cohen LM: Central and peripheral nervous systems in uremia, in Textbook of Nephrology, 4th Edition. Edited by Massry SG, Glassock R. Philadelphia, PA, Williams & Wilkins, 2001, pp 1279–1282

Levy NB, Wynbrandt GD: The quality of life on maintenance haemodialysis. Lancet 1:1328–30, 1975

Lockridge RS Jr, Spencer M, Craft V, et al: Nocturnal home hemodialysis in North America. Adv Ren Replace Ther 8: 250–256, 2001

Maher HS, Lamping DL, Dickinson CA, et al: Psychosocial aspects of hemodialysis. Kidney Int 23:S13, S50–S57, 1983

McBride P: The development of hemodialysis, in Clinical Dialysis, 2nd Edition. Edited by Nissenson AR, Fine RN, Gentile DE. Norwalk, CT, Appleton & Lang, 1990, p 20

McKenzie JK, Moss AH, Feest TG, et al: Dialysis decision making in Canada, the United Kingdom, and the United States. Am J Kidney Dis 31:12–18, 1998

Moss AH, Renal Physicians Association, American Society of Nephrology Working Group: A new clinical practice guideline on initiation and withdrawal of dialysis that makes explicit the role of palliative medicine. J Palliat Med 3:253–260, 2000

National Institutes of Health NIDDK/DKUHD: Excerpts from the United States Renal Data System 2000 Annual Data Report. Am J Kidney Dis 36 (suppl 2):S1–S239, 2000

Norris KC, Thornhill-Joyner M, Robinson C, et al: Cocaine use, hypertension, and end-stage renal disease. Am J Kidney Dis 38:523–529, 2001

O'Donnell K, Chung Y: The diagnosis of major depression in end-stage renal disease. Psychother Psychosom 66:38–43, 1997

Poppel D, Cohen L, Germain M: The renal palliative care initiative. J Palliat Med 6:321–326, 2003

Raj DSC: Role of APD in compliance with therapy. Semin Dial 15:434–436, 2002

Ries LA, Eisner MP, Kosary CL, et al: SEER Cancer Statistics Review, 1973–1999. National Cancer Institute, Bethesda, MD, 2002. Available at: http://seer.cancer.gov/csr/1973_1999/. Accessed July 2, 2003.

Roberts JC, Kjellstrand CM: Choosing death: withdrawal from chronic dialysis without medical reason. Acta Med Scand 223:181–186, 1988

Robinson MJ, Levenson JL: Psychopharmacology in transplant patients, in Biopsychosocial Perspectives on Transplantation. Edited by Rodrigues JR. New York, NY, Kluwer Academic, 2001, pp 151–172

Rosas ES, Wasserstein A, Kobrin S, et al: Preliminary observations of sildenafil treatment for erectile dysfunction in dialysis patients. Am J Kidney Dis 37:134–137, 2001

Rubin HR, Fink NE, Plantinga LC, et al: Patients' ratings of dialysis care with peritoneal dialysis vs. hemodialysis. JAMA 291:697–703, 2004

Sagawa M, Oka M, Chaboyer W: The utility of cognitive behavioural therapy on chronic haemodialysis patients' fluid intake: a preliminary examination. Int J Nurs Stud 40:367–373, 2003

Sakaguchi T, Akizawa T: Clinical guideline review: standards for initiation of chronic dialysis. Nippon Naika Gakkai Zasshi 91:1561–1569, 2002

Sekkarie MA, Moss AH: Withholding and withdrawing dialysis: the role of physician specialty and education and patient functional status. Am J Kidney Dis 31:464–472, 1998

Smith MD, Hong BA, Robson AM: Diagnosis of depression in patients with end stage renal disease. Am J Med 79:160–166, 1985

Sullivan M, LaCroix A, Russo J, et al: Depression in coronary heart disease: what is the appropriate diagnostic threshold? Psychosomatics 40:286–292, 1999

Surman OS: Psychiatric aspects of organ transplantation. Am J Psychiatry 146:872–882, 1989

Surman OS, Tolkoff-Rubin N: Use of hypnosis in patients receiving hemodialysis for end stage renal disease. Gen Hosp Psychiatry 6(1):31–35, 1984

U.S. Renal Data System: Treatment modalities for ESRD patients. Am J Kidney Dis 30:S54–S66, 1997a

U.S. Renal Data System: USRDS 1997 Annual Data Report. Bethesda, MD, National Institutes of Health, National Institute of Diabetes and Digestive and Kidney Diseases, 1997b, pp 49–67

U.S. Renal Data System: USRDS 2002 Annual Data Report: Atlas of End-Stage Renal Disease in the United Status. Bethesda, MD, National Institutes of Health, National Institute of Diabetes and Digestive and Kidney Diseases, 2002

U.S. Renal Data System: USRDS 2003 Annual Data Report. Bethesda, MD, National Institutes of Health, National Institute of Diabetes and Digestive and Kidney Diseases, 2003, p 48

Vamos M: Survivor guilt and chronic illness. Aust N Z J Psychiatry 31:592–596, 1997

Watnick S, Kirwin P, Mahnensmith R, et al: The prevalence and treatment of depression among patients starting dialysis. Am J Kidney Dis 41:105–110, 2003

Weisbord SD, Carmody SS, Bruns FJ, et al: Symptom burden, quality of life, advance care planning and the potential value of palliative care in severely ill haemodialysis patients. Nephrol Dial Transplant 18:1345–1352, 2003

Wolfe R, Ashley V, Milford E, et al: Comparison of mortality in all patients on dialysis, patients on dialysis awaiting transplantation, and recipients of a first cadaveric transplant. N Engl J Med 341:1725–1730, 1999

Self-Assessment Questions

Select the single best response for each question.

1. Regarding end-stage renal disease (ESRD) in the United States, which of the following statements is *true?*

    A. Each year nearly 80,000 Americans develop ESRD.
    B. More than 340,000 patients are being treated for kidney failure.
    C. Nearly 240,000 individuals are receiving maintenance dialysis.
    D. Approximately 100,000 people have a functioning kidney transplant.
    E. All of the above.

2. In a review of psychiatric illness involving 200,000 U.S. dialysis patients, it was reported that

    A. Nearly 10% had been hospitalized with a psychiatric diagnosis.
    B. Dementia was the most common psychiatric illness.
    C. Compared with other medical illnesses, the primary diagnosis of depression was higher in patients with ischemic heart disease than in patients with renal failure.
    D. A and C.
    E. A, B, and C.

3. Noncompliance with dialysis treatment is associated with all of the following variables *except*

    A. Hostility toward authority.
    B. Memory impairment.
    C. Ethnic barriers.
    D. Financial problems.
    E. Anxiety.

4. According to recently published U.S. guidelines (Moss et al. 2000), which of the following conditions is *not* an appropriate reason to withhold dialysis?

    A. End-stage cancer.
    B. Permanent unconsciousness (as in a persistent vegetative state).
    C. Severe delirium.
    D. Severe, continued, and unrelenting pain.
    E. Multiple organ system failure in a hospitalized patient.

5. Which of the following forms of psychotherapy has been shown to be helpful in treating patients with end-stage renal disease?

    A. Behavioral contracting and weekly telephone contacts.
    B. Hypnosis.
    C. Behavioral interventions.
    D. Group therapy.
    E. All of the above.

6 Endocrine Disorders

Ann Goebel-Fabbri, Ph.D.

Gail Musen, Ph.D.

Caitlin R. Sparks, B.A.

Judy A. Greene, M.D.

James L. Levenson, M.D.

Alan M. Jacobson, M.D.

THE ONSET, COURSE, and outcomes of endocrine disorders have traditionally been linked to psychological and social factors. A growing body of neuroendocrine research has begun to illuminate important biological mechanisms underlying the interplay of psyche and soma, and there are important clinical ramifications of these connections. This chapter focuses primarily on these latter pragmatic issues.

Diabetes

Type 1 Diabetes

Type 1 diabetes is a chronic, autoimmune disease that affects an estimated 500,000 to 1 million people in the United States. It is most commonly diagnosed in children and young adults but can occur at older ages. It appears that genetic and environmental factors trigger an autoimmune response, which attacks the insulin-producing beta cells of the pancreas. Prolonged hyperglycemia can lead to the severe macro- and microvascular complications of diabetes, such as cardiovascular disease, retinopathy, nephropathy, and peripheral and autonomic neuropathy.

The 9-year Diabetes Control and Complications Trial (DCCT) established that improvement in glycemic control delays the onset and slows the progression of diabetic complications (Diabetes Control and Complications Trial Research Group

1993). The DCCT's findings have informed and increased the complexity of what is now the standard treatment for type 1 diabetes. Treatment is aimed at lowering and stabilizing blood glucose to near normal levels through dietary control, exercise, blood glucose monitoring, and multiple daily insulin injections. This usually entails three or more insulin injections per day (or the use of a continuous insulin infusion pump)—with the goal of mirroring as closely as possible the physiological patterns of insulin release and near-normal blood glucose levels. Hemoglobin A_{1c}, reflective of average blood glucose concentrations over a 2- to 3-month period, is used as the standard measure of diabetes self-care success and treatment effectiveness.

Type 2 Diabetes

Approximately 90%–95% (20 million in the United States) of all people with diabetes have type 2 diabetes, which encompasses a variety of abnormalities involving blood glucose metabolism. The hallmark of the disease is insulin resistance, in which the body requires progressively increased pancreatic insulin production to achieve normal glycemia. However, beta cell mass decreases, so hyperglycemia results. Risk factors for type 2 diabetes include obesity and sedentary lifestyle. Onset of type 2 diabetes is typically during middle age, but with growing rates of obesity at younger ages, children and adolescents are starting to develop the disease at higher rates. Because they decrease insulin resistance, prescribed weight loss and regular exercise are first-line treatments for type 2 diabetes (Beaser 2004).

The United Kingdom Prospective Diabetes Study (UKPDS), the largest and longest prospective study of type 2 diabetes to date, found that for every 1-point reduction in hemoglobin A_{1c}, there was a corresponding 35% reduction in risk of diabetes complications. Successfully treating hypertension led to similar or greater reduction in cardiovascular complications (Krentz 1999; Matthews 1999; UK Prospective Diabetes Study Group 1998a, 1998b).

Stress and Diabetes

There is conflicting evidence on whether stress directly affects the onset of diabetes or its course (Mooy et al. 2000; Wales 1995). Stress hormones are involved in the body's counterregulatory response to insulin, so it is likely that stress plays a role in increasing blood glucose. A number of studies have shown that glycemic control is poorer in people with diabetes who report more stress (Garay-Sevilla et al. 2000). However, it is not clear whether stress directly influences metabolic regulation or whether people under stress change their self-care behaviors. Some laboratory studies have suggested that psychological stress can impair glucose control in both type 1 (Moberg et al. 1994) and type 2 (Goetsch et al. 1993) diabetes; other studies have not demonstrated this effect (Kemmer et al. 1986).

Psychiatric Disorders and Diabetes Management

In both type 1 and type 2 diabetes, psychiatric disorders have been linked to treatment nonadherence, worse blood glucose control, and ultimately greater prevalence of micro- and macrovascular complications. Because disease outcomes in diabetes are so dependent on patient behaviors, attitudes, and cognitions, optimal treatment is multidisciplinary, including psychiatrists and other mental health professionals. Treatment should take into account the psychology of individual patients, their support systems, and doctor–patient relationships.

Depression and Diabetes

The prevalence of depression in diabetes is two to three times higher than that found in the general population (Anderson et al. 2001). Several studies suggest that patients with depressive disorders appear to develop worse glycemic control and have a heightened risk of diabetes complications such as retinopathy, nephropathy, hypertension, cardiac disease, and sexual dysfunction (M. de Groot et al. 2001). However, it remains unclear if depression is a cause or an effect of poorer outcomes in diabetes. Lustman et al. (2000a), in a comprehensive meta-analytic review, reported a consistently strong association between elevated hemoglobin A_{1c} values (indicating chronic hyperglycemia) and depression. The relationship may be reciprocal, with hyperglycemia being provoked by depression as well as independently contributing to the exacerbation of depression.

Although depression may also result from complications and disease duration, it has been found to occur relatively early in the course of illness before the onset of complications (Jacobson et al. 2002). Therefore, it does not appear that the increased rate of depression in diabetes can be explained solely by emotional reactions to a chronic disease with complications.

Studies of type 2 diabetes are less clear with regard to the development of psychiatric disorders (Talbot and Nouwen 2000). The increased rates of depression seen in patients with type 2 diabetes appear in some instances to precede the onset of illness, thereby raising an entirely different hypothesis about the etiological relationship—that is, that depressive disorders themselves may place patients at risk for developing type 2 diabetes (Musselman et al. 2003). Both direct physiological and social factors could come into play. Depressed patients also decrease physical activity and increase cardiovascular risk factors by smoking and eating high-caloric and fatty foods, which place them at higher risk for developing type 2 diabetes (Marcus et al. 1992).

Some investigators have suggested that the metabolic problems of diabetes (increased rates of hypoglycemia and hyperglycemia) could themselves play a causal role in the development of depression. There is increasing evidence that diabetes leads to changes in white and gray matter in the brain (Dejgaard et al. 1991; Musen et al. 2006). These abnormalities, if present in regions of the brain involved in affect regulation (e.g., the limbic system), may play a causal role in the development of depression (Jacobson et al. 2000).

Diabetes-specific measures of quality of life, such as the Problem Areas in Diabetes Scale (PAID) (Polonsky et al. 1995; Welch et al. 1997, 2003) and the Diabetes Quality of Life Measure (DQOL) (Jacobson 1996; Jacobson et al. 1994), may be useful in screening patients who are overburdened by the demands of self-care and risk of complications and may be at increased risk for depression.

Two controlled studies have demonstrated that cognitive-behavioral therapy, nortriptyline, and fluoxetine are effective treatments for depression in diabetes (Lustman et al. 1997, 1998, 2000b). Thus, whatever the causal links between depression and diabetes, psychiatric treatment can improve psychological and biomedical outcomes of diabetes (Jacobson and Weinger 1998).

Bipolar Disorder, Schizophrenia, and Diabetes

A number of studies have demonstrated a significantly increased prevalence of diabetes (mainly type 2) in patients with bipolar disorder and schizophrenia (Dixon et al. 2000; Ruzickova et al. 2003). Much of the association appears to be related to more obesity, which is associated with, but not fully accounted for by, weight gain–associated psychotropic drugs (Buse 2002; McElroy et al. 2002). The added risk may reflect the generally poor lifestyle choices of individuals with schizophrenia.

With several of the atypical antipsychotics, the onset of diabetes may occur suddenly and dramatically, with emergent ketoacidosis or hyperosmolar coma (Buse 2002). It is believed that antagonism of serotonin 5-HT$_{1A}$ receptors may play a role in decreasing levels of insulin and increasing hyperglycemia (Wirshing et al. 2003).

Because sudden and dramatic presentation of hyperglycemia may occur in some cases, glucose intolerance should be assessed when treatment with antipsychotics is initiated and should be monitored regularly. Unfortunately, fasting blood glucose is a relatively insensitive method, so when there is a high index of suspicion (e.g., history of gestational diabetes, family history of diabetes, presence of obesity), postprandial blood glucose testing may be warranted. In patients with known diabetes, antipsychotics least likely to cause weight gain and glucose intolerance (e.g., aripiprazole and ziprasidone) should be favored.

Eating Disorders and Diabetes

A negative aspect of intensive diabetes management is weight gain (Diabetes Control and Complications Trial Research Group 1988, 2001). Heightened attention to food portions, blood sugars, and risk of weight gain in intensive diabetes management might place women with diabetes at heightened risk for developing eating disorders. Moreover, insulin manipulation (i.e., administering reduced insulin doses or omitting necessary doses altogether) can be used as a means of caloric purging. Intentionally induced glycosuria is a powerful weight loss behavior and a symptom of eating disorders unique to type 1 diabetes.

There appears to be an increased risk of eating disorders among female patients with type 1 diabetes (Jones et al. 2000). Intermittent insulin omission or dose reduction for weight loss purposes is common among women with type 1 diabetes. Polonsky et al. (1994) found that 31% reported intentional insulin omission. Rates of omission peaked in late adolescence and early adulthood. This behavior, even at a subclinical level of severity, places women at heightened risk for medical complications of diabetes (Polonsky et al. 1994). In a longitudinal study, Rydall et al. (1997) reported that after 4 years, 86% of patients classified as having high levels of eating disorders had retinopathy, as compared with 43% and 24% of women with moderate or no reported eating disturbance, respectively. The chronic hyperglycemia found in women with diabetes who intentionally omit or reduce their insulin doses also places these women at much greater risk for frequent episodes of diabetic ketoacidosis.

Because such patients may not use other means of purging (such as self-induced vomiting or laxative abuse), their eating disorders may go undiagnosed. Questions about omission behaviors are helpful in screening for insulin omission, especially when patients present with persistently elevated hemoglobin A$_{1c}$ levels or unexplained diabetic ketoacidosis.

Because obesity is a significant risk factor in type 2 diabetes, recurrent binge eating may increase the chances of developing it, in part because of significantly higher body mass index (BMI) (Striegel-Moore et al. 2000).

A multidisciplinary team approach, including an endocrinologist or diabetologist, nurse educator, nutritionist with eating disorder and diabetes training, and mental health practitioner, is ideal for the treatment of comorbid eating disorders and diabetes (Mitchell et al. 1997). Psychopharmacological evaluation and treatment can be useful.

Intensive glycemic management of diabetes is not an appropriate target for a person with diabetes and an eating disorder. The first goal should focus on medical stabilization. Gradually, the team can build toward increasing doses of insulin, increases in food intake, greater flexibility of meal plans, regularity of eating routine, and more frequent blood glucose monitoring.

Diabetes and Cognitive Functioning

Adolescents and children with onset of diabetes before age 6 experience some cognitive difficulties (Kaufman et al. 1999; Northam et al. 2001; Rovet and Ehrlich 1999; Rovet et al. 1987; Ryan et al. 1985). Equivocal results have been obtained as to the role of repeated hypoglycemic events on cognition in adults. Indeed, the DCCT suggested no deficits in cognition (Diabetes Control and Complications Trial Research Group 1996). However, long-term exposure to hyperglycemia and related micro- and macrovascular damage have also been posited to heighten risk of cognitive decline and dementia in diabetes in older patients. This increased risk may be mediated by an increase in vascular disease in diabetes (Gregg and Brown 2003), as well as other metabolic effects of diabetes on the brain (Musen et al. 2006).

Hypoglycemia in Diabetic and Nondiabetic Individuals

Hypoglycemia has been a popular explanation for anxiety symptoms, especially panic attacks, with past widespread use of 5-hour glucose tolerance tests for diagnosis and recommendations for dietary management with multiple small meals. This practice is no longer commonly recommended by physicians, but hypoglycemia is still a popular diagnosis among alternative medicine practitioners and many patients. Symptomatic hypoglycemia rarely occurs except in diabetic (mainly insulin-dependent) patients and patients with insulinomas. Although marked hypoglycemia does cause symptoms of adrenergic hyperactivity, they usually can be reliably distinguished by patients from panic attacks (Uhde et al. 1984).

However, insulin-induced hypoglycemia is an aversive experience, which has been reported to cause phobic anxiety—that is, a fear of hypoglycemia—in diabetic patients, leading to poorer diabetic control (Green et al. 2000).

Thyroid Disorders

Hyperthyroidism

The most common cause of hyperthyroidism (or thyrotoxicosis) is Graves' disease. Graves' disease is an autoimmune disorder that results in hyperthyroidism when thyroid-stimulating immunoglobulins (TSIs) bind to thyroid-stimulating hormone (TSH) receptors and mimic TSH. TSIs thereby stimulate the synthesis of hormones (T_4 and T_3), while serum TSH levels are very low or undetectable (Porterfield 1997). Patients with type 1 diabetes are at increased risk for Graves' disease. There is some evidence that stress can precipitate Graves' disease (Santos et al. 2002) and aggravate treated disease (Fukao et al. 2003).

Patients with Graves' disease often present with anxiety, hypomania, irritability, depression, and/or cognitive difficulties. Both physiological and psychiatric symptoms correlate poorly with thyroid hormone levels (Trzepacz et al. 1989). These symptoms typically resolve with antithyroid therapy (Kathmann et al. 1994) or with use of beta-blockers such as propranolol (Trzepacz et al. 1988b). Graves' disease patients have been reported to have difficulties with sustained attention, visuomotor speed tasks, and memory and concentration (MacCrimmon et al. 1979). It is possible that the memory and concentration difficulties appear only after long-term thyroid dysregulation. We do know that without treatment for Graves' disease, psychiatric symptoms such as major depressive disorder, generalized anxiety disorder, and hypomania will persist (Trzepacz et al. 1988a). Affective psychosis (e.g., depression and mania) can also result from thyrotoxicosis (Brownlie et al. 2000). Although thyroid disorders are known to affect behavior, the relationship between thyroid hormones per se and brain functions has not been well studied.

Antithyroid therapy should be the first course of action in treating depression in hyperthyroid patients (Kathol et al. 1986). However, treatment for depression may be indicated if the symptoms are sufficiently problematic or persistent. Hyperthyroidism may present differently depending on the age of the patient. In younger patients, hyperthyroidism typically presents as hyperactivity or anxious dysphoria, whereas in the elderly, it can present as apathy or depression (Bailes 1999).

Hypothyroidism

Hypothyroid patients often experience weakness, fatigue, somnolence, cold intolerance, constipation, stiffness, and muscle aches (Kornstein et al. 2000). Physical signs of hypothyroidism include weakness, bradycardia, facial puffiness, weight gain, hair loss, hoarseness, and slowed speech. The most common cause of hypothyroidism is autoimmune thyroiditis (Hashimoto's thyroiditis). Hypothyroidism can also occur as a side effect of lithium. Radioactive iodine, the most commonly used modality for treating hyperthyroidism (such as in Graves' disease), may cause hypothyroidism, which may go undiagnosed for several years after treatment for hyperthyroidism.

The symptoms of hypothyroidism overlap with retarded depression, and the diagnosis is easy to miss in patients already diagnosed as depressed. The best screening test for hypothyroidism is measurement of serum TSH concentration, but an elevated TSH should be followed by a free T_4 determination to confirm the diagnosis. A serum TSH determination will be misleading in the patient with secondary hypothyroidism caused by pituitary or hypothalamic disease. In such a patient, a free T_4 measurement will usually allow the clinician to make the appropriate diagnosis.

Hypothyroidism can be divided into three grades (Haggerty and Prange 1995). Grade 1 refers to patients with *overt* hypothyroidism who are usually symptomatic and have elevated serum TSH and low serum free T_4 concentrations. Patients with *subclinical* hypothyroidism are classified as having grade 2 or 3; these patients typically have either mild or no symptoms of thyroid hormone deficiency. The laboratory features of grade 2 hypothyroidism are an elevated serum TSH level and a serum free T_4 level within the normal range. Patients with grade 3 hypothyroidism have normal TSH and free T_4 levels, and the diagnosis can only be confirmed by an exaggerated serum TSH response to thyrotropin-releasing hormone (TRH). Subclinical hypothyroidism is fairly common, affecting 5%–10% of the population (mainly women) and occurs in 15%–20% of women over the age of 45. Subclinical hypothyroidism is particularly common in elderly women.

Cognition, Depression, and Psychosis

Overt hypothyroidism can impair memory function and other cognitive functions, independent of secondary depression. Even patients with subclinical hypothyroidism show subtle signs of cognitive dysfunction on tests of memory, which may improve after treatment (Jensovsky et al. 2002).

Hypothyroidism is a known cause of secondary depression. Almost all patients with hypothyroidism have some concurrent symptoms of depression (Haggerty and Prange 1995). In the early stages of hypothyroidism, circulating T_4 levels drop while T_3 levels often remain in the normal range. The brain preferentially uses T_4, as compared with other body tissues, and is thus more sensitive than other areas of the body to lower levels of T_4. This imbalance in thyroid hormones may contribute to mood disorder, and subclinical hypothyroidism is now recognized as a potential risk factor for depression (Haggerty and Prange 1995).

Patients with bipolar disorder with either rapid cycling or mixed episodes have particularly high rates of subclinical hypothyroidism. Every patient with rapid-cycling bipolar disorder should be evaluated for (subclinical) hypothyroidism and receive thyroxine if TSH levels are elevated. Some patients may benefit even if they are euthyroid (Haggerty and Prange 1995).

Untreated hypothyroidism can result in psychosis, so-called myxedema madness. This condition was fairly common—reported in up to 5% of all hypothyroid patients (Kudrjavcev 1978)—before the widespread use of modern thyroid function tests, but it is now rare. Psychotic symptoms typically remit when TSH levels return to normal, although cognitive dysfunction may continue. The syndrome can be difficult to diagnose because of confusion between hypothyroidism and primary Axis I psychopathology (Darko et al. 1988). Another rare possibility in hypothyroid patients is Hashimoto's encephalopathy, a delirium with psychosis, seizures, and focal neurological signs; associated with high serum antithyroid antibody concentrations, it is responsive to corticosteroids and is thought to be an autoimmune disorder (Chong et al. 2003).

Congenital Hypothyroidism

Congenital hypothyroidism usually occurs as a result of thyroid agenesis or dysgenesis, although inherited defects in thyroid hormone synthesis may also play a role. From a global perspective, iodine deficiency is the most common cause of congenital hypothyroidism. Newborns with untreated hypothyroidism develop the syndrome of cretinism, characterized by mental retardation, short stature, poor motor development, and characteristic puffiness of the face and hands. Because early treatment is essential to prevent permanent mental retardation, all infants born in the United States are screened for hypothyroidism at birth (Kooistra et al. 1996). Treatment with thyroid hormones before age 3 months can result in normal intellectual development in the majority of infants.

Parathyroidism

Hyperparathyroidism

Hyperparathyroidism can cause bone disease, kidney stones, and hypercalcemia via oversecretion of parathyroid hormone. Symptoms of hypercalcemia include anorexia, thirst, frequent urination, lethargy, fatigue, muscle weakness, joint pain, constipation, and, when severe, depression and eventually coma.

The prevalence of hyperparathyroidism is 0.1%. It is three times greater in women than in men, and its prevalence increases with age. Hyperparathyroidism may occur as a consequence of radiation therapy to head and neck or lithium therapy (Bendz et al. 1996).

With mild hypercalcemia, patients may show personality changes, lack of spontaneity, and lack of initiative. Moderate hypercalcemia (serum calcium concentration 10–14 mg/dL) may cause dysphoria, anhedonia, apathy, anxiety, irritability, and impairment of concentration and recent memory. In severe hypercalcemia (serum calcium concentration >14 mg/dL), confusion, disorientation, catatonia, agitation, paranoid ideation, delusions, auditory and visual hallucinations, and lethargy progressing to coma may occur (Kornstein et al. 2000). Verbal memory and logical abilities are also impaired (Reus 1986). After treatment of hypercalcemia, psychotic and cognitive symptoms disappear in most patients. However, psychosis has also been reported postparathyroidectomy, possibly because of the rapid decrease in serum calcium concentrations (Reus 1986).

Hypoparathyroidism

Patients with hypoparathyroidism present with hypocalcemia causing increased neuromuscular irritability. Typical symptoms include paresthesias, muscle cramps, carpopedal spasm, and, rarely, facial grimacing. Psychiatric symptoms may include anxiety and emotional irritability and lability (Kornstein et al. 2000). Severe hypocalcemia causes tetany and seizures. Hypoparathyroidism is caused by inadequate parathyroid hormone secretion, usually as a result of parathyroid or thyroid surgery.

Kowdley et al. (1999) showed that cognitive and neurological deficits are often present in patients with long-standing hypoparathyroidism (≥9 years). These deficits are thought to be related to the presence of intracranial calcification and thus irreversible (Kowdley et al. 1999).

Adrenal Gland Disorders

Cushing's Syndrome

Cushing's syndrome (CS) results from abnormally high levels of cortisol and other glucocorticoids. The most common cause is the pharmacological use of corticosteroids, followed by excessive adrenocorticotropic hormone (ACTH) secretion (most commonly by a pituitary tumor, referred to as Cushing's disease) and adrenal

tumors (Porterfield 1997). Symptoms and signs of CS include truncal obesity and striae, diabetes, hypertension, hyperglycemia, muscle weakness, osteopenia, skin atrophy and bruising, increased susceptibility to infections, and gonadal dysfunction.

CS patients commonly experience a range of psychiatric symptoms (Kornstein et al. 2000). Depression is the most prevalent psychiatric disturbance associated with CS. A full depressive syndrome has been reported in up to 50%–70% of cases (Sonino et al. 1998). Mental symptoms often precede physical changes. There is support in the literature for two possible mechanisms linking CS and depression: 1) depression in patients with Cushing's disease may be caused by hypothalamic dysfunction, and 2) elevated cortisol levels may directly cause depression in CS (Sonino et al. 1998).

Anxiety has been reported frequently (Loosen et al. 1992). Hypomania can also occur (Kelly et al. 1996).

The neocortex and the hippocampus are rich in glucocorticoid receptors (Starkman et al. 2001), so it is not surprising that learning and memory are affected in CS. Cushing's disease causes reduction in hippocampal volume, reversible after cortisol levels return to normal.

There is a small body of research suggesting that patients with Cushing's disease (but not other forms of CS) experience more stressful events in the year before diagnosis compared to patients with pituitary tumors secreting growth hormone and prolactin (Mazet et al. 2003; Sonino and Fava 2001).

Adrenal Insufficiency: Addison's Disease and ACTH Deficiency

Insufficient production of adrenal corticosteroids can be caused by a number of mechanisms. Primary adrenal insufficiency, or Addison's disease, results in deficient secretion of mineralocorticoids and glucocorticoids. The major causes of Addison's disease are autoimmune destruction of the adrenal cortex, tuberculosis, and HIV (Kornstein et al. 2000). The most common cause of secondary adrenal insufficiency is suppression of ACTH secretion by chronic glucocorticoid administration. Hypotension and hypoglycemia are common with stress or fasting. Although electrolytes can be normal in mild Addison's disease, hyponatremia and hyperkalemia are typical (Kornstein et al. 2000). Water intoxication with hyponatremia can occur if a water load is given, because cortisol deficiency impairs the ability to increase free water clearance. Other manifestations of adrenal insufficiency include anemia, anorexia, nausea, vomiting, diarrhea, abdominal pain, weight loss, and muscle weakness.

There has been no formal study of psychiatric symptoms. Apathy, social withdrawal, fatigue, anhedonia, poverty of thought, and negativism have been reported in up to 60%–90% of patients with Addison's disease (Popkin and Mackenzie 1980). Some form of depression has been observed in 30%–50% of patients (Kornstein et al. 2000). Cognitive impairment, especially memory loss, is often present but ephemeral and varying in severity. During Addisonian crisis, patients may experience delirium, disorientation, confusion, and even psychosis (Kornstein et al. 2000). Adrenal insufficiency is particularly likely to be misdiagnosed as primary major depression in patients with chronic medical illness previously treated with high doses of corticosteroids, resulting in unrecognized secondary adrenal insufficiency.

Although the diagnosis of adrenal insufficiency may be suspected on the basis of a low serum cortisol in the morning, definitive diagnosis requires an ACTH stimulation test. This is typically performed using cosyntropin, a synthetic ACTH analogue. An increase in the serum cortisol concentration to greater than 20 ng/dL following cosyntropin injection excludes the diagnosis of adrenal insufficiency.

The cause of depression in patients with Addison's disease is not clear. Regardless of the etiology of adrenal insufficiency, urgent treatment is indicated. Both glucocorticoid and mineralocorticoid replacement are usually necessary in the treatment of Addison's disease, whereas glucocorticoid replacement alone is sufficient in secondary adrenal insufficiency.

Adrenal insufficiency is also a feature in adrenoleukodystrophy, a rare, X-linked inherited metabolic disease, which also leads to leukoencephalic myeloneuropathy. Adult onset is rare but commonly presents with psychiatric symptoms, including mania, psychosis, and cognitive dysfunction (Garside et al. 1999).

Acromegaly

Acromegaly is a disease of excess growth hormone (GH) secretion. The most common cause of acromegaly is a GH-secreting adenoma of the anterior pituitary. These benign tumors account for 30% of all hormone-secreting pituitary adenomas (L.J. DeGroot et al. 2001). Clinical manifestations of acromegaly include headache, cranial nerve palsies, acral enlargement (frontal bossing), increased hand and foot size, prognathism, soft tissue overgrowth (macroglossia), glucose intolerance, and hypertension (Melmed 2001).

The literature to date does not conclusively support any particular increase in psychopathology in acromegaly (Abed et al. 1987).

Treatment of acromegaly may include surgery, medication, and radiation (Turner et al. 1984). A GH receptor antagonist, pegvisomant, has become available as another option for patients for whom surgery fails, and it has few adverse effects (Clemmons et al. 2003).

Pheochromocytoma

Pheochromocytomas are rare catecholamine-secreting tumors derived from the adrenal medulla and sympathetic ganglia. The clinical signs and symptoms result from the release of catecholamines, leading to increased heart rate and blood pressure, myocardial contractility, vasoconstriction, headache, profuse sweating, palpitations, apprehension, and a sense of impending doom (Melmed 2001). The symptoms may mimic anxiety disorders (especially panic), migraine or cluster headaches, amphetamine or cocaine abuse, alcohol withdrawal, brain tumors, subarachnoid hemorrhage, neuroblastoma in children, or temporal lobe seizures (L.J. DeGroot et al. 2001). Both tricyclic antidepressants (TCAs) and serotonin reuptake inhibitors have unmasked silent pheochromocytomas (Korzets et al. 1997). Monoamine oxidase inhibitors (MAOIs) would be expected to be even more hazardous.

The diagnosis of pheochromocytoma can be made by measurement of 24-hour urine to document increased excretion of catecholamines or catecholamine metabolites, including vanillylmandelic acid (VMA) and metanephrines. Plasma metanephrine determinations have an extremely high sensitivity, approaching 99%, and overall specificity in the 85%–90% range (Lenders et al. 2002). Urinary VMA levels can be elevated by physiological stress and with ingestion of foods high in vanillin, including vanilla extract, bananas, coffee, nuts, and citrus fruits (Sheps et al. 1990). Elevated urinary VMA levels are the least specific indicator of pheochromocytoma, whereas elevated metanephrines are the most sensitive (Stern and Cremens 1998). Misdiagnosis of pheochromocytoma has been reported in patients with hypertension and raised urinary catecholamines who were taking clozapine (Krentz et al. 2001) or selegiline (Cook and Katritsis 1990). Multiple cases of factitious pheochromocytoma due to vanilla extract ingestion and other causes have been reported.

The rare possibility of a pheochromocytoma should be considered in patients with panic attacks, headaches, and labile hypertension, particularly those who do not respond to treatment. It is not necessary to screen for pheochromocytoma in patients who only have psychiatric symptoms; elevated catecholamines are common and likely to be false positives. Some psychotropic drugs may cause hypertensive reactions that mimic pheochromocytoma, and in other cases, the drugs may be unmasking an unsuspected pheochromocytoma.

Hyperprolactinemia

Hyperprolactinemia is the most common pituitary hormone hypersecretion syndrome (Melmed 2001). The differential diagnosis of hyperprolactinemia includes pituitary adenomas, physiological causes (pregnancy and lactation), medication effects, chronic renal failure (via decreased peripheral prolactin clearance), primary hypothyroidism, and lesions of the pituitary stalk and the hypothalamus (e.g., hypothalamic tumors). Clinical signs in women include galactorrhea, menstrual irregularities, infertility, and decreased libido. Men present with diminished libido and rarely with galactorrhea.

Numerous studies and case reports demonstrate an association between hyperprolactinemia and depression and anxiety, as well as resolution of symptoms with treatment of hyperprolactinemia (e.g., Cohen

1995; Fava et al. 1987; Reavley et al. 1997). However, the link between hyperprolactinemia and depression has been disputed because of small sample sizes and different inclusion criteria across studies (Merritt 1991).

Medication-induced hyperprolactinemia has been associated with antipsychotics and, to a lesser extent, antidepressants. Conventional antipsychotic drugs block dopamine D_2 receptors on lactotroph cells and thus remove the main inhibitory influence on prolactin secretion (Wieck and Haddad 2003). Serum prolactin levels in patients taking therapeutic doses of typical neuroleptics are increased 6- to 10-fold from mean baseline prolactin levels (Arvanitis and Miller 1997). Atypical antipsychotics vary with respect to their effects on prolactin. Clozapine, quetiapine, and olanzapine either cause no increase in prolactin secretion or increase prolactin transiently (Tollefson and Kuntz 1999), but sustained hyperprolactinemia can occur in patients taking risperidone (Becker et al. 2003). Haloperidol raises the serum prolactin concentration by an average of 17 ng/mL, whereas risperidone may raise it by 45–80 ng/mL, with larger increases in women than in men (David et al. 2000).

Antidepressants with serotonergic activity, including SSRIs, MAOIs, and some TCAs, can cause modest elevations of prolactin (Haddad et al. 2001) and may further elevate prolactin levels in patients also taking prolactin-elevating antipsychotics (Wieck and Haddad 2003).

Women taking psychiatric medications that chronically elevate prolactin levels are at risk for premature bone loss secondary to hypoestrogenism. Patients taking prolactin-elevating antipsychotics should be educated about—and regularly monitored for—signs and symptoms of hyperprolactinemia (Haddad et al. 2001). In patients with affective disorders who both are unresponsive to treatment and have galactorrhea and/or amenorrhea, hyperprolactinemia should be considered as a causal factor.

Gonadal Disorders

Polycystic Ovary Syndrome

Polycystic ovary syndrome (PCOS) is a common disorder, affecting 5%–10% of women of childbearing age. Clinical manifestations include amenorrhea or oligomenorrhea, infrequent or absent ovulation, increased levels of testosterone, infertility, truncal obesity or weight gain, alopecia, hirsutism, acanthosis nigricans, hypertension, and insulin resistance. The cause of the disorder is unknown. There is some evidence that valproate is associated with PCOS (McIntyre et al. 2003).

Women with PCOS may complain they feel "abnormal or freakish" (Kitzinger and Willmott 2002), related to hirsutism, obesity, and altered reproductive function. A study using standardized self-report measures found that social phobia, anxiety, and depression may occur in one-third to two-thirds of women with PCOS (Barth et al. 1993). Psychological problems have been commonly reported in women with hirsutism of any cause (Sonino et al. 1993). Although these physical abnormalities may affect feelings of self-worth and femininity, some research suggests that psychological morbidity, such as depression, may be caused by hormonal shifts in PCOS, not psychosocial factors (Derogatis et al. 1993). Although the causal linkage between psychological symptoms and PCOS is not resolved, their frequency points to the importance of screening all PCOS patients for psychiatric syndromes, especially depression (Rasgon et al. 2003).

Testosterone Deficiency

Testosterone deficiency in men can result from diseases affecting the testes, pituitary gland, or hypothalamus. Testosterone production declines naturally with age, so that a relative testosterone deficiency occurs in older males. Hypogonadal disorders of the testes (primary hypogonadism) are most commonly caused by Klinefelter's syndrome, mumps orchitis, trauma, tumor, cancer chemotherapy, or immune testicular failure. Pituitary lesions caused by tumors, hemochromatosis, sarcoidosis, or cranial irradiation can lead to secondary hypogonadism. Hypogonadism in childhood is characterized by failure of normal secondary sexual characteristics to develop and diminished muscle mass. In adult men, typical complaints are sexual dysfunction, diminished energy, decreased beard and body hair, muscle loss, and breast enlargement.

Although it has been suggested that decreasing testosterone levels as men age may be associated with changes in mood and cognition, there is no clear relationship between psychiatric syndromes and testosterone level (Shores et al. 2004; Sternbach 1998). The concept of a male climacteric and related mood, anxiety, and cognitive disorders is controversial (Sternbach 1998).

Patients with Klinefelter's syndrome (XYY) are reported to have higher rates of mental retardation and a wide variety of psychiatric and behavioral symptoms, but these are a consequence primarily of the chromosomal abnormality rather than hypogonadism (Swanson and Stipes 1969).

Questions remain about the value of testosterone replacement in age-related testosterone decline as well as in the treatment of depressive disorder in hypogonadal men. Testosterone appears to improve mood, as well as sexual dysfunction and muscle strength, in hypogonadal men (Wang et al. 2000). However, a placebo-controlled trial of intramuscular testosterone in hypogonadal men with major depressive disorder whose depression did not respond to SSRIs demonstrated no antidepressant benefits (Seidman and Rabkin 1998). The potential serious side effects of testosterone should be carefully considered before initiating replacement therapy in men with age-related low testosterone levels (Nolten 2000).

Testosterone deficiency in women can cause impaired sexual function, low energy, and depression, but what level represents deficiency and the indications, risks, and benefits of replacement are even less well defined than in men (Padero et al. 2002).

Conclusion

Endocrine disorders frequently occur in conjunction with common psychiatric conditions. The causal linkages and mechanisms vary widely. In some situations, the endocrine state manifests in part as a psychiatric condition. In other instances, the psychiatric condition may be a complex biopsychosocial and/or biological response to the endocrine disorder. Psychiatric conditions and their treatment may also increase risk of endocrine disorders. Moreover, treatment with psychotropic drugs can induce endocrinopathies. Consequently, understanding the ways in which these disorders intersect represents an important facet of knowledge for the practitioners treating patients with psychiatric and/or endocrine disorders.

References

Abed RT, Clark J, Elbadawy MH, et al: Psychiatric morbidity in acromegaly. Acta Psychiatr Scand 75:635–639, 1987

Anderson R, Freedland KE, Clouse RE, et al: The prevalence of comorbid depression in adults with diabetes. Diabetes Care 24:1069–1078, 2001

Arvanitis LA, Miller BG: Multiple fixed doses of "Seroquel" (quetiapine) in patients with acute exacerbation of schizophrenia: a comparison with haloperidol and placebo. The Seroquel Trial 13 Study Group. Biol Psychiatry 42:233–246, 1997

Bailes BK: Hypothyroidism in elderly patients. AORN J 69: 1026–1030, 1999

Barth JH, Catalan J, Cherry CA, et al: Psychological morbidity in women referred for treatment of hirsutism. J Psychosom Res 37:615–619, 1993

Beaser RS: Joslin's Diabetes Deskbook: A Guide for Primary Care Providers, Revised Edition. Boston, MA, Joslin Diabetes Center, 2004

Becker D, Liver O, Mester R, et al: Risperidone, but not olanzapine, decreases bone mineral density in female premenopausal schizophrenia patients. J Clin Psychiatry 64:761–766, 2003

Bendz H, Sjodin I, Toss G, et al: Hyperparathyroidism and long-term lithium therapy—a cross-sectional study and the effect of lithium withdrawal. J Intern Med 240:357–365, 1996

Brownlie BE, Rae AM, Walshe JW, et al: Psychoses associated with thyrotoxicosis—"thyrotoxic psychosis." A report of 18 cases, with statistical analysis of incidence. Eur J Endocrinol 142:438–444, 2000

Buse JB: Metabolic side effects of antipsychotics: focus on hyperglycemia and diabetes. J Clin Psychiatry 63 (suppl 4): 37–41, 2002

Chong JY, Rowland LP, Utiger RD: Hashimoto encephalopathy: syndrome or myth? Arch Neurol 60:164–171, 2003

Clemmons DR, Chihara K, Freda PU, et al: Optimizing control of acromegaly: integrating a growth hormone receptor antagonist into the treatment algorithm. J Clin Endocrinol Metab 88:4759–4767, 2003

Cohen AJ: Bromocriptine for prolactinoma-related dissociative disorder and depression. J Clin Psychopharmacol 15:144–145, 1995

Cook RF, Katritsis D: Hypertensive crisis precipitated by a monoamine oxidase inhibitor in a patient with phaeochromocytoma. BMJ 300:614, 1990

Darko DF, Krull A, Dickinson M, et al: The diagnostic dilemma of myxedema and madness, Axis I and Axis II: a longitudinal case report. Int J Psychiatry Med 18:263–270, 1988

David SR, Taylor CC, Kinon BJ, et al: The effects of olanzapine, risperidone, and haloperidol on plasma prolactin levels in patients with schizophrenia. Clin Ther 22:1085–1096, 2000

DeGroot LJ, Jameson JL, Burger, HG, et al: Endocrinology, 4th Edition. Philadelphia, PA, WB Saunders, 2001

de Groot M, Anderson RJ, Freedland KE, et al: Association of depression and diabetes complications: a meta-analysis. Psychosom Med 63:619–630, 2001

Dejgaard A, Gade A, Larsson H, et al: Evidence for diabetic encephalopathy. Diabet Med 8:162–167, 1991

Derogatis LR, Rose LI, Shulman LH, et al: Serum androgens and psychopathology in hirsute women. J Psychosom Obstet Gynaecol 14:269–282, 1993

Diabetes Control and Complications Trial Research Group: Weight gain associated with intensive therapy in the diabetes control and complications trial. Diabetes Care 11:567–573, 1988

Diabetes Control and Complications Trial Research Group: The effect of intensive treatment of diabetes on the development and progression of long-term complications in insulin-dependent diabetes mellitus. N Engl J Med 329: 977–986, 1993

Diabetes Control and Complications Trial Research Group: Effects of intensive diabetes therapy on neuropsychological function in adults in the Diabetes Control and Complications Trial. Ann Intern Med 124:379–388, 1996

Diabetes Control and Complications Trial Research Group: Influence of intensive diabetes treatment on body weight and composition of adults with type 1 diabetes in the Diabetes Control and Complications Trial. Diabetes Care 24:1711–1721, 2001

Dixon L, Weiden P, Delahanty J, et al: Prevalence and correlates of diabetes in national schizophrenia samples. Schizophr Bull 26:903–912, 2000

Fava M, Fava GA, Kellner R, et al: Depression and hostility in hyperprolactinemia. Prog Neuropsychopharmacol Biol Psychiatry 6:479–482, 1982

Fukao A, Takamatsu J, Murakami Y, et al: The relationship of psychological factors to the prognosis of hyperthyroidism in antithyroid drug-treated patients with Graves' disease. Clin Endocrinol (Oxf) 58:550–555, 2003

Garay-Sevilla ME, Malacara JM, Gonzalez-Contreras E, et al: Perceived psychological stress in diabetes mellitus type 2. Rev Invest Clin 52:241–245, 2000

Garside S, Rosebush PI, Levinson AJ, et al: Late-onset adrenoleukodystrophy associated with long-standing psychiatric symptoms. J Clin Psychiatry 60:460–468, 1999

Goetsch VL, VanDorsten B, Pbert LA, et al: Acute effects of laboratory stress on blood glucose in noninsulin-dependent diabetes. Psychosom Med 55:492–496, 1993

Green L, Feher M, Catalan J: Fears and phobias in people with diabetes. Diabetes Metab Res Rev 16:287–293, 2000

Gregg E, Brown A: Cognitive and physical disabilities and aging-related complications of diabetes. Clinical Diabetes 21:113–116, 2003

Haddad PM, Helleweil JS, Wieck A: Antipsychotic induced hyperprolactinaemia: a series of illustrative case reports. J Psychopharmacol 15:293–295, 2001

Haggerty JJ Jr, Prange AJ: Borderline hypothyroidism and depression. Annu Rev Med 46:37–46, 1995

Jacobson AM: The psychological care of patients with insulin-dependent diabetes mellitus. N Engl J Med 334:1249–1253, 1996

Jacobson AM, Weinger K: Treating depression in diabetic patients: is there an alternative to medications? Ann Intern Med 129:656–657, 1998

Jacobson AM, de Groot M, Samson JA: The evaluation of two measures of quality of life in patients with type I and type II diabetes. Diabetes Care 17:267–274, 1994

Jacobson AM, Weinger K, Hill TC, et al: Brain functioning, cognition and psychiatric disorders in patients with type 1 diabetes. Diabetes 49 (suppl 1):537, 2000

Jacobson AM, Samson JA, Weinger K, et al: Diabetes, the brain, and behavior: is there a biological mechanism underlying the association between diabetes and depression? Int Rev Neurobiol 51:455–479, 2002

Jensovsky J, Ruzicka E, Spackova N, et al: Changes of event related potential and cognitive processes in patients with subclinical hypothyroidism after thyroxine treatment. Endocr Regul 36:115–122, 2002

Jones JM, Lawson ML, Daneman D, et al: Eating disorders in adolescent females with and without type 1 diabetes: cross sectional study. BMJ 320:1563–1566, 2000

Kathmann N, Kuisle U, Bommer M, et al: Effects of elevated triiodothyronine levels on cognitive performance and mood in healthy subjects. Neuropsychobiology 29:136–142, 1994

Kathol RG, Turner R, Delahunt J: Depression and anxiety associated with hyperthyroidism: response to antithyroid therapy. Psychosomatics 27:501–505, 1986

Kaufman FR, Epport K, Engilman R, et al: Neurocognitive functioning in children diagnosed with diabetes before age 10 years. J Diabetes Complications 13:31–38, 1999

Kelly WF, Kelly MJ, Faragher B: A prospective study of psychiatric and psychological aspects of Cushing's syndrome. Clin Endocrinol (Oxf) 45:715–720, 1996

Kemmer FW, Bisping R, Steingruber HJ, et al: Psychological stress and metabolic control in patients with type I diabetes mellitus. N Engl J Med 314:1078–1084, 1986

Kitzinger C, Willmott J: "The thief of womanhood": women's experience of polycystic ovarian syndrome. Soc Sci Med 54: 349–361, 2002

Kooistra L, van de Meere JJ, Vulsma T, et al: Sustained attention problems in children with early treated congenital hypothyroidism. Acta Paediatr 85:425–429, 1996

Kornstein SG, Sholar EF, Gardner DG: Endocrine disorders, in Psychiatric Care of the Medical Patient, 2nd Edition. Edited by Stoudemire A, Fogel BS, Greenberg D. New York, Oxford University Press, 2000, pp 801–819

Korzets A, Floro S, Ori Y, et al: Clomipramine-induced pheochromocytoma crisis: a near fatal complication of a tricyclic antidepressant. J Clin Psychopharmacol 17:428–430, 1997

Kowdley KV, Coull BM, Orwoll ES: Cognitive impairment and intracranial calcification in chronic hypoparathyroidism. Am J Med Sci 317:273–277, 1999

Krentz AJ: UKPDS and beyond: into the next millennium. United Kingdom Prospective Diabetes Study. Diabetes Obes Metab 1:13–22, 1999

Krentz AJ, Mikhail S, Cantrell P, et al: Pseudophaeochromocytoma syndrome associated with clozapine. BMJ 322:1213, 2001

Kudrjavcev T: Neurologic complications of thyroid dysfunction. Adv Neurol 19:619–636, 1978

Lenders JW, Pacak K, Walther MM, et al: Biochemical diagnosis of pheochromocytoma: which test is best? JAMA 287: 1427–1434, 2002

Loosen PT, Chambliss B, DeBold CR, et al: Psychiatric phenomenology in Cushing's disease. Pharmacopsychiatry 25: 192–198, 1992

Lustman PJ, Griffith LS, Clouse RE, et al: Effects of nortriptyline on depression and glycemic control in diabetes: results of a double-blind, placebo-controlled trial. Psychosom Med 59:241–250, 1997

Lustman PJ, Griffith LS, Freedland KE, et al: Cognitive behavior therapy for depression in type 2 diabetes mellitus: a randomized, controlled trial. Ann Intern Med 129:613–621, 1998

Lustman PJ, Anderson RJ, Freedland KE, et al: Depression and poor glycemic control: a meta-analytic review of the literature. Diabetes Care 23:934–942, 2000a

Lustman PJ, Freedland KE, Griffith LS, et al: Fluoxetine for depression in diabetes: a randomized double-blind placebo-controlled trial. Diabetes Care 23:618–623, 2000b

MacCrimmon DJ, Wallace JE, Goldberg WM, et al: Emotional disturbance and cognitive deficits in hyperthyroidism. Psychosom Med 41:331–340, 1979

Marcus MD, Wing RR, Guare J, et al: Lifetime prevalence of major depression and its effect on treatment outcome in obese type II diabetic patients. Diabetes Care 15:253–255, 1992

Matthews DR: The natural history of diabetes-related complications: the UKPDS experience. United Kingdom Prospective Diabetes Study. Diabetes Obes Metab 1 (suppl 2): S7–S13, 1999

Mazet P, Simon D, Luton J, et al: Syndrome de Cushing: Symptomatologie psychique et personalité de 50 malades. Nouv Presse Med 1988:2565–2570, 2003

McElroy SL, Frye MA, Suppes T, et al: Correlates of overweight and obesity in 644 patients with bipolar disorder. J Clin Psychiatry 63:207–213, 2002

McIntyre RS, Mancini DA, McCann S, et al: Valproate, bipolar disorder and polycystic ovarian syndrome. Bipolar Disord 5:28–35, 2003

Melmed S: Disorders of the anterior pituitary and hypothalamus, in Principles of Internal Medicine, 15th Edition. Edited by Braunwald E, Fauci AS, Kasper DL, et al. New York, McGraw-Hill, 2001, pp 2029–2051

Merritt DF: Hyperprolactinemia and depression. JAMA 266: 2004, 1991

Mitchell JE, Pomeroy C, Adson DE: Managing medical complications, in Handbook for Treatment of Eating Disorders. Editor by Garner D, Garfinkel P. New York, Guilford, 1997, pp 383–393

Moberg E, Kollind M, Lins PE, et al: Acute mental stress impairs insulin sensitivity in IDDM patients. Diabetologia 37: 247–251, 1994

Mooy JM, de Vries H, Grootenhuis PA, et al: Major stressful life events in relation to prevalence of undetected type 2 diabetes: the Hoorn Study. Diabetes Care 23:197–201, 2000

Musen G, Lyoo IK, Sparks CR, et al: Effects of type 1 diabetes on gray matter density as measured by voxel-based morphometry. Diabetes 55:326–333, 2006

Musselman DL, Betan E, Larsen H, et al: Relationship of depression to diabetes types 1 and 2: epidemiology, biology, and treatment. Biol Psychiatry 54:317–329, 2003

Nolten WE: Androgen deficiency in the aging male: when to evaluate and when to treat. Curr Urol Rep 1:313–319, 2000

Northam EA, Anderson PJ, Jacobs R, et al: Neuropsychological profiles of children with type 1 diabetes 6 years after disease onset. Diabetes Care 24:1541–1546, 2001

Padero MC, Bhasin S, Friedman TC: Androgen supplementation in older women: too much hype, not enough data. J Am Geriatr Soc 50:1131–1140, 2002

Polonsky WH, Anderson BJ, Lohrer PA, et al: Insulin omission in women with IDDM. Diabetes Care 17:1178–1185, 1994

Polonsky WH, Anderson BJ, Lohrer PA, et al: Assessment of diabetes-related distress. Diabetes Care 18:754–760, 1995

Popkin MK, Mackenzie TB: Psychiatric presentations of endocrine dysfunction, in Psychiatric Presentations of Medical Illness. Edited by Hall RCW. New York, Spectrum Publications, 1980, pp 139–156

Porterfield SP: Endocrine Physiology. St Louis, MO, Mosby-Year Book, 1997

Rasgon NL, Rao RC, Hwang S, et al: Depression in women with polycystic ovary syndrome: clinical and biochemical correlates. J Affect Disord 74:299–304, 2003

Reavley A, Fisher AD, Owen D, et al: Psychological distress in patients with hyperprolactinaemia. Clin Endocrinol (Oxf) 47:343–348, 1997

Reus VI: Behavioral disturbances associated with endocrine disorders. Annu Rev Med 37:205–214, 1986

Rovet JF, Ehrlich RM: The effect of hypoglycemic seizures on cognitive function in children with diabetes: A 7-year prospective study. J Pediatr 134:503–506, 1999

Rovet JF, Ehrlich RM, Hoppe M: Intellectual deficits associated with early onset of insulin-dependent diabetes mellitus in children. Diabetes Care 10:510–515, 1987

Ruzickova M, Slaney C, Garnham J, et al: Clinical features of bipolar disorder with and without comorbid diabetes mellitus. Can J Psychiatry 48:458–461, 2003

Ryan C, Vega A, Drash A: Cognitive deficits in adolescents who developed diabetes early in life. Pediatrics 75:921–927, 1985

Rydall AC, Rodin GM, Olmsted MP, et al: Disordered eating behavior and microvascular complications in young women with insulin-dependent diabetes mellitus. N Engl J Med 336:1849–1854, 1997

Santos AM, Nobre EL, Garcia e Costa, et al: Graves' disease and stress [in Portuguese]. Acta Med Port 15:423–427, 2002

Seidman SN, Rabkin JG: Testosterone replacement therapy for hypogonadal men with SSRI-refractory depression. J Affect Disord 48:157–161, 1998

Sheps SG, Jiang NS, Klee GG, et al: Recent developments in the diagnosis and treatment of pheochromocytoma. Mayo Clin Proc 65:88–95, 1990

Shores MM, Sloan KL, Matsumoto AM, et al: Increased incidence of diagnosed depressive illness in hypogonadal older men. Arch Gen Psychiatry 61:162–7, 2004

Sonino N, Fava GA: Psychiatric disorders associated with Cushing's syndrome. Epidemiology, pathophysiology and treatment. CNS Drugs 15:361–373, 2001

Sonino N, Fava GA, Mani E, et al: Quality of life of hirsute women. Postgrad Med J 69:186–189, 1993

Sonino N, Fava GA, Raffi AR, et al: Clinical correlates of major depression in Cushing's disease. Psychopathology 31:302–306, 1998

Starkman MN, Giordani B, Berent S, et al: Elevated cortisol levels in Cushing's disease are associated with cognitive decrements. Psychosom Med 63:985–993, 2001

Stern TA, Cremens CM: Factitious pheochromocytoma. Psychosomatics 39:283–287, 1998

Sternbach H: Age-associated testosterone decline in men: clinical issues for psychiatry. Am J Psychiatry 155:1310–1318, 1998

Striegel-Moore RH, Wilfley DE, Pike KM, et al: Recurrent binge eating in black American women. Arch Fam Med 9:83–87, 2000

Swanson DW, Stipes AL: Psychiatric aspects of Klinefelter's syndrome. Am J Psychiatry 126:82–90, 1969

Talbot F, Nouwen A: A review of the relationship between depression and diabetes in adults: is there a link? Diabetes Care 23:1556–1562, 2000

Tollefson GD, Kuntz AJ: Review of recent clinical studies with olanzapine. Br J Psychiatry 174 (suppl 37) 30–35, 1999

Trzepacz PT, McCue M, Klein I, et al: A psychiatric and neuropsychological study of patients with untreated Graves' disease. Gen Hosp Psychiatry 10:49–55, 1988a

Trzepacz PT, McCue M, Klein I, et al: Psychiatric and neuropsychological response to propranolol in Graves' disease. Biol Psychiatry 23:678–688, 1988b

Trzepacz PT, Klein I, Roberts M, et al: Graves' disease: an analysis of thyroid hormone levels and hyperthyroid signs and symptoms. Am J Med 87:558–561, 1989

Turner TH, Cookson JC, Wass JA, et al: Psychotic reactions during treatment of pituitary tumours with dopamine agonists. Br Med J (Clin Res Ed) 289:1101–1103, 1984

Uhde TW, Vittone BJ, Post RM: Glucose tolerance testing in panic disorder. Am J Psychiatry 141:1461–1463, 1984

UK Prospective Diabetes Study (UKPDS) Group: Effect of intensive blood-glucose control with metformin on complications in overweight patients with type 2 diabetes (UKPDS 34). Lancet 352:854–865, 1998a

UK Prospective Diabetes Study (UKPDS) Group: Intensive blood-glucose control with sulphonylureas or insulin compared with conventional treatment and risk of complications in patients with type 2 diabetes (UKPDS 33). Lancet 352:837–853, 1998b

Wales JK: Does psychological stress cause diabetes? Diabet Med 12:109–112, 1995

Wang C, Swedloff R, Iranmanesh A, et al: Transdermal testosterone gel improves sexual function, mood, muscle strength, and body composition parameters in hypogonadal men. Testosterone Gel Study Group. J Clin Endocrinol Metab 2839–2853, 2000

Welch GW, Jacobson AM, Polonsky WH: The Problem Areas in Diabetes Scale. An evaluation of its clinical utility. Diabetes Care 20:760–766, 1997

Welch G, Weinger K, Anderson B, et al: Responsiveness of the Problem Areas in Diabetes (PAID) questionnaire. Diabet Med 20:69–72, 2003

Wieck A, Haddad PM: Antipsychotic-induced hyperprolactinaemia in women: pathophysiology, severity and consequences. Selective literature review. Br J Psychiatry 182:199–204, 2003

Wirshing DA, Pierre JM, Erhart SM, et al: Understanding the new and evolving profile of adverse drug effects in schizophrenia. Psychiatr Clin North Am 26:165–190, 2003

Self-Assessment Questions

Select the single best response for each question.

1. The psychiatric care of diabetes mellitus (DM) poses several challenges for both psychiatric illness management and patients' global levels of health and functioning. Specifically, mood disorders are a significant problem in this population. All of the following are true *except*

   A. Psychiatric disorders are associated with treatment noncompliance and vascular complications in type 1, but not type 2, diabetes.
   B. The prevalence of depression in diabetic patients is two to three times higher than that in the general population.
   C. Lustman et al. (2000) have postulated that depression and poor glycemic control are reciprocally linked.
   D. Depression in diabetes mellitus typically antedates the development of vascular complications.
   E. It does not appear that the increased rate of depression in diabetes can be explained solely by emotional reactions to a chronic disease with complications.

2. Besides depressive disorders, other psychiatric illnesses are of clinical importance in diabetes. Which of the following statements is *true?*

   A. The high risk of diabetes in bipolar disorder patients primarily relates to type 1 diabetes.
   B. In bipolar disorder patients with type 2 diabetes, any excess weight is accounted for by weight gain from psychotropic medications.
   C. The onset of diabetes rarely occurs suddenly or dramatically with several of the atypical antipsychotics.
   D. It is believed that antagonism of 5-HT_{1A} receptors may lead to decreased levels of insulin and increased blood glucose in schizophrenic patients treated with atypical antipsychotics.
   E. Atypical antipsychotics least likely to cause weight gain and glucose intolerance include risperidone and quetiapine.

3. Hyperthyroidism is a useful clinical model for psychiatric illness arising from metabolic disturbance. The symptoms of hyperthyroidism converge with those of several psychiatric illness groups. All of the following are true *except*

   A. Presence and severity of psychiatric symptoms in Graves' disease correlate directly with thyroid hormone levels.
   B. The most common cause of hyperthyroidism is Graves' disease.
   C. Patients with Graves' disease often present with anxiety, hypomania, irritability, depression, and/or cognitive difficulties.
   D. Antithyroid therapy is associated with improvement in psychiatric symptoms.
   E. Hyperthyroidism with anxious dysphoria is more common in younger, rather than older, patients.

4. Hypothyroidism offers another model of an endocrinologically based psychiatric illness. Regarding hypothyroidism and psychiatric illness, which of the following statements is *true?*

   A. An elevated serum thyroid-stimulating hormone (TSH) concentration serves both to screen for and to confirm hypothyroidism.
   B. Grade 1 hypothyroidism involves overt clinical symptoms, elevated TSH, and low serum thyroxine (T$_4$) concentrations.
   C. Subclinical hypothyroidism is equally common in men and women.
   D. The most common cause of hypothyroidism is from lithium treatment.
   E. Subclinical hypothyroidism infrequently occurs in elderly women.

5. Various antipsychotic agents are associated with increased serum prolactin and resultant systemic complications. Which of the following atypical antipsychotic agents carries the highest risk of increased prolactin?

   A. Clozapine.
   B. Olanzapine.
   C. Ziprasidone.
   D. Risperidone.
   E. Quetiapine.

7 Oncology

Mary Jane Massie, M.D.
Donna B. Greenberg, M.D.

CANCER IS A major public health problem in developed nations. Although there has been a decline in death rates from many cancers, as the death rate decreases and the population ages, there will be more people living with cancer. In Europe, the most common cancers are lung, colorectal, and breast cancer, and the most common causes of cancer deaths are lung cancer followed by colorectal, stomach, and breast cancer (Boyle and Ferlay 2005).

In this chapter, we review psychological factors in cancer risk and progression, the most frequently encountered psychiatric disorders (depression, anxiety, and delirium) in adult cancer patients, psychiatric issues in specific cancers, psychiatric aspects of cancer treatments, psychiatric interventions in cancer patients, survivor issues, and cancer patients' use of complementary and alternative medicine treatments. See Chapter 17, "Pediatrics," for additional coverage of cancer in children.

Psychological Factors Affecting Cancer Risk and Progression

The role of psychological factors in cancer onset and progression is controversial and remains to be clarified (Levenson and Mc-Donald 2002). Depression may directly affect the course of illness in patients with cancer because it results in poorer pain control (Glover et al. 1995), poorer compliance (Ayres et al. 1994), and less desire for life-sustaining therapy (Lee and Ganzini 1992).

Psychiatric Disorders in Cancer Patients

A person's ability to manage a cancer diagnosis and treatment commonly changes over the course of the illness and depends on medical, psychological, and social factors: the disease itself (i.e., site, symptoms, clinical course, prognosis, type of treatments required); prior level of adjustment; the threat that cancer poses to attaining age-appropriate developmental tasks and goals (i.e., adolescence, career, family, retirement); cultural, spiritual, and religious attitudes; the presence of emotionally supportive persons; the potential for physical and psychological rehabilitation; the patient's own personality and coping style; and prior experience with loss.

Depression

Depressive symptoms may represent a normal reaction, a psychiatric disorder, or a somatic consequence of cancer or its treatment. Many depressed patients adhere poorly to treatment schedules and other recommendations; some may have a reduced chance of survival (Faller and Bülzebruck 2002; Watson et al. 1999).

Cancer, exclusive of site, is associated with a rate of depression that is higher than that in the general population and at least as high as the rate associated with other serious medical illnesses (Massie 2004). Many research groups have assessed depression in cancer patients, with widely variable reported prevalence (major depression, 0%–38%; depression spectrum syndromes, 0%–58%) in more than 150 studies (Massie 2004). Cancer types highly associated with depression include oropharyngeal (22%–57%), pancreatic (33%–50%), breast (1.5%–46%), and lung (11%–44%).

Depression in cancer patients results from 1) stress related to the cancer diagnosis and treatment; 2) medications; 3) underlying neurological or medical problems, such as nutritional deficiencies (e.g., folate, B_{12}), endocrine disturbances (e.g., thyroid abnormalities, adrenal insufficiency), brain metastases, and lepto-

meningeal disease; or 4) recurrence of a preexisting affective disorder. Clinical diagnosis rests on psychological symptoms: social withdrawal; anhedonia; dysphoric mood; feelings of hopelessness, helplessness, worthlessness, or guilt; poor self-esteem; or suicidality. Cancer patients likely at higher risk for depression are those in poor physical condition and in the advanced stages of illness who have inadequately controlled pain, a history of depression, or other significant life stresses or losses (Massie and Popkin 1998; Newport and Nemeroff 1998). An increased risk of depression has also been associated with pancreatic, head and neck, and lung cancers (Ginsburg et al. 1995; Holland et al. 1986).

Oncologists often underestimate the level of depressive symptoms and do not prescribe adequate treatment or assess the response (Passik et al. 1998). They tend to recognize low mood, pain, and anxiety, but they do not ask about suicidal ideation. When physicians are uncertain of the correct psychiatric treatment or its benefit, they are less apt to ask, and patients, not wanting to appear weak or to risk abandonment, are less apt to reveal their discouragement to oncologists (Greenberg 2004). Not infrequently, the psychiatric consultant is asked to evaluate a "depressed" cancer patient who really has a hypoactive delirium, poorly controlled pain, fatigue, or anorexia–cachexia syndrome.

Cancer-Related Suicide

Although few cancer patients commit suicide, they may be at a somewhat greater risk than the general population (Fox et al. 1982; Louhivuori and Hakama 1979; Massie and Popkin 1998). Passive suicidal thoughts are relatively common and may provide a sense of control in those overwhelmed by suffering, uncertainty, and helplessness. Both patients and doctors struggle to understand the degree to which noncompliance with or refusal of treatment represents a deliberate decision to end life (Nuland 1994).

An increased risk of suicide in cancer patients is associated with male gender, advanced stage of disease, poor prognosis, delirium with poor impulse control, inadequately controlled pain, depression, history of psychiatric illness, current or previous alcohol or substance abuse, previous suicide attempts, physical and emotional exhaustion, social isolation, and extreme need for control. Recognition of suicidal thoughts should lead to emergent psychiatric evaluation with frank discussion.

Anxiety

Anxiety is a normal response to threat, uncertainty, and loss of control. It is common as patients face the existential plight of cancer and the specific threats of deformity, abandonment, pain, or death. The diagnosis and treatment of cancer is stressful and often traumatic. After the initial shock and disbelief of diagnosis, patients typically feel anxious and irritable. They may experience anorexia, insomnia, and difficulty with concentration because they are distracted by intrusive thoughts about their prognosis. Often this acute anxiety dissipates as a treatment plan is established and prognosis clarified. Anxiety is common at crisis points such as the start of a new treatment or the diagnosis of recurrence or illness progression, but it also occurs before routine follow-up visits without evidence of disease. In a cross-sectional observational study of 178 patients with cancer, almost half had significant anxiety, but the rate of anxiety disorder and its subtypes was 18%, comparable to that in the normal population (Stark et al. 2002).

Specific syndromes of anxiety can prevent the patient from accepting appropriate medical treatment. Patients with claustrophobia have difficulty tolerating magnetic resonance imaging (MRI) scans, radiation therapy, or placement in isolation because of neutropenia. Needle phobia and other health-related phobias may interfere with chemotherapy and surgery, and radiation phobia can make some patients reluctant to accept radiation treatment. Also, anticipatory anxiety may prevent patients from following up with diagnostic or treatment visits.

In recent years, improved antiemetic treatments have reduced the number of patients who vomit with chemotherapy, but nausea is still common (Hickok et al. 2003). The nausea and vomiting with treatment are aversive stimuli that may condition anxious responses to reminders of treatment. Younger patients, patients with more emetic treatments, and those with trait anxiety are more prone to conditioning (Andrykowski 1990). Survivors of leukemia who had anticipatory nausea and vomiting during treatment are more apt to have a visceral reaction to reminders of treatment (Greenberg et al. 1997).

Evaluation of acute anxiety in cancer patients includes consideration of conditions that mimic anxiety disorders. Antiemetic phenothiazines (prochlorperazine, perphenazine, promethazine) or metoclopramide, especially when given intravenously, may cause restlessness or severe akathisia. The inner feeling of restlessness is frequently misdiagnosed as anxiety. The abrupt onset of anxiety and dyspnea may signal pulmonary emboli, which are common among cancer patients. The experience of severe, intermittent, or uncontrolled pain is associated with acute and chronic anxiety, and the patient's confidence that he or she has the analgesics to control pain alleviates anxiety. Furthermore, anxiety amplifies pain, and the momentum behind additional requests for analgesia may be anxiety rather than somatic pain.

Reminders of the traumas of cancer can provoke anxiety and physiological arousal. The prevalence of cancer-related posttraumatic stress disorder (PTSD) in women treated for breast cancer varies from 3% to 10% (Green et al. 1998). Younger age, less education, and lower income are associated with more PTSD symptoms (Cordova et al. 1995) as well as more advanced disease and lengthier hospitalizations (Jacobsen et al. 1998). Medical sequelae of cancer treatment (e.g., paresthesias because of peripheral nerve injury) may act as a trigger for memories of treatment (Kornblith et al. 2004).

Treatment of Anxiety Disorders

The management of anxiety symptoms begins with the provision of emotional support and information for the patient and family. Many patients are helped through behavioral techniques such as relaxation, distraction, and cognitive reframing (Fawzy et al. 1995). In addition to behavioral interventions, individual psychotherapy and group interventions can reduce anxiety in cancer patients. A group intervention that included education, emotional support, and behavioral training reduced tension and phobias in cancer patients (Spiegel et al. 1989).

Mania

In cancer patients, corticosteroid medications are the most common reason for hypomania or mania. Steroids are commonly given as a component of chemotherapy for lymphoma, as an antiemetic or to prevent hypersensitivity reactions with chemotherapy, or to prevent edema in the central nervous system (CNS) during radiation therapy. Psychotic mania secondary to steroids may be misdiagnosed as delirium. Interferon has also been associated with mania and mixed affective syndromes (Greenberg et al. 2000). Diencephalic tumors are a rare cause of secondary mania.

Delirium

Delirium is common in cancer as a result of metabolic sequelae of the disease and treatment, medications, metastatic tumors in the brain, and, more rarely, paraneoplastic syndromes. The prevalence of delirium in cancer patients has been reported as 5%–30% and is substantially higher (40%–85%) in terminal stages of illness (Fleishman et al. 1993). Delirium is associated with greater morbidity and mortality in patients and greater distress in patients, their families, and caregivers.

In addition to the general causes of delirium, there are particular diagnoses to consider in cancer patients. Primary brain tumor and brain metastases (especially common with lung and breast cancer) can cause delirium. Immunosuppressed cancer patients, especially those with hematological malignancies, are at high risk for opportunistic infection. Head and neck cancer patients undergoing surgery are at high risk for delirium because of their older age and high prevalence of alcohol abuse and withdrawal. Several antineoplastic agents (e.g., cytarabine, methotrexate, ifosfamide, asparaginase, procarbazine, fluorouracil) and immunotherapeutic agents (e.g., interferon and interleukins) can cause delirium and other changes in mental status (Table 7–1) (Brown and Stoudemire 1998). Some antibiotics (e.g., quinolones) and antifungals (e.g., amphotericin B), as well as opioids, anticholinergics, and nutritional deficiencies, can cause delirium. Hypercalcemia causes delirium in patients with bone metastases or ectopic hormone production. Hyperviscosity syndrome with lymphoma, Waldenström's macroglobulinemia, and myeloma are unusual causes of delirium. There are also rare autoimmune encephalopathies resulting from paraneoplastic syndromes (Lieberman and Schold 2002) that manifest with cognitive impairment and delirium. Limbic encephalopathy is a specific

---

TABLE 7–1.   **Neuropsychiatric side effects of common chemotherapeutic agents**

Hormones
  Corticosteroids
    Mild to severe insomnia, hyperactivity, anxiety, depression, psychosis with prominent
      affective and manic-like features
  Tamoxifen
    Sleep disorder, irritability

Biologicals
  Cytokines
    Encephalopathy
  Interferon
    Depression, mania, psychosis
    Delirium, akathisia
  Interleukin-2
    Dysphoria, delirium, psychosis

Chemotherapy agents
  L-Asparaginase
    Somnolence, lethargy, delirium
  Cisplatin
    Encephalopathy (rare), sensory neuropathy
  Cytarabine
    Delirium
    Leukoencephalopathy: syndrome of personality change, drowsiness, dementia,
      psychomotor retardation, ataxia
  5-Fluorouracil
    Fatigue, rare seizure or confusion, cerebellar syndrome
  Gemcitabine
    Fatigue
  Ifosfamide
    Lethargy, seizures, drunkenness, cerebellar signs, delirium, hallucinations
  Methotrexate
    Intrathecal regimens can cause leukoencephalopathy (acute and delayed forms)
    High dose can cause transient delirium
  Procarbazine
    Somnolence, depression, delirium, psychosis
  Taxanes
    Sensory neuropathy, fatigue
  Thalidomide
    Fatigue
  Vincristine, vinblastine, vinorelbine
    Depression, fatigue, encephalopathy

---

type of autoimmune encephalopathy (see Chapter 15, "Neurology and Neurosurgery") that presents with impaired memory, fluctuating mood, and seizures (Kung et al. 2002).

Cancer-Related Fatigue

Fatigue is a sign of illness in patients who have certain tumors (e.g., lymphoma) or extensive liver metastases. Both chemotherapy and radiation treatment are asso-

TABLE 7–2. Causes of cancer-related fatigue

Cancer treatment
  Interferon
  Chemotherapy
  Irradiation
Pain
Anemia
Nutritional deficits
Hormonal imbalance
  Thyroid
  Estrogen
  Androgens
Immune response
Cytokine release
Drug effects
  Opioids
  Sedatives
Psychiatric disorders
  Sleep disruption
  Depression

TABLE 7–3. Causes of cancer anorexia–cachexia syndrome

Gastrointestinal dysfunction
  Mechanical obstruction from tumors of
    mouth, esophagus, stomach,
    gastrointestinal tract
  Extrinsic pressure from metastatic disease
Anticancer treatment
  Change in food smell or taste (food
    aversions): dysosmia, dysgensia
  Nausea, vomiting, mucositis
Altered (hyper) metabolism
  Carbohydrate
  Lipid
  Protein
Host response to cancer
  Cytokine production
    Tumor necrosis factor, interleukin-1,
      interleukin-6, interferon
Psychological conditions
  Depression
  Anxiety
  Preexisting eating disorder
  Conditioned responses

ciated with predictable periods of fatigue following treatment. Causes of cancer-related fatigue are listed in Table 7–2. Psychiatrists play an important role in the treatment of depression and sleep disorders, and these common conditions may be more important as a cause of fatigue than the cancer or its treatment. Hypnotics and other psychotropic drugs may also contribute to fatigue. Patients who have persistent fatigue with progressive disease or cancer treatment may respond well to low-dose psychostimulants.

Anorexia–Cachexia Syndrome

Cachexia in cancer patients is debilitating and life-threatening. It is associated with anorexia, fat and muscle wasting, decreased quality of life, and psychological distress. The causes of cachexia are gastrointestinal dysfunction, altered metabolism and host response to cancer (cytokine production), hormone production by tumors, and anticancer treatments (Inui 2002) (see Table 7–3).

Anorexia may be the result of depression or anxiety. Preexisting eating disorders complicate nutritional management in cancer patients. Treatments of anorexia and cachexia in cancer patients are shown in Table 7–4.

Psychiatric Issues in Specific Cancers

Prostate Cancer

In general, the reaction of men with prostate cancer depends on age, marital status, recent losses, and social support. Older men are less likely to seek or accept intervention for emotional distress.

The recent increased incidence of prostate cancer directly relates to improved detection with the serum prostate specific antigen test (PSA). False-positive results can be seen with prostatitis and benign pros-

---

TABLE 7–4.   Treatment of cancer anorexia–cachexia syndrome

Educational and behavioral approaches

Hypercaloric feeding (enteral and parenteral nutrition)
  Does not increase skeletal muscle mass
  Useful for nutritional support for patients with potentially therapy-responsive cancer

Drugs
  Amino acids; ATP
  Corticosteroids
      Increase sense of well-being
      Useful adjunct for pain control
      Decrease nausea
      May cause osteoporosis, muscle weakness, immunosuppression, delirium
      Have no demonstrated effects on body weight
  Progestational drugs
      Megestrol acetate
      • Increases body weight (fat) gain
      • Increases appetite and sense of well-being
      • Can cause thromboembolic phenomena, edema, hyperglycemia, hypertension,
        adrenal insufficiency (abrupt discontinuation)
      Medroxyprogesterone acetate
      • Increases appetite and body weight
      • Available in depot and oral suspension
  Antiserotonergic drugs
      Cyproheptadine
      • Increases appetite; does not prevent weight loss
      Ondansetron
      • Does not prevent weight loss
  Prokinetic drugs
      Metoclopramide
      • Treatment for chemotherapy-induced emesis
      • May relieve anorexia
      Cannabinoids
      • Dronabinol (Marinol)
      • May improve mood and appetite
      • Minimally effective in increasing body weight in cancer
      • Can cause euphoria, dizziness
  Emerging drugs
      Melatonin, thalidomide
      Nonsteroidal anti-inflammatory drugs (prostaglandin inhibitors)
      Testosterone

---

tatic hypertrophy, as well as with manipulation of the prostate. Distress surrounding each PSA test has been dubbed "PSA anxiety" (Roth and Passik 1996) and may be even greater in spouses than in patients (Kornblith et al. 1994).

It is difficult to distinguish indolent forms of prostate cancer that will not impact the quality or quantity of a patient's survival from more lethal varieties. It is also difficult to assess the relative risk of treatment complications that may significantly impair quality of life. Controversy among clinicians about primary treatment (surgery vs. radiation) or "watchful waiting" creates uncertainty and makes treatment decisions difficult. Counseling assists patients with these choices, based on the extent of disease, age of patient, life expectancy, expense, and geography (Harlan et al. 1995), and the choices are often based on the potential side effects (e.g., impotence, urinary incontinence, and bowel problems). In general, men undergoing surgery, older men, and men with less serious disease have less mental distress (Litwin et al. 2002).

In prostate cancer patients, the most important risk factor for depression is a past history of depression (Ingram et al. 2003; Pirl et al. 2002). Androgen deprivation therapy (ADT) by orchiectomy or chronic administration of gonadotropin-releasing hormone agonists may cause hot flashes, loss of sexual interest, fatigue, anemia, decreased muscle mass, and osteoporosis. Men with prostate cancer who received ADT reported poorer quality of life compared with men who underwent any prostate cancer treatment without hormonal treatment (Wei et al. 2002). Antidepressant medications may treat depression and hot flashes and improve sleep.

Breast Cancer

More than 85% of women diagnosed with stage I (small cancers confined to the breast) cancers will be alive 5 years later. Survival drops dramatically when cancers are diagnosed at later stages.

Although only 5% of breast cancer occurs in women younger than 40 years, a disproportionately large number of younger women seek psychiatric consultation to consider treatment options; sexual side effects of treatments; fertility; self-image and body image; prophylactic contralateral mastectomy; genetic testing; and

the effects of cancer on relationships, children, and career.

Chemotherapy with alkylating agents can cause alopecia, ovarian failure, premature menopause, and weight gain. Taxanes can cause painful and disabling peripheral neuropathy. Antiestrogen therapy is prescribed over a period of years and may cause insomnia, hot flashes, irritability, and depression in some women (Duffy et al. 1999). Many women undergoing chemotherapy report difficulty with concentration and memory, but these reports do not correlate consistently with persistent deficits on neuropsychological testing.

Psychological distress is common at the conclusion of cancer treatment. Women feel vulnerable and less protected when not being seen regularly by their oncologist (Rowland and Massie 2004). Ganz et al. (1996) found that survivors appear to attain maximum recovery from the physical and emotional trauma at 1 year after breast surgery. Sexual problems are important to address after acute treatment.

Genetics

The two most significant risk factors for breast cancer are increasing age and family history. The hereditary breast or ovarian cancer syndrome accounts for 5%–7% of all breast cancer cases and 10% of all ovarian cancer cases, and is attributed to germ-line mutations in *BRCA1* and *BRCA2* genes (Robson et al. 2001). Now that gene testing is available, women may be referred for consultation with a clinical geneticist, which includes preparing a pedigree, documenting cancer diagnoses, estimating cancer risks, and discussing options for genetic testing and cancer screening and prevention (Robson and Offit 2002). Women at high risk will face decisions about risk reduction by taking hormones or having prophylactic mastectomy (PM) or prophylactic oophorectomy (PO). The woman who tests positive for a gene mutation faces unique psychological challenges. The psychiatrist may help the patient deal with the emotional challenge of explaining the genetics and its implications to mothers, sisters, daughters, and granddaughters.

The psychiatric evaluation of a woman who is considering prophylactic surgery includes a review of the woman's family and personal psychiatric history (e.g., body dysmorphic disorder, depressive disorder, personality disorder); family history of all cancers; perception of cancer risk and anxiety associated with perceptions; understanding of actual risk; satisfaction with previous plastic surgery(ies); litigation history; history of abuse, rape, or assault; sexual, pregnancy, and breast-feeding history; desire to have (more) children and planned timing of PM and PO in relationship to future pregnancies; and the feasibility of child rearing with uncertainty about the future. A partner's role in considering the decision to have PM or PO is explored. Patients have an opportunity to clarify information, discuss decisions and the decision-making process, and obtain psychological understanding and support. Regardless of whether PM and PO will be selected as an option, strategies to reduce anxiety are discussed. Some women at high risk choose to have PM or PO in the absence of genetic testing. In this case, psychiatric evaluation should be a standard component of the surgical evaluation. The women who later express regret about having had prophylactic mastectomy are those who feel that the decision to have surgery was driven by their surgeon (Payne et al. 2000).

Colorectal Cancer

Some patients who are diagnosed with colon cancer feel guilty that they were not screened by colonoscopy. Only 36% of colorectal cancers are diagnosed at an early stage, and surgical resection is the only curative therapy. A patient's adjustment is closely related to the type and extent of surgery, the presence or absence of a stoma and ostomy, and the partner's adjustment. Concerns about body image, sexual functioning, fatigue, pain, and odor can lead to social withdrawal (Bernhard et al. 1999; Sahay et al. 2000). Confusion occurs in 1% of colon cancer patients in the last 6 months of life but in 28% in the last 3 days. Significant financial burden occurs in the 3–6 months before death (McCarthy et al. 2000).

A recent survey of colorectal cancer survivors demonstrated that they had a relatively uniform and high quality of life, irrespective of stage at and time from diagnosis. Noncancer comorbid disorders and low-income status had more influence on quality of life than stage or time since diagnosis. Compared with an age-matched population, long-term survivors reported higher quality-of-life scores, but they had higher rates of depression. Frequent bowel movements and chronic recurrent diarrhea were a problem for many (Ramsey et al. 2002) (see Chapter 13, "Surgery," for a discussion of ostomies). There are many self-help groups that provide vital education and coping skills for these patients and their families.

Lung Cancer

Although it is the most preventable of all cancers, with 87% of cases linked to cigarette smoking, lung cancer is difficult to diagnose early.

Depressive symptoms and difficulty concentrating are more common at diagnosis of small cell lung cancer than non–small cell lung cancer (NSCLC). Small cell lung cancer, more than any other tumor, is associated with paraneoplastic syndromes such as Cushing's syndrome, hyponatremia, and autoimmune encephalopathy. Because pulmonary emboli are common during treatment, dyspnea and anxiety should be evaluated carefully. Hypoxia due to preexisting chronic obstructive pulmonary disease and postradiation hypothyroidism may contribute to cognitive dysfunction. Postthoracotomy neuralgic pain is common.

In lung cancer, there is a substantial risk of brain metastases. Isolated lesions may be removed surgically, but cranial radiation is common once the metastasis is noted. Patients with small cell lung cancer often receive prophylactic cranial radiation because the risk of brain metastases is 50% over 2 years. Some cognitive deficits have been noted in long-term survivors of small cell cancer whether or not they received cranial radiation. Leukoencephalopathy has occurred after treatment for small cell cancer as a result of the combination of chemotherapy and radiation, but changes in chemotherapy have decreased this risk.

In one recent study of 145 survivors of NSCLC who were 5 or more years disease free, most were hopeful. Half viewed the cancer experience as contributing to positive life changes (Sarna et al. 2002).

Many smokers with cancer experience guilt, but many continue to smoke. Continued smoking is associated with decreased survival, development of a secondary primary cancer, and increased risk of developing or exacerbating other medical conditions. Chemotherapy and radiation are likely to produce more complications and greater morbidity among smokers than among nonsmokers (Sanderson et al. 2002). Although some health care providers are hesitant to raise the issue of smoking cessation during the stress of initial diagnosis, the literature supports early antismoking intervention with patients and their family members (Sanderson et al. 2002). But in terminal lung cancer, if the patient derives pleasure from smoking, cessation interventions are not indicated.

For further review of lung cancer, see Chapter 3, "Lung Disease."

Ovarian Cancer

Patients with ovarian cancer often present with advanced disease.

Because CA 125 levels often rise before symptoms appear, patients' emotions often rise and fall with the report of the CA 125 level (Fertig and Hayes 1998). Kornblith and colleagues found that more than 60% of ovarian cancer patients were worried, tired, feeling sad, and in pain (Kornblith et al. 1995).

Living with chronic ovarian cancer is a challenge. Cancer treatment decisions must be made on the course of the cancer, not on the course of anxiety. A psychiatrist can help the patient cope with anxiety so that she receives the best cancer care.

Patients report difficulties with sexual desire, response, and communication after gynecological cancer treatment (Schover 1997). Infertility concerns are vital for younger women, who require information about fertility and emotional support to make treatment decisions and to cope with those choices.

Melanoma

Melanoma is a very variable tumor. Fawzy and associates reported that a short-term focused psychological treatment could diminish distress and prolong survival (Fawzy et al. 2003). The intervention was associated with survival benefit after 6 years, but the benefit weakened after 10 years.

Patients with advanced disease are currently treated with a 12-month protocol of interferon-alfa, the side effects of which include fatigue, anxiety, insomnia, depression, and, rarely, mania (Kirkwood et al. 2002). Paroxetine started at the time interferon-alfa is started has been shown to reduce the incidence of depression (Musselman et al. 2001). Brain metastases are always a consideration in advanced disease.

Head and Neck Cancers

Head and neck cancers carry the risks of facial deformity and loss of speech. These tumors are most frequent in patients with a history of alcohol abuse and smoking. Treatment is daunting and leads to mucositis, pain, dysphagia, and dry mouth or sticky saliva, all of which make eating difficult. Feeding tubes and tracheotomies are often necessary (List et al. 1997). Hypothyroidism is common following radiation treatment to the neck (Mercado et al. 2001). Because these tumors are more common among isolated men with a history of substance abuse, the risk of suicide has been thought to be high, but one study suggested that the rate of suicide remains low (Henderson and Ord 1997).

Pancreatic Cancer

Depression, anxiety, restlessness, and insomnia have been thought to be common first signs of pancreatic cancer, before physical signs appear, and physicians have wondered whether pancreatic hormones or neuropeptides might be responsible (Alter 1996; Fras et al. 1967; Green and Austin 1993; Joffe et al. 1986; Krech and Walsh 1991). One clinical study reported that depressive thoughts were more common in people with pancreatic cancer than in those with gastric cancer (Holland et al. 1986), and a recent epidemiological study found that depression preceded pancreatic cancer more often than other GI malignancies (odds ratio 4.6) (Carney et al. 2003). In a depressed patient, clues to the diagnosis of pancreatic cancer include abdominal symptoms and weight loss out of proportion to the degree of psychological symptoms. However, the symptoms of pancreatic cancer are typically vague and nonspecific. Symptoms of upper abdominal disease occur in 25% of patients 6 months before diagnosis. Anorexia, early satiety, and back pain are features of progressive disease.

Diabetes may also be present (DiMagno 1999). One study of 130 patients presenting with pancreatic cancer found 38% had scores above 15 on the Beck Depression Inventory. Depression was more common in those who had pain (Kelsen et al. 1995).

Following diagnosis, patients come to surgical evaluation, but few have surgically treatable disease. Finding that the tumor is not resectable is an additional psychological blow. Management of pain and discomfort includes pancreatic enzymes to relieve the cramps of fat malabsorption, octreotide for diarrhea, prevention of constipation, narcotics, and sometimes celiac block, as well as antidepressants for depression.

Psychiatric Aspects of Cancer Treatments

Chemotherapy

The neuropsychiatric side effects of common chemotherapeutic agents are listed in Table 7–1. The effects of chemotherapy on cognition are under investigation, but there are no definitive findings thus far (Phillips and Bernhard 2003). For the most part, there are no significant clinical interactions between cancer drugs and antidepressant medications, antipsychotic medications, and benzodiazepines. Procarbazine, a weak monoamine oxidase (MAO) inhibitor, is an exception. Alcohol may lead to an Antabuse-like reaction, and antidepressant medications should be prescribed only with consideration of possible MAO inhibition in mind.

Radiation

Radiation treatment usually requires a patient to remain absolutely still on a flat table for 5–10 minutes daily, 5 days a week, so that a prescribed dose can be applied to a specific site over 2–9 weeks. Patients worry that they cannot remain still either because of claustrophobia or because of inadequate pain control. Fatigue continues to increase during the month following radiation treatment but then begins to diminish. Nausea and vomiting from radiation treatment, more severe when viscera are irradiated, are reduced by serotonin 5-HT$_3$ antagonists like ondansetron. Brain irradiation causes more profound fatigue than treatment of other sites. Concomitant dexamethasone reduces cerebral edema, but late sequelae of brain radiation may occur, including radiation necrosis in focal areas or leukoencephalopathy. Newer methods to reduce the volume of brain that requires radiation may reduce these risks.

Bone Marrow Transplantation

Bone marrow transplantation (BMT) is used to treat acute and chronic leukemia, aplastic anemia, lymphomas, some solid tumors, and immunological deficiency states. There is no correlation between type of transplant and psychological morbidity (Leigh et al. 1995). In a prospective longitudinal cohort study of 319 adults (94 completed 5-year follow-up) who had myeloablative hematopoietic cell transplantation, 22% of patients had symptoms of clinical depression and 31% had mild depression. The authors reported that higher levels of depression, lower levels of physical function, and less satisfaction with social support before transplantation increased the risk of impaired physical and emotional recovery post transplant (Syrjala et al. 2004).

The psychological stress of BMT begins when transplant is first considered. It offers a chance of cure but carries significant risk of morbidity and mortality. In one study of BMT candidates, one-third reported depression (Baker et al. 1997); in another study, two-thirds reported a high level of anxiety (Keogh et al. 1998).

An important part of the pretransplant planning is to evaluate and shore up the patient's social support. Parents making this decision for a child may show depressive symptoms pretransplant and develop mental and physical exhaustion as the process continues (Pot-Mees and Zeitlin 1987). Some family members have alterations in immune status at various phases of the transplant (Futterman et al. 1996) and overall report distress similar to that of patients (Siston et al. 2001). In one prospective longitudinal study of 101 adults who underwent BMT, which included pretransplant data, the greatest emotional distress occurred after hospital admission and prior to bone marrow infusion. The authors concluded that perceived personal control may be a potential indicator of vulnerability to secondary psychosocial morbidity (Fife et al. 2000).

During high-dose chemotherapy and irradiation, visitors are limited to avoid infection. Patients often experience nausea, vomiting, and fatigue. During this time, psychiatric disorders are extremely common, especially adjustment disorder with anxiety and depression. In a study of 220 patients that included a psychiatric assessment on admission and weekly thereafter until discharge or death, higher psychiatric morbidity was associated with longer length of stay for transplant. The prevalence of psychiatric disorders was 44.1%; nearly 23% had an adjustment disorder, 14% had a mood disorder (mostly major depression), 8% had an anxiety disorder, and 7.3% had delirium (Prieto et al. 2002). Graft-versus-host disease is not generally associated with occurrence of mental disorders (Sasaki et al. 2000), although when severe, it may result in delirium.

The transplant itself (a brief intravenous infusion of several packets of concentrated bone marrow) is anticlimactic compared to the pretransplant regimen and the anxious recovery period waiting for platelet and red and white blood cell counts to "come back," the evidence of hematological recovery. Hypervigilant patients keep charts of their cell counts, anticipating the day of "probable" recovery; others request medications to "sleep through the experience," a passive attitude antithetical to caregivers who want the patient to participate in self-care. In one study, half of the adult patients ($N=90$) who underwent hematopoietic stem cell transplantation had an episode of delirium during the 4-week posttransplantation period (Fann et al. 2002).

After a prolonged period of dependence, patients are often very fearful as they anticipate hospital discharge and must assume greater roles in self-care. Persistent fatigue is a major problem when patients resume normal activities at home and work (Hann et al. 1997). Chronic anxiety and depression are the most common psychiatric sequelae, and psychological adjustment is particularly difficult for those patients who have delayed or disrupted important developmental life tasks.

In general, successful adaptation to BMT is associated with the ability to use information about illness and treatment, coupled with the ability to delegate control and authority temporarily and to trust the staff (Lesko and Holland 1998). A study of adults undergoing allogeneic BMT for acute leukemia found three variables affected outcome: illness status, presence of depressed mood, and the extent of perceived social support (Colon et al. 1991). Depressed mood pretransplant is associated with poorer survival (Colon et al. 1991; Loberiza et al. 2002), perhaps suggesting the potential benefit of early psychiatric intervention.

Long-term survivors of BMT for acute leukemia show no difference in psychological and social functioning than those who received standard chemotherapy (Wellisch et al. 1996). A decrease in sexual frequency

and satisfaction is seen in women (Mumma et al. 1992).

Bone marrow transplant recipients are at increased risk for developing CNS toxicity such as neuropsychological impairment, including compromised motor and cognitive test performance (Tschuschke et al. 2001). In a study of 40 progression-free, long-term adult survivors (>2 years) of BMT, mild to moderate cognitive impairment was found in 60% of patients (Harder et al. 2002).

Surgery

See Chapter 13, "Surgery," for a full discussion of the emotional aspects of surgery.

Psychiatric Interventions in Cancer

Psychotherapy

Psychotherapy can often help patients to accept the diagnosis of cancer; sort out treatment options; overcome fear, depression, or denial; and enhance patients' ability to cope with cancer treatment (Weisman 1979). Suffering is intensified by lack of meaning, and some interventions for cancer patients have focused on the maintenance of morale and the search for meaning (Frankl 1946; Greenstein and Breitbart 2000; Weisman 1993). Chochinov (2002) has developed methods to support patients' desire for dignity at the end of life.

Psychosocial interventions can reduce distress, facilitate problem-solving strategies, and augment a sense of control. Cognitive and behavioral models can be tailored to the specific tumor type. Educational and behavioral training, in either group or individual psychotherapy, are the best-documented approaches to reducing distress in cancer patients (Fawzy et al. 1995; Newell et al. 2002).

Group therapy and self-help groups allow cancer patients to receive support from others who are coping with similar problems. In a group setting, patients can glean practical tips and see the range of normal reactions to illness, as well as adaptive coping styles and strategies that make adjustment to illness easier. Group therapy helps to decrease the sense of isolation and alienation as the patient and family see that they are not alone adjusting to illness. Groups are often disease specific or targeted for patients at the same stage of illness. Past concerns about having dying patients in a group with those recently diagnosed or whose prognosis was good have been dispelled.

Spiegel et al. (1989) developed supportive expressive group psychotherapy led by trained professionals for women with breast cancer. The goal of supportive-expressive psychotherapy is to help patients with existential concerns and disease-related emotions as well as to deepen social support and physician relationships and provide symptom control. The therapist challenges patients' tendency to withdraw from the implications of having metastatic breast cancer. Such groups relieve distress while reducing avoidance of the implications of the diagnosis. This strategy improves mood and pain perception, especially in the most distressed (Goodwin et al. 2001).

Studies of psychosocial interventions in hopes of prolonging survival have had a mixed outcome. Spiegel and colleagues' report of greater longevity in a small number of women with advanced breast cancer undergoing group supportive-expressive psychotherapy was not replicated in larger studies (Goodwin et al. 2001; Spiegel et al. 1989). Fawzy and colleagues' study of a structured psychoeducational intervention for patients with early-stage melanoma showed a modest survival benefit at 6 years that weakened at 10-year follow-up (Fawzy

et al. 1993, 2003). Patients can be told that group support contributes to living better, not necessarily longer.

Psychopharmacology

Patients commonly ask whether psychiatric drugs increase cancer risk or render antineoplastics ineffective. There is no evidence for either belief (Steingart and Cotterchio 1995; Theoharides and Konstantinidou 2003).

Depression

The selective serotonin reuptake inhibitors (SSRIs) are the first-line antidepressants prescribed in cancer settings because they are effective, have few sedative and autonomic side effects, and have few drug interactions. A small minority of cancer patients experience transient weight loss when starting an SSRI; however, weight usually returns to baseline level, and the anorectic properties of these drugs are usually not a limiting factor in those with cancer anorexia–cachexia. Ondansetron can be used to block initial serotonin-mediated nausea. Antidepressants like mirtazapine that can cause weight gain may be advantageous in anorexic–cachectic cancer patients but are not a good choice in those who are gaining weight from steroids or from chemotherapy (Theobald et al. 2002). If recurrent periods of inability to eat and drink tend to interrupt the antidepressant regimen, then fluoxetine, with its longer half-life, has an advantage. The SSRIs and venlafaxine reduce both the number and the intensity of hot flashes and night sweats in nondepressed women who become menopausal after chemotherapy for breast cancer or who have a recurrence of vasomotor symptoms when they discontinue hormone replacement therapy (Duffy et al. 1999; Loberiza et al. 2002; Stearns et al. 2000; Weitzner et al. 2002). Hot flashes are also an issue for men on androgen deprivation treatment regimens.

Bupropion's stimulating properties make it useful in lethargic patients, but because of its association with increased seizure risk, it should be used with caution in patients who are malnourished or who have a history of seizures or brain tumor. Bupropion may assist in smoking cessation, especially in patients with lung or head and neck cancers.

The tricyclic antidepressants (TCAs) are used to treat both depression and the neuropathic pain syndromes caused by chemotherapy and surgery. Nortriptyline and desipramine have more favorable side-effect profiles compared with amitriptyline, with fewer anticholinergic symptoms.

Psychostimulants (i.e., dextroamphetamine and methylphenidate) can promote a sense of well-being, treat depression, decrease fatigue, stimulate appetite, and improve cognitive function. Psychostimulants are used as an adjuvant to potentiate the analgesic effects of opioid analgesics and are commonly used to counteract opioid-induced sedation (Rozans et al. 2002). Psychostimulants offer clear benefits, especially in terminally ill patients, because there may be an improvement in symptoms within hours to days.

In patients with primary bipolar disorder, mood stabilizers and neuroleptics can be continued. Lithium tends to increase the patient's white blood count and usually can be continued during cancer treatment. However, complications of chemotherapy, including vomiting, diarrhea, dehydration, and renal insufficiency, may raise lithium levels, and symptoms of toxicity, nausea, diarrhea, and confusion may be misattributed to chemotherapy.

Anxiety

Prior to treatment with a benzodiazepine, all patients should be screened for depressive symptoms as well as for specific anxiety disorders such as PTSD and obsessive-compulsive disorder. When anxiety is a manifestation of a primary depressive disorder, treatment should be an antidepressant with, or instead of, a benzodiazepine. The experience of cancer treatment may reawaken problems in patients who were the victims of earlier traumas, increasing their risk of anxiety and depressive symptoms (Baider et al. 2000).

Benzodiazepines are frequently given to patients for acute anxiety and are often prescribed to augment antiemetics during chemotherapy. Dosing depends on the patient's tolerance and the drug's duration of action. Lorazepam and alprazolam are favored in the acute setting because of their rapid onset of action and benefit on an "as-needed" basis. Buspirone and antidepressants are alternatives for longer treatment of anxiety. Low doses of neuroleptics are useful in patients who are unresponsive to or intolerant of benzodiazepines or in patients with severe anxiety and agitation. If patients have been taking a benzodiazepine chronically, they may suffer withdrawal if the dose is not tapered.

Electroconvulsive Therapy

Although the use of electroconvulsive therapy (ECT) in patients with brain tumor was once believed to be contraindicated because of the risk of brain herniation, there are numerous case reports describing safe and effective use of ECT in such patients (Patkar et al. 2000).

Survivor Issues

Advances in cancer treatment over the past 30 years have led to a rapidly growing population of long-term survivors, many of them children and young adults. The long-term adjustment of many appears to be largely unimpaired (Kornblith et al. 2004). Some cured cancer patients have delayed medical complications (i.e., organ failure, CNS dysfunction, sterility, secondary malignancies, and decreased physical stamina) and psychiatric concerns, including fears of termination of treatment; preoccupation with the threat of disease recurrence and a sense of greater vulnerability to illness; pervasive awareness of mortality and difficulty with reentry into normal life; persistent guilt (the survivor syndrome); difficult adjustment to physical losses and handicaps that lead to problems with peer acceptance and social integration; diminished self-esteem or confidence; perceived loss of job mobility; and fear of job and insurance discrimination. The survivor's intellectual functioning is also a major concern. Children and adults with brain tumors or CNS involvement, and those undergoing bone marrow transplant, are at risk from both the disease and the treatment. Most have residual deficits, with neuropsychological impairment including compromised motor and cognitive test performance (Anderson et al. 2001; Bhatia 2003; Phipps et al. 2000).

Complementary and Alternative Medicine

Some 80% of cancer patients use complementary and alternative medicine (CAM) treatments. Some alternative treatments (acupuncture; relaxation; yoga; meditation; massage; tai chi; biofeedback; music, art, movement, and aroma therapies) are offered as adjuncts to traditional cancer care aimed at increasing quality of life and decreasing symptoms with no promise of cure. Other therapies such as shark cartilage, colonics, herbal remedies, and high-dose vitamin therapies do not improve quality of life and may be harmful. Some remedies are highly toxic (Markman 2002). Laetrile, now banned in the United States, contains cyanide; chaparral tea causes liver damage; Ma huang contains ephedrine, a CNS stimulant. No CAM technique or preparation has been demonstrated to cause tumor regression.

A study of women with newly diagnosed early-stage breast cancer found that 28% used alternative medicine (Burstein et al. 1999). Interestingly, the use of alternative medicine was independently associated with depression, fear of recurrence of cancer, lower scores for mental health and sexual satisfaction, and more physical symptoms, suggesting that those who seek alternative medicine therapies may be experiencing more anxiety, depression, or physical symptoms. Those taking alternative medications may be more in need of but less open to psychiatric consultation.

Most patients who elect to use untried or unproven therapies do so in a desperate search for a cure or for a more acceptable quality of life. The clinician has to find a balance between condoning unproven or harmful treatment and preserving the patient's hope.

References

Alter C: Palliative and supportive care in patients with pancreatic cancer. Sem Oncol 23:229–240, 1996

Anderson DM, Rennie KM, Ziegler RS, et al: Medical and neurocognitive late effects among survivors of childhood center nervous system tumors. Cancer 92:2709–2719, 2001

Andrykowski MA: The role of anxiety in the development of anticipatory nausea in cancer chemotherapy: a review and synthesis. Psychosom Med 52:458–475, 1990

Ayres A, Hoon PW, Franzoni JB, et al: Influence of mood and adjustment to cancer on compliance with chemotherapy among breast cancer patients. J Psychosom Res 38:393–402, 1994

Baider L, Peretz R, Hadani Pe, et al: Transmission of response to trauma? Second-generation Holocaust survivors' reaction to cancer. Am J Psychiatry 157:904–910, 2000

Baker F, Marcellus D, Zabora J, et al: Psychological distress among adult patients being evaluated for bone marrow transplantation. Psychosomatics 38:10–19, 1997

Bernhard J, Hurny C, Maibach R, et al: Quality of life as subjective experience: reframing of perception in patients with colon cancer undergoing radical resection with or without adjuvant chemotherapy. Ann Oncol 10:775–782, 1999

Bhatia S: Late effects among survivors of leukemia during childhood and adolescence. Blood Cells Mol Dis 31:84–92, 2003

Boyle P, Ferlay J: Cancer incidence and mortality in Europe, 2004. Ann Oncol 16:481–488, 2005

Brown TM, Stoudemire A: Antineoplastic agents, in Psychiatric Side Effects of Prescription and Over-the-Counter Medications. Edited by Brown TM, Stoudemire A. Washington DC, American Psychiatric Press, 1998, pp 239–261

Burstein HJ, Gelber S, Guadagnoli E, et al: Use of alternative medicine by women with early stage breast cancer. N Engl J Med 340:1733–1739, 1999

Carney CP, Jones L, Woolson RF, et al: Relationship between depression and pancreatic cancer in the general population. Psychosom Med 65:884–888, 2003

Chochinov HM: Dignity-conserving care—a new model for palliative care: helping the patient feel valued. JAMA 287: 2253–2260, 2002

Colon EA, Callier AL, Popkin MJ, et al: Depressed mood and other variables related to bone marrow transplantation survival in acute leukemia. Psychosomatics 32:420–425, 1991

Cordova MJ, Andrykowski MA, Kenady DE, et al: Frequency and correlates of posttraumatic-stress-disorder-like symptoms after treatment for breast cancer. J Consult Clin Psychol 63:981–986, 1995

DiMagno EP: Pancreatic cancer: clinical presentation, pitfalls and early clues. Ann Oncol 4:S140–S142, 1999

Duffy LS, Greenberg DB, Younger J, et al: Iatrogenic acute estrogen deficiency and psychiatric syndromes in breast cancer patients. Psychosomatics 40:304–308, 1999

Faller H, Bülzebruck H: Coping and survival in lung cancer: a 10-year follow-up. Am J Psychiatry 159:2105–2107, 2002

Fann JR, Roth-Roemer S, Burington BE, et al: Delirium in patients undergoing hematopoietic stem cell transplantation. Cancer 95:1971–1981, 2002

Fawzy FI, Fawzy N, Hun CS, et al: Malignant melanoma: effects of an early structured psychiatric intervention, coping and affective state on recurrence and survival 6 years later. Arch Gen Psychiatry 50:681–689, 1993

Fawzy FI, Fawzy NW, Arndt LA, et al: Critical review of psycho-social interventions in cancer care. Arch Gen Psychiatry 52:100–113, 1995

Fawzy FI, Canada AL, Fawzy NW: Effects of a brief, structured psychiatric intervention on survival and recurrence at 10-year follow-up. Arch Gen Psychiatry 60:100–103, 2003

Fertig DL, Hayes DF: Psychological responses to tumor markers, in Psycho-oncology. Edited by Holland, JC. New York, Oxford University Press, 1998, pp 1147–1160

Fife BL, Huster GA, Cornetta KG, et al: Longitudinal study of adaptation to the stress of bone marrow transplantation. J Clin Oncol 18:1539–1549, 2000

Fleishman S, Lesko L, Breitbart WS: Treatment of organic mental disorders in cancer patients, in Psychiatric Aspects of Symptom Management in Cancer Patients. Edited by Breitbart WS, Holland JC. Washington DC, American Psychiatric Press, 1993, pp 23–47

Fox BH, Stanek EJ III, Boldy SC, et al: Suicide rates among cancer patients in Connecticut. J Chronic Dis 35:85–100, 1982

Frankl V: Man's Search for Meaning. Boston, MA, Beacon, 1946

Fras I, Litin EM, Pearson JS: Comparison of psychiatric symptoms in carcinoma of the pancreas with those in some other intra-abdominal neoplasms. Am J Psychiatry 123:1553–1562, 1967

Futterman AD, Wellisch DK, Zighelboim J, et al: Psychological and immunological reactions of family members to patients undergoing bone marrow transplantation. Psychom Med 58:472–480, 1996

Ganz PA, Coscarelli A, Fred C, et al: Breast cancer survivors: Psychosocial concerns and quality of life. Breast Cancer Res Treat 38:183–199, 1996

Ginsburg ML, Quirt C, Ginsburg AD, et al: Psychiatric illness and psychological concerns of patients with newly diagnosed lung cancer. CMAJ 1:152:701–708, 1995

Glover J, Dibble SL, Dood MJ, et al: Mood states of oncology outpatients: does pain make a difference? J Pain Symptom Manage 10:120–128, 1995

Goodwin PJ, Leszcz M, Ennis M, et al: The effects of group psychosocial support on survival in metastatic breast cancer. N Engl J Med 345:1719–1726, 2001

Green AI, Austin CP: Psychopathology of pancreatic cancer. A psychobiological probe (review). Psychosomatics 34:208–221, 1993

Green BL, Rowland JH, Krupnick JL, et al: Prevalence of posttraumatic stress disorder in women with breast cancer. Psychosomatics 39:102–111, 1998

Greenberg DB: Barriers to the treatment of depression in cancer patients. J Natl Cancer Inst Monogr 32:127–135, 2004

Greenberg DB, Kornblith AB, Herndon JE, et al: Quality of life of adult leukemia survivors treated on clinical trials of the Cancer and Leukemia Group B from 1971–1988: predictors for later psychological distress. Cancer 80:1936–1944, 1997

Greenberg DB, Jonasch E, Gadd MA, et al: Adjuvant therapy of melanoma with interferon alpha 2b associated with mania and bipolar syndromes. Cancer 89:356–362, 2000

Greenstein M, Breitbart WS: Cancer and the experience of meaning: a group psychotherapy program for people with cancer. Am J Psychother 54:486–500, 2000

Hann DM, Jacobsen PB, Martin SC, et al: Fatigue in women treated with bone marrow transplantation for breast cancer: a comparison with women with no history of cancer. Support Care Cancer 5:44–52, 1997

Harder H, Cornelissen JJ, Van Gool AR, et al: Cognitive functioning and quality of life in long-term adult survivors of bone marrow transplantation. Cancer 95:183–192, 2002

Harlan L, Brawley O, Pommerenke F, et al: Geographic, age, and racial variation in the treatment of local/regional carcinoma of the prostate. J Clin Oncol 13:93–100, 1995

Henderson JM, Ord RA: Suicide in head and neck cancer patients. J Oral Maxillofac Surg 55:1217–1221; (discussion) 1221–1222, 1997

Hickok JT, Roscoe JA, Morrow GR, et al: Nausea and emesis remain significant problems of chemotherapy despite prophylaxis with 5-hydroxytryptamine-3 antiemetics. Cancer 97:2880–2886, 2003

Holland JC, Korzun AH, Tross S, et al: Comparative psychological disturbance in patients with pancreatic and gastric cancer. Am J Psychiatry 143:982–986, 1986

Ingram D, Browne G, Reyno L, et al: Prevalence, correlates and cost of anxiety and affective disorder in men with prostate cancer one year after initial assessment (abstract #523). Psychooncology 12:S1–S277, 2003

Inui A: Cancer Anorexia-cachexia syndrome. CA Cancer J Clin 52:72–91, 2002

Jacobsen PB, Widows MR, Hann DM, et al: Posttraumatic stress disorder symptoms after bone marrow transplantation for breast cancer. Psychosom Med 62:366–371, 1998

Joffe RT, Rubinow DR, Denicoff KD, et al: Depression and carcinoma of the pancreas. Gen Hosp Psychiatry 8:241–245, 1986

Kelsen DP, Portenoy RK, Thaler HT, et al: Pain and depression in patients with newly diagnosed pancreas cancer. J Clin Oncol 13:748–755, 1995

Keogh F, O'Riordan J, McNamara C, et al: Psychosocial adaptation of patients and families following bone marrow transplantation: a prospective, longitudinal study. Bone Marrow Transplant 22:905–911, 1998

Kirkwood JM, Bender C, Agarwala S, et al: Mechanisms and management of toxicities associated with high-dose interferon alfa-2b therapy. J Clin Oncol 20:3703–3718, 2002

Kornblith AB, Herr HW, Ofman US, et al: Quality of life of patients with prostate cancer and their spouses. The value of a database in clinical care. Cancer 73:2791–2802, 1994

Kornblith AB, Thaler HT, Wong G, et al: Quality of life of women with ovarian cancer. Gynecol Oncol 59:231–242, 1995

Kornblith AB, Herndon JE II, Weiss RB, et al: Long-term adjustment of survivors of early stage breast carcinoma, 20 years after adjuvant chemotherapy. Cancer 98:679–689, 2004

Krech RL, Walsh D: Symptoms of pancreatic cancer. J Pain Symptom Manage 6:360–367, 1991

Kung S, Mueller PS, Yonas EG, et al: Delirium resulting from paraneoplastic limbic encephalitis caused by Hodgkin's disease. Psychosomatics 43:498–501, 2002

Lee MA, Ganzini L: Depression in the elderly: effect on patient attitudes toward life-sustaining therapy. J Am Geriatr Soc 40:983–988, 1992

Leigh S, Wilson KC, Burns R, et al: Psychosocial morbidity in bone marrow transplant recipients: a prospective study. Bone Marrow Transplant 16:635–640, 1995

Lesko LM, Holland JC: Psychosocial issues in patients with hematological malignancies, in Supportive Care in Cancer Patients (Vol. 108 in Recent Results in Cancer Research series). Edited by Senn HJ, Claus A, Schmid L. Berlin, Germany, Springer-Verlag, 1998, pp 109–243

Levenson JL, McDonald MK: The role of psychological factors in cancer onset and progression: a critical appraisal, in The Psychoimmunology of Cancer, 2nd Edition. Edited by Lewis CE, O'Brien R, Barraclough J. New York, Oxford University Press, 2002, pp 149–163

Lieberman FS, Schold SC: Distant effects of cancer on the nervous system. Oncology 16:1539–1548, 2002

List MA, Mumby P, Haraf D, et al: Performance and quality of life outcome in patients completing concomitant chemoradiotherapy protocols for head and neck cancer. Qual Life Res 6:274–284, 1997

Litwin MS, Lubeck DP, Spitalny GM, et al: Mental health in men treated for early stage prostate carcinoma. Cancer 95:54–60, 2002

Loberiza FR Jr, Rizzo JD, Bredeson CN, et al: Association of depressive syndrome and early deaths among patients after stem-cell transplantation for malignant diseases. J Clin Oncol 20:2118–2126, 2002

Louhivuori KA, Hakama M: Risk of suicide among cancer patients. Am J Epidemiol 109:59–65, 1979

Markman M: Safety issues in using complementary and alterative medicine. J Clin Oncol 20:S39–S41, 2002

Massie MJ: Prevalence of depression in patients with cancer. J Natl Cancer Inst Monogr 32:57–71, 2004

Massie MJ, Popkin M: Depressive disorders, in Psycho-Oncology. Edited by Holland JC. New York, Oxford University Press, 1998, pp 518–540

McCarthy EP, Phillips RS, Zhong Z, et al: Dying with cancer: patients' function, symptoms, and care preferences as death approaches. J Am Geriatr Soc 48:S110-S121, 2000

Mercado G, Adelstein DJ, Saxton JP, et al: Hypothyroidism, a frequent event after radiotherapy and after radiotherapy with chemotherapy for patients with head and neck carcinoma. Cancer 92:2892–2897, 2001

Mumma GH, Mashberg D, Lesko LM: Long-term psychosexual adjustment of acute leukemia survivors: impact of marrow transplantation versus conventional chemotherapy. Gen Hosp Psychiatry 14:43–55, 1992

Musselman DL, Lawson DH, Gumnick JF, et al: Paroxetine for the prevention of depression induced by high-dose interferon alfa. N Engl J Med 344:961–966, 2001

Newell SA, Sanson-Fisher RW, Savolainen NJ: Systematic review of psychological therapies for cancer patients: overview and recommendations for future research. J Natl Cancer Inst 94:558–584, 2002

Newport DJ, Nemeroff CB: Assessment and treatment of depression in the cancer patient. J Psychosom Res 45:215–237, 1998

Nuland SB: How We Die: Reflections on Life's Final Chapter. New York, Knopf, 1994

Passik SD, Dugan W, McDonald MV, et al: Oncologists' recognition of depression in their patients with cancer. J Clin Oncol 16:1594–1600, 1998

Patkar AA, Hill KP, Weinstein SP, et al: ECT in the presence of brain tumor and increased intracranial pressure: evaluation and reduction of risk. J ECT 16:189–197, 2000

Payne DK, Biggs C, Tran KN, et al: Women's regrets after bilateral prophylactic mastectomy. Ann Surg Oncol 7:150–154, 2000

Phillips K-A, Bernhard J: Adjuvant breast cancer treatment and cognitive function: current knowledge and research directions. J Natl Cancer Inst 95:190–197, 2003

Phipps S, Dunavant M, Srivastava DK, et al: Cognitive and academic functioning in survivors of pediatric bone marrow transplantation. J Clin Oncol 18:1004–1011, 2000

Pirl WF, Siegel GI, Goode MJ, et al: Depression in men receiving androgen deprivation therapy for prostate cancer: a pilot study. Psychooncology 11:518–523, 2002

Pot-Mees CC, Zeitlin H: Psychosocial consequences of bone marrow transplantation in children: a preliminary communication. Journal of Psychosocial Oncology 5:73–78, 1987

Prieto JM, Blanch J, Atala J, et al: Psychiatric morbidity and impact on hospital length of stay among hematologic cancer patients receiving stem-cell transplantation. J Clin Oncol 20:1907–1917, 2002

Ramsey SD, Berry K, Moinpour C, et al: Quality of life in long term survivors of colorectal cancer. Am J Gastroenterol 97:1228–1234, 2002

Robson ME, Offit K: Considerations in genetic counseling for inherited breast cancer predisposition. Semin Radiat Oncol 12:362–370, 2002

Robson ME, Boyd J, Borgen PI, et al: Hereditary breast cancer. Curr Probl Surg 38:377–480, 2001

Roth A, Passik SD: Anxiety in men with prostate cancer may interfere with effective management of the disease. Primary Care and Cancer 16:30, 1996

Rowland JR, Massie MJ: Psychosocial issues and interventions, in Diseases of the Breast, 3rd Edition. Edited by Harris JR, Lippman ME, Morrow M, et al. Philadelphia, PA, Lippincott Williams & Wilkens, 2004, pp 1419–1452

Rozans M, Dreisbach A, Lertora JJ, et al: Palliative uses of methylphenidate in patients with cancer: a review. J Clin Oncol 20:335–339, 2002

Sahay TB, Gray RE, Fitch M: A qualitative study of patient perspectives on colorectal cancer. Cancer Pract 8:38–44, 2000

Sanderson L, Patten CH, Ebbert JO: Tobacco use outcomes among patients with lung cancer treated for nicotine dependence. J Clin Oncol 20:3461–3469, 2002

Sarna L, Padilla G, Holmes C, et al: Quality of life of long-term survivors on non-small-cell lung cancer. J Clin Oncol 20: 2920–2929, 2002

Sasaki T, Akaho R, Sakamaki H, et al: Mental disturbances during isolation in bone marrow transplant patients with leukemia. Bone Marrow Transplant 25:315–318, 2000

Schover LR: Sexuality and Fertility After Cancer. New York, Wiley, 1997

Siston AK, List MA, Daugherty CK, et al: Psychosocial adjustment of (40) patients and (39) caregivers prior to allogenic bone marrow transplant. Bone Marrow Transplant 27:1181–1188, 2001

Spiegel D, Bloom JR, Kramer HJC, et al: Effect of psychosocial treatment on survival of patients with metastatic breast cancer. Lancet 14:88–89, 1989

Stark D, Kiely M, Smith A, et al: Anxiety disorders in cancer patients: their nature, associations, and relation to quality of life. J Clin Oncol 20:3137–3148, 2002

Stearns V, Isaacs C, Rowland J, et al: A pilot trial assessing the efficacy of paroxetine hydrochloride (Paxil) in controlling hot flashes in breast cancer survivors. Ann Oncol 11:17–22, 2000

Steingart AB, Cotterchio M: Do antidepressants cause, promote, or inhibit cancers. J Clin Epidemiol 48:1407–1412, 1995

Syrjala KL, Langer SL, Abrams JR, et al: Recovery and long-term function after hematopoietic cell transplantation for leukemia and lymphoma. JAMA 291:2335–2343, 2004

Theobald DE, Kirsh KL, Holtsclas E, et al: An open-label, crossover trial of mirtazapine (15 and 30 mg) in cancer patients with pain and other distressing symptoms. J Pain Symptom Manage 23:7–8, 2002

Theoharides T, Konstantinidou A: Antidepressants and risk of cancer: a case of misguided associations and priorities. J Clin Psychopharmacol 23:1–4, 2003

Tschuschke V, Hertenstein B, Arnold R, et al: Associations between coping and survival time of adult leukemia patients receiving allogeneic bone arrow transplantation: results of a prospective study. J Psychosom Res 50:277–285, 2001

Watson M, Haviland JS, Greer S, et al: Influence of psychological response on survival in breast cancer: a population-based cohort study. Lancet 354:1331–1336, 1999

Wei JT, Dunn RL, Sandler HM, et al: Comprehensive comparison of health related quality of life after contemporary therapies for localized prostate cancer. J Clin Oncol 20: 557–566, 2002

Weisman AD: Coping with Cancer. New York, McGraw-Hill, 1979

Weisman AD: Vulnerable Self. New York, Plenum, 1993

Weitzner MA, Moncello J, Jacobsen PB, et al: A pilot trial of paroxetine for the treatment of hot flashes and associated symptoms in women with breast cancer. J Pain Symptom Manage 23:337–345, 2002

Wellisch DK, Centeno J, Guzman J, et al: Bone marrow transplantation vs. high-dose cytarabine-based consolidation chemotherapy for acute myelogenous leukemia. A long-term follow-up study of quality of life measures of survivors. Psychosomatics 37:144–154, 1996

Self-Assessment Questions

Select the single best response for each question.

1. Many research groups have assessed depression in cancer patients. Cancer types highly associated with depression include all of the following *except*

   A. Breast cancer.
   B. Lymphoma.
   C. Lung cancer.
   D. Oropharyngeal cancer.
   E. Pancreatic cancer.

2. An increased risk of suicide in cancer patients is associated with all of the following *except*

   A. Advanced stage of disease.
   B. Inadequately controlled pain.
   C. Social isolation.
   D. Female gender.
   E. History of psychiatric illness.

3. Common causes of cancer-related fatigue include which of the following cancer treatments?

   A. Interferon.
   B. Chemotherapy.
   C. Irradiation.
   D. All of the above.
   E. None of the above.

4. In general, which of the following variables is associated with *less* mental distress in men with prostate cancer?

   A. More serious disease.
   B. Undergoing radiation treatment.
   C. Younger age.
   D. Undergoing surgery.
   E. None of the above.

5. Neuropsychiatric side effects of chemotherapeutic agents are common and need to be addressed by the clinician. Which of the following is associated with the triad of depression, fatigue, and encephalopathy:

   A. Cisplatin.
   B. 5-Fluorouacil.
   C. Taxanes.
   D. Thalidomide.
   E. Vincristine.

8 Rheumatology

Chris Dickens, M.B.B.S., Ph.D.

James L. Levenson, M.D.

Wendy Cohen, M.D.

IN THE FOLLOWING chapter, we describe aspects of the rheumatological disorders that are likely to be relevant to a clinician working in the field of psychosomatic medicine. Most of the chapter is devoted to rheumatoid arthritis (RA) and systemic lupus erythematosus (SLE), because these disorders are likely to be encountered most commonly; other disorders, including osteoarthritis, Sjögren's syndrome, systemic sclerosis, temporal arteritis, polymyositis, polyarteritis nodosa, and Behçet's disease, are mentioned briefly. Issues relating to psychiatric problems resulting from treatments are dealt with at the end of the chapter.

General Principles of Diagnosis and Assessment

Detecting CNS Involvement in Rheumatological Disorders

Mental Status Examination and Neuropsychological Testing

The mental status examination is the most sensitive, most available, and least expensive tool for detecting and tracking neuropsychiatric status in rheumatological disorders. Neuropsychological testing provides a more detailed, sensitive assessment of cognitive function, but it is not specific.

Laboratory Tests

Laboratory studies help rule out infection and confirm the presence of rheumatological disease activity. High disease activity increases the likelihood of primary central nervous system (CNS) involvement, because the pathogenesis is shared; however, the absence of systemic disease activity does not preclude CNS involvement.

When rheumatology patients have neuropsychiatric symptoms, lumbar puncture is indicated to rule out CNS infection and assess the degree of disease activity in the CNS. In patients without CNS infection, cerebrospinal fluid (CSF) pleocytosis and increased CSF protein are suggestive of CNS involvement by lupus or other rheumatological disease (West 1994). In addition, CSF studies should include oligoclonal bands, which are present in only a small number of disorders, including neurosyphilis, Lyme disease, multiple sclerosis, Sjögren's syndrome, and CNS SLE.

Electroencephalogram

In patients with rheumatological disorders who also have neuropsychiatric symptoms, the electroencephalogram (EEG) is often abnormal but seldom useful (Waterloo et al. 1999), except in diagnosing subclinical seizure activity or differentiating hypoactive delirium (diffuse slowing on EEG) from depression (normal EEG).

Neuroimaging

Although magnetic resonance imaging (MRI) is the best available imaging technique for identifying focal structural neurological lesions in patients with rheumatological disorders and neuropsychiatric symptoms, MRI is limited because it cannot reliably differentiate active from chronic lesions resulting from a previous neuropsychiatric insult (Sabbadini et al. 1999).

Detecting, Diagnosing, and Quantifying Psychiatric Symptoms and Disorders

Psychiatric disorders remain mostly unrecognized and undertreated in patients with rheumatological disorders due partly to a tendency to focus on the physical aspects of disease. This is exacerbated by a misconception that because depression is understandable, occurring secondary to the pain and disability, treatment of the depression is not necessary (Rifkin 1992). Furthermore, diagnosing depression in patients with rheumatological disorders is complicated because there is an overlap in symptoms of depression and rheumatological disorders (e.g., fatigue, weight loss, insomnia, and lack of appetite) (Rifkin 1992).

Scales that have little somatic content, such as the Geriatric Depression Scale (Sheikh and Yesavage 1989), the Hospital Anxiety and Depression Scale (HADS) (Zigmond and Snaith 1983), or disease-specific instruments (Smedstad et al. 1995) may aid accurate diagnosis of depression in such patients. These self-rated questionnaires may be used by rheumatologists or specialist nurses to identify probable cases of psychiatric disorder.

Complex cases will require more detailed assessment by a psychosomatic medicine specialist. In addition to assessing the patient's current mental state, the specialist psychiatrist should explore the development of psychiatric symptoms and how these relate to the recent disease state and to changes in management, availability of social support, psychosocial stresses resulting from pain and disability, and stresses independent of the illness. Inquiries about maladaptive coping strategies to physical symptoms (e.g., "I just lie down and wait for my symptoms to ease"; "I simply avoid activities that cause me pain") can identify fruitful targets for psychological interventions. Assessing past psychiatric history and family history will help identify which patients are most vulnerable to developing depression and other psychiatric disorders. Finally, investigating the patient's personal beliefs about the illness, such as the perceived causes, possible outcomes, and likelihood of controlling disease progression through treatment, can identify psychological mechanisms by which psychiatric problems have arisen.

General Principles of Treatment

Primary Neuropsychiatric Involvement

When rheumatological diseases affect the CNS, the primary treatment is *corticoster-*

oids when the pathophysiology is thought to be neuronal injury or inflammation resulting from autoantibodies, and *anticoagulants* when hypercoagulability is involved (e.g., the anticardiolipin antibody syndrome). When corticosteroids are ineffective, other immunosuppressive agents may be helpful.

Primary Psychiatric Disorders

Intervention studies have shown that psychological treatments, mostly cognitive and behavioral, are effective in reducing psychological distress and improving coping in subjects with rheumatological disorders (Bradley et al. 1987; Sharpe et al. 2001). Such therapies may also reduce pain and improve functioning, though it is unclear whether any of these effects are mediated by changes to the inflammatory state (Bradley et al. 1987; Sharpe et al. 2001).

In addition, there is a wide choice of antidepressants currently available to clinicians. Although the majority of these drugs have not undergone assessment of efficacy in patients with physical illness, current evidence from studies in psychiatric and other chronic pain patient populations indicates that antidepressants, when given in appropriate therapeutic doses, have roughly equal efficacy in the treatment of depression (Anderson et al. 2000). However, they do differ in their analgesic efficacy, tolerability, and profile of drug interactions.

Tricyclic antidepressants (TCAs) with the least specific receptor activity, such as amitriptyline, appear to have the greatest analgesic efficacy (Onghena and Van Houdenhove 1992), even at low doses (e.g., 25 mg of amitriptyline) and independent of whether depression is present or not (Bromm et al. 1986). In higher doses, tolerability and safety are poor, particularly in the elderly. Newer drugs have comparable antidepressant efficacy, al-

though their analgesic efficacy has yet to be established, and they are more expensive. In general, selective serotonin reuptake inhibitors (SSRIs), such as fluoxetine or citalopram, in doses up to recommended maxima, should be considered as first-line treatment for depression in RA (Anderson et al. 2000). Combined use of TCAs and SSRIs greatly increases the risk of adverse events and should be avoided unless under expert guidance. Drug interactions may occur, although this is not a problem with current first- and second-line treatments for RA.

Rheumatoid Arthritis

RA is a chronic disorder characterized by persistent inflammatory synovitis. The disease typically involves peripheral small joints in a symmetrical pattern. Inflammation of the synovium can result in destruction of joint cartilage and bony erosions, which can eventually result in destruction of the joint. Extra-articular manifestations are common, with some degree of extra-articular involvement being found in most patients. These extra-articular manifestations can involve the CNS.

Neuropsychiatric Disorders in Rheumatoid Arthritis

Epidemiology

Neuropsychiatric disorders are common in patients with RA, as they are in most chronic illness populations. Conservative figures, obtained by using standardized research interviews, indicate that about one-fifth of patients with RA have a psychiatric disorder. Using the Present State Examination, Murphy and colleagues (1988) interviewed a mixed group of inpatients and outpatients with definite or classic RA and found that 21% of subjects had a psychiatric disorder: 12.5% were depressed, and the remainder were anxious. This study also revealed that a population of RA patients of approximately equal size (19%) had psychiatric symptoms, although they did not meet the criteria for a psychiatric disorder. These prevalence figures are consistent with those from other studies that used standardized research interviews (Frank et al. 1988).

Etiology

Neuropsychiatric manifestations in RA can arise through four processes: 1) direct CNS involvement, 2) secondary effects of the illness or its treatments, 3) emotional reactions to chronic illness, and 4) comorbid primary psychiatric illness.

Involvement of the Central Nervous System in Rheumatoid Arthritis

Despite its multisystem manifestations, neurological complications in RA are not common. When present, the most common is peripheral neuropathy due to entrapment resulting from synovial proliferation or vasculitis. Direct involvement of the CNS is rare. Atlanto-axial subluxation may occur, resulting in transverse myelitis, and is the most widely recognized CNS complication of RA.

Vasculitis in RA can involve cerebral vessels, resulting in cerebral ischemia or infarction, and has been associated with acute and chronic brain syndromes (Ando et al. 1995). Treatment with corticosteroids can usually alleviate vasculitis and edema, with resultant improvement in symptoms, but impairment from the infarction is permanent.

Psychiatric Disorders as a Reaction to Illness

The vast majority of psychiatric disorders in patients with RA are emotional reactions to having RA. Patients experience life stress because of the burden not only of chronic physical symptoms but also of personal losses resulting from RA and associated disability. Albers et al. (1999) found that in 89% of RA patients, the disease adversely affected at least one domain of socioeconomic functioning (work, income, required rest time during day, leisure activity, transport mobility, housing, and social dependency), with 58% experiencing adverse effects in at least three domains. Other social impacts to consider are loss of personal ambitions, loss of social role, loss of future financial security, relationship disturbances, and body image concerns. Social support that might help to offset the stress of RA may be less available because of limited mobility. Furthermore, RA patients may have fewer coping resources available to deal with comorbid illnesses and stresses unrelated to RA. The evidence for the associations of emotional reactions and the various aspects of RA are dealt with next.

Psychological Symptoms and Clinical State

A large number of studies have examined the associations of depression with the physical symptoms of RA. Cross-sectional studies using self-report measures have shown that levels of depressive symptoms are associated with the severity of the pain experienced and the degree of functional disability.

Few longitudinal studies have examined whether changes in depression correlate with changes in the severity of RA symptoms. Wolfe and Hawley (1993) found that changes in depression were associated with changes in pain and disability, although only 17% of the variance in depression was accounted for by these two variables, indicating that the degree of association was weak. Katz and Yelin (1995) performed a detailed prospective study of women with RA and found that a 10% loss in activities that the individuals had identified as being important to them resulted in a sevenfold increase in depression in the subsequent year.

A large longitudinal study over 18 years found depression to be an independent risk factor for mortality in RA (Ang et al. 2005).

Role of Cognitive Factors

The way RA patients think about their illness is crucial to understanding the association of depression with pain and disability. Depression is associated with increased worry about illness and conviction of severe disease (Pilowsky 1993). Depressed RA patients perceive their illness as being more serious and feel hopeless about a cure compared with nondepressed RA patients (Murphy et al. 1999). Furthermore, depressed patients are more likely to have cognitive distortions relating to the RA (Smith et al. 1988). Depression is associated with impairment of general coping, especially at high levels of pain (Brown et al. 1989; Hurwicz and Berkanovic 1993). These associations remain significant in RA patients even after the extent of disease and pain levels are controlled, indicating that the association between depression and negative appraisals of health status is not simply the result of depressed people having more severe illness.

Other Psychosocial Factors

A number of other psychosocial factors that may predispose any RA patient to psychiatric problems have been suggested.

Neuroticism

Some individuals are predisposed to experience and react to stress, including health stress, in a negative way. In a prospective study, RA patients completed daily reports on joint pain and mood for a period of 75 days. Those scoring higher on neuroticism experienced more chronic distress, regardless of their pain intensity (Affleck et al. 1992).

Social Support

It is recognized that social support is associated with health and good quality of life in the general population (S. Cohen and Wills 1985). A number of studies have demonstrated that social support benefits patients with RA (Goodenow et al. 1990). In patients with RA, social support and its actual or perceived availability have been shown to be associated with use of more adaptive coping strategies (Manne and Zautra 1989), greater perception of ability to control the disease (Spitzer et al. 1995), and less psychological distress (Evers et al. 1997, 1998).

Rheumatoid arthritis has an adverse effect on the availability of social support to its patients, however. Patients with RA have been shown to have reduced social networks and social support (Fyrand et al. 2000). This disruption of social support appears to be greatest in those with disease of greatest duration with most severe functional disability, possibly caused by a significant reduction in the availability of important others to patients with RA (Murphy et al. 1988).

Social Stresses

As indicated previously, in addition to the burden of the symptoms, RA patients experience considerable hardship in association with their chronic illness. Social stresses independent of those of RA are also likely to contribute to the development of depression in RA patients, however. In fact, among ambulatory outpatients, the stresses independent of RA may well have a greater importance in predicting depression than the RA-related stresses (Dickens et al. 2003).

Impact of Mental Disorders

The mechanisms by which depression influences pain and disability are also poorly understood. Although depression and psychological stress have been shown to result in immune dysfunction (Herbert and Cohen 1993), there is no evidence to suggest that depression increases the pain and disability of RA by changing the underlying inflammatory activity. Studies suggesting that depression increases disease activity or that psychological treatment reduces RA activity have mostly relied on clinical assessments of disease activity such as counting tender joints (Bradley et al. 1987). Such clinical assessments rely on patient reports of tenderness and are vulnerable to the effects of depression, including pessimistic self-perception and the negative way patients react to their illness.

As mentioned previously, psychiatric disorders, particularly anxiety and depression, are associated with more negative illness cognitions in RA. As a result of these negative illness cognitions, health-seeking behaviors and health care utilization may increase as they do in other medical patients (Macfarlane et al. 1999; Manning and Wells 1992; Wells et al. 1989). Depressed RA patients are more likely to report physical symptoms (Murphy et al. 1999), less likely to be reassured by a doctor (Pilowsky 1993), and less likely to comply with medications (DiMatteo et al. 2000).

Osteoarthritis

Osteoarthritis (OA) is the most common joint disease, with the idiopathic form being the most prevalent. Secondary OA arises most frequently as the result of trauma (acute or chronic), although it also may occur in a variety of metabolic and endocrine disorders.

Direct involvement of the CNS is not a feature of primary OA, and one can conclude that psychological disorders in patients with this disorder arise either as a reaction to the pain, disability, and life difficulties related to the OA or for reasons independent of the OA.

In a study of patients with a variety of musculoskeletal disorders who were attending a secondary care facility, patients with OA of the knee or hand tended to have slightly lower scores on a standardized assessment of depression compared with patients with other musculoskeletal disorders (Hawley and Wolfe 1993). These results indicate that OA is less closely associated with depression than is RA, although studies of patients with more advanced disease are required.

When depression does occur in patients with OA, it has been shown to be associated with a number of factors: younger age, less education, higher pain, and greater self-reported impact of the OA (Dexter and Brandt 1994; van Baar et al. 1998; Zautra and Smith 2001). Other psychological factors such as anxiety and hopelessness have been shown to be associated with functional disability (Creamer et al. 2000).

Intervention studies suggest that improvement in depression is associated with reduced pain and disability from the disease (Calfas et al. 1992; Lin et al. 2003).

Systemic Lupus Erythematosus

SLE is an autoimmune disorder of unknown cause characterized by immune dysregulation with tissue damage caused by pathogenic autoantibodies, immune complexes, and T lymphocytes. Approximately 90% of cases are in women, usually of childbearing age. At onset, SLE may involve one or multiple organ systems. Common clinical manifestations include cutaneous lesions (photosensitivity, malar or discoid rash, oral ulcers), constitutional symptoms (fatigue, weight loss, fevers), arthralgias and frank arthritis, serositis (pericarditis or pleuritis), renal disease, neuropsychiatric disorders, and hematological disorders (anemia, leukopenia). Autoantibodies are detectable at presentation in most cases.

Psychiatric Manifestations

CNS involvement is a major cause of morbidity in SLE, second only to renal failure as a cause of mortality. Neuropsychiatric manifestations vary from stroke, seizures, headaches, neuropathy, transverse myelitis, and movement disorders to cognitive deficits, depression, mania, anxiety, psychosis, and delirium.

Pathogenesis of Neuropsychiatric Manifestations

Psychiatric syndromes in SLE can be caused by 1) direct CNS involvement; 2) infection, other systemic illness, or drug-induced side effects; 3) reaction to chronic illness; or 4) comorbid primary psychiatric illness (Hanly 2005).

Direct Pathophysiological CNS Effects

Two major antibody-mediated mechanisms of CNS injury have been proposed: neuronal injury and microvasculopathy (Scolding and Joseph 2002). Autoantibodies may directly damage neurons by either causing cell death or transiently and reversibly impairing neuronal function. Antineuronal antibodies have been associated with psychosis, depression, delirium, coma, and cognitive dysfunction (West et al. 1995). In contrast, antiphospholipid antibodies (e.g., anticardiolipin) cause focal deficits (strokes) and cognitive dysfunction (Levine et al. 2002; Menon et al. 1999; West et al. 1995). Antibody-mediated microvasculopathy seems to involve two processes: either endothelial damage (Wierzbicki 2000) or coagulation disturbances resulting from the prothrombotic effects of antiphospholipid (including anticardiolipin) antibodies (Gharavi 2001), both culminating in ischemia or infarction. These two pathogenic mechanisms may be mutually reinforcing, perpetuating the disease process. Microvascular endothelial injury in the CNS may increase the permeability of the blood-brain barrier, leading to influx of autoantibodies and further CNS damage.

With the possible exception of cognitive dysfunction, all the major psychiatric manifestations of SLE (i.e., psychosis, depression, mania, anxiety, and delirium) exhibit a degree of reversibility, as does coma. Even the cognitive deficits sometimes respond to corticosteroids (Denburg et al. 1994). Because psychiatric syndromes tend to resolve within 2–3 weeks with corticosteroid treatment (Denburg et al. 1994), they are probably caused by reversible or transient mechanisms rather than irreversible neuronal death. Most focal neurological events are irreversible and are associated with fixed lesions on neuroimaging. In some patients, the progressive nature of cognitive impairment, often with cerebral atrophy, suggests cumulative irreversible CNS damage.

Risk factors for direct CNS involvement in SLE include cutaneous vasculitis and antiphospholipid syndrome and its manifestations, especially arterial thromboses (Karassa et al. 2000).

Psychological Impact

Psychological reactions to having SLE are common and include grief, depression, anxiety, regression, denial, and invalidism. A feeling of isolation is reinforced by public ignorance about lupus. People with SLE may become socially withdrawn, especially if they are self-conscious about their appearance. The most prevalent fears of SLE patients are worsening disease, disability, and death. In particular, patients fear cognitive impairment, stroke, renal failure, and becoming a burden on their families (Liang et al. 1984). Although negative reactions to having SLE are common, at least 50% of patients experience positive reactions at some point during their illness (Liang et al. 1984).

Stress and SLE

Although stress may cause a lupus flare, it is also likely, if not inevitable, that lupus flares cause stress. Several studies have provided support for stress-induced immune dysregulation in SLE (Ferstl et al. 1992; Hinrichsen et al. 1989; Jacobs et al. 2001; Pawlak et al. 2003).

Whether stress precipitates onset or exacerbation of SLE symptoms has received relatively little study. There is only one controlled study demonstrating that 20 patients hospitalized for SLE had significantly greater stress prior to the onset of their illness than did the seriously ill hospitalized control subjects (Otto and Mackay 1967).

Classification of Psychiatric Disorders in Systemic Lupus Erythematosus

The American College of Rheumatology (ACR) convened a committee to develop a standardized nomenclature for neuropsychiatric SLE, and guidelines were published in 1999 (American College of Rheumatology Ad Hoc Committee 1999). The guidelines defined neuropsychiatric lupus as "the neurological syndromes of the central, peripheral, and autonomic nervous systems, and the psychiatric syndromes observed in patients with SLE in which other causes have been excluded." Psychiatric disorders included psychosis, acute confusional state, cognitive dysfunction, anxiety disorder, and mood disorders. A fundamental problem with the ACR classification system, however, is that it is difficult to apply clinically. To diag-

nose neuropsychiatric SLE as the cause of the psychiatric symptoms, one must exclude a primary psychiatric disorder. Whereas medical disorders and substance use can be easily excluded, there are no clinical criteria or laboratory tests for excluding primary psychiatric disorders.

Cognitive dysfunction is the most common neuropsychiatric disorder in patients with SLE, occurring in up to 80% of patients (Ainiala et al. 2001a; Denburg et al. 1994). On neuropsychological testing, even patients who have never had overt neuropsychiatric symptoms are often found to have cognitive impairment. Patients with anticardiolipin antibodies have a three- to fourfold increased risk of cognitive impairment, which is often progressive (Hanly et al. 1997; Menon et al. 1999). Cognitive impairment may be associated with lymphocytotoxic antibodies, CSF antineuronal antibodies, and pathological findings such as microinfarcts and cortical atrophy.

Depression is the second most common neuropsychiatric disorder in SLE. Using structured interviews, the prevalence of depression in SLE has been approximately 50% (Giang 1991). Diagnosing depression in SLE is confounded by the overlap between depressive symptoms and those associated with SLE or its treatment. Hypothyroidism should be ruled out, because it can mimic depression and is more common in SLE than in the general population.

Anxiety is quite common in SLE patients, often as a reaction to the illness. In patients with SLE, the most common cause of mania is corticosteroid therapy. Psychosis in SLE patients can be a manifestation of direct CNS involvement, and in some but not all studies, it has been linked to antiribosomal P antibodies. Delirium, referred to as "acute confusional state" in the ACR criteria, is common in severe SLE and is a result of CNS lupus,

TABLE 8–1. Secondary medical and psychiatric causes of neuropsychiatric symptoms in systemic lupus erythematosus and other rheumatological disorders

CNS infections
Systemic infections
Renal failure (e.g., due to lupus nephritis or vasculitis involving the renal artery)
Fluid/electrolyte disturbance
Hypertensive encephalopathy
Hypoxemia
Fever
CNS tumor (e.g., cerebral lymphoma because of immunosuppression)
Medication side effects (see Table 8–2)
Comorbid medical illness
Psychiatric symptoms in reaction to illness
Comorbid psychiatric illness

Note. CNS = central nervous system.

medication, or medical disorders, as shown in Table 8–1. Personality changes have been reported in SLE patients whose disease has damaged the frontal or temporal lobes, and symptoms are typical of those resulting from pathology in those brain regions.

Prevalence of Neuropsychiatric Disorders

Using the ACR nomenclature, two studies, a cross-sectional Finnish population-based study (Ainiala et al. 2001b) and a cohort study of predominantly Mexican Americans (Brey et al. 2002), examined the prevalence of neuropsychiatric syndromes in outpatients with SLE. Overall, 80%–91% of patients had at least one neuropsychiatric disorder, and the prevalence rates in the two studies were similar for individual neuropsychiatric syndromes. Cognitive dysfunction was the most common neuropsychiatric condition, occurring in 79%–80% of patients; however, less than a third of those

patients had moderate to severe impairment. Major depression occurred in 28%–39%; mania or mixed episodes, in 3%–4%; anxiety, in 13%–24%; and psychosis, in 0%–5%. Acute confusional state occurred in 7% of the Finnish patients with SLE; it was not reported in the Mexican American cohort. Although comparable prevalence studies have not been reported for acutely ill inpatients with neuropsychiatric SLE, the incidence of psychosis and delirium is likely to be substantially higher. Neuropsychiatric manifestations are also common in juvenile-onset SLE (Olfat et al. 2004).

Detection of CNS Systemic Lupus Erythematosus

The general principles of assessment discussed earlier in this chapter are applicable to neuropsychiatric SLE, but there are also relevant laboratory tests specific to SLE. In SLE, complement levels (C3, C4, CH50) and anti-DNA antibodies are elevated during disease flares (West et al. 1995). Serum antinuclear antibody (ANA) titers need not be obtained in SLE because they do not seem to correlate with systemic or CNS lupus activity. Testing for antiphospholipid antibodies (including lupus anticoagulant and anticardiolipin) is crucial, particularly in patients with focal symptoms, because the results may determine treatment and prognosis (Gharavi 2001; Levine et al. 2002). Patients with antiphospholipid syndrome are treated primarily with anticoagulation rather than corticosteroid or cytotoxic therapy. Antiribosomal-P antibodies have been linked to psychosis, but their usefulness is limited by their low positive predictive value: 13%–16% for psychosis and depression (Arnett et al. 1996). Other serum autoantibodies, including antineuronal, antineurofilament, and antiganglioside antibodies, have not proven to be diagnostic markers for CNS lupus.

Corticosteroid-Induced Psychiatric Symptoms

Distinguishing corticosteroid-induced psychiatric reactions from a flare of CNS lupus is one of the most challenging aspects of treating SLE (Kohen et al. 1993). Given the risk of untreated CNS lupus, and the likelihood that corticosteroids will alleviate such flares and only temporarily exacerbate corticosteroid-induced psychiatric reactions, an empirical initiation or increase of corticosteroids is often the most prudent intervention (Denburg et al. 1994; McCune 1988). (Corticosteroid-induced psychiatric reactions are discussed in depth later in this chapter.)

Pregnancy in Women With Systemic Lupus Erythematosus

Women may be at increased risk of SLE flares (usually mild) during pregnancy, especially in the second and third trimesters, and during the postpartum period (Khamashta et al. 1997; Ruiz-Irastorza et al. 1996). Some patients with antiphospholipid syndrome have been advised to forgo reproduction because of the risk of thrombosis, preeclampsia, and fetal demise (now uncommon because of anticoagulation therapy).

Differential Diagnosis of Psychiatric Disorders

Other Medical Disorders

A wide variety of diseases can mimic neuropsychiatric SLE. One group of diseases, associated with a medium to high ANA titer (>1:160), includes Sjögren's syndrome and mixed or undifferentiated connective tissue disease. A second group of diseases, associated with a low ANA titer (<1:160), includes multiple sclerosis and, less commonly, ANA-positive rheumatoid arthritis, sarcoidosis, and hepatitis C. A third group of diseases, characterized by a negative ANA, may also be mistaken for CNS lupus.

This group includes polyarteritis nodosa, microscopic angiitis, Wegener's granulomatosis, chronic fatigue syndrome, fibromyalgia, temporal arteritis, and Behçet's disease.

Psychotropic Drug–Induced Positive ANA

Patients who are receiving antipsychotic drugs, particularly phenothiazines such as chlorpromazine, may have positive ANAs and antiphospholipid antibodies (Canoso et al. 1990; Yannitsi et al. 1990). Drug-induced lupus has also been reported with other psychotropic drugs, including carbamazepine, divalproex, other anticonvulsants, and lithium (Wallach 2000). In drug-induced lupus, CNS manifestations are rare (Stratton 1985). If the offending drug is discontinued, the lupus symptoms typically resolve within weeks, although the ANA may remain positive for over a year.

Somatization Disorder ("Psychogenic Pseudolupus")

SLE can be misdiagnosed in "somatizing" patients with multisystem complaints and mildly positive tests for ANAs, which are common in young women.

Factitious Systemic Lupus Erythematosus

Factitious SLE appears to be rare, but several cases have been reported (Tlacuilo-Parra et al. 2000). Patients have simulated hematuria by pricking their finger surreptitiously to add trace amounts of blood to urine specimens, injected themselves with feces or other contaminants to cause infections, or applied rouge to their cheeks to simulate a malar rash. One patient feigned proteinuria by inserting a packet of protein into her bladder. These patients had no serological evidence of an autoimmune disorder.

Sjögren's Syndrome

The nature of CNS involvement in Sjögren's syndrome can be focal (cerebellar ataxia, vertigo, ophthalmoplegia, cranial nerve involvement) or diffuse (encephalopathy, aseptic meningoencephalitis, dementia or psychiatric manifestations). Focal lesions are visible on MRI scanning and most frequently involve the white matter (periventricular and subcortical) in the frontal and temporal lobes (Alexander et al. 1988). Cognitive deficits were found to be common, with more than 80% of subjects with primary Sjögren's syndrome reporting subjective cognitive deficits (Alexander et al. 1988). Objective cognitive deficits were confirmed in 85% of those with subjective problems: impairment in attention and concentration were most common (63% of subjects with neuropsychiatric involvement), with deficits in short-term memory and verbal fluency also being detected. Of those with recognized neuropsychiatric manifestations, 25% had progressive dementia, although it should be recognized that the number of subjects was small, and subjects were recruited based on having neuropsychiatric symptoms.

Psychiatric manifestations do occur and usually take the form of affective disturbance (depression, hypomania, anxiety) and somatization (Alexander et al. 1988; Stevenson et al. 2004). The exact prevalence of psychiatric complications is not clear because most studies have investigated small populations with unreliable questionnaire assessments.

Systemic Sclerosis (Scleroderma)

Of all the connective tissue disorders, systemic sclerosis is considered to be the least likely to cause CNS damage (Hietaharju et al. 1993). In one study, all patients with a diagnosis of systemic sclerosis in an area of Finland over an 11-year period were traced, and 16% were found to have neurological involvement (Hietaharju et al. 1993).

Psychiatric symptoms are common, with up to half of patients reporting symptoms of depression and about 20% scoring in the moderate to severe range on the Beck Depression Inventory (BDI) (Roca et al. 1996). Body image dissatisfaction is common in these patients and is likely to increase distress and psychosocial impairment in this group (Benrud-Larson et al. 2003).

Temporal (Giant Cell) Arteritis

Neuropsychiatric manifestations of temporal arteritis arise because of the involvement of arteries supplying blood to the CNS. The insults to the CNS in temporal arteritis can be ischemic (either permanent or transient) or hemorrhagic. The clinical characteristics of the presentation depend on the nature and extent of the brain areas affected. Resultant impairments can be focal (e.g., cerebrovascular accidents leading to specific motor or sensory deficit) or diffuse, resulting in impairment of consciousness. Other neuropsychiatric manifestations include affective symptoms (Johnson et al. 1997). Visual hallucinations have been reported as occurring in up to 80% of patients, who progress to develop permanent visual loss (Nesher et al. 2001).

Treatment with high-dose steroids is commenced as soon as the diagnosis is made on clinical grounds, before results of arterial biopsy are available, to prevent progression of the disease resulting in irreversible blindness or other serious CNS damage.

Polymyositis

Vasculitis can occur in polymyositis, affecting the CNS and resulting in neuropsychiatric manifestations. As with SLE and temporal arteritis, the clinical features of neuropsychiatric involvement secondary to vasculitis depend on the site and extent of the vasculitic lesions.

Polyarteritis Nodosa

Polyarteritis nodosa (PAN) is a systemic necrotizing arteritis affecting small and medium-sized vessels, often related to hepatitis B virus infection. Although multiple organ systems can be damaged in this disease, direct involvement of the CNS is rare and usually occurs after the disease is well established. Small cerebral infarcts are the most common neuroradiological findings, although intracranial aneurysms and intracranial hemorrhage have been reported (Oran et al. 1999).

Behçet's Disease

Neuropsychiatric involvement occurs in 10%–20% of cases of Behçet's disease. Acutely, aseptic meningitis or meningoencephalitis may occur. Later manifestations include personality change, meningoencephalitis, and motor signs. Depression and anxiety are common (Calikoglu et al. 2001). In terminal Behçet's, one-third of patients have dementia (Kaklamani et al. 1998).

Secondary Causes of Neuropsychiatric Symptoms in Rheumatological Disorders

Infection, Other CNS or Systemic Illness, and Drug-Induced Side Effects

A number of the rheumatological disorders or their treatments can be associated with immune dysregulation or immunosuppression; these disorders predispose individuals to CNS and systemic infec-tions. These infections can simulate direct involvement of the CNS by the primary disease process as in, for example, neuropsychiatric lupus (West et al. 1995). Infections causing these secondary neuropsychiatric complications include cryptococcal, tubercular, and meningococcal infections and Listeria meningitis; herpes encephalitis; neurosyphilis; CNS nocardiosis; toxoplasmosis; brain abscesses; and progressive multifocal leukoencephalopathy (see also Chapter 10, "Infectious Diseases"). Other etiologies of neuropsychiatric manifestations in rheumatological disorders include uremia, hypertensive encephalopathy, cerebral lymphoma, and medication side effects, as well as comorbid medical or psychiatric disorders and psychological reactions to illness (see Tables 8–1 and 8–2).

Corticosteroid-Induced Psychiatric Syndromes

Mood disorders, including mania, are the most common psychiatric reaction to corticosteroids. Patients may experience both mania and depression during a single course of corticosteroid therapy. Affective symptoms are often accompanied by psychotic symptoms. The psychiatric symptoms induced by corticosteroids most often resemble those of bipolar disorder (Brown and Suppes 1998). Delirium and psychosis (without mood symptoms) are less common. Cognitive dysfunction also has been reported and may be attributable to corticosteroid-induced cortical atrophy and loss of hippocampal neurons.

The incidence of corticosteroid-induced psychiatric symptoms is dose-related: 1.3% in patients receiving less than 40 mg/day of prednisone, 4.6% in those receiving 41–80 mg/day, and 18.4% in those receiving greater than 80 mg/day (Boston Collaborative Drug Surveillance Program 1972). For the majority of patients, the onset of psychiatric symptoms

TABLE 8–2. Psychiatric side effects of medications used in treating systemic lupus erythematosus

Medication	Psychiatric side effects
NSAID (high dose)	Depression, anxiety, paranoia, hallucinations, hostility, confusion, delirium, ↓ concentration
Sulfasalazine	Insomnia, depression, hallucinations
Corticosteroids	Mood lability, euphoria, irritability, anxiety, insomnia, mania, depression, psychosis, delirium, cognitive disturbance
Gold salts	None reported
Penicillamine	None reported
Leflunomide	Anxiety
Azathioprine	Delirium
Mycophenolate mofetil	Anxiety, depression, sedation (all rare)
Cyclophosphamide	Delirium (at high doses) (rare)
Methotrexate	Delirium (at high doses) (rare)
Cyclosporine	Anxiety, delirium, visual hallucinations
Tacrolimus	Anxiety, delirium, insomnia, restlessness
Immunoglobulin (intravenous)	Delirium, agitation
LJP-394[a]	None reported
Hydroxychloroquine	Confusion, psychosis, mania, depression, nightmares, anxiety, aggression, delirium

Note. NSAID = nonsteroidal anti-inflammatory drug.
[a]B-cell tolerogen–anti-anti-double-stranded DNA antibodies.

is within the first 2 weeks (and in 90%, within the first 6 weeks) of initiating or increasing corticosteroid treatment.

The preferred treatment for corticosteroid-induced psychiatric reactions is tapering of corticosteroids, if possible, resulting in greater than 90% response rate. However, rapid tapering or discontinuation of corticosteroids can also induce psychiatric reactions by precipitating a flare of the rheumatological disease, iatrogenic adrenal insufficiency, or possibly corticosteroid withdrawal syndrome. Corticosteroid withdrawal syndrome is manifested by headache, fever, myalgias, arthralgias, weakness, anorexia, nausea, weight loss, and orthostatic hypotension and sometimes depression, anxiety, agitation, or psychosis (Wolkowitz 1989). Symptoms respond to an increase or resumption of corticosteroid dosage. Adjunctive treatment with antipsychotics, antidepressants, and mood stabilizers can be helpful, depending on the particular psychiatric symptom constellation.

Other drugs used in treating rheumatological disorders may also cause psychiatric side effects, especially hydroxychloroquine (see Table 8–2).

References

Affleck G, Tennen H, Urrows S, et al: Neuroticism and the pain-mood relation in rheumatoid arthritis: insights from a prospective daily study. J Consult Clin Psychol 60:119–126, 1992

Ainiala H, Loukkola J, Peltola J, et al: The prevalence of neuropsychiatric syndromes in systemic lupus erythematosus. Neurology 57:496–500, 2001a

Ainiala H, Hietaharju A, Loukkola J, et al: Validity of the American College of Rheumatology criteria for neuropsychiatric lupus syndromes: a population-based evaluation. Arthritis Care Res 45:419–423, 2001b

Albers JM, Kuper HH, van Riel PL, et al: Socio-economic consequences of rheumatoid arthritis in the first years of the disease. Rheumatology (Oxf) 38:423–430, 1999

Alexander EL, Beall SS, Gordon B, et al: Magnetic resonance imaging of cerebral lesions in patients with Sjögren's syndrome. Ann Intern Med 108:815–823, 1988

American College of Rheumatology Ad Hoc Committee on Neuropsychiatric Lupus Nomenclature: Nomenclature and case definitions for neuropsychiatric lupus syndromes. Arthritis Rheum 42:599–608, 1999

Anderson IM, Nutt DJ, Deakin JF: Evidence-based guidelines for treating depressive disorders with antidepressants: a revision of the 1993 British Association for Psychopharmacology guidelines. J Psychopharmacol 14:3–20, 2000

Ando Y, Kai S, Uyama E, et al: Involvement of the central nervous system in rheumatoid arthritis: its clinical manifestations and analysis by magnetic resonance imaging. Intern Med 34:188–191, 1995

Ang DC, Choi H, Kroenke K, et al: Comorbid depression is an independent risk factor for mortality in patients with rheumatoid arthritis. J Rheumatol 32:1013–1019, 2005

Arnett FC, Reveille JD, Moutsopoulos HM, et al: Ribosomal P autoantibodies in systemic lupus erythematosus: frequencies in different ethnic groups and clinical and immunogenetic associations. Arthritis Rheum 39:1833–1839, 1996

Benrud-Larson LM, Heinburg LJ, Boling C, et al: Body image dissatisfaction among women with scleroderma and relationship to psychosocial function. Health Psychol 22:130–139, 2003

Boston Collaborative Drug Surveillance Program: Acute adverse reactions to prednisone in relation to dosage. Clin Pharmacol Ther 13:694–698, 1972

Bradley LA, Young LD, Anderson KO, et al: Effects of psychological therapy on pain behavior of rheumatoid arthritis patients. Treatment outcome and six-month follow-up. Arthritis Rheum 30:1105–1114, 1987

Brey RL, Holliday SL, Saklad AR, et al: Neuropsychiatric syndromes in lupus: prevalence using standardized definitions. Neurology 58:1214–1220, 2002

Bromm B, Meier W, Scharein E: Imipramine reduces experimental pain. Pain 25:245–257, 1986

Brown ES, Suppes T: Mood symptoms during corticosteroid therapy: a review. Harv Rev Psychiatry 5:239–246, 1998

Brown GK, Nicassio PM, Wallston KA: Pain coping strategies and depression in rheumatoid arthritis. J Clin Psychol 57: 652–657, 1989

Calfas KJ, Kaplan RM, Ingram RE: One year evaluation of cognitive behavioral intervention in osteoarthritis. Arthritis Care and Research 5:202–209, 1992

Calikoglu E, Onder M, Cosar B, et al: Depression, anxiety levels and general psychological profile in Behçet's disease. Dermatology 203:238–240, 2001

Canoso RT, de Oliveira RM, Nixon RA: Neuroleptic-associated autoantibodies. A prevalence study. Biol Psychiatry 27:863–870, 1990

Cohen S, Wills TA: Stress, social support and the buffering hypothesis. Psychol Bull 98:310–357, 1985

Creamer P, Lethbridge-Cejku M, Hochberg MC: Factors associated with functional impairment in symptomatic knee osteoarthritis. Rheumatology 39:490–496, 2000

Denburg SD, Carbotte RM, Denburg JA: Corticosteroids and neuropsychological functioning in patients with systemic lupus erythematosus. Arthritis Rheum 37:1311–1320, 1994

Dexter P, Brandt K: Distribution and predictors of depressive symptoms in osteoarthritis. Journal of Rheumatology 21: 279–286, 1994

Dickens C, Jackson J, Tomenson B, et al: Associations of depression in rheumatoid arthritis. Psychosomatics 44:209–215, 2003

DiMatteo MR, Lepper HS, Croghan TW: Depression is a risk factor for noncompliance with medical treatment: meta-analysis of the effects of anxiety and depression on patient adherence. Arch Intern Med 160: 2101–2107, 2000

Evers AW, Kraaimaat FW, Geenen R, et al: Determinants of psychological distress and its course in the first year after diagnosis in rheumatoid arthritis patients. J Behav Med 20: 489–504, 1997

Evers AW, Kraaimaat FW, Geenen R, et al: Psychosocial predictors of functional change in recently diagnosed rheumatoid arthritis patients. Behav Res Ther 36:179–193, 1998

Ferstl R, Niemann T, Biehl G, et al: Neuropsychological impairment in auto-immune disease. Eur J Clin Invest 20 (suppl 1):16–20, 1992

Frank RG, Beck NC, Parker JC, et al: Depression in rheumatoid arthritis. J Rheumatol 15:920–925, 1988

Fyrand L, Moum T, Wichstrom L, et al: Social network size of female patients with rheumatoid arthritis compared to healthy controls. Scand J Rheumatol 29:38–43, 2000

Gharavi AE: Anticardiolipin syndrome: antiphospholipid syndrome. Clin Med 1:14–17, 2001

Giang DW: Systemic lupus erythematosus and depression. Neuropsychiatry Neuropsychol Behav Neurol 4:78–82, 1991

Goodenow C, Reisine ST, Grady KE: Quality of social support and associated social and psychological functioning in women with rheumatoid arthritis. Health Psychol 9:266–284, 1990

Hanly JG: Neuropsychiatric lupus. Rheum Clin North Am 31:273–298, 2005

Hanly JG, Cassell K, Fisk JD: Cognitive function in systemic lupus erythematosus: results of a 5-year prospective study. Arthritis Rheum 40:1542–1543, 1997

Hawley DJ, Wolfe F: Depression is not more common in RA: a 10 year longitudinal study of 6,153 patients with rheumatic disease. Journal of Rheumatology 20:2025–2031, 1993

Herbert TB, Cohen S: Stress and immunity in humans: a meta-analytic review. Psychosom Med 55:364–379, 1993

Hietaharju A, Jaaskelainen S, Hietarinta M, et al: Central nervous system involvement and psychiatric manifestations in systemic sclerosis: clinical and neurophysiological involvement. Acta Neurol Scand 87:382–387, 1993

Hinrichsen H, Barth J, Ferstl R, et al: Changes of immunoregulatory cells induced by acoustic stress in patients with systemic lupus erythematosus, sarcoidosis, and in healthy controls. Eur J Clin Invest 19:372–377, 1989

Hurwicz ML, Berkanovic E: The stress process in rheumatoid arthritis. J Rheumatol 20:1836–1844, 1993

Jacobs R, Pawlak CR, Mikeska E, et al: Systemic lupus erythematosus and rheumatoid arthritis patients differ from healthy controls in their cytokine pattern after stress exposure. Rheumatology 40:868–875, 2001

Johnson H, Bouman W, Pinner G: Psychiatric aspects of temporal arteritis: a case report and review of the literature. J Geriatr Psychiatry Neurol 10:142–145, 1997

Kaklamani VG, Vaiopoulos G, Kaklamanis PG: Behçet's disease. Semin Arthritis Rheum 27:197–217, 1998

Karassa FB, Ioannidis JPA, Touloumi G, et al: Risk factors for central nervous system involvement in systemic lupus erythematosus. QJM 93:169–174, 2000

Katz PP, Yelin EH: The development of depressive symptoms among women with rheumatoid arthritis. The role of function. Arthritis Rheum 38:49–56, 1995

Khamashta MA, Ruiz-Irastorza G, Hughes GR: Systemic lupus erythematosus flares during pregnancy. Rheum Dis Clin North Am 23:15–30, 1997

Kohen M, Asheron RA, Gharavi AE, et al: Lupus psychosis: differentiation from the steroid-induced state. Clin Exp Rheumatol 11:323–326, 1993

Levine JS, Branch DW, Rauch J: The antiphospholipid syndrome. N Engl J Med 346:752–763, 2002

Liang MH, Rogers M, Larson M, et al: The psychosocial impact of systemic lupus erythematosus and rheumatoid arthritis. Arthritis Rheum 27:13–19, 1984

Lin E, Katon, W, Von Korff M, et al: Effects of improving depression care on pain and functional outcomes among older adults with arthritis. JAMA 290:2428–2434, 2003

Macfarlane GJ, Morris S, Hunt IM, et al: Chronic widespread pain in the community: the influence of psychological symptoms and mental disorder on health care seeking behavior. J Rheumatol 26:413–419, 1999

Manne SL, Zautra AJ: Spouse criticism and support: their association with coping and psychological adjustment among women with rheumatoid arthritis. J Pers Soc Psychol 56:608–617, 1989

Manning WG Jr, Wells KB: The effects of psychological distress and psychological well-being on use of medical services. Med Care 30:541–553, 1992

McCune WJ: Neuropsychiatric lupus. Rheum Dis Clin N Am 14:149–167, 1988

Menon S, Jameson-Shortall E, Newman SP, et al: A longitudinal study of anticardiolipin antibody levels and cognitive functioning in systemic lupus erythematosus. Arthritis Rheum 42:735–741, 1999

Murphy H, Dickens C, Creed F, et al: Depression, illness perception and coping in rheumatoid arthritis. J Psychosom Res 46:155–164, 1999

Murphy S, Creed F, Jayson MI: Psychiatric disorder and illness behaviour in rheumatoid arthritis. Br J Rheumatol 27:357–363, 1988

Nesher G, Nesher R, Rozenman Y, et al: Visual hallucinations in giant cell arteritis: association with visual loss. J Rheumatol 28:2046–2048, 2001

Olfat MO, Al-Mayouf SM, Muzaffer MA: Pattern of neuropsychiatric manifestations and outcome in juvenile systemic lupus erythematosus. Clin Rheumatol 23:395–399, 2004

Onghena P, Van Houdenhove B: Antidepressant-induced analgesia in chronic nonmalignant pain: a meta-analysis of 39 placebo-controlled studies. Pain 49: 205–219, 1992

Oran I, Memis A, Paridar M, et al: Multiple intracranial aneurysms in polyarteritis nodosa: MRI and angiography. Neuroradiology 41:436–439, 1999

Otto R, Mackay IR: Psycho-social and emotional disturbance in systemic lupus erythematosus. Med J Aust 2:488–493, 1967

Pawlak C, Witte T, Heiken H, et al: Flares in patients with systemic lupus erythematosus are associated with daily psychological stress. Psychother Psychosom 72:159–165, 2003

Pilowsky I: Dimensions of illness behaviour as measured by the Illness Behaviour Questionnaire. J Psychosom Res 37:53–62, 1993

Rifkin A: Depression in physically ill patients. Postgrad Med 92:147–154, 1992

Roca RP, Wigley FM, White B: Depressive symptoms associated with scleroderma. Arthritis Rheum 39:1035–1040, 1996

Ruiz-Irastorza G, Lima F, Alves J, et al: Increased rate of lupus flare during pregnancy and the puerperium: a prospective study of 78 pregnancies. Br J Rheumatol 35:133–138, 1996

Sabbadini MG, Manfredi AA, Bozzolo E, et al: Central nervous system involvement in systemic lupus erythematosus patients without overt neuropsychiatric manifestations. Lupus 8:1–2, 1999

Scolding NJ, Joseph FG: The neuropathology and pathogenesis of systemic lupus erythematosus. Neuropathol Appl Neurobiol 28:173–189, 2002

Sharpe L, Sensky T, Timberlake N, et al: A blind, randomized, controlled trial of cognitive-behavioural intervention for patients with recent onset rheumatoid arthritis: preventing psychological and physical morbidity. Pain 89:275–283, 2001

Sheikh JI, Yesavage J: Geriatric Depression Scale (GDS): recent evidence and development of a shorter version. Clin Gerontol 9:37–43, 1989

Smedstad LM, Vaglum P, Kvien TK, et al: The relationship between self-reported pain and sociodemographic variables, anxiety, and depressive symptoms in rheumatoid arthritis. J Rheumatol 22:514–520, 1995

Smith TW, Peck JR, Milano RA, et al: Cognitive distortion in rheumatoid arthritis: relation to depression and disability. J Consult Clin Psychol 56:412–416, 1988

Spitzer A, Bar-Tal Y, Golander H: Social support: how does it really work? J Adv Nurs 22:850–854, 1995

Stevenson HA, Jones ME, Rostron JL, et al: UK patients with primary Sjögren's syndrome are at increased risk from clinical depression. Gerodontology 21:141–145, 2004

Stratton MA: Drug induced systemic lupus erythematosus. Clin Pharm 4:657–663, 1985

Tlacuilo-Parra JA, Guevara-Gutierrez E, Garcia-De La Torre I: Factitious disorders mimicking systemic lupus erythematosus. Clin Exp Rheumatol 18:89–93, 2000

van Baar ME, Dekker J, Lemmens JA, et al: Pain and disability in patients with osteoarthritis of the hip or knee: the relationship with articular, kinesiological and psychological characteristics. Journal of Rheumatology 25:125–133, 1998

Wallach J: Interpretation of Diagnostic Tests, 7th Edition. Baltimore, MD, Lippincott, 2000

Waterloo K, Omdal R, Jacobsen EA, et al: Cerebral computed tomography and electroencephalography compared with neuropsychological findings in systemic lupus erythematosus. J Neurol 246:706–711, 1999

Wells KB, Stewart A, Hays RD, et al: The functioning and well-being of depressed patients. Results from the Medical Outcomes Study. JAMA 262:914–919, 1989

West SG: Neuropsychiatric lupus. Rheum Dis Clin N Am 20:129–158, 1994

West SG, Emlen W, Wener MH, et al: Neuropsychiatric lupus erythematosus: a prospective study on the value of diagnostic tests. Am J Med 99:153–163, 1995

Wierzbicki AS: Lipids, cardiovascular disease and atherosclerosis in systemic lupus erythematosus. Lupus 9:194–201, 2000

Wolfe F, Hawley DJ: The relationship between clinical activity and depression in rheumatoid arthritis. J Rheumatol 20: 2032–2037, 1993

Wolkowitz OM: Long-lasting behavioral changes following prednisolone withdrawal. JAMA 261:1731–1732, 1989

Yannitsi SG, Manoussakis MN, Mavridis AK, et al: Factors related to the presence of autoantibodies in patients with chronic mental disorders. Biol Psychiatry 27:747–756, 1990

Zautra AJ, Smith BW: Depression and reactivity to stress in older women with rheumatoid arthritis and osteoarthritis. Psychosom Med 63:687–696, 2001

Zigmond AS, Snaith RP: The Hospital Anxiety and Depression Scale. Acta Psychiatr Scand 67:361–370, 1983

Self-Assessment Questions

Select the single best response for each question.

1. Depression is a common problem in rheumatoid arthritis. However, consideration of the specific needs and complexity of these patients is important. Which is the recommended first-line pharmacological management strategy for depression in rheumatoid arthritis?

    A. Selective serotonin reuptake inhibitors (SSRIs), with doses limited to one-half the usual adult dose.
    B. SSRIs, in typical adult doses.
    C. Tricyclic antidepressants (TCAs), limited to low doses only.
    D. TCAs in low doses, routinely combined with SSRIs.
    E. Full-dose TCAs.

2. Regarding central nervous system (CNS) or psychiatric complications in rheumatoid arthritis, which of the following statements is *not* true?

    A. Neurological complications are common in rheumatoid arthritis due to direct CNS involvement.
    B. Psychiatric illness in rheumatoid arthritis most commonly occurs as emotional reactions to having a serious systemic illness.
    C. Depressive symptoms correlate with levels of physical pain in rheumatoid arthritis.
    D. Social stresses independent of those of rheumatoid arthritis are likely to contribute to the development of depression.
    E. Neuroticism in rheumatoid arthritis patients is associated with more distress, regardless of pain levels.

3. Which of the following is *not* associated with greater risk of depression in osteoarthritis?

    A. Older age.
    B. Lower level of education.
    C. Greater self-reported impact of osteoarthritis on patient's life.
    D. More pain.
    E. Objective measures of functional disability.

4. Among the neuropsychiatric syndromes in systemic lupus erythematosus (SLE) specified by the American College of Rheumatology (1999), which of the following is the most common?

    A. Mood disorders.
    B. Anxiety disorders.
    C. Psychosis.
    D. Cognitive dysfunction.
    E. Acute confusional state/delirium.

5. Confusion, psychosis, mania, aggression, depression, nightmares, anxiety, and delirium have all been associated with which of the following medications for SLE?

   A. Gold salts.
   B. Penicillamine.
   C. Azathioprine.
   D. Leflunomide.
   E. Hydroxychloroquine.

9

Chronic Fatigue and Fibromyalgia Syndromes

Michael C. Sharpe, M.A., M.D.

Patrick G. O'Malley, M.D., M.P.H.

IN THIS CHAPTER, we review two symptom-defined somatic syndromes: chronic fatigue syndrome (CFS) and fibromyalgia syndrome (FMS). The central feature of CFS is the symptom of severe chronic, disabling fatigue that is typically exacerbated by exertion and unexplained by any other medical condition. The central feature of FMS is widespread pain with localized tenderness that similarly is unexplained by any other diagnosis. Although these syndromes have different historical origins, it is increasingly recognized that they have much in common (Sullivan et al. 2002). Therefore, in this chapter we consider them together.

CFS, FMS, and other symptom-defined somatic syndromes are conditions whose homes in medicine (as functional syndromes) and in psychiatry (as somatoform disorders) are both rather temporary structures located in unfashionable areas of their respective communities. These functional disorders (Wessely et al. 1999) are, however, of central concern to psychosomatic medicine. Other functional or medically unexplained syndromes are covered elsewhere in this volume.

We are grateful to the following for helpful comments on earlier versions of the chapter: Dr. Peter White, Dr. Leslie Arnold, Professor Simon Wessely, Professor Gijs Belijenberg, Professor Dan Clauw, and Dr. Robert Perry.

General Issues

Organic or Psychogenic?

The history of CFS and FMS has been notable for its vigorous disputes about whether these disorders are organic or psychogenic (Asbring and Narvanen 2003). The extreme organic position argues that they eventually will be found to be as firmly based in disease pathology as any other medical condition. Attempts to establish a conventional pathology (e.g., inflammation in muscles in fibromyalgia and chronic infection in CFS) have not yet succeeded, however. An extreme psychogenic view is that these syndromes are pseudodiseases, not rooted in biology but rather representing social constructions based on psychological amplification of normal somatic sensations such as tiredness and pain. Neither of these extreme positions is sustained by the evidence or helpful for patients. An etiologically neutral and integrated perspective that recognizes these functional disorders as real and that also acknowledges the likely contribution of biological, psychological, and social factors is the best basis for clinical practice (Engel 1977).

Medical or Psychiatric Diagnosis?

In parallel with the debate about etiology is an argument about whether these conditions are most appropriately regarded as medical or as psychiatric. For the same symptoms, the medical diagnosis is CFS (chronic fatigue and immune dysfunction syndrome; myalgic encephalomyelitis or encephalopathy—see "History" subsection in the following section "The Syndromes") or FMS, and the psychiatric diagnosis is often an anxiety, mood, or somatoform disorder. However, it can be argued that neither alone is adequate. Proper use of the DSM-IV-TR (American Psychiatric Association 2000) axes allows the patient to be given both a medical (Axis III) and a psychiatric (Axis I) diagnosis. The final diagnosis may be, for example, FMS and generalized anxiety disorder (GAD). Ultimately, a classification that avoids two diagnoses being given for the same symptoms is required. This is a task for the authors of the forthcoming DSM-V (Mayou et al. 2003).

The Syndromes

Chronic Fatigue Syndrome

History

It has been convincingly argued that CFS is not a new illness. A very similar, if not identical, condition was described as *neurasthenia* more than 100 years ago and probably much earlier (Wessely 1990). The term *chronic fatigue syndrome* was coined in 1988 to describe a condition characterized by chronic disabling fatigue, with many other somatic symptoms and strict psychiatric exclusions (Holmes et al. 1988). The authors of this early definition anticipated that a specific disease cause, possibly infectious, would be found, but this has never been established.

The term *chronic fatigue syndrome* subsumed a multitude of previous terms used to describe patients with similar symptoms. These include *chronic Epstein-Barr virus infection* (see Chapter 10, "Infectious Diseases"), *myalgic encephalomyelitis, neurasthenia* (still a specific diagnosis in ICD-10 [World Health Organization 1992]), and *postviral fatigue syndrome*. Arguments persist about the similarity of these conditions to CFS. Patient advocacy groups in particular have been very vocal and politically active in arguing that CFS is an inadequate description of their illness and that a name such as *myalgic encephalomyelitis* or *encephalopathy* or *chronic fatigue and immune dysfunction syndrome*, which emphasizes a biological pathology, is

---

TABLE 9–1. Diagnostic criteria for chronic fatigue syndrome

Inclusion criteria

1. Clinically evaluated, medically unexplained fatigue of at least 6 months' duration that is
   - Of new onset (not lifelong)
   - Not the result of ongoing exertion
   - Not substantially alleviated by rest
   - Associated with a substantial reduction in previous level of activities

2. The occurrence of four or more of the following symptoms:
   - Subjective memory impairment
   - Sore throat
   - Tender lymph nodes
   - Muscle pain
   - Joint pain
   - Headache
   - Unrefreshing sleep
   - Postexertional malaise lasting more than 24 hours

Exclusion criteria

- Active, unresolved, or suspected medical disease
- Psychotic, melancholic, or bipolar depression (but not uncomplicated major depression)
- Psychotic disorders
- Dementia
- Anorexia or bulimia nervosa
- Alcohol or other substance misuse
- Severe obesity

Source. Adapted from Fukuda et al. 1994.

---

more appropriate. The new terminology of CFS did, however, have the important advantage for researchers of being clearly operationally defined and provided a basis for replicable scientific research.

Definition

The most recent diagnostic criteria (shown in Table 9–1) were based on an international consensus and were published in 1994. These remain the most widely used (Fukuda et al. 1994) and have been recently clarified (Reeves et al. 2003).

Clinical Features

The clinical presentation of the individuals whose symptoms meet the criteria for CFS (Fukuda et al. 1994; see Table 9–1) is heterogeneous, although the core symptoms of fatigue exacerbated by exercise, subjective cognitive impairment, and disrupted and

unrefreshing sleep are almost universally described, and some degree of widespread pain is common. Patients often report marked fluctuations in fatigue that occur from week to week and even from day to day. Most patients are not so disabled that they cannot attend an outpatient consultation, although some describe difficulty walking or cannot attend an outpatient consultation without the aid of wheelchairs and other appliances. Other patients who remain bedridden and unable to visit the clinic represent an important and neglected group.

Fibromyalgia

History

In 1904, Gowers first coined the term *fibrositis* to describe a chronic widespread pain thought to be caused by inflammation of muscles. However, as with CFS, specific

---

TABLE 9–2.   American College of Rheumatology 1990 criteria for fibromyalgia

1. History of widespread pain of at least 3 months' duration. "Widespread" means: pain in the right and left side of the body, pain above and below the waist, and axial skeletal pain (cervical spine or anterior chest or thoracic spine or low back). In this definition, shoulder and buttock pain is considered as pain for each involved side. "Low back" pain is considered lower-segment pain.

2. Pain, on digital palpation, must be present in at least 11 of 18 specified tender point sites. Digital palpation should be performed with an approximate force of 4 kg. For a tender point to be considered "positive," the patient must state that the palpation was painful.

Source.   Adapted from Wolfe et al. 1990.

---

disease pathology in muscle has not subsequently been confirmed. In 1990, the American College of Rheumatology (ACR) adopted the operationally defined and descriptive term *fibromyalgia* as an alternative to *fibrositis* (Wolfe et al. 1990). Other terms have been used, such as *chronic widespread pain* and *myofascial pain syndrome.* As with CFS, the new definition facilitated replicable research and has been widely adopted.

Definition

A variety of different diagnostic criteria for fibromyalgia have been proposed. The ACR criteria published in 1990 are the most widely accepted (Wolfe et al. 1990). These specify widespread pain of at least 3 months' duration and tenderness at 11 or more of 18 specific sites on the body. The ACR criteria are shown in Table 9–2.

A particular feature of the FMS criteria is the specification of examination findings as well as of symptoms. A standardized method of eliciting these "tender points" has been defined (i.e., the application of pressure with the thumb pad perpendicular to each defined site with increasing force by approximately 1 kg/second until 4 kg of pressure is achieved, which usually leads to whitening of the thumbnail bed). Despite the apparent precision of this clinical sign, both the specificity of the locations and the uniqueness of the proposed tender points to FMS have been questioned (Croft et al. 1996; Wolfe 1997).

Clinical Features

The core clinical features of fibromyalgia are chronic widespread pain and musculoskeletal tenderness (muscles, ligaments, and tendons). Pain occurs typically in all four quadrants of the body and the axial skeleton but also can be regional. Fatigue, sleep disturbance, and subjective cognitive impairment (memory and concentration) are common associations. As with CFS, the report of pain is essentially a subjective phenomenon and may not be reflected in attempts to assess physical and mental performance objectively.

Same or Different?

Many studies have shown an overlap in the symptoms of patients with a diagnosis of FMS and those with a diagnosis of CFS if these are specifically asked about. Put simply, CFS is fatigue with pain, and FMS is pain with fatigue. A latent class analysis of the symptoms of more than 600 patients failed to identify separate syndromes (Sullivan et al. 2002). Not only are the symptoms similar, but a patient who has received the diagnosis of one of these conditions is also likely to meet the diagnostic criteria for the other. Of 163 consecutive female patients with CFS enrolled at a tertiary care clinic, more than a third also met criteria for FMS (Ciccone and Natelson 2003). Consequently, most authorities now accept that important similarities exist between CFS and FMS (Aaron and Buchwald

2003; Wessely et al. 1999). One potential difference between FMS and CFS is the presence of so-called tender points in the former. However, tender points also are often found in patients with CFS. Whether they will be found ultimately to be distinct entities, overlapping conditions, or aspects of the same condition remains both unclear and controversial.

Association With Other Symptom-Defined Syndromes

Studies that have assessed the comorbidity of FMS and CFS with other symptom-defined syndromes (also known as medically unexplained symptoms or functional somatic syndromes) also have found high rates of migraine, irritable bowel syndrome, pelvic pain, and temporomandibular joint pain. These syndromes, like CFS and FMS, are also associated with high lifetime rates of comorbid mood and anxiety disorders (Hudson and Pope 1994). Other similarities are also seen between FMS, CFS, and these disorders, including a female predominance, association with childhood abuse, and response to similar treatments. This observation raises the possibility not only that CFS and FMS are similar but also that all the functional syndromes have more in common than previously thought by the specialists who diagnose each (Sullivan et al. 2002; Wessely et al. 1999). It has been further suggested that these syndromes, along with mood and anxiety disorders, share a common psychological and central nervous system (CNS) pathophysiology (Clauw and Chrousos 1997).

Association With Psychiatric Disorders

In clinical practice, many but not all patients with CFS and FMS can be given a psychiatric diagnosis. Most will meet criteria for a depression or an anxiety syndrome. Those who do not are likely to meet DSM criteria for a somatoform disorder or merit an ICD-10 diagnosis of neurasthenia (Sharpe 1996). The more somatic symptoms the patient has, the more likely a diagnosis of depression or anxiety is (Skapinakis et al. 2003). Precise prevalence rates of psychiatric disorder do, however, depend on the nature of the patient population studied and the diagnostic criteria used.

Depression

Fatigue is strongly associated with depression. The international World Health Organization (WHO) study of more than 5,000 primary care patients in several countries (Sartorius et al. 1993) found that 67% of the patients with CFS (defined from survey data) also had an ICD-10 depressive syndrome (Skapinakis 2000). Studies of clinic attenders with CFS reported that more than 25% have a current DSM major depression diagnosis, and 50%–75% have a lifetime diagnosis (Afari and Buchwald 2003). Population studies also find an elevated prevalence, although a lower rate than in some clinic studies (Taylor and Jason 2003).

Chronic pain is also strongly associated with depression in the general population (Ohayon and Schatzberg 2003) (see also Chapter 19, "Pain"). In FMS, a study of attenders at a specialist clinic reported that 32% had a depressive disorder (22% major depression) (Epstein et al. 1999). An increased prevalence of lifetime and family history of major depression also has been reported in FMS (Hudson and Pope 1996). As with CFS, the prevalence of depression is probably lower in patients with FMS in the general population (Clauw and Crofford 2003).

GAD, Panic Disorder, and Posttraumatic Stress Disorder

Anxiety disorders have been relatively neglected in association with CFS and FMS.

One study reported GAD in as many as half of the clinic patients with CFS or FMS when the hierarchical rules that subsume it under major depression were suspended (Fischler et al. 1997).

Panic disorder is especially common in patients with medically unexplained symptoms. A prevalence of 7% has been reported in clinic patients with FMS (Epstein et al. 1999), and the prevalence was 13% in one study of CFS (Manu et al. 1991). Panic should be suspected when symptoms are markedly episodic.

The prevalence of posttraumatic stress disorder (PTSD) has been reported to be higher in patients with CFS (Taylor and Jason 2003) and FMS (Cohen et al. 2002) than in the general population, and PTSD is associated with a report of previous abuse (see "Abuse" subsection in the "Etiology" section later in this chapter).

Somatoform Disorders

Somatoform disorders are descriptive diagnoses primarily defined by somatic symptoms not explained by a medical condition. Hence, replacing a diagnosis of CFS or FMS with a somatoform one may simply be relabeling. Furthermore, the choice of diagnosis depends on one's beliefs about the nature of these conditions. If one regards CFS and FMS as medical conditions, then the symptoms will not be counted toward a diagnosis of a somatoform disorder, whereas if one regards CFS and FMS as medically unexplained syndromes, then they will be counted toward a diagnosis of a somatoform disorder (Johnson et al. 1996). Some patients will meet the criteria for hypochondriasis because of persistent anxious concern about the nature of their illness. Others may meet the criteria for somatization disorder because of a long history of multiple symptoms. Patients with FMS are likely to meet the criteria for somatoform pain disorder.

Most patients with CFS and FMS who do not meet the criteria for anxiety, depression, or these more specific disorders will fit the undemanding criteria for a diagnosis of undifferentiated somatoform disorder.

Summary

Depressive and anxiety disorders are relatively common in patients with CFS and FMS. There is some suggestion that anxiety is associated more with pain, and depression with fatigue (Kurtze and Svebak 2001). This association with psychiatric disorders appears not to be explained simply by overlapping symptoms, because it remains high even when fatigue is excluded from the diagnostic criteria for major depression (Kruesi et al. 1989). The occurrence of depression or anxiety disorders in patients with CFS or FMS cannot be attributed entirely to referral bias because the rate is still elevated, although less so, in community cases. Also, it does not appear that depression can be explained entirely as a reaction to disability, because it has been found to be more common than in patients with disabling rheumatoid arthritis (Katon et al. 1991; Walker et al. 1997a). However, many patients with CFS and FMS do not have depressive and anxiety syndromes, even after detailed assessment (Henningsen et al. 2003). Whether these patients are given appropriate diagnoses of a somatoform disorder is controversial.

The relation between symptom syndromes defined by psychiatry and those of CFS and FMS is an intimate and complex one. It can be conceived of either as psychiatric comorbidity with a medical condition or as different perspectives on the same condition. Whichever view one takes, the importance of making the psychiatric diagnosis in patients with CFS and FMS lies in its implications for treatment.

Epidemiology

Prevalence of Fatigue and Chronic Fatigue Syndrome

Fatigue is common, but CFS as currently defined is relatively rare. A large survey of 90,000 residents in Wichita, Kansas, which used rigorous assessment and exclusion criteria, found that 6% of the population had fatigue of more than 1 month's duration, but only 235 per 100,000 (or 0.2%) had CFS (Reyes et al. 2003). It should be noted, however, that the application of current diagnostic criteria (Fukuda et al. 1994; Table 9–1) excluded numerous patients, mainly because of diagnoses of rheumatoid arthritis and psychiatric disorder.

Prevalence of Pain and Fibromyalgia Syndrome

The studies of prevalence of pain and FMS have reported similar findings (Makela 1999). Chronic pain is common and has been reported in as many as 10% of the general population (Croft et al. 1993). However, FMS defined according to the ACR criteria has an estimated prevalence of only 2% (Wolfe et al. 1995) to 4% (K.P. White et al. 1999). The observation that FMS appears to be more common than CFS (Bazelmans et al. 1997) may indicate that chronic pain states are more common than chronic fatigue states but also may simply reflect the requirement in the CFS diagnostic criteria for a longer duration and greater disability from the condition (see Tables 9–1 and 9–2).

Associations

Gender

Both CFS and FMS are more common in women. The female-to-male ratio for CFS has been reported to be about 4:1 (Reyes et al. 2003) and for FMS, 8:1 (Wolfe et al.

1995), although this increased female preponderance in FMS may be primarily associated with tender points rather than with pain (Clauw and Crofford 2003).

Age

The most common age at onset for both CFS and FMS is between 30 and 50 years. However, patients who present with FMS are on average 10 years older (Reyes et al. 2003; K.P. White et al. 1999). These syndromes are also diagnosed, although controversially, in children. A recent epidemiological study from the United Kingdom found a prevalence of CFS of only 0.002% in 5- to 15-year-olds (Chalder et al. 2003). CFS and FMS are also diagnosed in the elderly, but the frequency of other chronic medical conditions complicates the differential diagnosis.

Socioeconomic Status

Both CFS and FMS are more prevalent in persons of lower socioeconomic status and in those who have received less education (Jason et al. 1999; K.P. White et al. 1999). CFS is 50% more common in semiskilled and unskilled workers than in professionals.

International and Cross-Cultural Studies

It is often noted that the diagnoses of CFS and FMS are almost entirely restricted to Western nations, whereas the symptoms of fatigue and pain are universal. It is unclear to what extent this reflects differing epidemiology or simply different diagnostic practice.

Disability and Work

FMS and CFS are both associated with substantial self-reported loss of function and substantial work disability (Assefi et al. 2003). Unemployment in patients with CFS and FMS attending specialist services in the United States is as high as 50% (Bombardier and Buchwald 1996).

TABLE 9–3.   Etiological factors to consider in a formulation of chronic fatigue

Type	Predisposing	Precipitating	Perpetuating
Biological	Genetics	Acute infection, disease, or injury	Deconditioning Sleep disorder Neuroendocrine changes
Psychological	Personality Childhood abuse	Perceived stress	Depression Illness beliefs Avoidance of activity
Social	Lack of support Low social status	Life events	Information from others Lack of acceptance of illness Occupational and financial factors

Prognosis

The prognosis for patients with CFS or FMS is variable and typically has a chronic but fluctuating course. Rehabilitative therapy improves outcome (see subsection "Specialist Nonpharmacological Treatments" later in this chapter).

Prospective studies of CFS and FMS in the general population report that in about half the cases, the syndrome is in partial or complete remission at 2–3 years (Granges et al. 1994; Nisenbaum et al. 2003). Poor outcome in CFS and FMS is predicted by longer illness duration, more severe symptoms, older age, depression, and lack of social support (McBeth et al. 2001; van der Werf et al. 2002), and in CFS, by a strong belief in physical causes (Joyce et al. 1997). Severely disabled patients attending specialist clinics have a particularly poor prognosis for recovery (Hill et al. 1999; Wolfe et al. 1997).

Etiology

The precise etiology of CFS and FMS remains unknown. A wide range of etiological factors have been proposed, but none has been unequivocally established. The available evidence may be summarized as suggesting that a combination of environ-mental factors and individual vulnerability initiates a series of biological, psychological, and social processes that lead to the development of CFS or FMS (see Table 9–3). These factors are discussed in the following subsections as predisposing, precipitating, and perpetuating factors.

Predisposing Factors

Biological Factors

Genetics.   Modest evidence from family and twin studies suggests that genetic factors play a part in predisposing individuals to CFS and to FMS.

Psychological and Social Factors

Personality and activity.   Clinicians often claim a predisposing "obsessional" personality type, but this theory has been little studied.

Abuse.   Childhood and adult neglect, abuse, and maltreatment have been reported by some, but not all, studies to be more common in both FMS and CFS groups than in medical comparison groups (Van Houdenhove et al. 2001). In FMS, a particular association with abuse in adulthood has been noted (Walker et al. 1997b).

Social status.   Low social status and lower levels of education are risk factors for both

CFS and FMS (see subsection "Socioeconomic Status" in the "Epidemiology" section earlier in this chapter).

Precipitating Factors

Precipitating factors trigger the illness in vulnerable persons.

Biological Factors

Infection.   Some evidence indicates that infection can precipitate CFS, and some, but less, evidence indicates that infection also may trigger FMS (Rea et al. 1999). Specific infections have been found to be associated with the subsequent development of CFS in 10%–40% of patients. These infections are Epstein-Barr virus (P.D. White et al. 2001), Q fever (Ayres et al. 1998), viral meningitis (Hotopf et al. 1996), and viral hepatitis (Berelowitz et al. 1995).

Injury.   The role of physical injury in the etiology of CFS and FMS has been controversial, in part because of the implications for legal liability and compensation. Limited evidence indicates that both conditions may be precipitated by injury, particularly to the neck. If a link exists, it is stronger for FMS (Al Allaf et al. 2002).

Psychological and Social Factors

Life stress.   Clinical experience indicated that patients often report the onset of CFS and FMS as occurring during or after a stressful period in their lives. The evidence for life stress or life events being a precipitant of FMS and CFS is, however, both limited and retrospective (Anderberg et al. 2000; Theorell et al. 1999).

Perpetuating Factors

Perpetuating factors are those that maintain a condition once it is established. They are clinically the most important because they are potential targets for treatment.

Biological Factors

Chronic infection.   There has been much interest in the potential role of ongoing infection and in associated immunological factors, especially in CFS. It was previously thought that chronic Epstein-Barr virus was a cause of CFS, but that hypothesis has been rejected. There have been numerous reports of evidence of chronic infection with other agents in both CFS and FMS, but none has been substantiated.

Immunological factors.   Immunological factors, especially cytokines, also have been much investigated in CFS and FMS, not only because of the possible triggering effect of infection but also because administration of immune active agents, such as interferons, is recognized as a cause of fatigue and myalgia (Vial and Descotes 1994). However, a recent systematic review found no evidence of any consistent immune abnormality in CFS (Lyall et al. 2003).

Muscular abnormalities and physiological deconditioning.   The bulk of evidence indicates that there are no proven pathological or biochemical abnormalities of muscle or muscle metabolism, either at rest or with exercise, other than those associated with deconditioning. *Deconditioning* describes the physiological changes that lead to the loss of tolerance of activity after prolonged rest (e.g., as a result of pain). It has been found in many, but not all, patients with CFS (Bazelmans et al. 2001; Fulcher and White 2000) and also in patients with FMS (Valim et al. 2002).

Sleep disorder.   Patients with CFS and FMS typically complain of unrefreshing and broken sleep, a symptom that has been objectively confirmed with polysomnography. Abnormalities in sleep have been claimed to be of major etiological importance, especially in FMS. Early work (Moldofsky et al. 1975) reported a specific sleep electroencephalogram abnormality of alpha wave intrusion into slow wave sleep (so-called alpha-delta sleep) and suggested that this was a cause of the myalgia. However, attempts to replicate this finding in both FMS and CFS have produced inconsistent results, and its specificity to chronic pain remains unclear (Rains and Penzien 2003).

Neuroendocrine changes. One of the best-supported biological abnormalities reported to be associated with both CFS and FMS is changes in neuroendocrine stress hormones. A repeated observation has been of a tendency to low blood levels of cortisol and a poor cortisol response to stress (Parker et al. 2001). This finding differs from what would be expected in depression (in which blood levels of cortisol are typically elevated) but is similar to that reported in other stress-induced and anxiety states. It is not known whether this is a primary abnormality or merely a consequence of inactivity or sleep disruption, however.

Patients with FMS also have an elevated level of substance P in their cerebrospinal fluid (Russell et al. 1994). A similar finding has been made in patients with other chronic pain syndromes such as osteoarthritis. However, elevated substance P has not been found in CFS patients (Evengard et al. 1998).

Blood pressure regulation. Failure to maintain blood pressure when assuming erect posture (orthostatic intolerance) and particularly a pattern in which the heart rate increases abnormally (postural orthostatic tachycardia syndrome) have been reported in both CFS (Rowe et al. 1995) and FMS (Bou-Holaigah et al. 1997). These findings have been interpreted as indicating abnormal autonomic nervous system function. However, postural hypotension occurs after prolonged inactivity (Sandler

and Vernikos 1986), and its specificity to CFS and FMS is unclear.

CNS structure. The brains of patients with CFS and FMS are probably structurally normal, although minor abnormalities have been reported in a minority of patients with CFS (Cook et al. 2001). A small proton magnetic resonance imaging study has suggested a deficiency of brain choline in CFS patients compared with healthy control subjects (Puri et al. 2002).

CNS function. It seems likely that these conditions are associated with changes in brain function, rather than structure. The use of functional brain imaging has great potential to elucidate the biology of these conditions but remains in its infancy.

Psychological and Social Factors
There is good evidence that psychological and behavioral factors play a major role in perpetuating CFS and FMS.

Depression. Depressive disorder is common in patients with CFS and fibromyalgia and is associated with persistence of symptoms (Joyce et al. 1997; McBeth et al. 2001). There is also some evidence that treatment for depression may improve outcome (see the later subsection Antidepressants, under Pharmacological Therapies).

Illness beliefs. Some of the striking aspects of CFS and FMS are the concern, and often strong beliefs, of many patients about the causes of such illnesses. Three categories of illness beliefs are considered here: 1) cause (attributions), 2) significance of symptoms (catastrophizing), and 3) what one is able to do despite symptoms (self-efficacy).

Although the cause of CFS and FMS is unknown, many patients, and especially those seen in specialist clinics, strongly attribute their symptoms to a physical disease (Neerinckx et al. 2000). A systematic review of prognostic studies in CFS found that such strong attributions predicted a poorer outcome (Joyce et al. 1997). The mechanism of this effect is unclear.

Catastrophizing is a tendency to make excessively negative predictions about symptoms, such as "If I do more, my pain or fatigue will keep getting worse and worse." Catastrophizing has been observed in patients with CFS (Petrie et al. 1995) and FMS (Hassett et al. 2000) and is associated with increased symptom vigilance, avoidance of activity, and more severe disability. Furthermore, a reduction in the belief that activity is damaging is associated with recovery during rehabilitative therapy (Deale et al. 1998), suggesting that it may be a critical psychological target for effective rehabilitation.

Self-efficacy—the belief that one can do something, despite symptoms—has been found to be low and to be associated with more severe disability in patients with CFS (Findley et al. 1998), FMS (Buckelew et al. 1996), and chronic pain (Asghari and Nicholas 2001). Achieving an increase in self-efficacy is another potential target for treatment that aims to improve function.

Behavioral factors. Patients cope with their symptoms in different ways. The way in which a patient copes will be influenced by his or her illness beliefs (Silver et al. 2002). Of particular interest is coping by avoiding any activity that the patient fears will exacerbate symptoms. This fear–avoidance phenomenon is well established in chronic pain patients (Philips 1987) and also has been observed in CFS (Afari et al. 2000) and in FMS (Davis et al. 2001).

Another potentially important coping behavior is the focusing of attention on symptoms—so-called symptom focusing or symptom vigilance (Roelofs et al. 2003). This behavior is, not surprisingly, associated with catastrophizing beliefs and

greater perceived symptom intensity; it offers another target for treatment.

Social factors. Patients' beliefs about their illness and associated coping behavior will be influenced by information received from others. A striking social aspect of CFS and FMS is the high level of activity in patient support and advocacy organizations, mainly over the Internet (Ross 1999). Studies from the United Kingdom have reported that patients who are members of a support group have a poorer outcome, despite similar illness duration and disability (Sharpe et al. 1992), and a poorer response to rehabilitation (Bentall et al. 2002). Perhaps unsurprisingly, the acquisition of a disability pension is also associated with a worse prognosis (Wigers 1996).

Summary

In summary, the evidence suggests that patients are predisposed to develop CFS and FMS by some combination of genetics, previous experience, and possibly lack of social support. Many patients with CFS have a history of preceding infection, and many patients with FMS point to an accident, injury, or trauma as the triggering event. Others can identify no precipitant. Most research has been into factors associated with established illness, so-called perpetuating factors, because these are both clearly more accessible to study and more relevant to treatment of established cases. Many biological factors have been investigated, with interest initially being directed at peripheral nerves and muscles and subsequently focusing on the CNS and its neuroendocrine and autonomic outputs. Also, some tantalizing findings have suggested but not yet established the role of immune factors. The physiological effects of inactivity seem to be important. Substantial evidence indicates the importance of psychological and behavioral factors, especially the fear of exacerbating symptoms and the associated avoidance of activity in both FMS and CFS. Social factors are more difficult to study but often are of striking importance clinically.

Models of Chronic Fatigue and Fibromyalgia Syndromes

The findings discussed in the previous section can be amalgamated into models. Three main models can be discerned that correspond approximately to biological, psychological, and social perspectives, although, in reality, all three are probably relevant.

Biological Model

It is well known that the immune system and the CNS and endocrine system interact and also have reciprocal relations with sleep and activity. It is thus possible to construct a tentative biological model in which these systems interact to perpetuate the illness (Moldofsky 1995). There seems to be stronger evidence for the role of infection in triggering CFS and for the role of trauma and changes in central pain processing in FMS. However, it is unclear whether these represent real differences or simply differences in the hypotheses pursued by researchers.

Cognitive-Behavioral Model

Whatever the biological aspects of these conditions, cognitive-behavioral models assume that the symptoms and disability are perpetuated, at least in part, by psychological, behavioral, and social factors. Biological factors are assumed to be either only partially responsible for the illness or largely reversible (Surawy et al. 1995). The cognitive-behavioral models for chronic pain and CFS have much in common (Philips

1987). Both emphasize the importance of fear of symptoms leading to a focusing on the symptoms, helplessness, and avoidance of activity. This model provides the rationale for behavioral and cognitive-behavioral approaches to rehabilitation (see section "Management" later in this chapter).

Social Model

The social model emphasizes the role of social factors in shaping the illness. A fight for the legitimacy of the syndrome as a chronic medical condition is central (Banks and Prior 2001). Patient advocacy has been strongly hostile to psychological and psychiatric involvement, probably because it is seen as undermining the legitimacy of the illness as a genuine medical condition. The social model proposes that patient organizations, while providing valuable social support, can also shape patients' illness beliefs, medical care, and disability payment seeking in ways that are not conducive to recovery (Shorter 1997).

Diagnostic Evaluation

Effective management of patients with possible CFS or FMS requires that 1) alternative medical and psychiatric diagnoses are considered and 2) the patient receives a comprehensive assessment so that collaborative management may be planned.

Identifying Medical and Psychiatric Conditions

Medical Differential Diagnosis

The medical differential diagnosis for CFS and FMS is a long one because many diseases present with pain and/or fatigue (Sharpe and Wilks 2002; Yunus 2002) (Table 9–4). Both a physical and a mental status examination must be performed in every case to determine any alternative medical and psychiatric diagnoses. As with many chronic diseases, particularly rheumatological conditions, time is often the principal arbiter because the conditions evolve clinically.

Routine investigations.   Initial investigation depends on the clinical signs, symptoms, and temporal nature of symptoms. When symptoms exceed 4–6 weeks, an initial basic screening workup is appropriate. If there are no specific indications for special investigations, the following have been found to be adequate as screening tests: thyrotropin, erythrocyte sedimentation rate (sensitive for any condition with systemic inflammation), complete blood count, basic chemistries, and withdrawal of some medications (particularly statins or 3-hydroxy-3-methylglutaryl coenzyme A reductase inhibitors; typical resolution of symptoms in 4–6 weeks).

Special investigations.   Special investigations should be carried out only if clearly indicated by history or examination. Immunological and virological tests are generally unhelpful as routine investigations and remain research tools. Sleep studies can be useful in excluding other diagnoses, especially when the fatigue is characterized by sleepiness. Diagnoses include sleep apnea, narcolepsy, nocturnal myoclonus, and periodic leg movements during sleep.

Medical misdiagnosis.   Those concerned about missing a serious medical diagnosis can be reassured that in most cases, the primary care physician's initial judgment in this regard is likely to be accurate (Khan et al. 2003). However, some evidence shows that CFS and FMS may be overdiagnosed by primary care physicians (Fitzcharles and Boulos 2003), and psychiatrists should feel able to request second medical opinions.

Psychiatric Differential Diagnosis

Underdiagnosis of psychiatric disorders is particularly common (Torres-Harding et al. 2002), probably reflecting a focus of the initial medical assessment on somatic symptoms and a tendency to disregard mood changes as simply being a consequence of these symptoms. The most important psychiatric diagnoses to consider are depressive and anxiety disorders because of their frequency and their implications for treatment. Depression may be masked and require expert assessment if it is to be detected. Panic attacks with agoraphobia may cause intermittent severe fatigue and disability. Somatoform disorders are common but have fewer implications for management. A diagnosis of somatization disorder indicates a poorer prognosis, and hypochondriasis indicates special attention to repeated reassurance seeking, which may perpetuate fears of undiagnosed disease (Sharpe and Williams 2001).

Assessment of the Illness

Other than to make diagnoses, the aims of the assessment are to 1) establish a collaborative relationship with the patient, 2) elicit the patient's own understanding of his or her illness and how he or she copes with it, and 3) identify current family and social factors such as employment and litigation that may complicate management. It is important to inquire fully about the patient's understanding of his or her illness (e.g., "What do you think is wrong with you?" or "What do you think the cause is?"). Patients may be fearful that their symptoms indicate a progressive, as yet undiagnosed, disease or that exertion will cause a long-term worsening of their condition. A formulation that identifies potential predisposing, precipitating, and perpetuating factors (see Table 9–3) is valuable both in providing an individualized explanation to the patient and for targeting interventions.

TABLE 9–4.   Medical differential diagnosis for patients with chronic fatigue syndrome (CFS) and fibromyalgia syndrome (FMS)

Relative frequency	Diagnoses	Syndrome	Differentiating clinical features	Initial workup
Very common (~1 per 100)	Thyroid disorders	CFS, FMS	Hypothyroidism: cold intolerance, slowed relaxation phase of reflexes, weight gain, elevated cholesterol Hyperthyroidism: heat intolerance, tremor, weight loss	Thyrotropin
	Medications (statins)	CFS, FMS	Symptom resolution with withdrawal of medication	Creatine kinase, aldolase
	Sleep apnea	CFS, FMS	Daytime somnolence, motor vehicle accidents, witnessed nighttime apnea and snoring, hypertension	Sleep study
	Spinal stenosis	FMS	History of osteoarthritis, degenerative disc disease, back pain with radiculopathy, sensory and/or motor deficits, pseudoclaudication	Nerve conduction study, electromyogram, magnetic resonance imaging of spine if neurological deficits
	Anemia	CFS	Pallor	Complete blood cell count
Common (~1 per 1,000)	Chronic infection: HIV, hepatitis C, endocarditis, osteomyelitis, Lyme disease, occult abscess	CFS, FMS	Infection-specific risk factors and signs (e.g., sexual habits, diabetes, fevers, murmur)	Serology, erythrocyte sedimentation rate, liver function tests, serial blood cultures, bone scan, indium scan
	Polymyalgia rheumatica	FMS	>60 years old	Erythrocyte sedimentation rate
	Cancer	CFS	Pallor, anemia, anorexia, weight loss, cachexia	Complete blood cell count, albumin, age-appropriate cancer screening studies
	Pulmonary condition: asthma, obstructive lung disease, interstitial lung disease	CFS	Shortness of breath, prominent exertional symptoms, smoking history, hypoxia	Chest X ray, pulmonary function tests, oxygenation saturation with exercise

TABLE 9–4. Medical differential diagnosis for patients with chronic fatigue syndrome (CFS) and fibromyalgia syndrome (FMS) *(continued)*

Relative frequency	Diagnoses	Syndrome	Differentiating clinical features	Initial workup
Common (~1 per 1,000) *(continued)*	Symptomatic hyperparathyroidism	CFS	Bone pain, nephrolithiasis, pancreatitis, renal insufficiency	Serum calcium and parathyroid hormone
Uncommon (~1 per 2,500–100,000)	Systemic lupus	FMS	Malar rash, joint pain	Antinuclear antibody, double-stranded DNA
	Rheumatoid arthritis	FMS	Symmetric synovitis, morning stiffness	Rheumatoid factor
	Polymyositis, dermatomyositis, myopathy	CFS, FMS	Proximal muscle weakness	Antinuclear antibody, creatine kinase, aldolase
	Myasthenia gravis, multiple sclerosis	CFS	Neurological findings: extinguishing strength with repetitive movements, ptosis, swallowing difficulties, optic neuritis, sensory deficits	Tensilon test, acetylcholine receptor antibodies, magnetic resonance imaging of brain
	Narcolepsy	CFS	Drop attacks, falling asleep during daily activities	Sleep study
	Inflammatory bowel disease (Crohn's)	CFS	Diarrhea, weight loss, fever, anemia	Serial fecal occult blood with endoscopy if positive

Management

Diagnosis, Formulation, and Management Plan

Forming a Therapeutic Relationship With the Patient

The patient often will have seen many other doctors and will have experienced problematic interactions with them (Asbring and Narvanen 2003). Other doctors may have offered overly biomedical or overly psychological explanations or even dismissed the patient completely.

Explaining Psychiatric Involvement

Psychiatrists' involvement in management may be interpreted by the patient as indicating that his or her condition is considered to be "all in his or her head." It is often best therefore to begin with a somatic assessment and to introduce discussion of psychological factors later. This can be done in a nonblaming and normalizing way. For example, "You have clearly had a terrible time made worse by not being believed. It is entirely understandable that this has gotten you down." It is generally unhelpful to force a psychiatric diagnosis on an unwilling patient. It is also important to explain how treatments commonly associated with psychiatry (particularly antidepressants and cognitive-behavioral therapy [CBT]) do not necessarily imply that the person is mentally ill. Rather, they can be explained as ways of normalizing brain and bodily function in conditions that are exacerbated by stress (Sharpe and Carson 2001).

Giving the Diagnosis

It is important to give the patient a positive diagnosis supplemented with an etiological formulation. Some controversy exists about whether giving patients a di-agnosis of CFS or FMS is helpful or harmful (Finestone 1997). Some who believe that a diagnosis is helpful argue that it enables patients to both conceptualize their illness and communicate about it with others (Sharpe 1998). Others who are concerned about the potentially harmful effect of diagnosis argue that it medicalizes and pathologizes symptoms in a way that can exacerbate social and occupational disability (Hadler 1996). It is our clinical experience that a positive diagnosis linked to an explanation of the potential reversibility of symptoms and a management plan to achieve this is an essential starting point for effective management.

Offering an Explanation

The explanation ideally should be scientifically accurate, acceptable to the patient, and congruent with the management plan. It can be explained that although the specific causes of CFS or FMS remain unknown, a combination of vulnerability and environmental stress likely to involve the brain and endocrine system is most likely. One such explanation is that the illness is a disorder of brain *function* rather than *structure*—that is, a functional nervous disorder (Stone et al. 2002).

Explaining the Management Plan

The management plan should be explained to the patient as following from the formulation, focusing on illness perpetuating factors and consisting of elements to 1) relieve symptoms such as depression, pain, and sleep disturbance with agents such as antidepressants; 2) assist the patient's efforts at coping by stabilizing activity and retraining the body to function effectively (graded exercise, CBT); and 3) assist the patient in managing the social and financial aspects of his or her illness and, when possible, remaining in or returning to employment (problem solving).

General Measures

Providing Advice on Symptom Management

One of the most important interventions the clinician can make is to encourage and guide patients in active self-management of the illness. Such advice will include the importance of being realistic about what they are able to accomplish without giving up hope for improvement in the future. It should involve advice on the pros and cons of self-medication, particularly with analgesics, and also might require a discussion of the potential benefits and risks of iatrogenic harm associated with seeking treatment from other practitioners, both conventional and alternative. The overall aim is to encourage the patients to feel that they can do things to manage the condition themselves, to accept the reality of their illness while still planning positively for the future, and to be cautious about seeking potentially harmful and expensive treatments. There are several evidence-based self-help books available (for example, Campling and Sharpe 2000, 2006).

Managing Activity and Avoidance

Once activity is stabilized and large fluctuations between excessive rest and unsustainable activity are reduced, gradual increases in activity can be advised. It is critical, however, to distinguish between carefully graded increases carried out in collaboration with the patient and a forced or an overambitious exercise regimen.

Managing Occupational and Social Factors

Patients who continue working may be overstressed by the effort of doing this. Those who have left work may have become inactive and demoralized and may not wish to return to the same job. These situations require a problem-solving approach to consider how to manage work demands, achieve a graded return to work, or plan an alternative career. Ongoing litigation is potentially a complicating factor because it reinforces (and may reward) the patient for remaining symptomatic and disabled.

Pharmacological Therapies

Most pharmacological treatment studies in CFS and FMS have focused on antidepressants, although various other agents have been advocated.

Antidepressants

Antidepressant drug treatment is indicated by the fact that 1) many patients with CFS or FMS have depressive and anxiety syndromes and 2) these agents reduce pain and improve sleep, even in the absence of depression. However, the evidence that antidepressants lead to an overall improvement in CFS and FMS is mixed, with the evidence being better for FMS (O'Malley et al. 2000) than for CFS (Reid et al. 2003).

The tricyclic antidepressants (TCAs) are probably more effective than the selective serotonin reuptake inhibitors (SSRIs) for relieving pain (Fishbain 2003) and for inducing sleep. Small doses (e.g., 25–50 mg of amitriptyline) are often adequate for these purposes (Arnold et al. 2000; O'Malley et al. 2000), but full doses are required to treat major depression.

Cyclobenzaprine, a tricyclic agent chemically similar to amitriptyline but used as a "muscle relaxant" rather than as an antidepressant, has been found to be effective in improving symptoms in FMS, especially pain and sleep disturbance (Tofferi et al. 2004).

SSRIs are generally better tolerated than TCAs. In CFS, fluoxetine was found in a large trial to be no more effective than placebo (Vercoulen et al. 1996). In FMS, one recent study found that patients who received fluoxetine (mean dose 45 mg) experienced a greater reduction in pain, fatigue, and depressed mood than did those who received placebo (Arnold et al. 2002); however, in a small previous trial, fluoxetine at a dosage of 20 mg/day did not have the same effect (Wolfe et al. 1994).

Other antidepressant agents also have been tried. Venlafaxine, a dual serotonin-norepinephrine reuptake inhibitor (SNRI), is useful for pain and has been reported as showing initial promise in both FMS (Dwight et al. 1998) and CFS (Goodnick 1996). A trial of duloxetine provided provisional evidence for the short-term efficacy of this agent in patients with fibromyalgia also (Arnold et al. 2005). Moclobemide, a reversible inhibitor of monoamine oxidase A, has been reported to be of no benefit in FMS but of some value in increasing energy in CFS (Hickie et al. 2000).

Other Pharmacological Agents

Patients with FMS and CFS frequently use nonsteroidal anti-inflammatory drugs (NSAIDs) to relieve pain. No evidence from clinical trials indicates that NSAIDs are effective when used alone, although they may be of some benefit in FMS when combined with amitriptyline (Goldenberg et al. 1986).

Opiates are occasionally used for pain in FMS and CFS. However, no trials of their use have been done, and a major concern is the development of dependence.

As with opiates, great caution is required with benzodiazepines because of the risk of dependence in patients with chronic conditions. TCAs are probably preferable to benzodiazepines for treating insomnia, and the chronic use of benzodiazepines should be reserved for patients with intractable anxiety.

Given the finding of low serum levels of cortisol, it is not surprising that corticosteroids have been tried. Prednisone was found to be ineffective in FMS (Clark et al. 1985). Hydrocortisone was reported to produce some benefit in CFS but was not recommended because of the long-term risks of adrenal suppression (Cleare et al. 1999). In CFS, fludrocortisone has been used in patients with orthostatic hypotension but has not been found to be of value (Rowe et al. 2001).

Serotonin$_3$ receptor antagonists (e.g., ondansetron and tropisetron) have analgesic effects (Kranzler et al. 2002). A randomized, placebo-controlled, double-blind trial in FMS found short-term benefit only with the lowest dosage (5 mg/day) (Farber et al. 2001). Trials of longer duration are needed.

Gabapentin has substantial analgesic effects, but its mechanism of action is unknown. There are only anecdotal reports of its successful use in FMS. Pregabalin, a drug still in clinical development that has pharmacological properties similar to those of gabapentin, also may have potential efficacy.

Amphetamines have been used in CFS with some evidence of short-term efficacy (Olson et al. 2003) but are not widely used because of the risk of dependence. In one small randomized crossover trial ($N=60$), the stimulant methylphenidate (10 mg twice daily for 4 weeks) was associated with improved fatigue, concentration, and functional status, at the cost of an increased incidence of dry mouth.

Summary

It is wise to exercise caution when prescribing pharmacological therapy for CFS and FMS. The mainstay of therapy continues to be the so-called antidepressant drugs, which may be helpful for mood, pain, and sleep but have limited effect on overall outcome. TCAs are preferred for nighttime sedation and pain, but an SSRI or an SNRI may be preferable as first-line treatment because of greater tolerability. In current clinical practice, although patients often receive low doses of antidepressants, higher doses may be required to achieve a therapeutic response. The increased interest in pharmacological treatment of functional syndromes in the past few years will likely expand treatment options, and several medications in clinical development show promise, including duloxetine, milnacipran, and pregabalin. However, the available evidence suggests that drug therapy has a limited role in the management of these conditions.

Specialist Nonpharmacological Treatments

If the patient does not respond to, or requires more active treatment than, the general and pharmacological management described above, referral for specialist therapy should be considered. For most patients, a rehabilitative outpatient program based on appropriately managed increases in activity, either as graded exercise therapy (GET) or as CBT, is indicated. Some patients may require inpatient multidisciplinary rehabilitation, although evidence of its efficacy is inadequate (Karjalainen et al. 2000).

Graded Exercise Therapy

GET is a structured progressive exercise program administered and carefully monitored by an exercise therapist. It also may be given in individual or group form, but the evidence is best for individually administered treatment (Fulcher and White 1998).

GET has been found in systematic review to be of benefit in both CFS and FMS. In FMS, four high-quality aerobic training studies (total 227 patients) reported significantly greater improvements in aerobic performance, tender point pain pressure threshold, and pain with exercise than with comparison treatments (Busch et al. 2002). In CFS, three high-quality trials (total 340 patients) all found benefits over comparison treatments in symptoms and disability. However, the number of dropouts in one study was substantial (Whiting et al. 2001). Of particular interest is a trial of brief simple education about the physiology and rationale of exercise that found the education to be as effective as CBT (Powell et al. 2001).

Cognitive-Behavioral Therapy

There are a variety of types of CBT (Williams 2003). Here, we refer to a collaborative psychologically informed type of rehabilitation that aims to achieve both graded increases in activity and changes in unhelpful beliefs and concerns about symptoms. It also may include problem solving for life and occupational dilemmas. It can be given in an individual or a group form, although more evidence exists for the efficacy of individual therapy (Sharpe 1997).

In CFS, individually administered CBT has now been found to be effective in two systematic reviews, with approximately two-thirds of the patients showing significant improvement. Three high-quality trials (total 164 patients) found improvement in both symptoms and disability and concluded that CBT appears to be an effective and acceptable treatment for adult outpatients with CFS (Price and Couper 2003; Whiting et al. 2001).

Although CBT is an established treatment for chronic pain (Morley et al. 1999) (see also Chapter 19, "Pain"), in FMS, only group CBT has been adequately evaluated in randomized trials. One trial reported no benefit (Vlaeyen et al. 1996), but a more recent study did find a clear advantage of group CBT over usual medical care (Williams et al. 2002). Further evaluation of the intensive individual CBT shown to be effective in CFS is required in FMS.

Nonresponsive Patients

Most patients respond to some degree to rehabilitative therapies, but many will achieve only partial improvement, and some will fail to improve at all. In such cases, the management is the same as that for other chronic conditions—to maximize functioning and quality of life while minimizing the risk of iatrogenic harm.

Conclusion

Although peripheral to both internal medicine and psychiatry, somatic syndromes such as chronic fatigue syndrome and fibromyalgia are core to the practice of psychosomatic medicine. A willingness and ability to integrate biological, psychological, and social factors is essential to both an adequate understanding of these syndromes' etiology and their effective management. The challenge that these syndromes present to the more narrow paradigms of the biomedical and psychopathological perspectives makes them an effective Trojan horse for those who seek to persuade others of the benefits of much greater integration of medical and psychiatric theory and practice.

References

Aaron LA, Buchwald D: Chronic diffuse musculoskeletal pain, fibromyalgia and comorbid unexplained clinical conditions: Bailliere's best practice and research. Clin Rheumatol 17:563–574, 2003

Afari N, Buchwald D: Chronic fatigue syndrome: a review. Am J Psychiatry 160:221–236, 2003

Afari N, Schmaling KB, Herrell R, et al: Coping strategies in twins with chronic fatigue and chronic fatigue syndrome. J Psychosom Res 48:547–554, 2000

Al Allaf AW, Dunbar KL, Hallum NS, et al: A case-control study examining the role of physical trauma in the onset of fibromyalgia syndrome. Rheumatology (Oxford) 41:450–453, 2002

American Psychiatric Association: Diagnostic and Statistical Manual of Mental Disorders, 4th Edition, Text Revision. Washington, DC, American Psychiatric Association, 2000

Anderberg UM, Marteinsdottir I, Theorell T, et al: The impact of life events in female patients with fibromyalgia and in female healthy controls. Eur Psychiatry 15:295–301, 2000

Arnold LM, Keck PE Jr, Welge JA: Antidepressant treatment of fibromyalgia: a meta-analysis and review. Psychosomatics 41:104–113, 2000

Arnold LM, Hess EV, Hudson JI, et al: A randomized, placebo-controlled, double-blind, flexible-dose study of fluoxetine in the treatment of women with fibromyalgia. Am J Med 112:191–197, 2002

Arnold LM, Rosen A, Pritchett YL, et al: A randomized, double-blind, placebo-controlled trial of duloxetine in the treatment of women with fibromyalgia with or without major depressive disorder. Pain 119 5–15, 2005

Asbring P, Narvanen AL: Ideal versus reality: physicians' perspectives on patients with chronic fatigue syndrome (CFS) and fibromyalgia. Soc Sci Med 57:711–720, 2003

Asghari A, Nicholas MK: Pain self-efficacy beliefs and pain behaviour: a prospective study. Pain 94:85–100, 2001

Assefi NP, Coy TV, Uslan D, et al: Financial, occupational, and personal consequences of disability in patients with chronic fatigue syndrome and fibromyalgia compared to other fatiguing conditions. J Rheumatol 30:804–808, 2003

Ayres JG, Flint N, Smith EG, et al: Post-infection fatigue syndrome following Q fever. Q J Med 91:105–123, 1998

Banks J, Prior L: Doing things with illness: the micro politics of the CFS clinic. Soc Sci Med 52:11–23, 2001

Bazelmans E, Vercoulen JH, Galama JMD, et al: Prevalence of chronic fatigue syndrome and primary fibromyalgia syndrome (PFS) in the Netherlands. Ned Tijdschr Geneeskd 141:1520–1523, 1997

Bazelmans E, Bleijenberg G, Van der Meer JW, et al: Is physical deconditioning a perpetuating factor in chronic fatigue syndrome? A controlled study on maximal exercise performance and relations with fatigue, impairment and physical activity. Psychol Med 31:107–114, 2001

Bentall RP, Powell P, Nye FJ, et al: Predictors of response to treatment for chronic fatigue syndrome. Br J Psychiatry 181:248–252, 2002

Berelowitz GJ, Burgess AP, Thanabalasingham T, et al: Post-hepatitis syndrome revisited. J Viral Hepat 2:133–138, 1995

Blockmans D, Persoons P, Van Houdenhove B, et al: Does methylphenidate reduce the symptoms of chronic fatigue syndrome? Am J Med 119:167.e23–30, 2006

Bombardier CH, Buchwald D: Chronic fatigue, chronic fatigue syndrome, and fibromyalgia: disability and health-care use. Med Care 34:924–930, 1996

Bou-Holaigah I, Calkins H, Flynn JA, et al: Provocation of hypotension and pain during upright tilt table testing in adults with fibromyalgia. Clin Exp Rheumatol 15:239–246, 1997

Buckelew SP, Huyser B, Hewett JE, et al: Self-efficacy predicting outcome among fibromyalgia subjects. Arthritis Care Res 9:97–104, 1996

Busch A, Schachter CL, Peloso PM, et al: Exercise for treating fibromyalgia syndrome. Cochrane Database Syst Rev 3: CD003786, 2002

Campling F, Sharpe M: Chronic Fatigue Syndrome: The Facts. Oxford, UK, Oxford University Press, 2000

Campling F, Sharpe M: Living With a Long-Term Illness: The Facts. Oxford, UK, Oxford University Press, 2006

Chalder T, Goodman R, Wessely S, et al: Epidemiology of chronic fatigue syndrome and self reported myalgic encephalomyelitis in 5–15 year olds: cross sectional study. BMJ 327:654–655, 2003

Ciccone DS, Natelson BH: Comorbid illness in women with chronic fatigue syndrome: a test of the single-syndrome hypothesis. Psychosom Med 65:268–275, 2003

Clark SR, Tindall E, Bennett RM: A double blind crossover trial of prednisone versus placebo in the treatment of fibrositis. J Rheumatol 12:980–983, 1985

Clauw DJ, Chrousos GP: Chronic pain and fatigue syndromes: overlapping clinical and neuroendocrine features and potential pathogenic mechanisms. Neuroimmunomodulation 4:134–153, 1997

Clauw DJ, Crofford LJ: Chronic widespread pain and fibromyalgia: what we know, and what we need to know. Bailliere's best practice and research. Clin Rheumatol 17:685–701, 2003

Cleare AJ, Heap E, Malhi GS, et al: Low-dose hydrocortisone in chronic fatigue syndrome: a randomised crossover trial. Lancet 353:455–458, 1999

Cohen H, Neumann L, Haiman Y, et al: Prevalence of post-traumatic stress disorder in fibromyalgia patients: overlapping syndromes or post-traumatic fibromyalgia syndrome? Semin Arthritis Rheum 32:38–50, 2002

Cook DB, Lange G, DeLuca J, et al: Relationship of brain MRI abnormalities and physical functional status in chronic fatigue syndrome. Int J Neurosci 107:1–6, 2001

Croft P, Rigby AS, Boswell R, et al: The prevalence of chronic widespread pain in the general population. J Rheumatol 20: 710–713, 1993

Croft P, Burt J, Schollum J, et al: More pain, more tender points: is fibromyalgia just one end of a continuous spectrum? Ann Rheum Dis 55:482–485, 1996

Davis MC, Zautra AJ, Reich JW: Vulnerability to stress among women in chronic pain from fibromyalgia and osteoarthritis. Annals of Behavioural Medicine 23:215–226, 2001

Deale A, Chalder T, Wessely S: Illness beliefs and treatment outcome in chronic fatigue syndrome. J Psychosom Res 45: 77–83, 1998

Dwight MM, Arnold LM, O'Brien H, et al: An open clinical trial of venlafaxine treatment of fibromyalgia. Psychosomatics 39:14–17, 1998

Engel GL: The need for a new medical model: a challenge for biomedicine. Science 196:129–196, 1977

Epstein SA, Kay G, Clauw D, et al: Psychiatric disorders in patients with fibromyalgia: a multicenter investigation. Psychosomatics 40:57–63, 1999

Evengard B, Nilsson CG, Lindh G, et al: Chronic fatigue syndrome differs from fibromyalgia: no evidence for elevated substance P levels in cerebrospinal fluid of patients with chronic fatigue syndrome. Pain 78:153–155, 1998

Farber L, Stratz TH, Bruckle W, et al: Short-term treatment of primary fibromyalgia with the 5-HT3-receptor antagonist tropisetron: results of a randomized, double-blind, placebo-controlled multicenter trial in 418 patients. Int J Clin Pharmacol Res 21:1–13, 2001

Findley JC, Kerns R, Weinberg LD, et al: Self-efficacy as a psychological moderator of chronic fatigue syndrome. J Behav Med 21:351–362, 1998

Finestone AJ: A doctor's dilemma: is a diagnosis disabling or enabling? Arch Intern Med 157:491–492, 1997

Fischler B, Cluydts R, De Gucht Y, et al: Generalized anxiety disorder in chronic fatigue syndrome. Acta Psychiatr Scand 95:405–413, 1997

Fishbain DA: Analgesic effects of antidepressants. J Clin Psychiatry 64:96–97, 2003

Fitzcharles MA, Boulos P: Inaccuracy in the diagnosis of fibromyalgia syndrome: analysis of referrals. Rheumatology (Oxford) 42:263–267, 2003

Fukuda K, Straus SE, Hickie IB, et al: Chronic fatigue syndrome: a comprehensive approach to its definition and management. Ann Intern Med 121:953–959, 1994

Fulcher KY, White PD: Chronic fatigue syndrome: a description of graded exercise treatment. Physiotherapy 84:223–226, 1998

Fulcher KY, White PD: Strength and physiological response to exercise in patients with chronic fatigue syndrome. J Neurol Neurosurg Psychiatry 69:302–307, 2000

Goldenberg DL, Felson DT, Dinerman H: A randomized, controlled trial of amitriptyline and naproxen in the treatment of patients with fibromyalgia. Arthritis Rheum 29:1371–1377, 1986

Goodnick PJ: Treatment of chronic fatigue syndrome with venlafaxine (letter). Am J Psychiatry 153:294, 1996

Gowers WR: A lecture on lumbago: its lessons and analogues. BMJ 1:117–121, 1904

Granges G, Zilko P, Littlejohn GO: Fibromyalgia syndrome: assessment of the severity of the condition 2 years after diagnosis. J Rheumatol 21:523–529, 1994

Hadler NM: Fibromyalgia, chronic fatigue, and other iatrogenic diagnostic algorithms: do some labels escalate illness in vulnerable patients? Postgrad Med 102:161–162, 1996

Hassett AL, Cone JD, Patella SJ, et al: The role of catastrophizing in the pain and depression of women with fibromyalgia syndrome. Arthritis Rheum 43:2493–2500, 2000

Henningsen P, Zimmermann T, Sattel H: Medically unexplained physical symptoms, anxiety, and depression: a meta-analytic review. Psychosom Med 65:528–533, 2003

Hickie IB, Wilson AJ, Wright JM, et al: A randomized, double-blind placebo-controlled trial of moclobemide in patients with chronic fatigue syndrome. J Clin Psychiatry 61:643–648, 2000

Hill NF, Tiersky LA, Scavalla VR, et al: Natural history of severe chronic fatigue syndrome. Arch Phys Med Rehabil 80:1090–1094, 1999

Holmes GP, Kaplan JE, Gantz NM, et al: Chronic fatigue syndrome: a working case definition. Ann Intern Med 108:387–389, 1988

Hotopf MH, Noah N, Wessely S: Chronic fatigue and minor psychiatric morbidity after viral meningitis: a controlled study. J Neurol Neurosurg Psychiatry 60:504–509, 1996

Hudson JI, Pope HG: The concept of affective spectrum disorder: relationship to fibromyalgia and other syndromes of chronic fatigue and chronic muscle pain. Baillieres Clin Rheumatol 8:839–856, 1994

Hudson JI, Pope HG Jr: The relationship between fibromyalgia and major depressive disorder. Rheum Dis Clin North Am 22:285–303, 1996

Jason LA, Richman JA, Rademaker AW, et al: A community-based study of chronic fatigue syndrome. Arch Intern Med 159:2129–2137, 1999

Johnson SK, DeLuca J, Natelson BH: Assessing somatization disorder in the chronic fatigue syndrome. Psychosom Med 58:50–57, 1996

Joyce J, Hotopf M, Wessely S: The prognosis of chronic fatigue and chronic fatigue syndrome: a systematic review. Q J Med 90:223–233, 1997

Karjalainen K, Malmivaara A, van Tulder M, et al: Multidisciplinary rehabilitation for fibromyalgia and musculoskeletal pain in working age adults. Cochrane Database Syst Rev 2, 2000

Katon W, Buchwald DS, Simon GE, et al: Psychiatric illness in patients with chronic fatigue and rheumatoid arthritis. J Gen Intern Med 6:277–285, 1991

Khan AA, Khan A, Harezlak J, et al: Somatic symptoms in primary care: etiology and outcome. Psychosomatics 44:471–478, 2003

Kranzler JD, Gendreau JF, Rao SG: The psychopharmacology of fibromyalgia: a drug development perspective. Psychopharmacol Bull 36:165–213, 2002

Kruesi MJ, Dale JK, Straus SE: Psychiatric diagnoses in patients who have chronic fatigue syndrome. J Clin Psychiatry 50:53–56, 1989

Kurtze N, Svebak S: Fatigue and patterns of pain in fibromyalgia: correlations with anxiety, depression and co-morbidity in a female county sample. Br J Med Psychol 74:523–537, 2001

Lyall M, Peakman M, Wessely S: A systematic review and critical evaluation of the immunology of chronic fatigue syndrome. J Psychosom Res 55:79–90, 2003

Makela MO: Is fibromyalgia a distinct clinical entity? The epidemiologist's evidence. Baillieres Best Pract Res Clin Rheumatol 13:415–419, 1999

Manu P, Matthews DA, Lane TJ: Panic disorder among patients with chronic fatigue. South Med J 84:451–456, 1991

Mayou R, Levenson J, Sharpe M: Somatoform disorders in DSM-V. Psychosomatics 44:449–451, 2003

McBeth J, Macfarlane GJ, Hunt IM, et al: Risk factors for persistent chronic widespread pain: a community-based study. Rheumatology (Oxford) 40:95–101, 2001

Moldofsky H: Sleep, neuroimmune and neuroendocrine functions in fibromyalgia and chronic fatigue syndrome. Adv Neuroimmunol 5:39–56, 1995

Moldofsky H, Scarisbrick P, England R, et al: Musculoskeletal symptoms and Non-REM sleep disturbances in patients with fibrositis syndrome and healthy subjects. Psychosom Med 37:341–351, 1975

Morley S, Eccleston C, Williams A: Systematic review and meta-analysis of randomized controlled trials of cognitive behaviour therapy and behaviour therapy for chronic pain in adults, excluding headache. Pain 80:1–13, 1999

Neerinckx E, Van Houdenhove B, Lysens R, et al: Attributions in chronic fatigue syndrome and fibromyalgia syndrome in tertiary care. J Rheumatol 27:1051–1055, 2000

Nisenbaum R, Jones JF, Unger ER, et al: A population-based study of the clinical course of chronic fatigue syndrome. Health Qual Life Outcomes 1:49, 2003

Ohayon MM, Schatzberg AF: Using chronic pain to predict depressive morbidity in the general population. Arch Gen Psychiatry 60:39–47, 2003

Olson LG, Ambrogetti A, Sutherland DC: A pilot randomized controlled trial of dexamphetamine in patients with chronic fatigue syndrome. Psychosomatics 44:38–43, 2003

O'Malley PG, Balden E, Tomkins G, et al: Treatment of fibromyalgia with antidepressants: a meta-analysis. J Gen Intern Med 15:659–666, 2000

Parker AJ, Wessely S, Cleare AJ: The neuroendocrinology of chronic fatigue syndrome and fibromyalgia. Psychol Med 31:1331–1345, 2001

Petrie KJ, Moss-Morris R, Weinman J: The impact of catastrophic beliefs on functioning in chronic fatigue syndrome. J Psychosom Res 39:31–38, 1995

Philips HC: Avoidance behaviour and its role in sustaining chronic pain. Behav Res Ther 25:273–279, 1987

Powell P, Bentall RP, Nye FJ, et al: Randomised controlled trial of patient education to encourage graded exercise in chronic fatigue syndrome. BMJ 322:387–390, 2001

Price JR, Couper J: Cognitive behaviour therapy for chronic fatigue syndrome in adults. Cochrane Database Syst Rev 4, 2003

Puri BK, Counsell SJ, Zaman R, et al: Relative increase in choline in the occipital cortex in chronic fatigue syndrome. Acta Psychiatr Scand 106:224–226, 2002

Rains JC, Penzien DB: Sleep and chronic pain: challenges to the alpha-EEG sleep pattern as a pain specific sleep anomaly. J Psychosom Res 54:77–83, 2003

Rea T, Russo J, Katon W, et al: A prospective study of tender points and fibromyalgia during and after an acute viral infection. Arch Intern Med 159:865–870, 1999

Reeves WC, Lloyd A, Vernon SD, et al: Identification of ambiguities in the 1994 chronic fatigue syndrome research case definition and recommendations for resolution. BMC Health Serv Res 3:25, 2003

Reid S, Chalder T, Cleare A, et al: Chronic fatigue syndrome. Clin Evid 9:1172–1185, 2003

Reyes M, Nisenbaum R, Hoaglin DC, et al: Prevalence and incidence of chronic fatigue syndrome in Wichita, Kansas. Arch Intern Med 163:1530–1536, 2003

Roelofs J, Peters ML, McCracken L, et al: The pain vigilance and awareness questionnaire (PVAQ): further psychometric evaluation in fibromyalgia and other chronic pain syndromes. Pain 101:299–306, 2003

Ross SE: "Memes" as infectious agents in psychosomatic illness. Ann Intern Med 131:867–871, 1999

Rowe PC, Bou Holaigah I, Kan JS, et al: Is neurally mediated hypotension an unrecognised cause of chronic fatigue? Lancet 345:623–624, 1995

Rowe PC, Calkins H, DeBusk K, et al: Fludrocortisone acetate to treat neurally mediated hypotension in chronic fatigue syndrome: a randomized controlled trial. JAMA 285:52–59, 2001

Russell IJ, Orr MD, Littman B, et al: Elevated cerebrospinal fluid levels of substance P in patients with the fibromyalgia syndrome. Arthritis Rheum 37:1593–1601, 1994

Sandler H, Vernikos J: Inactivity: Physiological Effects. London, Academic Press, 1986

Sartorius N, Ustun TB, Costa e Silva JA, et al: An international study of psychological problems in primary care: preliminary report from the World Health Organization collaborative project on psychological problems in general health care. Arch Gen Psychiatry 50:819–824, 1993

Sharpe M: Chronic fatigue syndrome. Psychiatr Clin North Am 19:549–574, 1996

Sharpe M: Cognitive behavior therapy for functional somatic complaints: the example of chronic fatigue syndrome. Psychosomatics 38:356–362, 1997

Sharpe M: Doctors' diagnoses and patients' perceptions: lessons from chronic fatigue syndrome. Gen Hosp Psychiatry 20: 335–338, 1998

Sharpe M, Carson A: "Unexplained" somatic symptoms, functional syndromes, and somatization: do we need a paradigm shift? Ann Intern Med 134(9 Pt 2):926–930, 2001

Sharpe M, Wilks D: ABC of psychological medicine: fatigue. BMJ 325:480–483, 2002

Sharpe M, Williams A: Treating patients with hypochondriasis and somatoform pain disorder, in Psychological Approaches to Pain Management. Edited by Turk DC, Gatchel RJ. New York, Guilford, 2001, pp 515–533

Sharpe M, Hawton KE, Seagroatt V, et al: Patients who present with fatigue: a follow up of referrals to an infectious diseases clinic. BMJ 305:147–152, 1992

Shorter E: Somatization and chronic pain in historic perspective. Clin Orthop 336:52–60, 1997

Silver A, Haeney M, Vijayadurai P, et al: The role of fear of physical movement and activity in chronic fatigue syndrome. J Psychosom Res 52:485–493, 2002

Skapinakis P: Clarifying the relationship between unexplained chronic fatigue and psychiatric morbidity: results from a community survey in Great Britain. Am J Psychiatry 157: 1492–1498, 2000

Skapinakis P, Lewis G, Mavreas V: Unexplained fatigue syndromes in a multinational primary care sample: specificity of definition and prevalence and distinctiveness from depression and generalized anxiety. Am J Psychiatry 160:785–787, 2003

Stone J, Wojcik W, Durrance D, et al: What should we say to patients with symptoms unexplained by disease? The number needed to offend. BMJ 325:1449–1450, 2002

Sullivan PF, Smith W, Buchwald D: Latent class analysis of symptoms associated with chronic fatigue syndrome and fibromyalgia. Psychol Med 32:881–888, 2002

Surawy C, Hackmann A, Hawton KE, et al: Chronic fatigue syndrome: a cognitive approach. Behav Res Ther 33:535–544, 1995

Taylor RR, Jason LA: Chronic fatigue and sociodemographic characteristics as predictors of psychiatric disorders in a community-based sample. Psychosom Med 65:896–901, 2003

Theorell T, Blomkvist V, Lindh G, et al: Critical life events, infections, and symptoms during the year preceding chronic fatigue syndrome (CFS): an examination of CFS patients and subjects with a nonspecific life crisis. Psychosom Med 61:304–310, 1999

Tofferi J, Jackson JL, O'Malley PG: Treatment of fibromyalgia with cyclobenzaprine: a meta-analysis. Arthritis Rheum 51:9–13, 2004

Torres-Harding SR, Jason LA, Cane V, et al: Physicians' diagnoses of psychiatric disorders for people with chronic fatigue syndrome. Int J Psychiatry Med 32:109–124, 2002

Valim V, Oliveira LM, Suda AL, et al: Peak oxygen uptake and ventilatory anaerobic threshold in fibromyalgia. J Rheumatol 29:353–357, 2002

van der Werf SP, de Vree B, Alberts M, et al: Natural course and predicting self-reported improvement in patients with chronic fatigue syndrome with a relatively short illness duration. J Psychosom Res 53:749–753, 2002

Van Houdenhove B, Neerinckx E, Lysens R, et al: Victimization in chronic fatigue syndrome and fibromyalgia in tertiary care: a controlled study on prevalence and characteristics. Psychosomatics 42:21–28, 2001

Vercoulen JH, Swanink CM, Zitman FG, et al: Randomized, double-blind, placebo-controlled study of fluoxetine in chronic fatigue syndrome. Lancet 347:858–861, 1996

Vial T, Descotes J: Clinical toxicity of the interferons. Drug Saf 10:115–150, 1994

Vlaeyen JW, Teeken-Gruben NJ, Goossens ME, et al: Cognitive-educational treatment of fibromyalgia: a randomized clinical trial, I: clinical effects. J Rheumatol 23: 1237–1245, 1996

Walker EA, Keegan D, Gardner G, et al: Psychosocial factors in fibromyalgia compared with rheumatoid arthritis, I: sexual, physical, and emotional abuse and neglect. Psychosom Med 59:572–577, 1997a

Walker EA, Keegan D, Gardner G, et al: Psychosocial factors in fibromyalgia compared with rheumatoid arthritis, II: psychiatric diagnoses and functional disability. Psychosom Med 59:565–571, 1997b

Wessely S: Old wine in new bottles: neurasthenia and M.E. Psychol Med 20:35–53, 1990

Wessely S, Nimnuan C, Sharpe M: Functional somatic syndromes: one or many? Lancet 354:936–939, 1999

White KP, Speechley M, Harth M, et al: The London Fibromyalgia Epidemiology Study: the prevalence of fibromyalgia syndrome in London, Ontario. J Rheumatol 26:1570–1576, 1999

White PD, Thomas JM, Kangro HO, et al: Predictions and associations of fatigue syndromes and mood disorders that occur after infectious mononucleosis. Lancet 358:1946–1954, 2001

Whiting P, Bagnall A, Sowden A, et al: Interventions for the treatment and management of chronic fatigue syndrome: a systematic review. JAMA 286:1360–1368, 2001

Wigers SH: Fibromyalgia outcome: the predictive values of symptom duration, physical activity, disability pension, and critical life events—a 4.5 year prospective study. J Psychosom Res 41:235–243, 1996

Williams DA: Psychological and behavioural therapies in fibromyalgia and related syndromes. Baillieres Best Pract Res Clin Rheumatol 17:649–665, 2003

Williams DA, Cary MA, Groner KH, et al: Improving physical functional status in patients with fibromyalgia: a brief cognitive behavioral intervention. J Rheumatol 29:1280–1286, 2002

Wolfe F: The relation between tender points and fibromyalgia symptom variables: evidence that fibromyalgia is not a discrete disorder in the clinic. Ann Rheum Dis 56:268–271, 1997

Wolfe F, Smythe HA, Yunus MB, et al: The American College of Rheumatology 1990 criteria for the classification of fibromyalgia: report of the Multicenter Criteria Committee. Arthritis Rheum 33:160–172, 1990

Wolfe F, Cathey MA, Hawley DJ: A double-blind placebo controlled trial of fluoxetine in fibromyalgia. Scand J Rheumatol 23:255–259, 1994

Wolfe F, Ross K, Anderson JA, et al: The prevalence and characteristics of fibromyalgia in the general population. Arthritis Rheum 38:19–28, 1995

Wolfe F, Anderson J, Harkness D, et al: Health status and disease severity in fibromyalgia: results of a six-center longitudinal study. Arthritis Rheum 40:1571–1579, 1997

World Health Organization: International Statistical Classification of Diseases and Related Health Problems, 10th Revision. Geneva, World Health Organization, 1992

Yunus MB: A comprehensive medical evaluation of patients with fibromyalgia syndrome. Rheum Dis Clin North Am 28:201–205, 2002

Self-Assessment Questions

Select the single best response for each question.

1. All of the following psychiatric disorders are among the exclusion criteria for chronic fatigue syndrome *except*

   A. Dementia.
   B. Anorexia or bulimia nervosa.
   C. Unipolar depression without melancholia.
   D. Alcohol or substance misuse.
   E. Bipolar depression.

2. The American College of Rheumatology (ACR) has developed diagnostic criteria for fibromyalgia. Which of the following is/are included in the criteria?

   A. Widespread pain.
   B. Symptom duration of at least 1 year.
   C. Pain at 11 or more of 18 specific sites on the body.
   D. A and C.
   E. A, B, and C.

3. Which of the following psychiatric disorders is most commonly found in patients with chronic fatigue syndrome or fibromyalgia syndrome?

   A. Depression.
   B. Psychosis.
   C. Anxiety.
   D. A and C.
   E. A, B, and C.

4. Which of the following is one of the best-supported biological abnormalities reported to be associated with both chronic fatigue syndrome and fibromyalgia syndrome?

   A. Low blood levels of cortisol.
   B. High blood levels of cortisol.
   C. Low cerebrospinal fluid (CSF) levels of substance P.
   D. Elevated blood pressure.
   E. Abnormalities of muscle metabolism.

5. All of the following medical disorders are commonly found in patients evaluated for either chronic fatigue syndrome or fibromyalgia syndrome *except*

   A. Sleep apnea.
   B. Rheumatoid arthritis.
   C. Spinal stenosis.
   D. Anemia.
   E. Thyroid disorders.

10 Infectious Diseases

James L. Levenson, M.D.
Robert K. Schneider, M.D.

PSYCHIATRIC SYMPTOMS ARE part of the clinical presentation of many systemic and central nervous system (CNS) infectious processes. Rapid cultural and economic changes affecting regional and international mobility, sexuality, and other behaviors have led to worldwide spread of new epidemics (e.g., HIV, severe acute respiratory syndrome [SARS] [Cheng et al. 2004]) and more limited spread of previously geographically isolated diseases (e.g., cysticercosis) (Power and Johnson 2005). Infectious diseases have been considered as contributing to the pathogenesis of psychiatric disorders (e.g., viral antibodies in schizophrenia). Causal links between specific infections and a subset of psychiatric syndromes (e.g., pediatric autoimmune neuropsychiatric disorder associated with streptococcal infection [PANDAS]) provide intriguing models of etiology. Controversy surrounds some attributions of psychopathology to infectious pathophysiology (e.g., Lyme disease, Epstein-Barr virus [EBV]).

Consulting psychiatrists should carefully consider relevant aspects of patients' histories, including immune status, regions of origin and residence, travel, high-risk sexual behaviors, occupation, and recreational activities. Physicians must consider which infectious diseases are endemic in the practice area and in the areas where the patient has traveled or resided. Similar psychiatric symptoms might suggest possible Lyme disease in a hiker in the northeastern United States and neurocysticercosis in an immigrant from Central America.

Many brain diseases or injuries, as well as the effects of aging, render patients more vulnerable to neuropsychiatric effects of even limited infectious diseases. For example, a simple upper respiratory or bladder infection may cause only discomfort in an otherwise healthy individual but agitation, irritability, and frank delirium in the elderly, especially in patients who also have dementia. The reasons that older age and brain disease would make patients vulnerable to delirium with minor infections are not understood but may involve changes in immune function (Prio et al. 2002) and the blood-brain barrier.

Psychological factors may significantly affect the risk for and course of infectious diseases, with HIV as the most studied example. Psychological factors have been shown to influence other infectious diseases as well, including the common cold (Takkouche et al. 2000), pneumonia (Mehr et al. 2001), genital herpes (Levenson et al. 1987), hepatitis B and C infection (Osher et al. 2003), and recurrent urinary tract infections (Hunt and Waller 1992). Several studies have convincingly shown that psychological stress suppresses the secondary (but not primary) antibody response to immunization (Cohen et al. 2001).

This chapter covers bacterial, viral (except HIV/AIDS; see Chapter 11), fungal, and parasitic infections; psychiatric side effects of antimicrobial drugs and their interactions with psychotropic medications; and psychiatric aspects of immunization.

Occult Infections

Occult infections by definition are concealed, often requiring detective work. Such infections may occur essentially anywhere in the body (see Table 10–1). Psychiatric symptoms may result from even a small focus of chronic infection (e.g., Yamasaki et al. 1997). The most likely psychiatric symptoms are subtle cognitive dysfunction or mood change consistent with a mild encephalopathy, but depression, psychosis, and delirium also may occur.

The diagnosis is suggested by secondary signs of infection, specifically temperature dysregulation and increases in white blood cell count, granulocyte count, or sedimentation rate. A careful history and physical examination may identify overlooked clues to guide the search (e.g.,

TABLE 10–1.   Occult infections that may cause psychiatric symptoms

Sinusitis

Chronic otitis

Abscess (e.g., dental, lung, intra-abdominal, retroperitoneal, perirectal)

Bronchiectasis

Endocarditis

Cholecystitis

Parasitosis

Urinary tract infection

Pelvic inflammatory disease

Osteomyelitis

Subclinical systemic infections (e.g., HIV, tuberculosis)

chronic toothache or lymphadenopathy). If repeat history and physical examination are not fruitful, other studies may be needed.

Bacterial Infections

Bacteremia and Sepsis

Systemic symptoms of sepsis, including CNS symptoms, may result from bacterial toxins, release of cytokines, hyperthermia, shock, acute renal insufficiency, pulmonary failure, coagulopathy, disruption of the blood-brain barrier, and spread of the organism into the CNS and other organs. An acute change in mental status may be the first sign of impending sepsis and may precede the development of fever. Any patient who has an abrupt change in mental status in concert with a shaking chill should be presumed to have a high risk for impending sepsis.

Septic encephalopathy occurs more frequently than is generally assumed. Its severity is associated with the severity of overall illness, and it is often part of multiorgan failure (Zauner et al. 2002). Symptoms of posttraumatic stress disorder recently have been recognized as very common following septic shock (Schelling et al. 2001).

Toxic Shock Syndrome

Toxic shock syndrome (TSS) is typically caused by either *Staphylococcus aureus* or *Streptococcus pyogenes*, with the latter much more common currently. TSS generally manifests with rapid onset of fever, rash, and hypotension and is a multisystem disease with at least three organ systems involved, very often including the CNS. Most cases of TSS are associated with a wound and/or foreign body. Most staphylococcal TSS occurs in young menstruating white women (the proportion of menstrual cases has decreased following removal of superabsorbent tampons from the market) but can occur at any age, even in early childhood (Van Lierde et al. 1997). TSS should be suspected in any patient with a recent wound who acutely develops unexplained pain, lethargy, and confusion and may occur even when a surgical wound appears not to be inflamed.

There may be a prodromal period of 2–3 days of malaise, myalgia, and chills followed by confusion and lethargy. Confusion, weakness, and headache rapidly progress to hypotension and shock. CNS sequelae may persist for years and include deficits in memory, computation, and concentration (Rosene et al. 1982).

Pediatric Autoimmune Neuropsychiatric Disorder Associated With Streptococcal Infection

PANDAS is an autoimmune model of neuropsychiatric disease (Swedo and Grant 2005). PANDAS is not a diagnosis but an acronym for the clinical characteristics of a subgroup of children whose obsessive-compulsive and tic disorders seem to have been triggered by an infection with group A beta-hemolytic streptococci (GABHS). The syndrome is defined by early childhood onset of symptoms; an episodic course characterized by abrupt onset of symptoms with frequent relapses and remissions; associated neurological signs, especially tics; and temporal association with GABHS infections (most commonly pharyngitis) (Swedo et al. 1997). The best way to show the association between recent GABHS infection and PANDAS symptoms is to document a rapid rise in antistreptococcal (ASO) titers associated with symptom onset or exacerbation and a decrease in titers associated with symptom resolution or improvement. Children with PANDAS also may have behavioral symptoms (e.g., attention deficits and hyperactivity) (Perlmutter et al. 1998; Swedo et al. 1998). GABHS may play a role in Tourette's syndrome as well (Church et al. 2003). Adult onset of illness fulfilling criteria for PANDAS has been reported (Bodner et al. 2001).

In addition to ASO titers, a throat culture should be obtained (Swedo et al. 1998). Prompt antibiotic treatment may prevent the expected rise in ASO titers. Although PANDAS is conceptualized as an autoimmune disorder, antibiotics active against GABHS may be beneficial in reducing current symptoms (Snider et al. 2005). Children with uncomplicated strep infections treated with antibiotics appear to have no increased risk for PANDAS (Perrin et al. 2004).

Bacterial Endocarditis

Bacterial endocarditis may cause neuropsychiatric symptoms at all stages of the disease, via focal, systemic, and CNS disease processes. Osler first described the triad of fever, heart murmur, and cerebral infarction in 1885. Among causes, rheumatic heart disease has decreased, while senescent valvular disease, prosthetic valve placement, and intravenous drug use have increased. Malaise and fatigue may present before progression of the infection is evident. Neuropsychiatric deficits resulting from septic emboli will reflect which cerebral vessels have been affected (Singhal et al. 2002). The most common psychiatric symptoms are those of diffuse encephalopathy, which may occur at any stage of infection. Their onset may be insidious to acute, paralleling the course of the endocarditis.

Diagnosis is based on clinical history and physical examination, particularly looking for new or changing heart murmurs, signs of microembolism (splinter hemorrhages, retinal hemorrhages, microscopic hematuria), positive blood cultures, and echocardiography.

Rocky Mountain Spotted Fever

Rocky Mountain spotted fever (RMSF) is a tickborne rickettsial disease peaking May through September. Its name is misleading because in the United States half of the cases are in the South Atlantic region, and rickettsial spotted fevers occur worldwide. RMSF typically includes fever and a rash characterized by erythematous macules that later progress to maculopapular lesions with central petechiae. Initially appearing as a nonspecific severe febrile illness, the diagnosis is seldom suspected until the rash appears. CNS involvement, including lethargy, confusion, and occasionally fulminant delirium, occurs in 25% of cases. Subtle changes such as irritability, personality changes, and apathy may occur before the rash, particularly in children. While abnormalities on computed tomography or magnetic resonance imaging (MRI) of the brain may include infarctions or cerebral edema, 80% of RMSF patients with normal scans have symptoms of encephalopathy (Bonawitz et al. 1997). Cognitive dysfunction persisting months after resolution of the acute illness has been reported (Bergeron et al. 1997).

Typhus Fevers

Rickettsia bacteria also cause typhus. Mouse-borne typhus usually occurs in epidemics related to war or famine when communal hygiene deteriorates. Flea-borne typhus is associated with rodents. The annual disease frequency in the United States was 2,000–5,000 cases in the 1940s. It is now fewer than 100, with most in Texas, as a result of rat control programs. Clinical manifestations, diagnosis, and treatment of typhus are similar to RMSF. The psychiatric manifestations are confusion, lethargy, and particularly headache in a febrile illness with rash. The delirium of typhus and typhoid has been classically described as having a peculiar preoccupied nature, with patients picking at the bedclothes and imaginary objects (Verghese 1985). The word *typhus* in Greek means "cloud" or "mist," a term Hippocrates used to describe clouded mental status in patients with unremitting fevers.

Typhoid Fever

Typhoid fever is an enteric fever caused by salmonellae. The incidence of typhoid fever has steadily declined in the United States because of improved sanitation. Sixty percent of the cases in the United States are acquired outside the country, most often in Mexico and India.

Abdominal pain, headache, and fever are the classic presentation. However, when typhoid fever is endemic or not treated promptly, psychiatric symptoms appear. *Salmonella typhi* enters a bacteremic phase and can localize in the CNS. High fever and electrolyte imbalances may cause encephalopathy, with delirium reported in up to 75% of the cases in some parts of the world (Aghanwa and Morakinyo 2001). Mental symptoms such as indifference, listlessness, and dullness are common at presentation (Farmer and Graeme-Cook 1999), but psychosis remains a frequent complication (Parry et al. 2002). Most symptoms in survivors completely resolve following treatment.

Tetanus

Tetanus is uncommon in the United States but remains internationally significant. *Clostridium tetani* produces a potent neurotoxin called *tetanospasmin*, which is the cause of tetanus. The greatest risk factor for tetanus remains lack of up-to-date immunization. Infections generally occur because an open wound comes into contact with soil contaminated with spores from *C. tetani*.

The classic symptom is muscle stiffness, particularly in the muscles of mastication, thus the term *lockjaw*. If the muscle stiffness extends across the entire face, risus sardonicus occurs, an expression of continuous grimace. Stiffness may progress to the entire body if left untreated.

Tetanospasmin may enter the CNS, causing encephalopathic symptoms. On initial presentation, patients with tetanus have been given misdiagnoses of an anxiety or conversion disorder (Treadway and Prange 1967), although more commonly, a conversion disorder is mistakenly thought to be possible tetanus (Barnes and Ware 1993). If the patient has received neuroleptics or antiemetics, one may easily mistake the symptoms as drug-induced acute dystonia.

Brucellosis

Most human cases of brucellosis are acquired from consumption of unpasteurized dairy products from sheep or goats. It has become rare in developed countries but is likely underdiagnosed because of the nonspecificity of symptoms. Signs of acute brucellosis include fever, diaphoresis, headache, and myalgia. Chronic brucellosis is not always preceded by acute symptoms. Its manifestations include fatigue, depression, and multiple chronic pains, so it is not surprising that patients' symptoms can be misdiagnosed as primary psychiatric illness (Sacks and Van Rensbueg 1976). CNS involvement occurs in about 5% of cases and may present as meningitis, psychosis, or cranial nerve dysfunction (Al-Sous et al. 2004; Bodur et al. 2003).

Syphilis

Syphilis is a chronic systemic disease caused by the spirochetal bacterium *Treponema pallidum*. A hundred years ago, syphilis was the leading diagnosis in psychiatric inpatients; the incidence declined as the antibiotic era began. The rates of syphilis increased in the 1990s, probably linked to the global pandemic of HIV infection. A low point in incidence was reached in the United States in 2000, but rates have since climbed.

The clinical manifestations of syphilis are varied and mimic those of other diseases. In adults, syphilis passes through several stages. *Primary syphilis* occurs as a chancre. If left untreated, the chancre will disappear, but *secondary syphilis* occurs later and multiple organ systems, including the CNS, may become involved. Most symptoms are constitutional (malaise, fatigue, anorexia, and weight loss), but meningitis may occur.

Tertiary syphilis occurs years to decades after initial infection, and neurosyphilis is now the predominant form of tertiary syphilis (Gliatto and Caroff 2001).

The most common forms of tertiary neurosyphilis are meningeal, meningovascular, and general paresis (Conde-Sendin et al. 2004). Presenting symptoms of neurosyphilis include changes in memory and personality, psychosis, and seizures, but it also can mimic atherosclerotic disease (Timmermans and Carr 2004). General paresis is an insidious dementia that can include seizures and personality deterioration 15–20 years after infection, and if untreated it may be fatal. In our clinical experience, the infection has "burned out" in some patients; they manifest dementia, have positive cerebrospinal fluid (CSF) and serum serology, and yet show no clinical response to penicillin G.

Except in populations where syphilis is common, it is not cost-effective to screen all new psychiatric patients for syphilis (Banger et al. 1995; Roberts et al. 1992); screening should focus on patients with unexplained cognitive dysfunction or other neurological symptoms accompanying the psychopathology. In neurosyphilis, the Venereal Disease Research Laboratory (VDRL) test on serum is not specific and has a sensitivity of about 70%–75%. The serum fluorescent treponemal antibody absorption (FTA-ABS) test on serum is more specific and has a sensitivity of 99%. Tested on CSF, the VDRL is very specific but has a sensitivity of only 30%–70%. The FTA-ABS is very sensitive on CSF.

Lyme Disease

Lyme disease is caused by the spirochete *Borrelia burgdorferi*, transmitted by deer ticks. The risk of contracting Lyme disease from a single tick bite is 3% (Nadelman et al. 2001). Lyme disease occurs worldwide; it is the most common tickborne disease in the United States. Disease onset is marked by erythema migrans, a characteristic (in more than 90% of cases) rash with central clearing. Acute disseminated disease includes fatigue, arthralgia, headache, fever, and stiff neck. If untreated, Lyme disease may disseminate to other organs and produce subacute or chronic disease. Neurological symptoms occur in about 15% and may include cranial neuropathies (most often, the facial nerve), meningitis, or painful radiculopathy (Rahn and Evans 1998). If still untreated, patients may develop chronic neuroborreliosis, including a mild sensory radiculopathy, cognitive dysfunction, or depression. Typical symptoms of chronic Lyme encephalopathy include difficulty with concentration and memory, fatigue, daytime hypersomnolence, irritability, and depression. Rarely, Lyme disease has included chronic encephalomyelitis.

While these chronic syndromes are not distinctive, they are almost always preceded by the classic early symptoms of Lyme disease, such as erythema migrans, arthritis, cranial neuropathy, or radiculopathy (Rahn and Evans 1998).

Many different psychiatric symptoms have been reported to be associated with Lyme disease, including depression, mania, delirium, dementia, psychosis, obsessions or compulsions, panic attacks, catatonia, and personality change (Tager and Fallon 2001). However, association does not allow one to infer causation by Lyme. Although symptoms such as pain, fatigue, and difficulty with daily activities are common in patients who received treatment for Lyme disease years earlier, the frequencies of such symptoms are similar in control subjects without Lyme disease (Seltzer et al. 2000). Even in patients with classic symptomatic Lyme disease confirmed by serological testing, persisting symptoms are usually explained by some illness other than chronic borreliosis if these patients have received adequate antibiotic therapy (Kalish et al. 2001; Seltzer et al. 2000).

The differential diagnosis of neuroborreliosis in a patient presenting with fatigue, depression, and/or impaired cognition includes fibromyalgia, chronic fatigue syndrome, other infections, somatoform disorders, depression, autoimmune diseases, and multiple sclerosis (Tager and Fallon 2001).

Adverse consequences of overdiagnosis include reinforcement of somatization and the creation of invalidism. The diagnosis of an infection that can be treated with antibiotics can be very appealing to patients for whom depression or somatoform disorder is an unacceptable diagnosis.

Diagnosis is based on the characteristic clinical features. Serological testing can support the diagnosis but should never be the primary basis (Rahn and Evans 1998). False-negative and false-positive results are common. Even a true-positive test result simply indicates that the patient has had Lyme disease at some point in life, but no conclusion about current disease activity or extent of infection can be drawn. In chronic neuroborreliosis, increased CSF protein and antibody to the organism occur in more than 50% of the patients. Electroencephalograms (EEGs) are typically normal, whereas MRI shows nonspecific white matter lesions in about 25%. Neuropsychological assessment is useful in measuring cognitive dysfunction, but the findings are not specific (Ravdin et al. 1996).

Neither serological testing nor antibiotic treatment is cost-effective in patients who have a low probability of having the disease (i.e., nonspecific symptoms, low incidence region) (Nichol et al. 1998). Three controlled trials found no benefit of extended intravenous or oral antibiotics in patients with well-documented, previously treated Lyme disease who had persistent pain, neurocognitive symptoms, or dysesthesia, often with fatigue (Kaplan et al. 2003; Klempner et al. 2001).

Leptospirosis

Leptospirosis is another protean spirochetal disease occurring globally in rural and urban areas (Vinetz 2001), even in the American inner city (Vinetz et al. 1996). Most infections resemble influenza and are relatively benign, but severe multiorgan leptospirosis may cause meningoencephalitis or aseptic meningitis. Confusion and delirium are common, and mental status changes are the strongest predictor of mortality (Ko et al. 1999).

Bacterial Meningitis

Bacterial meningitis is an acute illness associated with significant morbidity and mortality. Psychiatric symptoms may result by several mechanisms, including toxic effects of the organism, mediators of inflammation, cerebral edema, and hypoxia.

The classic sign of meningeal inflammation is nuchal rigidity. Headache, nausea, vomiting, confusion, lethargy, and apathy also may occur. Psychiatric symptoms are the result of encephalopathy. As in other infections, encephalopathy may present subtle changes in personality, mood, motivation, or mentation. Symptom severity generally correlates with the magnitude of the host's immune response (Weinstein 1985). When the patient cannot mount a full inflammatory response, the classic symptoms may not occur. In infants, the elderly, or immunocompromised patients, the only clinical signs may be irritability or minor changes in mentation or personality (Segreti and Harris 1996).

Cat-Scratch Disease

Cat-scratch disease, which is caused by *Bartonella henselae*, usually presents as self-limiting lymphadenopathy following a cat scratch or bite. Encephalopathy, one of the common complications, manifests with combative behavior, lethargy, and seizures, though significant fever may be absent; almost all reported cases have been in children (Carithers and Margileth 1991).

Bacterial Brain Abscess

Brain abscesses frequently occur as a complication of bacterial meningitis, although they also are a complication of infective endocarditis. The classic triad of headache, fever, and focal neurological deficits has been described, but all three symptoms occur in fewer than half of the patients who have a brain abscess. Seizures are common. Various psychiatric symptoms may occur, depending on the size and location of the abscess, how irritating the organism is, and the extent of the inflammatory response. Disordered mood, cognitive dysfunction, psychosis, and aggression are the most common psychiatric complications (Chang et al. 1997; Douen and Bourque 1997).

Tuberculous Meningitis

Tuberculosis remains endemic in many developing countries and is the most common serious HIV-related complication worldwide. Where tuberculosis is not endemic, the diagnosis of tuberculous meningitis is often not considered because the clinical manifestations are often nonspecific. Early diagnosis of tuberculous meningitis is essential because delay in treatment is associated with high morbidity and mortality.

Early symptoms include low fever, generalized malaise, fatigue, and mild headache. Over the course of a week, there is progression to high fever, severe nuchal rigidity, confusion, and delirium. Persons with HIV, the elderly, substance abusers, and others with impaired immunity are more likely to present without nuchal rigidity and headache. In such patients, the symptoms will tend to be most nonspecific, with a higher risk of missing the correct diagnosis while attributing the symptoms to more common diagnoses such as alcohol withdrawal.

Early in the course, CSF glucose may be unchanged and protein only marginally elevated. As the disease progresses, glucose declines drastically, and protein becomes markedly elevated, with white blood cell counts typically between 50 and 200 per cubic millimeter (predominantly lymphocytes).

Viral Infections

The overwhelming majority of viral infections are asymptomatic or mild, but viruses can produce psychiatric symptoms by primary CNS involvement, from secondary effects of immune activation, or indirectly from systemic effects. One serious sequela of several viral infections is acute disseminated encephalomyelitis; patients with this condition can present with encephalopathy, acute psychosis, seizures, and other CNS dysfunction. Active demyelination is widespread, and the disease may be difficult to distinguish from multiple sclerosis (Nasr et al. 2000). Residual cognitive dysfunction may occur (Jacobs et al. 2004).

Epstein-Barr Virus

EBV, one of the herpesviruses, causes infectious mononucleosis ("mono"), common in children and young adults. The prodromal stage is characterized by headache, fatigue, and malaise, with progression to fever, sore throat, and lymphadenopathy. Diagnosis is based on the combination of typical clinical symptoms and a positive heterophil antibody test (Monospot) result. Fatigue commonly persists for a few months, but this can occur with other viral infections (White et al. 1998). Rarely, anemia, leukopenia, eosinophilia, thrombocytopenia, pneumonitis, heptosplenomegaly, uveitis, and an abnormal pattern of serum globulins occur.

In patients with chronic fatigue and malaise, the differential diagnosis may include depression or chronic EBV infection. Because EBV may persist lifelong in a latent state following acute infection, periodic reactivation may occur. Patients with latent EBV infection typically report overwhelming fatigue, malaise, depression, low-grade fever, lymphadenopathy, and other nonspecific symptoms. This resembles chronic fatigue syndrome, even though only a small fraction of chronic fatigue symptoms are attributable to EBV infection. In the past, patients with chronic fatigue caused by depression or somatoform disorder who resisted considering a psychiatric diagnosis (and sometimes their physicians) often pursued an explanation in chronic EBV infection. They found (erroneous) confirmation in a positive Monospot test result; it is erroneous because the test result remains positive long after complete resolution of uncomplicated infectious mononucleosis, often for life. With wider recognition of the limitations of Monospot testing, this misdiagnosis is now very infrequent.

As in other postviral syndromes, antidepressant therapy is often helpful if depression exists in the recovery phase of infectious mononucleosis.

Cytomegalovirus

Like EBV, cytomegalovirus (CMV) is a common herpesvirus, and most infections are subclinical. CMV infection occurs in a broader age group. CMV can produce a syndrome identical to infectious mononucleosis, except that heterophil antibody testing is negative in CMV, and a sore throat is usually absent. CMV also may cause hepatitis, retinitis, colonitis, and pneumonitis. In immunocompromised patients, CMV has been implicated as a cause of depression or dementia. CMV should be considered in the differential diagnosis of acute depression or cognitive dysfunction in the first few months after organ transplantation (Hibberd et al. 1995). Antidepressant therapy may be needed if the patient develops a postviral mood disorder.

Viral Meningoencephalitis

Most viruses that cause encephalitis cause meningitis as well. Enteroviruses, mumps, and lymphocytic choriomeningitis primarily affect the meninges, with enteroviruses responsible for most identifiable cases. Patients with viral meningitis (often referred to as *aseptic meningitis*) present with headache, fever, nuchal rigidity, malaise, drowsiness, nausea, and photophobia.

Arboviruses

Arboviruses (short for arthropod-borne viruses) are the most common worldwide cause of viral encephalitis. Of the arbovirus diseases, Japanese encephalitis is the most common worldwide. In the United States, the four major types are St. Louis encephalitis, eastern equine encephalomyelitis, western equine encephalomyelitis, and California encephalitis. Recently, West Nile virus has appeared in the United States (Solomon 2003). Most arboviruses are mosquito-borne. Arboviral encephalitis typically appears in the summer or fall, with abrupt onset of fever, headache, nausea, photophobia, and vomiting, and may be fatal. Reduced level of consciousness, flaccid paralysis resembling poliomyelitis, parkinsonism, and seizures are common (Solomon 2004). Occasionally, patients with viral encephalitis may present initially with psychopathology without neurological symptoms. Caroff et al. (2001) reviewed 108 published cases of psychiatric presentation, classified as psychosis (35%), catatonia (33%), psychotic depression (16%), or mania (11%). Patients in such cases often receive misdiagnosis and inappropriate treatment and may be more vulnerable to adverse effects of neuroleptics, including extrapyramidal side effects, catatonia, and neuroleptic malignant syndrome. Among those who survive, outcomes vary from complete recovery to serious neuropsychiatric sequelae.

Dengue

Dengue, another disease caused by an arbovirus, is transmitted by mosquitoes, endemic in 100 countries and encountered in temperate developed countries mainly in travelers and new immigrants (Castleberry and Mahon 2003). The virus causes the relatively more benign dengue fever, hemorrhagic dengue, and dengue shock syndrome; the latter two are rare in travelers.

However, neuropsychiatric symptoms were noted in 14% of the tourists who returned to France with dengue (Badiaga et al. 1999). In the more serious endemic dengue infections, meningoencephalitis is common, with confusion, delirium, and seizures (Pancharoen and Thisyakorn 2001).

Herpes Simplex Virus

Herpes encephalitis is caused by invasion of the brain by herpes simplex type 1 virus in 90% of herpes encephalitis cases. Symptoms may include personality change, dysphasia, seizures, autonomic dysfunction, ataxia, delirium, psychosis, and focal neurological symptoms. Herpes simplex virus (HSV) encephalitis differs from arboviral encephalitis by causing more unilateral and focal findings, with a predilection for the temporal lobes. HSV encephalitis is more likely to cause focal seizures, olfactory hallucinations, and personality change (Whitley et al. 1982). HSV is the most common identified cause of viral encephalitis simulating a primary psychiatric disorder (Caroff et al. 2001). EEG is a sensitive (but not specific) diagnostic test, showing periodic temporal spikes and slow waves as opposed to more diffuse changes usually seen in other forms of viral encephalitis (Smith et al. 1975). Rapid diagnosis is essential because only early treatment improves outcome. One possible sequela of HSV encephalitis is the Klüver-Bucy syndrome, which includes oral touching compulsions, hypersexuality, amnesia, placidity, agnosia, and hyperphagia (Hart et al. 1986).

Varicella/Herpes Zoster

The varicella/herpes zoster virus causes chickenpox in children and herpes zoster in adults. Most cases of encephalopathy in children with varicella infection have been due to Reye's syndrome, although the virus itself can cause encephalitis. The most common neurological sequela of herpes zoster is postherpetic neuralgia. Comorbid psychopathology, especially depression, is common in postherpetic neuralgia (Clark et al. 2000) and may influence the choice of treatment for the neuropathic pain (e.g., antidepressant vs. anticonvulsant). Weeks or months after recovery from herpes zoster, encephalitis or cerebral arteritis may appear. In immunocompetent hosts, it is usually a granulomatous arteritis affecting large vessels, producing strokelike symptoms. In immunosuppressed patients, the vasculitis mostly affects small vessels, producing headache, altered mental status, fever, seizures, and focal deficits (Gilden et al. 2000).

Postencephalitis Syndromes

Psychiatric sequelae are common following recovery from acute viral encephalitis and constitute a major cause of disability, especially mood disorders. Depression, hypomania, irritability, and disinhibition of anger, aggression, or sexuality have been frequently noted months after recovery, and psychosis occurs rarely (Caparros-Lefebvre et al. 1996). Depressive symptoms may respond to treatment with antidepressants or stimulants. Hypomania, irritability, and disinhibition have benefited from mood stabilizers, and behavior modification also may be helpful for aggressive and sexual behaviors (Boulais et al. 1976; Vallini and Burns 1987).

The global pandemic encephalitis in 1917–1929 known as *encephalitis lethargica* (von Economo's disease) had an acute encephalitic phase during which lethargy, psychosis, and catatonia were common. This period was followed by a chronic postencephalitic syndrome, including parkinsonism, mania, depression, and apathy in adults (Cummings et al. 2001) and conduct disorder, emotional lability, and tics in children, with relatively little cognitive impairment (Cummings et al. 2001). Sporadic similar cases continue to be reported (Dale et al. 2004).

Viral Hepatitis

Hepatitis C infection is very common in the chronically mentally ill (Dinwiddie et al. 2003; Osher et al. 2003). Fatigue, malaise, and anorexia are usually prominent in viral hepatitis and may lead to a misdiagnosis of depression. However, fatigue in chronic hepatitis is more closely correlated with depression and other psychological factors than is severity of hepatitis (McDonald et al. 2002). Depression is frequently comorbid in chronic hepatitis, but whether the etiology of depression is really viral has been questioned (Wessely and Pariante 2002). Subtle cognitive dysfunction not attributable to depression, substance abuse, or hepatic encephalopathy has been documented in hepatitis C infection, and the virus has been identified in brain, suggesting that cerebral infection also may occur (Morgello 2005). Complicating the diagnostic picture further, treatment with interferon causes depression itself in 20%–40% of patients (Dieperink et al. 2003). Depression has been the most common adverse effect leading to cessation of interferon treatment. Depression associated with hepatitis or interferon is amenable to treatment with antidepressants (Kraus et al. 2002), allowing continuation of interferon in most patients (Schaefer et al. 2003). Therefore, depression should not be considered a contraindication to interferon therapy.

Rabies

In the United States, rabies is rare but has been misdiagnosed as an anxiety disorder (Centers for Disease Control 1991) or alcohol withdrawal (Centers for Disease Control and Prevention 1998).

Initial symptoms include generalized anxiety, fever, depression, hyperesthesia, and dysesthesia. In one case, "mild personality changes" preceded more suggestive symptoms such as unsteady gait and slurred speech by more than a week (Centers for Disease Control and Prevention 2003). The rabies virus has a proclivity for attacking the limbic system, and delusions may result. The initial phase is followed by an excitatory phase, when the classic symptom of hydrophobia may occur. Hydrophobia is an aversion to swallowing liquids (not a phobia of water) secondary to the spasmodic contractions of the muscles of swallowing and respiration, resulting in pain and aspiration. The final phase is a progressive, general, flaccid paralysis that progresses relentlessly to death. Both rabies and the rabies vaccine may cause delirium (Leung et al. 2003).

Prion Diseases

Prions are proteinaceous agents that cause spongiform changes in the brain. Prion diseases are rare and universally fatal, with an incubation period of months to years—hence, the term *slow viruses*. Kuru occurs only in Papua New Guinea. It is spread by the cannibalistic consumption of dead relatives during mourning rituals.

Creutzfeldt-Jakob disease (CJD) occurs sporadically and sometimes familially in humans. It also has been transmitted by intracerebral electrodes, grafts of dura mater, corneal transplants, human growth hormone, and gonadotropin, but iatrogenic transmission is now rare (Ironside 1996; Tyler 2003). CJD is a severe dementia accompanied by psychosis, affective lability, and dramatic myoclonus that rapidly progresses to rigid mutism and then death.

In the last few years, mainly in Great Britain, "new-variant" CJD (nvCJD) has appeared, with distinct differences from CJD. nvCJD patients are younger than CJD patients (average age 26 vs. 60 years).

In most cases of nvCJD, psychiatric symptoms, including depression, irritability, anxiety, and apathy, appear several months before any neurological symptoms (Spencer et al. 2002; Tyler 2003). Although bovine spongiform encephalopathy ("mad cow disease") and nvCJD are temporally and geographically associated, a causative link has not been proven. EEG, MRI, and CSF all usually show abnormalities in both forms of CJD, but definitive diagnosis requires brain biopsy (Johnson et al. 2005).

Fungal Infections

The frequency of fungal infection has steadily increased over the last three decades, coincident with the growing number of immunosuppressed patients. Most fungi are opportunistic (as in aspergillosis, mucormycosis, and candidiasis), whereas others are pathogenic (as in coccidioidomycosis and cryptococcosis) irrespective of the host's defenses.

Aspergillosis

Aspergillus, an opportunistic organism, infects only debilitated patients. CNS involvement usually follows infection of the lungs or gastrointestinal tract. Symptoms of confusion, headache, and lethargy often accompany focal neurological signs.

Cryptococcosis

Cryptococcosis is an infection caused by *Cryptococcus*, which may act as a solo pathogen but in up to 85% of cases is associated with another illness, especially AIDS.

Cryptococcus is the most common form of fungal meningitis. It is typically insidious in onset and slowly progressive. Headache is present in up to 75% of the cases, varying from mild and episodic to progressively incapacitating and constant. Other signs include cerebellar, cranial

nerve, and motor deficits; irritability; psychosis; and lethargy, which may progress to coma. Remission and relapse are common.

Coccidioidomycosis

Coccidioidomycosis is restricted to warm, dry areas such as the southwestern United States, Mexico, and parts of South America. Dissemination beyond the lung is relatively rare. When it does occur, CNS infection is typically insidious in onset, 1–3 months after initial infection, with severe headache associated with confusion, restlessness, hallucinations, lethargy, and transient focal signs (Bañuelos et al. 1996).

Histoplasmosis

Histoplasmosis is a common respiratory infection throughout the world, especially common in the central United States. Most infections are asymptomatic and involve the lungs or the reticuloendothelial system. CNS involvement is rare but is of insidious onset. After a few weeks of irregular fever and persistent cough, extreme nervousness and irritability progress to marked lethargy and, if untreated, coma (Tan et al. 1992).

Mucormycosis

Mucormycosis is notorious for causing an acute fulminant infection in diabetic patients and patients with neutropenia. Any diabetic patient with a purulent, febrile infection of the face or nose should be emergently evaluated for mucormycosis, because it may rapidly erode into the orbit and cerebrum in a matter of hours. Early mild encephalopathy (Crowley and Wilcox 1996) may quickly progress to severe delirium.

Candidiasis

Disseminated candidiasis occurs only in immunocompromised patients. Psychiatric symptoms occur from the toxic effects of fungemia or from direct invasion of the CNS. *Candida* may cause meningitis, abscesses, or vasculitis in the CNS. The nonspecific signs include confusion, drowsiness, lethargy, and headache.

An alternative medicine belief is that occult systemic *Candida* infection is the cause of a wide array of somatic and psychological symptoms. There is no scientific support for this theory or its advocated treatments.

Parasitic Infections

Neurocysticercosis

One of the world's most common parasitic infections, neurocysticercosis (NCC) is an infection of the CNS by the larval form (cysticerci) of *Taenia solium*, also known as the pork tapeworm. Cysticercosis is endemic in the developing nations. In the United States, it is usually reported in immigrants from Latin America and has been reportedly found in 10% of the patients with seizures presenting to an emergency department in Los Angeles, California, and in 6% in an emergency department in New Mexico (Ong et al. 2002).

A high percentage of NCC infections remain asymptomatic. Cerebral involvement may produce seizures, stroke, or hydrocephalus (Wallin and Kurtzke 2004); NCC is the leading cause of seizures in adults in endemic areas. Psychiatric symptoms are frequently reported and include depression and psychosis (Mahajan et al. 2004). NCC is a common cause of dementia in developing nations (Jha and Patel 2004), though the cognitive decline may be reversible (Ramirez-Bermudez et al. 2005).

Between clinical history, neuroimaging, and serology, a presumptive diagnosis of NCC usually can be made (Pittella 1997a).

Toxoplasmosis

Toxoplasmosis is caused by *Toxoplasma gondii*, a parasite affecting all mammals, some birds, and probably some reptiles. Latent infection is common, but in immunosuppressed individuals, it may preferentially infect the CNS, resulting in a wide range of clinical presentations. Mass lesions mimicking tumor or abscess are most common, but psychosis has been reported as a presenting symptom (Donnet et al. 1991). It has been suggested that maternal toxoplasmosis exposure might be a risk factor for schizophrenia (Brown et al. 2005).

Trypanosomiasis

The family of protozoa Trypanosomatidae causes two different syndromes: African trypanosomiasis (sleeping sickness) and American trypanosomiasis (Chagas' disease). African trypanosomiasis is transmitted to humans and animals by the bite of the tsetse fly. The illness begins with a lesion at the site of the fly bite, headache, fever, malaise, weight loss, and myalgia and is often misdiagnosed as malaria. Patients with African trypanosomiasis often report excruciating pain after minor injuries (Kerandel's hyperesthesia) (Chimelli and Scaravilli 1997). Meningoencephalitis may develop with prominent somnolence—hence the name *sleeping sickness* (Villanueva 1993). Africans living in other countries have received misdiagnoses of primary psychiatric disorder (Bedat-Millet et al. 2000).

American trypanosomiasis, or Chagas' disease, is spread by insects (known as "kissing bugs" or "assassin bugs") in Latin America. Transmission is so inefficient that years of exposure are required to acquire the infection, and most infections are quiescent. Following immunosuppression, reactivated disease may present as meningoencephalitis.

TABLE 10–2. Psychiatric side effects of selected drugs for infectious diseases (excluding antiretroviral drugs)

Drug	Side effects
Antibacterial	
Procaine penicillin	Anxiety, psychosis (probably due to procaine)
Quinolones	Psychosis, agitation
Antituberculous	
Cycloserine	Agitation, depression, psychosis, anxiety
Antiviral	
Acyclovir	Psychosis, delirium
Amantadine	Psychosis
Interferon-alpha	Irritability, depression
Interleukin-2	Psychosis
Antiparasitic	
Antimalarials	Psychosis, mania, depression, anxiety
Antifungal	
Amphotericin	Delirium, psychosis, depression

Malaria

Malaria remains a major cause of morbidity in tropical nations, especially in young children and pregnant women. In other parts of the world, cases occur in immigrants and travelers to malarial areas. *Plasmodium* species are transmitted to humans by the bite of mosquitoes.

Relapsing fever typifies malaria, and with temperatures commonly in excess of 41°C (105°F), delirium is common. *Plasmodium falciparum* causes cerebral malaria, the most catastrophic complication of malaria, which begins with disorientation, mild stupor, or even psychosis (Thiam et al. 2002) and can rapidly progress to seizures and coma. Despite the severity and high fatality of cerebral malaria, those who recover usually have little or no persisting cognitive dysfunction. Although anxiety, depression, irritability, and personality change are common after recovery (Dugbartey et al. 1998; Varney et al. 1997), they are more likely a result of psychosocial stress (Weiss 1985). More severe neuropsychiatric signs, including psychosis in

fully recovered (aparasitemic) cerebral malaria, are most likely attributable to pharmacotherapy (Nguyen et al. 1996). Antimalarial drugs commonly cause psychiatric side effects (see Table 10–2).

Schistosomiasis

Schistosomiasis, infection by larval blood flukes, usually occurs from swimming in infected fresh water. It affects about 200 million people in 74 countries. Most infections are asymptomatic. CNS involvement is uncommon but may lead to increased intracranial pressure (e.g., headache, confusion, nausea, and papilledema) (Pittella 1997b).

Trichinosis

Trichinosis is a worldwide disease caused by the ingestion of *Trichinella* larvae, most commonly found in pork, but 150 species of mammals may be infected. Trichinosis has become rare in developed nations but still occurs in ethnic groups that prefer raw or undercooked pork or wild animals, such as polar bear or walrus. Typical symptoms include fever, myalgias, and diarrhea, accompanied by marked eosinophilia. CNS involvement occurs in 10%–20%, causing headache, delirium, insomnia, meningo-encephalitis, and seizures (Nikolic et al. 1998; Taratuto and Venturiello 1997). Residual cognitive dysfunction may occur (Harms et al. 1993).

Amebiasis

Primary amebic meningoencephalitis is produced by *Naegleria fowleri* in healthy, young individuals engaged in water sports. Its course is acute and fulminant, with headache, nausea, confusion, and stiff neck followed by coma and death within days. Granulomatous amebic encephalitis, caused by *Balamuthia mandrillaris* and some species of *Acanthamoeba*, usually occurs in debilitated, immunosuppressed, or malnourished individuals. The course is more chronic, with personality changes, confusion, and irritability, eventually progressing to seizures and death (Martinez and Visvesvara 1997).

Drugs for Infectious Diseases: Adverse Psychiatric Effects and Drug Interactions

That antibiotics can cause delirium and other psychiatric symptoms is not well appreciated. The best-documented psychiatric side effects of selected drugs for infectious diseases are listed in Table 10–2. Delirium and psychosis have been particularly associated with quinolones (e.g., ciprofloxacin), procaine penicillin, antimalarial and other antiparasitic drugs, and the antituberculous drug cycloserine. The most common adverse effect causing discontinuation of interferon is depression.

Selected well-established interactions between antimicrobial and psychotropic drugs are shown in Table 10–3. Drug interactions between antibiotics and non-

psychiatric drugs also may present risk in psychiatric practice. Erythromycin (and similar antibiotics like clarithromycin) and ketaconazole (and similar antifungals) may cause QT interval prolongation and ventricular arrhythmias when given to a patient taking other QT-prolonging drugs, including tricyclic antidepressants and many antipsychotics.

Fears of Infectious Disease

Infectious diseases historically have been, and remain, frightening. In the recent epidemic of SARS, both affected patients and health care workers experienced fears of the illness and fears of contagion to family and friends, sometimes resulting in posttraumatic stress disorder (Hawryluck et al. 2004; Sim et al. 2004). Quarantined patients struggle with loneliness, isolation, and stigmatization, and they fear the effect of their absence on those who depend on them (Maunder et al. 2003).

Feared, stigmatized infected individuals may delay seeking care and remain undetected (Person et al. 2004). Both individual and group reactions to real or imagined threats of infectious diseases also may include hysterical and phobic behaviors. Anxiety about acquiring a feared disease may lead to conversion symptoms, hypochondriacal preoccupation, and unnecessary avoidance behaviors. Contamination obsessions and washing compulsions are among the most frequent symptoms in obsessive-compulsive disorder (OCD). Delusional fears or beliefs that one is infected also occur in psychotic disorders, including schizophrenia, psychotic depression, and delusional disorder, somatic type (e.g., delusions of intestinal parasitosis) (Ford et al. 2001; Podoll et al. 1993); however, it is important to consider that a patient with a delusion of infection may actually be infected (Chigusa et al. 2000).

TABLE 10–3. Selected antimicrobial–psychotropic drug interactions

Antimicrobial	Effect on psychiatric drug
Antimalarials	Increase phenothiazine level
Azoles	Increase alprazolam, midazolam levels
	Increase buspirone level
Clarithromycin, erythromycin	Increase alprazolam, midazolam levels
	Increase carbamazepine level
	Increase buspirone level
	Increase clozapine level
Quinolones	Increase clozapine level
	Increase benzodiazepine level
	Decrease benzodiazepine effect via GABA receptor
Isoniazid	Increases haloperidol level
	Increases carbamazepine level
	With disulfiram, causes ataxia

Note. GABA=gamma-aminobutyric acid.
Source. Cozza KL, Armstrong SC, Oesterheld JR: *Concise Guide to Drug Interaction Principles for Medical Practice,* 2nd Edition. Washington, DC, American Psychiatric Publishing, 2003; Hansten PD, Horn JR: *Drug Interactions and Management.* Vancouver, WA, Applied Therapeutics, 1997.

Unrealistic fears of infection are especially likely with venereal diseases (particularly HIV), serious outbreaks (e.g., meningococcal meningitis on campus), and infectious threats given heavy media coverage (e.g., bacterial food contamination, bovine spongiform encephalopathy, SARS, anthrax, smallpox) (Logsdail et al. 1991; McEvedy and Basquille 1997; Vuorio et al. 1990; Weir 2001).

At times, mass outbreaks of symptoms occur, falsely attributed to a supposed toxic exposure (e.g., bacterial food poisoning or toxic fumes) or infectious disease. There have been hundreds of reports in the literature of such outbreaks of "mass psychogenic" or "mass sociogenic" illness, and they tend to follow trends in societal concerns (e.g., bioterrorism) (Bartholomew and Wessely 2002). They are most likely to occur in groups of young people in close quarters, such as students at schools (Jones et al. 2000) or military recruits (Struewing and Gray 1990). Some aspects of "germ panic" have become socially normative (Tomes 2000)—for example, inappropriate

use of antibiotics (such as ciprofloxacin during the anthrax scare), and the widespread overuse of antiseptic soaps, mouthwashes, sprays, and cleaning agents. A related phobia of fever in their children remains prevalent among parents (Crocetti et al. 2001).

Psychiatric Aspects of Immunizations

Mass outbreaks of psychogenic symptoms similar to those described earlier in this chapter have been reported several times following vaccinations (Kharabsheh et al. 2001). In developed countries, the public's fears of vaccine-preventable diseases have waned, and awareness of potential adverse effects of the vaccines has increased, which is threatening vaccine acceptance (Amanna and Slifka 2005; Epstein 2005). Much misinformation has been disseminated about vaccination risks, adding to the tendency toward phobic avoidance of immunization. Rare serious CNS adverse effects, including acute disseminated encephalomyelitis, can occur after a variety of vaccinations. However, recent studies have found no basis for the widely publicized fears that measles-mumps-rubella vaccination causes encephalitis, aseptic meningitis, or autism (Chen et al. 2004; Madsen et al. 2002).

Finally, it should be kept in mind that the chronically mentally ill often do not receive basic preventive medical care (Folsom et al. 2002). Psychiatrists can help ensure that their patients receive important immunizations.

References

Aghanwa HS, Morakinyo O: Correlates of psychiatric morbidity in typhoid fever in a Nigerian general hospital setting. Gen Hosp Psychiatry 23:158–162, 2001

Al-Sous MW, Bohlega S, A-Kawi MZ, et al: Neurobrucellosis: clinical and neuroimaging correlation. AJNR Am J Neuroradiol 25:395–401, 2004

Amanna I, Slifka MK: Public fear of vaccination: separating fact from fiction. Viral Immunol 18:307–315, 2005

Badiaga S, Delmont J, Brouqui P, et al: Imported dengue: study of 44 cases observed from 1994 to 1997 in 9 university hospital centers. Infectio-Sud-France group [in French]. Pathol Biol (Paris) 47:539–542, 1999

Banger M, Olbrich HM, Fuchs S, et al: Cost-effectiveness of syphilis screening in a clinic for general psychiatry [in German]. Nervenarzt 66:49–53, 1995

Bañuelos AF, Williams PL, Johnson RH, et al: Central nervous system abscesses due to coccidioides species. Clin Infect Dis 22:240–250, 1996

Barnes V, Ware MR: Tetanus, pseudotetanus, or conversion disorder: a diagnostic dilemma? South Med J 86:591–592, 1993

Bartholomew RE, Wessely S: Protean nature of mass sociogenic illness: from possessed nuns to chemical and biological terrorism fears. Br J Psychiatry 180:300–306, 2002

Bedat-Millet AL, Charpentier S, Monge-Strauss MF, et al: Psychiatric presentation of human African trypanosomiasis: overview of diagnostic pitfalls, interest of difluoromethylornithine treatment and contribution of magnetic resonance imaging. Rev Neurol (Paris) 156:505–509, 2000

Bergeron JW, Braddom RL, Kaelin DL: Persisting impairment following Rocky Mountain spotted fever: a case report. Arch Phys Med Rehabil 78:1277–1280, 1997

Bodner SM, Morshed SA, Peterson BS: The question of PANDAS in adults. Biol Psychiatry 49:807–810, 2001

Bodur H, Erbay A, Akinci E, et al: Neurobrucellosis in an endemic area of brucellosis. Scand J Infect Dis 35:94–97, 2003

Bonawitz C, Castillo M, Mukherji SK: Comparison of CT and MR features with clinical outcome in patients with Rocky Mountain spotted fever. Am J Neuroradiol 18:459–464, 1997

Boulais P, Delcros J, Signoret JL, et al: Subacute excitation caused by probable herpetic encephalitis: favorable effects of lithium. Ann Med Interne (Paris) 127:345–352, 1976

Brown AS, Schaefer CA, Quesenberry CP Jr, et al: Maternal exposure to toxoplasmosis and risk of schizophrenia in adult offspring. Am J Psychiatry 162:767–773, 2005

Caparros-Lefebvre D, Girard-Buttaz I, Reboul S, et al: Cognitive and psychiatric impairment in herpes simplex virus encephalitis suggest involvement of the amygdalo-frontal pathways. J Neurol 243:248–256, 1996

Carithers HA, Margileth AM: Cat-scratch disease: acute encephalopathy and other neurologic manifestations. Am J Dis Child 145:98–101, 1991

Caroff SN, Mann SC, Glittoo MF, et al: Psychiatric manifestations of acute viral encephalitis. Psychiatr Ann 31:193–204, 2001

Castleberry JS, Mahon CR: Dengue fever in the Western Hemisphere. Clin Lab Sci 16:34–38, 2003

Centers for Disease Control: Human rabies—Texas, Arkansas, and Georgia, 1991. MMWR Morb Mortal Wkly Rep 40: 765–769, 1991

Centers for Disease Control and Prevention: Human rabies: Texas and New Jersey, 1997. MMWR Morb Mortal Wkly Rep 47:1–5, 1998

Centers for Disease Control and Prevention: First human death associated with raccoon rabies—Virginia, 2003. MMWR Morb Mortal Wkly Rep 52:1102–1103, 2003

Chang CZ, Wang CJ, Howng SL: Epidural abscess presented with psychiatric symptoms. Kaohsiung J Med Sci 13:578–582, 1997

Chen W, Landau S, Sham P, et al: No evidence for links between autism, MMR and measles virus. Psychol Med 34:543–553, 2004

Cheng SK, Tsang JS, Ku KH, et al: Psychiatric complications in patients with severe acute respiratory syndrome (SARS) during the acute treatment phase: a series of 10 cases. Br J Psychiatry 184:359–360, 2004

Chigusa Y, Shinonaga S, Koyama Y, et al: Suspected intestinal myiasis due to Dryomyza formosa in a Japanese schizophrenic patient with symptoms of delusional parasitosis. Med Vet Entomol 14:453–457, 2000

Chimelli L, Scaravilli F: Trypanosomiasis. Brain Pathol 7:599–611, 1997

Church AJ, Dale RC, Lees AJ, et al: Tourette's syndrome: a cross sectional study to examine the PANDAS hypothesis. J Neurol Neurosurg Psychiatry 74:602–607, 2003

Clark MR, Heinberg LJ, Haythornthwaite JA, et al: Psychiatric symptoms and distress differ between patients with postherpetic neuralgia and peripheral vestibular disease. J Psychosom Res 48:51–57, 2000

Cohen S, Miller GE, Rabin BS: Psychological stress and antibody response to immunization: a critical review of the human literature. Psychosom Med 63:7–18, 2001

Conde-Sendin MA, Amela-Peris R, Aladro-Benito Y, et al: Current clinical spectrum of neurosyphilis in immunocompetent patients. Eur Neurol 52:29–35, 2004

Crocetti M, Moghbeli N, Serwint J: Fever phobia revisited: have parental misconceptions about fever changed in 20 years? Pediatrics 107:1241–1246, 2001

Crowley P, Wilcox JA: Cerebral mucormycosis presenting as psychiatric distress. Psychosomatics 37:164–165, 1996

Cummings JL, Chow T, Masterman D: Encephalitis lethargica: lessons for neuropsychiatry. Psychiatr Ann 31:165–169, 2001

Dale RC, Church AJ, Surtees RA, et al: Encephalitis lethargica syndrome: 20 new cases and evidence of basal ganglia autoimmunity. Brain 52:29–35, 2004

Dieperink E, Ho SB, Thuras P, et al: A prospective study of neuropsychiatric symptoms associated with interferon-alpha-2b and ribavirin therapy for patients with chronic hepatitis C. Psychosomatics 44:104–112, 2003

Dinwiddie SH, Shicker L, Newman T: Prevalence of hepatitis C among psychiatric patients in the public sector. Am J Psychiatry 160:172–174, 2003

Donnet A, Harle JR, Cherif AA, et al: Acute psychiatric pathology disclosing subcortical lesion in neuro-AIDS. Encephale 17:79–81, 1991

Douen AG, Bourque PR: Musical auditory hallucinosis from Listeria rhombencephalitis. Can J Neurol Sci 24:70–72, 1997

Dugbartey AT, Dugbartey MT, Apedo MY: Delayed neuropsychiatric effects of malaria in Ghana. J Nerv Ment Dis 186: 183–186, 1998

Epstein RA: It did happen here: fear and loathing on the vaccine trail. Health Aff (Millwood) 24:740–743, 2005

Farmer PE, Graeme-Cook FM: Case records of the Massachusetts General Hospital. Weekly clinicopathological exercises. Case 8—1999. A 28-year-old man with gram-negative sepsis of uncertain cause. N Engl J Med 340:869–876, 1999

Folsom DP, McCahill M, Bartels SJ, et al: Medical comorbidity and receipt of medical care by older homeless people with schizophrenia or depression. Psychiatr Serv 53:1456–1460, 2002

Ford EB, Calfee DP, Pearson RD: Delusions of intestinal parasitosis. South Med J 94:545–547, 2001

Gilden DH, Klienschmidt-DeMasters BK, LaGuardia JJ, et al: Neurologic complications of the reactivation of varicella-zoster virus. N Engl J Med 342:635–645, 2000

Gliatto MF, Caroff SN: Neurosyphilis: a history and clinical review. Psychiatr Ann 31:153–161, 2001

Harms G, Binz P, Feldmeier H, et al: Trichinosis: a prospective controlled study of patients ten years after acute infection. Clin Infect Dis 17:637–643, 1993

Hart RP, Kwentus JA, Frazier RB, et al: Natural history of Kluver-Bucy syndrome after the treatment of herpes encephalitis. South Med J 79:1376–1378, 1986

Hawryluck L, Gold WL, Robinson S, et al: SARS control and psychological effects of quarantine, Toronto, Canada. Emerg Infect Dis 10:1206–1012, 2004

Hibberd PL, Surman OS, Bass M, et al: Psychiatric disease and cytomegalovirus viremia in renal transplant recipients. Psychosomatics 36:561–563, 1995

Hunt JC, Waller G: Psychological factors in recurrent uncomplicated urinary tract infection. Br J Urol 69:460–464, 1992

Ironside JW: Review: Creutzfeldt-Jakob disease. Brain Pathol 6:379–388, 1996

Jacobs RK, Anderson VA, Neale JL, et al: Neuropsychological outcome after acute disseminated encephalomyelitis: impact of age at illness onset. Pediatr Neurol 31:191–197, 2004

Jha S, Patel R: Some observations on the spectrum of dementia. Neurol India 52:213–214, 2004

Johnson RT, Gonzalez RG, Frosch MP: Case 27-2005: an 80-year-old man with fatigue, unsteady gait, and confusion. N Engl J Med 353:1042–1050, 2005

Jones TF, Craig AS, Hoy D, et al: Mass psychogenic illness attributed to toxic exposure at a high school. N Engl J Med 342:96–100, 2000

Kalish RA, Kaplan RF, Taylor E, et al: Evaluation of study patients with Lyme disease: 10–20 year follow-up. J Infect Dis 183:453–460, 2001

Kaplan RF, Trevino RP, Johnson GM, et al: Cognitive function in post-treatment Lyme disease: do additional antibiotics help? Neurology 60:1916–1922, 2003

Kharabsheh S, Al-Otoum H, Clements J, et al: Mass psychogenic illness following tetanus-diphtheria toxoid vaccination in Jordan. Bull World Health Organ 79:764–770, 2001

Klempner MS, Hu LT, Evans J, et al: Two controlled trials of antibiotic treatment in patients with persistent symptoms and a history of Lyme disease. N Engl J Med 344:85–92, 2001

Ko AI, Galvao RM, Ribeiro D, et al: Urban epidemic of severe leptospirosis in Brazil. Salvador Leptospirosis Study Group. Lancet 354:820–825, 1999

Kraus MR, Schafer A, Faller H, et al: Paroxetine for the treatment of interferon-alpha-induced depression in chronic hepatitis C. Aliment Pharmacol Ther 16:1091–1099, 2002

Leung AM, Kennedy R, Levenson JL: Rabies exposure and psychosis. Psychosomatics 44:336–338, 2003

Levenson JL, Hamer RM, Myers T, et al: Psychological factors predict symptoms of severe recurrent genital herpes infection. J Psychosom Res 31:153–159, 1987

Logsdail S, Lovell K, Warwick H, et al: Behavioural treatment of AIDS-focused illness phobia. Br J Psychiatry 159:422–425, 1991

Madsen KM, Hviid A, Vestergaard M, et al: A population-based study of measles, mumps, and rubella vaccination and autism. N Engl J Med 347:1477–1482, 2002

Mahajan SK, Machhan PC, Sood BR, et al: Neurocysticercosis presenting with psychosis. J Assoc Physicians India 52:663–665, 2004

Martinez AJ, Visvesvara G: Free-living, amphizoic and opportunistic amebas. Brain Pathol 7:583–598, 1997

Maunder R, Hunter J, Vincent L, et al: The immediate psychological and occupational impact of the 2003 SARS outbreak in a teaching hospital. CMAJ 168:1245–1251, 2003

McDonald J, Jayasuriya J, Bindley P, et al: Fatigue and psychological disorders in chronic hepatitis C. J Gastroenterol Hepatol 17:171–176, 2002

McEvedy CJ, Basquille J: BSE, public anxiety and private neurosis. J Psychosom Res 42:485–486, 1997

Mehr DR, Binder EF, Kruse RL, et al: Predicting mortality in nursing home residents with lower respiratory tract infection: the Missouri LRI Study. JAMA 286:2427–2436, 2001

Morgello S: The nervous system and hepatitis C virus. Semin Liv Dis 118–121, 2005

Nadelman RB, Nowakowski J, Fish D, et al: Prophylaxis with single-dose doxycycline for the prevention of Lyme disease after an Ixodes scapularis tick bite. N Engl J Med 345:79–84, 2001

Nasr JT, Andriola MR, Coyle PK: ADEM: literature review and case report of acute psychosis presentation. Pediatr Neurol 22:8–18, 2000

Nguyen TH, Day NP, Ly VC, et al: Post-malaria neurological syndrome. Lancet 348:917–921, 1996

Nichol G, Dennis DT, Steere AC, et al: Test-treatment strategies for patients suspected of having Lyme disease: a cost-effectiveness analysis. Ann Intern Med 128:37–48, 1998

Nikolic S, Vujosevic M, Sasic M, et al: Neurologic manifestations in trichinosis. Srp Arh Celok Lek 126:209–213, 1998

Ong S, Talan DA, Moran GJ, et al: Neurocysticercosis in radiographically imaged seizure patients in U.S. emergency departments. Emerg Infect Dis 8:608–613, 2002

Osher FC, Goldberg RW, McNary SW, et al: Substance abuse and the transmission of hepatitis C among persons with severe mental illness. Psychiatr Serv 54:842–847, 2003

Pancharoen C, Thisyakorn U: Neurological manifestations in dengue patients. Southeast Asian J Trop Med Public Health 32:341–345, 2001

Parry CM, Hien TT, Dougan G, et al: Typhoid fever. N Engl J Med 347:1770–1782, 2002

Perlmutter SJ, Garvey M, Castellanos X, et al: A case of pediatric autoimmune neuropsychiatric disorders associated with streptococcal infections. Am J Psychiatry 155:1592–1598, 1998

Perrin EM, Murphy ML, Casey JR, et al: Does group A beta-hemolytic streptococcal infection increase risk for behavioral and neuropsychiatric symptoms in children? Arch Pediatr Adolesc Med 158:848–856, 2004

Person B, Sy F, Holton K, et al: Fear and stigma: the epidemic within the SARS outbreak. Emerg Infect Dis 10:358–363, 2004

Pittella JEH: Neurocysticercosis. Brain Pathol 7:681–693, 1997a

Pittella JEH: Neuroschistosomiasis. Brain Pathol 7:649–662, 1997b

Podoll K, Bofinger F, von der Stein B, et al: Delusional parasitosis in a patient with endogenous depression [in German]. Fortschr Neurol Psychiatr 61:62–66, 1993

Power C, Johnson RT (eds): Emerging Neurological Infections. Boca Raton, FL, Taylor & Francis, 2005

Prio TK, Bruunsgaard H, Roge B, et al: Asymptomatic bacteriuria in elderly humans is associated with increased levels of circulating TNF receptors and elevated numbers of neutrophils. Exp Gerontol 37:693–699, 2002

Rahn DW, Evans J (eds): Lyme Disease. Philadelphia, PA, American College of Physicians, 1998

Ramirez-Bermudez J, Higuera J, Sosa AL, et al: Is dementia reversible in patients with neurocysticercosis? J Neurol Neurosurg Psychiatry 7:1164–1166, 2005

Ravdin LD, Hilton E, Primeau M, et al: Memory functioning in Lyme borreliosis. J Clin Psychiatry 57:281–286, 1996

Roberts MC, Emsley RA, Jordaan GP: Screening for syphilis and neurosyphilis in acute psychiatric admissions. S Afr Med J 82:16–18, 1992

Rosene KA, Copass MK, Kastner LS, et al: Persistent neuropsychological sequelae of toxic shock syndrome. Ann Intern Med 96:865–870, 1982

Sacks N, Van Rensbueg AJ: Clinical aspects of chronic brucellosis. S Afr Med J 50:725–728, 1976

Schaefer M, Schmidt F, Folwaczny C, et al: Adherence and mental side effects during hepatitis C treatment with interferon alfa and ribavirin in psychiatric risk groups. Hepatology 37:443–451, 2003

Schelling G, Briegel J, Roozendaal B, et al: The effect of stress doses of hydrocortisone during septic shock on posttraumatic stress disorder in survivors. Biol Psychiatry 50:978–985, 2001

Segreti J, Harris AA: Acute bacterial meningitis. Infect Dis Clin North Am 10:797–809, 1996

Seltzer EG, Gerber MA, Cartter ML, et al: Long-term outcomes of persons with Lyme disease. JAMA 283:609–616, 2000

Sim K, Chong PN, Chan YU, et al: Severe acute respiratory syndrome-rated psychiatric and posttraumatic morbidities and coping responses in medical staff within a primary health care setting in Singapore. J Clin Psychiatry 65:1120–1127, 2004

Singhal AB, Topcuoglu MA, Buonanno FS: Acute ischemic stroke patterns in infective and nonbacterial thrombotic endocarditis: a diffusion-weighted magnetic resonance imaging study. Stroke 33:1267–1273, 2002

Smith JB, Westmoreland BF, Reagan TJ, et al: A distinctive clinical EEG profile in herpes simplex encephalitis. Mayo Clin Proc 50:469, 1975

Snider LA, Lougee L, Slattery M, et al: Antibiotic prophylaxis with azithromycin or penicillin for childhood-onset neuropsychiatric disorders. Biol Psychiatry 57:788–792, 2005

Solomon T: Recent advances in Japanese encephalitis. J Neurovirol 9:274–283, 2003

Solomon T: Flavivirus encephalitis. N Engl J Med 351:370–378, 2004

Spencer MD, Knight RS, Will RG: First hundred cases of variant Creutzfeldt-Jakob disease: retrospective case note review of early psychiatric and neurological features. BMJ 324:1479–1482, 2002

Struewing JP, Gray GC: An epidemic of respiratory complaints exacerbated by mass psychogenic illness in a military recruit population. Am J Epidemiol 132:1120–1129, 1990

Swedo SE, Grant PJ: Annotation: PANDAS: a model for human autoimmune disease. J Child Psychol Psychiatry 46:227–234, 2005

Swedo SE, Leonard HL, Mittleman BB, et al: Identification of children with pediatric autoimmune neuropsychiatric disorders associated with streptococcal infections by a marker associated with rheumatic fever. Am J Psychiatry 154:110–112, 1997

Swedo SE, Susan E, Leonard HL, et al: Pediatric autoimmune neuropsychiatric disorders associated with streptococcal infections: clinical description of the first 50 cases. Am J Psychiatry 155:264–271, 1998

Tager FA, Fallon BA: Psychiatric and cognitive features of Lyme disease. Psychiatr Ann 31:172–181, 2001

Takkouche B, Regueira C, Gestal-Otero JJ: A cohort study of stress and the common cold. Epidemiology 12:345–349, 2001

Tan V, Wilkins P, Badve S, et al: Histoplasmosis of the central nervous system. J Neurol Neurosurg Psychiatry 55:619–622, 1992

Taratuto AL, Venturiello SM: Trichinosis. Brain Pathol 7:663–672, 1997

Thiam MH, Diop BM, Dieng Y, et al; Mental disorders in cerebral malaria. Dakar Med 47(2)122–127, 2002

Timmermans M, Carr J: Neurosyphilis in the modern era. J Neurol Neurosurg Psychiatry 75:1727–1730, 2004

Tomes N: The making of a germ panic, then and now. Am J Public Health 90:191–198, 2000

Treadway CR, Prange AJ Jr: Tetanus mimicking psychophysiologic reaction: occurrence after dental extraction. JAMA 200:891–892, 1967

Tyler KL: Creutzfeldt-Jakob disease. N Engl J Med 348:681–682, 2003

Vallini AD, Burns RL: Carbamazepine as therapy for psychiatric sequelae of herpes simplex encephalitis. South Med J 80: 1590–1592, 1987

Van Lierde S, van Leeuwen WJ, Ceuppens J, et al: Toxic shock syndrome without rash in a young child: link with syndrome of hemorrhagic shock and encephalopathy? Pediatrics 13:130–134, 1997

Varney NR, Roberts RJ, Springer JA, et al: Neuropsychiatric sequelae of cerebral malaria in Vietnam veterans. J Nerv Ment Dis 185:695–703, 1997

Verghese A: The "typhoid state" revisited. Am J Med 79:370–372, 1985

Villanueva MS: Trypanosomiasis of the central nervous system. Semin Neurol 13:209–218, 1993

Vinetz JM: Leptospirosis. Curr Opin Infect Dis 14:527–538, 2001

Vinetz JM, Glass GE, Flexner CE, et al: Sporadic urban leptospirosis. Ann Intern Med 125:794–798, 1996

Vuorio KA, Aarela E, Lehtinen V: Eight cases of patients with unfounded fear of AIDS. Int J Psychiatry Med 20:405–411, 1990

Wallin MT, Kurtzke JF: Neurocysticercosis in the United States: review of an important emerging infection. Neurology 63:1559–1564, 2004

Weinstein L: Bacterial meningitis. Specific etiologic diagnosis on the basis of distinctive epidemiologic, pathogenetic, and clinical features. Med Clin North Am 69:219–229, 1985

Weir E: Anthrax: walking the fine line between precaution and panic. CMAJ 165:1528, 2001

Weiss MG: The interrelationship of tropical disease and mental disorder: conceptual framework and literature review (Part I: malaria). Cult Med Psychiatry 9:121–200, 1985

Wessely S, Pariante C: Fatigue, depression and chronic hepatitis C infection. Psychol Med 32:1–10, 2002

White PD, Thomas JM, Amess J, et al: Incidence, risk and prognosis of acute and chronic fatigue syndromes and psychiatric disorders after glandular fever. Br J Psychiatry 173:475–481, 1998

Whitley RJ, Soong SJ, Linneman C Jr, et al: Herpes simplex encephalitis: clinical assessment. JAMA 247:317–320, 1982

Yamasaki K, Morimoto N, Gion T, et al: Delirium and a subclavian abscess. Lancet 350:1294, 1997

Zauner C, Gendo A, Kramer L, et al: Impaired subcortical and cortical sensory evoked potential pathways in septic patients. Crit Care Med 30:1136–1139, 2002

Self-Assessment Questions

Select the single best response for each question.

1. Pediatric autoimmune neuropsychiatric disorder associated with streptococcal infection (PANDAS) offers a compelling model for infectious disease–induced psychiatric illness. All of the following are true regarding PANDAS *except*

   A. PANDAS frequently has an episodic course characterized by abrupt onset of symptoms with frequent relapses and remissions.
   B. PANDAS consists of obsessive-compulsive and tic symptoms that occur following group A beta-hemolytic streptococcus (GABHS) infection.
   C. The infection most commonly implicated is pharyngitis.
   D. Antistreptolysin-O (ASO) titers rise with GABHS infections, and levels covary with symptoms.
   E. Because of the high specificity of ASO titers in evaluation, throat cultures are not necessary.

2. Rocky Mountain spotted fever (RMSF) is another infectious disease that is associated with neuropsychiatric complications. Which of the following statements is *true?*

   A. The incidence of RMSF peaks in October through April.
   B. Central nervous system (CNS) involvement is seen in 25% of RMSF cases and includes lethargy, confusion, and delirium.
   C. Irritability, personality changes, and apathy may occur commonly in elderly individuals before the rash in RMSF.
   D. Encephalopathy in RMSF is rare unless computed tomography (CT) or magnetic resonance imaging (MRI) scans are abnormal.
   E. Over 50% of U.S. RMSF cases occur in the mountainous west.

3. Viral hepatitis is a common clinical problem with psychiatric implications. Which of the following statements is *true?*

   A. Depression is a contraindication to interferon therapy.
   B. Fatigue in chronic hepatitis is more closely related to disease severity than to depression or social factors.
   C. Depression is uncommon in hepatitis C and B infections.
   D. Depression is induced in 20%–40% of patients treated with interferon.
   E. Depression induced by interferon is not responsive to selective serotonin reuptake inhibitors (SSRIs).

4. Meningoencephalitis with prominent somnolence, colloquially known as sleeping sickness, is associated with which of the following infections?

   A. Neurocysticercosis.
   B. Toxoplasmosis.
   C. Trypanosomiasis.
   D. Malaria.
   E. Schistosomiasis.

5. Which of the following drugs has been associated with irritability and depression?

    A. Procaine penicillin.

    B. Quinolones.

    C. Acyclovir.

    D. Interferon-alpha.

    E. Interleukin-2.

11 HIV/AIDS

Niccolò D. Della Penna, M.D.
Glenn J. Treisman, M.D., Ph.D.

SOON AFTER THE human immuno-deficiency virus (HIV) epidemic began in the early 1980s, neurologists described several HIV-related central nervous system (CNS) syndromes. Two decades later, it is apparent that psychiatric issues play a central role in the HIV epidemic. HIV is transmitted almost entirely by specific risk behaviors and in high-risk populations targeted for education and prevention since the mid-1980s. Because of this, HIV, at least in the developed countries, has become a condition predominantly of vulnerable people with certain risk factors. Psychiatric disorders also can adversely affect the treatment of HIV infection primarily through undermining adherence, and taking medications as prescribed is critical to successful treatment.

In this chapter, we address those conditions commonly seen in HIV, including those that increase risk for HIV or are barriers to HIV treatment. The introductory part of the chapter is a medical overview of HIV disease; the second part considers neuropsychiatric and medical complications associated with HIV; and the third part includes psychiatric conditions associated with HIV. Additional details regarding psychiatric disorders and treatment issues can be found in the American Psychiatric Association's "Practice Guideline for the Treatment of Patients With HIV/AIDS" (American Psychiatric Association 2000).

Overview of HIV Infection and AIDS

HIV was originally recognized through a series of cases of young homosexual men with *Pneumocystis carinii* pneumonia in the early 1980s. Current global statistics suggest that 750,000 infants are born each year with HIV infection, and some estimate that 16,000 new infections occur each day, with one individual being infected about every 10 seconds (UNAIDS Joint United Nations Programme on HIV/AIDS Update 2000).

In the United States, as of December 31, 2001, 807,075 adults and adolescents had been reported as having AIDS, with current estimates suggested around 1 million. Of these, 462,653 (57%) have died. As of the end of 2002, 42 million people were estimated to be living with HIV/AIDS worldwide (Centers for Disease Control and Prevention 2001). An estimated 20 million individuals have died from HIV worldwide. Some populations within the United States are at increased risk for infection. Homosexual men have reduced their risk substantially but as a group continue to have high seroprevalence. Blood product screening has made transfusion risk negligible. Vertical transmission risk from mother to fetus is influenced by delivery type, severity of HIV disease, and the availability of preventive antiviral treatment.

Unfortunately, psychiatric disorders continue to make many vulnerable patients unable to access or benefit from prevention efforts. Patients who are likely to have poor adherence and therefore fail treatment may be excluded from treatment. The primary reason for excluding them from antiretroviral drug treatment is that inconsistent adherence breeds viral resistance, rendering treatment ineffective and increasing public health risk. Additionally, resources are often scarce in HIV clinics, and patients who are less likely to remain adherent are the least likely to receive effective treatment. Psychiatric disorders compromise the ability to take medications, adhere to treatment, practice safer sexual behaviors, and stop using intravenous drugs.

Neuropsychiatric and Medical Complications of HIV Infection

Opportunistic infections are covered in Chapter 10, "Infectious Diseases," but here we review some specifics related to HIV infection.

Toxoplasmosis

Infection with *Toxoplasma gondii* generally occurs in patients with fewer than 200 CD4 cells/mm^3. In AIDS patients, toxoplasmosis is the most common reason for intracranial masses, affecting between 2% and 4% of the AIDS population. Symptoms of CNS infection are fever, change in level of alertness, headache, focal neurological signs, and partial or generalized seizures. Computed tomography (CT) and magnetic resonance imaging (MRI) scans usually show multiple ring-enhancing lesions in the basal ganglia or at the gray–white matter junction.

Cytomegalovirus

Cytomegalovirus (CMV) infection is found at autopsy in about 30% of brains from HIV-infected patients. However, the development of clinically evident CMV encephalitis is fairly rare and most often occurs in patients with CD4 cell counts less than 50 cells/mm^3. CMV encephalitis in AIDS may progress gradually as a dementia with focal deficits (Holland et al. 1994) or rapidly as a fatal delirium (Kalayjian et al. 1993).

Cryptococcal Meningitis

Meningitis caused by *Cryptococcus neoformans* occurs in approximately 8%–10% of AIDS patients and may be devastating. Patients generally present with fever and delirium. Seizures and focal neurological deficits occur in about 10% of patients, and intracranial pressure is elevated in about 50% of patients.

Progressive Multifocal Leukoencephalopathy

Progressive multifocal leukoencephalopathy (PML) is a demyelinating disease of white matter in immunocompromised patients. The causative agent is the JC virus, and its transmission route is unclear but may be respiratory. The prevalence of PML in AIDS is between 1% and 10%, and AIDS patients account for almost three-quarters of PML cases reported in the United States. Typically, PML affects AIDS patients with fewer than 100 CD4 cells/mm^3.

The clinical syndrome consists of multiple focal neurological deficits, such as mono- or hemiparetic limb weakness, dysarthria, gait disturbances, sensory deficits, and progressive dementia, with eventual coma and death. Occasionally, seizures or visual losses may occur.

MRI is more useful than CT in diagnosis; multiple areas of attenuated signal are seen on T2 images, primarily in the white matter of brain, although gray matter, brain stem, cerebellar, and spinal cord lesions are possible. Cerebrospinal fluid (CSF) studies may reveal the presence of JC virus, which is sensitive and specific.

Central Nervous System Neoplasms

Lymphoma is the most common neoplasm seen in AIDS patients, affecting between 0.6% and 3%. AIDS is the most common condition associated with primary CNS lymphoma. The patient is generally afebrile; may develop a single lesion with focal neurological signs or small, multifocal lesions; and most commonly presents with mental status change. Seizures occur in about 15% of these patients.

CT scan of the brain may be normal or show multiple hypodense or patchy, nodular enhancing lesions. MRI generally shows enhanced lesions that may be difficult to differentiate from CNS toxoplasmosis. CSF studies may be normal or show a moderate monocytosis; cytology studies report lymphoma cells in fewer than 5% of patients. Brain biopsy is required for confirmation of the diagnosis of CNS lymphoma. The differential diagnosis of CNS neoplasm also includes metastatic Kaposi's sarcoma and primary glial tumors.

Fatigue in HIV

Fatigue is a very common symptom in HIV-infected patients. It is associated with poor quality of life and impaired physical functioning (Breitbart et al. 1998; Darko et al. 1992; Hoover et al. 1993; Longo et al. 1990; Vlahov et al. 1994). Estimates of prevalence of fatigue in patients infected with HIV range from 10% to 30% in early cases to 40% to 50% in AIDS cases (Anderson and Grady 1994; Crocker 1989; Miller et al. 1991; Revicki et al. 1994; Richman et al. 1987). Fatigue is a nonspecific symptom and may have a single or multifactorial etiology. In a sample of ambulatory AIDS patients, fatigue significantly correlated with anemia and pain (Breitbart et al. 1998). In addition to disease causes, fatigue may be a side effect of medications, including HAART. Fatigue is one of the most common side effects of protease inhibitors and may be a reason for nonadherence (Duran et al. 2001).

Fatigue also may be the result of substance abuse, and HIV patients with major depression are much more likely to complain of fatigue than are patients without depression (Ferrando et al. 1998a; Perkins et al. 1995). HIV wasting syndrome, chronic diarrhea, and testosterone deficiency are all associated with fatigue. Low serum testosterone has been found among symptomatic AIDS patients, especially those with HIV wasting syndrome (Berger et al. 1998; Dobs et al. 1996; Grinspoon et al. 1998; Laudat et al. 1995; Muurahainen and Mulligan 1998). Hypotestosteronism is most likely in advanced AIDS (Kopicko et al. 1999) but also may be due to medications (e.g., fluconazole, ketoconazole, or ganciclovir) (Wagner et al. 1995).

Testosterone may be a successful treatment for fatigue in HIV-infected men, even when depressive symptoms are present (Wagner et al. 1998). More activating antidepressants may be better tolerated by fatigued depressed patients. Some authors have reported that stimulants may be useful in treating fatigue and depression in HIV, as discussed later in this chapter.

Psychiatric Conditions Associated With HIV

Delirium

Delirium occurs frequently in patients with advanced HIV infection (Bialer et al. 1991; Fernandez et al. 1989). One study found that 46% of the AIDS patients at a skilled nursing facility had at least one episode of delirium (Uldall and Berghuis 1997). In addition, delirium has been shown to be a marker for decreased survival in patients with AIDS (Uldall et al. 2000a, 2000b).

The clinical presentation of delirium in HIV patients is the same as in non-HIV-infected individuals and is characterized by inattention, disorganized thinking or confusion, and fluctuations in level of consciousness. Emotional changes are common and often unpredictable, and hallucinations and delusions are frequently seen. The syndrome has an acute or a subacute onset and remits fairly rapidly once the underlying etiology is treated.

Aside from general risk factors such as older age, multiple medical problems, multiple medications, impaired visual acuity, and previous episodes of delirium, patients with HIV-associated dementia are at increased risk to develop delirium. The cause of delirium should be aggressively sought. The approach to determining cause is similar to that for delirium in general. Particular considerations in HIV patients include hypoxia with *Pneumocystis* pneumonia, malnutrition, CNS infections and neoplasms, systemic infections (e.g., mycobacteria, CMV, bacterial sepsis), HIV nephropathy, substance intoxication

and withdrawal, medication toxicity, and deliriant medications. Variations in hydration or electrolyte status also may profoundly affect patients with HIV who already have cerebral compromise. HIV infection itself also may produce an acute encephalopathy similar to that reported with CMV (Bialer et al. 2000).

Treatment

Management of delirium in HIV is very similar to that for delirium in general, including identification and removal of the underlying cause (when possible), non-pharmacological reorientation and environmental interventions, and pharmacotherapy. Low doses of high-potency antipsychotic agents usually are effective. Newer, atypical antipsychotics are currently being used with some success, but those with more anticholinergic activity may worsen the condition. Benzodiazepines should be used with caution because they may contribute to delirium in some patients but are of particular use in alcohol or benzodiazepine withdrawal deliria. Physical restraint may be necessary if the patient becomes violent but should be used only when alternatives are inadequate, because restraint may worsen delirium.

Treatment with antipsychotic medication requires awareness of the higher susceptibility of patients with HIV to neuroleptic-induced extrapyramidal symptoms (EPS), even with exposure to drugs with low potential for inducing EPS (Edelstein and Knight 1987; Hollander et al. 1985; Hriso et al. 1991). Increased susceptibility to EPS has been particularly notable with use of conventional neuroleptic medications and has limited the dosage that can be used to treat patients (Maj 1990; Sewell et al. 1994b). Extreme sensitivity to EPS is encountered in patients with HIV dementia (Fernandez et al. 1989). To date, only one randomized controlled trial in delirious patients with AIDS has documented efficacy of low-dose haloperidol and chlorpromazine (Breitbart et al. 1996). If indicated, typical neuroleptic medications should be used at the lowest dosage and for the briefest duration possible. Atypical antipsychotics are generally preferred because of lower risk for EPS.

Dementia

Prevalence

Early in the AIDS epidemic, some patients presented with rapidly progressing neurocognitive disturbances. A subset of patients remained for which no identifiable pathogen could be found, and it was deduced that HIV itself was the causative factor behind the dementia. It appears that basal ganglia and nigrostriatal structures are affected early in the dementia process, with diffuse neuronal losses following. Typical late findings show an approximate 40% reduction in frontal and temporal neurons.

In 1986, HIV-associated dementia was reported in up to two-thirds of AIDS patients (Navia et al. 1986), but it is less frequent now in patients receiving HAART. It has become one of the leading causes of dementia in persons younger than 60 (McArthur et al. 1993). However, its frequency among patients with otherwise asymptomatic HIV infection or CD4 cell count greater than 500 cells/mm^3 is probably less than 5% in a community sample (Handelsman et al. 1992; Krikorian et al. 1990; Maj et al. 1994; McKegney et al. 1990; Wilkie et al. 1990). For hospitalized HIV-infected patients seen in psychiatric consultation, the rate of HIV-associated dementia has been measured at 7%–25% (Buhrich and Cooper 1987; Dilley et al. 1985). In the Multicenter AIDS Cohort Study (Sacktor et al. 1999a), the incidence of HIV-associated dementia declined 50% from 1990–1992 to 1996–1998, a period during which effective antiretroviral therapy was used (Sacktor et al. 1999a). HIV-

associated dementia is generally seen in late stages of HIV illness, usually in patients who have had a CD4 cell count nadir of less than 200/mm^3.

Risk factors associated with eventual development of HIV dementia include higher HIV RNA viral load, lower educational level, older age, anemia, illicit drug use, and female sex. High CSF HIV RNA levels may be present in patients with relatively low serum HIV RNA levels and may correlate more directly with severity of neurological deficits (McArthur et al. 1997).

Assessment

Clinically, HIV dementia presents with the typical triad of symptoms seen in other subcortical dementias—memory and psychomotor speed impairments, depressive symptoms, and movement disorders. Initially, patients may notice slight problems with reading, comprehension, memory, and mathematical skills, but these symptoms are subtle, so they may be overlooked or discounted as being caused by fatigue and illness. The Modified HIV Dementia Scale is a very useful bedside screen and can be administered serially to document disease progression (Davis et al. 2002). Later, patients develop more global dementia, with marked impairments in naming, language, and praxis.

Motor symptoms are also often subtle in the early stages and include occasional stumbling while walking or running, as well as slowing of fine repetitive movements. Patients will have impaired saccadic eye movements, dysdiadochokinesia, hyperreflexia, and, especially in later stages, frontal release signs. In late stages, motor symptoms may be quite severe, with marked difficulty in smooth limb movements. Rate of progression is variable and may cause mild dysfunction over a long period or rapid progression with severe impairment (Price and Brew 1988). Parkinsonian features are common in HIV-associated dementia, and clinical correlates between HIV and parkinsonism have been identified (Koutsilieri et al. 2002; Mirsattari et al. 1998).

Apathy is a common early symptom of HIV-associated dementia, often causing noticeable withdrawal by the patient from social activity. A frank depressive syndrome also commonly develops, typically with irritable mood and anhedonia instead of sadness and crying spells. Sleep disturbances and weight loss are common. Restlessness and anxiety may occur. Psychosis develops in a significant number of patients, typically with paranoid thoughts and hallucinations. Overall, HIV-associated dementia is rapidly progressive, usually ending in death within 2 years. Because of impulsive behavior and emotional lability, HIV-associated dementia has been suggested as a strong risk factor for suicide (Alfonso and Cohen 1994).

Diagnosis

Typical findings on MRI of patients with advanced HIV-associated dementia include significant white matter lesions, as well as cortical and subcortical atrophy (Dal Pan et al. 1992; Jarvik et al. 1988; Stout et al. 1998). MRI also has been suggested to be of utility in monitoring HIV-associated dementia treatment with HAART (Thurnher et al. 2000).

Increased brain activation on functional MRI during working memory was found in patients with early HIV cognitive disturbance (Chang et al. 2001). Further studies showed increased activation on functional MRI in HIV-positive patients that predated clinical signs or deficits on cognitive tests (Ernst et al. 2002).

Recent evidence suggests that HIV-associated dementia may develop in the presence of milder immunosuppression (Dore et al. 1999). Rates of HIV-associated dementia have declined, but not to the same extent that other AIDS-defining illnesses have declined. In the Multicenter AIDS Cohort Study (1990–1998; Sacktor et al. 2001), the proportion of cases of HIV-associated dementia in patients with CD4 cell counts of 201–350 cells/mm^3 was higher in 1996–1998 compared with the early 1990s. This suggests that screening for HIV-associated dementia should be extended to patients with CD4 cell counts less than 350 cells/mm^3 (Sacktor et al. 1999b, 2001). The extended survival that antiretroviral regimens have offered patients also may increase their vulnerability to developing dementia rather than dying secondary to other fulminant complications (Lopez et al. 1999).

Treatment

Intensification of antiretroviral therapy and associated control of viral load are associated with significantly lower risk for progression to HIV-associated dementia (Childs et al. 1999). The AIDS Clinical Trial Groups trial compared high doses of zidovudine with placebo but was stopped sooner than planned after preliminary data showed dramatic cognitive improvement in those receiving zidovudine (Sidtis et al. 1993). A sharp decline in the incidence of HIV-associated dementia was observed following widespread use of zidovudine (Chiesi et al. 1990, 1996; Portegies et al. 1989), and HIV-associated dementia became rare in patients receiving continued zidovudine treatment (Portegies et al. 1989). More recent studies showed efficacy of HAART in improving cognitive impairment in patients with HIV-associated dementia (Ferrando et al. 1998b; Giesen et al. 2000; Halman and Rourke 2000; Letendre et al. 2000; Price et al. 1999; Tozzi et al. 1999, 2001).

The long-term effect of HAART on the course of HIV-associated dementia remains undetermined, with some evidence of ongoing HIV-related cognitive damage despite more than 3 years of potent antiretroviral treatment (Tozzi et al. 2001). The only other controlled trial of antiretroviral drugs compared effective antiviral therapy with and without added high-dose abacavir (Brew et al. 1998), but the study did not detect further cognitive improvement.

At first, it was believed that only antiretroviral agents with good penetration into the CNS would be useful in treating HIV-associated dementia with associated reduction of CSF HIV RNA levels (Halman and Rourke 2000), but later efforts indicated that HAART in many different combinations, including those with poor CNS levels, could provide some relief. Despite these theoretical considerations, little evidence suggests an improved outcome for any particular antiretroviral regimen (Clifford 2000).

Use of dopamine receptor agonists in pediatric patients with HIV and parkinsonian features has led to improvement in motor function (Mintz et al. 1996), yet results of similar medications in adults have been less fruitful (Kieburtz et al. 1991a). Psychostimulants have been shown to improve cognitive performance in patients with HIV (Brown 1995; Hinkin et al. 2001), but others have noted apparent acceleration of HIV-associated dementia following psychostimulant use (Czub et al. 2001; Nath et al. 2001).

Quality care for patients with HIV-associated dementia is to ensure an optimal HAART regimen and to treat associated symptoms aggressively. Depression can be treated with standard antidepressants, and, in some cases, methylphenidate or other stimulants may be useful in treatment of apathy.

Minor Cognitive-Motor Disorder

HIV-associated dementia is a late-stage disorder, whereas minor cognitive-motor disorder (or mild neurocognitive disorder) is a less severe syndrome seen in earlier HIV infection. Patients with this disorder may present with a singular minor complaint, such as taking longer to read a novel, dysfunction when performing fine motor tasks such as playing the piano, an increased tendency to stumble or trip, or making more mistakes when balancing the checkbook. Minor cognitive-motor disorder is now regarded as part of the spectrum of HIV-associated dementia.

Prevalence data for minor cognitive-motor disorder are variable, often suggesting up to 60% prevalence by late-stage AIDS. Whether minor cognitive-motor disorder inevitably leads to HIV-associated dementia is uncertain.

Treatment

No controlled treatment data are available specifically for minor cognitive-motor disorder.

Major Depression

Depression is a significant problem among persons with HIV and AIDS. The question of whether the incidence or prevalence of major depression is increased in HIV-infected patients has been a controversial topic (Ciesla and Roberts 2001). First, identification of major depressive disorder rather than depressive symptoms is a methodological barrier to cross-sample comparison. Additionally, populations at risk for HIV infection, including homosexual men and patients with substance use disorders, have elevated rates of major depression. A recent meta-analysis of 10 studies comparing HIV-positive and at-risk HIV-negative patients found a twofold increase in the prevalence of major depression in patients infected with HIV (Ciesla and Roberts 2001).

Lyketsos and Treisman reported an association between depression and HIV infection as early as 1993 and speculated that major depression was a risk factor for developing HIV (Lyketsos et al. 1993a). Studies have shown prevalence rates of major depression among individuals with HIV of 15%–40%, depending on the setting and risk group studied (American Psychiatric Association 2000; Atkinson et al. 1988; Perkins et al. 1994; Treisman et al. 1998). However, the prevalence exceeds 50% in persons with HIV seeking psychiatric treatment (American Psychiatric Association 2000). Major depression is a risk factor for HIV infection (McDermott et al. 1994) by virtue of its effect on behavior, intensification of substance abuse, exacerbation of self-destructive behaviors, and promotion of poor partner choice in relationships. HIV-negative persons with higher scores on screening instruments for general psychological distress were found to have increased risk behaviors for HIV acquisition (Hartgers et al. 1992).

Major depression also is a risk factor for various behavioral disturbances that may increase exposure to HIV infection (Regier et al. 1990). In this way, depression can be seen as a vector of HIV transmission (Angelino and Treisman 2001; Treisman et al. 1998). Depression not only serves as a risk for perpetuation of the HIV epidemic (Morrill et al. 1996; Nyamathi 1992; Orr et al. 1994) but also is a complication preventing effective treatment. It has been clearly shown to hinder effective treatment of HIV infection (van Servellen et al. 2002). Patients with major depression are at increased risk for disease progression and mortality (Ickovics et al. 2001).

HIV increases the risk of developing major depression through a variety of mechanisms, including direct injury to subcortical areas of brain, chronic stress, worsening social isolation, and intense demoralization. Direct evidence for a relation between worsening HIV disease and the development of major depression is limited, but several studies support this link, particularly the Multicenter AIDS Cohort Study. This study showed that rates of depression increased 2.5-fold as CD4 cells declined to fewer than 200/mm^3 just before patients developed AIDS (Lyketsos et al. 1996a), suggesting that lower CD4 cell counts predict increased rates of depression.

Patients with AIDS have been recognized as a group with a high risk for psychological distress (Lyketsos et al. 1996b). High prevalence rates of suicide have been reported among HIV-infected patients (Cournos et al. 1991; L. Grassi 1996; Pugh et al. 1993; Sacks et al. 1992; Weinhardt and Carey 1995). Factors associated with HIV and suicide include depression, hopelessness, alcohol abuse, poor social support, low self-esteem, and history of psychiatric disorder (Fawcett 1992; Murphy 1977). Recent diagnosis of HIV or presence of pain also is associated with increased suicidal thoughts (Louhivuori and Hakama 1979; Steer et al. 1994). The course of HIV has been purported to affect the prevalence of suicidal thoughts and behavior (Rabkin et al. 1993), and stage of HIV infection also may alter the potential for suicidal behavior and other psychiatric symptoms (Lyketsos et al. 1994).

Differential Diagnosis

The differential diagnosis of depression in HIV includes nonpathological states of grief and mourning (sometimes made quite severe by the vulnerabilities of the person) and a variety of psychological and physiological disturbances. Patients with complaints of depressive syndromes can have dysthymia, dementia, delirium, demoralization, intoxication, withdrawal, CNS injury or infection, malnutrition, wasting syndromes, medication side effects, and a variety of other conditions. HIV-associated dementia and other HIV-related CNS conditions can produce a flat, apathetic state that is often misdiagnosed as depression. Cocaine withdrawal produces a depressive syndrome, and hypoactive delirium can be mistaken for depression.

HIV-infected patients with major depression frequently present to internists and family practitioners with multiple somatic symptoms and may also report slowed thought processes, with impairments in concentration and short-term memory and occasionally generalized confusion. Nonspecific somatic symptoms are often the result of depression rather than HIV infection in patients whose infection is early and asymptomatic. Care should be taken in distinguishing between major depression and demoralization (i.e., adjustment disorder) in patients with HIV. Approximately one-half of the patients presenting to an urban HIV clinic with depressive complaints were found to have demoralization alone (Lyketsos et al. 1994). The ability to report feeling fairly normal when distracted from thinking about the precipitating event or circumstance causing distress is a hallmark of demoralization.

Worsening of fatigue and insomnia at 6-month follow-up was highly correlated with worsening depression but not with CD4 cell count, change in CD4 cell count, or disease progression by Centers for Disease Control and Prevention category (Perkins et al. 1995). These findings support the notion that somatic symptoms generally suggestive of depression should trigger a full psychiatric evaluation.

Certain HIV-related medical conditions can cause depressive symptoms, including CNS infections and hypotestosteronism (Rabkin et al. 1999b). Several drugs used in patients with HIV, including efavirenz, interferon, metoclopramide, clonidine, propranolol, sulfonamides, anabolic steroids, and corticosteroids, have been reported to produce depression. These depressive symptoms often respond to withdrawal of the offending drug; when they do not respond to withdrawal of the drug or when the drug must be continued, the symptoms should be treated as major depression with appropriate antidepressant medication.

Treatment

Treatment with HAART was associated with significant improvement in symptoms of depression but did not necessarily have a causal relationship (Brechtl et al. 2001). Several studies reported efficacy of various antidepressants in HIV-infected patients, but no single antidepressant has been found superior in treating HIV-infected patients as a group. As with all depressed patients, nonadherence is the most common reason for ineffective drug treatment, and adverse effects are the most common reason for nonadherence. Antidepressants should be started at subtherapeutic dosage and raised slowly.

For a detailed review of the pharmacological treatment of major depression in HIV, see Ferrando and Wapenyi (2002). Early controlled trials of imipramine showed good response compared with placebo, but dropout with imipramine was frequent (Manning et al. 1990; Rabkin et al. 1994a). Open-label trials of fluoxetine, sertraline, and paroxetine in various stages of HIV illness reported response rates (including affective and somatic depressive symptoms) of 70%–90%, and all the medications were well tolerated (Ferrando et al. 1997; Rabkin et al. 1994a, 1994b). One double-blind, placebo-controlled study of fluoxetine found significant response (Rabkin et al. 1999a). Another similarly designed trial in HIV-infected users of intravenous cocaine and opioids showed significant reduction in depressive symptoms with fluoxetine compared with placebo (Batki et al. 1993).

Supportive group psychotherapy and fluoxetine were found to be superior to placebo plus group therapy for a population of homosexual or bisexual men with HIV, and patients with more severe symptoms tended to achieve greater benefits from medication (Zisook et al. 1998). In a comparison of paroxetine and imipramine, both drugs were superior to placebo in patients with HIV and major depression (Elliott et al. 1998). Small open-label trials of venlafaxine, mirtazapine, and nefazodone in patients with major depression and HIV found that response rates were higher than 70% and there were few side effects (Elliott and Roy-Byrne 2000; Elliott et al. 1999; Fernandez and Levy 1997).

In a comparison between fluoxetine and desipramine in women with AIDS, rates of response were 53% and 75%, respectively (Schwartz and McDaniel 1999). A separate trial comparing women taking fluoxetine and sertraline showed response rates of 78% and 75%, respectively (Ferrando et al. 1999).

Major depression in HIV-positive men with testosterone deficiency has been effectively treated with intramuscular testosterone in an open trial (with 79% response in mood symptoms) (Rabkin et al. 1999b) and was replicated in a double-blind, controlled trial (Rabkin et al. 2000b). Dehydroepiandrosterone, a precursor to testosterone, improved mood symptoms during an open-label phase but not during a placebo-controlled discontinuation phase (Rabkin et al. 2000a).

Psychostimulants also have been evaluated for treatment of fatigue, cognitive impairment, and depression in patients with HIV. Open-label trials report an 85% mood response rate in patients with HIV-associated dementia taking methylphenidate (V.F. Holmes et al. 1989) and a 95% mood response rate in men with AIDS taking dextroamphetamine (Wagner et al. 1997). A double-blind trial showed a significant response to dextroamphetamine compared with placebo in patients with

AIDS and major depression, subthreshold major depression, or dysthymia (Wagner and Rabkin 2000). Double-blind comparison of methylphenidate, pemoline, and placebo in patients with HIV (most with AIDS) found improvement in both depressive symptoms and fatigue (Breitbart et al. 2001). Others have reported similar outcomes in treating fatigue and depression in HIV (Fernandez et al. 1995; Masand and Tesar 1996; White et al. 1992).

St. John's wort is often used by patients as alternative antidepressant treatment, but it may lower serum levels of protease inhibitors ("St. John's Wort and HAART" 2000), and patients receiving any HIV treatment should be advised not to take it.

The side effects of certain antidepressants can render them advantageous or disadvantageous in particular patients with HIV. For example, selective serotonin reuptake inhibitors are best avoided in patients with chronic diarrhea. Sedating antidepressants should be avoided in patients with weakness, lethargy, orthostasis, or other risk for falls. Tricyclic antidepressants should be avoided with oral candidiasis because of the aggravating effect of dry mouth on thrush. In cases of anorexia or cachexia, antidepressants with appetite-stimulating effects are preferred.

An important issue is the interaction of antidepressants and HAART medications. Particularly because depression is associated with reductions in adherence to HAART, the risks of untreated depression must be measured against those of potential medication interactions. Clinical significance of these drug–drug interactions has not yet been clearly established (i.e., dose adjustments are probably not required). This is likely because both antidepressants and HAART, unlike drugs such as warfarin or digoxin, have wide therapeutic indices. No evidence indicates that antidepressants cause fluctuations in CD4 cell counts (Wagner et al. 1996).

Psychotherapy. The literature on the use of psychotherapy for treatment of depression in HIV-infected patients is extensive, but clinical trial data are sparse. One study showed that interpersonal psychotherapy and supportive psychotherapy with adjunctive use of imipramine were superior to cognitive-behavioral therapy (CBT) or supportive psychotherapy without antidepressants in treating symptoms of depression and improving Karnofsky performance scores (Markowitz et al. 1998). Group CBT used alone or in combination with medication also has shown efficacy for HIV-infected patients. Improvements have been reported as well for HIV-positive patients receiving group CBT either as a single treatment modality or combined with medication (Antoni et al. 1991; Chesney et al. 1996; J. Kelly 1998; Lutgendorf et al. 1997a).

Supportive psychotherapy can help patients with major depression who interpret their suffering to be a sign of weakness in the face of adversity. Education about the disease and nature of their depression, encouragement, and therapeutic optimism all may be helpful. Other issues that arise in psychotherapy include guilt over acquiring HIV; guilt over infecting others; and anger at the source of disease, or at oneself. The diagnosis of HIV infection may lead to precipitous revelation of hidden sexual or drug abuse behavior, eliciting shame and self-loathing. The stigma of HIV may lead to rejection or abandonment by loved ones, and shunning by wider society. Despite the development of HAART, some patients become hopeless and nihilistic and forgo HIV treatment.

Bipolar Disorder

Patients with preexisting bipolar disorder may experience exacerbations because of the stresses of HIV illness. Numerous case reports and case series have described mania in HIV-infected patients (Boccellari et al. 1988; Halman et al. 1993; Hoffman 1984; Kieburtz et al. 1991b; Lyketsos et al. 1993b, 1997).

The prevalence of mania has been found to be increased in patients with AIDS when compared with the general population (Halman et al. 1993; Kieburtz et al. 1991b). One report indicated a 17-month prevalence of 1.4% in those with HIV and 8.0% in patients with AIDS, which was 10 times the expected 6-month prevalence in the general population (Lyketsos et al. 1993b). In this group, late-onset patients were less likely to have a personal or family history of mood disorder. Another study among inpatients reported a 29-month prevalence of secondary mania of 1.2% in patients with HIV and 4.3% in those with AIDS (Ellen et al. 1999).

Some have suggested that mania should be subdivided into primary and secondary types, with patients who have the secondary type showing close temporal proximity to an organic insult, no prior history of mania, essentially negative family history, and late age at onset (Krauthammer and Klerman 1978). Secondary mania includes those cases due to HIV brain disease itself (Gabel et al. 1986; Kermani et al. 1985; Perry and Jacobsen 1986; Schmidt and Miller 1988), those due to antiretroviral drugs (Brouillette et al. 1994; Maxwell et al. 1988; O'Dowd and McKegney 1988; Wright et al. 1989), and those due to other HIV-related conditions (e.g., cryptococcal meningitis) or medications (Fichtner and Braun 1992; V.F. Holmes and Ficchione 1989; Johannessen and Wilson 1988; Nightingale et al. 1995; Pickles and Spelman 1996). An increased risk of HIV-associated dementia and cognitive slowing was found in one group of patients with secondary HIV mania, with cognitive decline prior to onset of mania (Lyketsos et al. 1997). In addition, the secondary mania associated with HIV was found to be associated with low CD4 cell count (Ellen et al. 1999; Lyketsos et al. 1993b), often lower than 100 cells/mm^3. The incidence of secondary mania, like that of HIV-associated dementia, appears to have declined since the widespread use of HAART (Ferrando and Wapenyi 2002).

AIDS mania seems to have a clinical profile somewhat different from that of primary mania (Ellen et al. 1999; Lyketsos et al. 1993b, 1997). Irritable mood is often a prominent feature, but elevated mood can be observed. Sometimes prominent psychomotor slowing accompanying the cognitive slowing of AIDS dementia will replace the expected hyperactivity of mania, which complicates the differential diagnosis. AIDS mania is usually quite severe in its presentation and malignant in its course. Late-onset patients may be more commonly irritable and less commonly hyperverbal. AIDS mania seems to be more chronic than episodic, with infrequent spontaneous remissions, and usually relapses with cessation of treatment.

One presentation of mania, either early or late, is the delusional belief that one has discovered a cure for HIV or has been cured. Although this belief may serve to cheer otherwise demoralized patients, it also may result in the resumption of high-risk behavior and lead to the spread of HIV and exposure to other infections.

Treatment

Treatment of secondary HIV or AIDS mania has not been systematically studied to date, and the optimal treatment remains unclear. The treatment of mania in early-stage HIV infection is not substantially different from the standard treatment of bipolar disorder with mood stabilizers and antipsychotics. As HIV infection advances, with lower CD4 cell counts, more medical complications, more CNS involvement, and greater overall physiological vulnerability, changes in treatment may be required.

Treatment with traditional antimanic agents can be very difficult in patients with advanced disease. AIDS mania patients may respond to monotherapy with antipsychotic agents (Ellen et al. 1999). Late-stage patients are sensitive to side effects of antipsychotics, especially EPS.

Lithium use has been problematic for several reasons, including side effects of cognitive slowing, nausea, diarrhea, and polyuria resulting in dehydration, all of which may already plague HIV-infected patients. The major problem with lithium in AIDS patients has been rapid fluctuations in blood level, especially in the hospital despite previously stable doses. Anecdotal reports describe problems with administering lithium and valproic acid because of subsequent delirium (Angelino and Treisman 2001).

A study of valproic acid in the treatment of HIV-associated mania reported that it was well tolerated and led to significant improvement in manic symptoms, with doses up to 1,750 mg/day and serum levels greater than 50 µg/L (Halman et al. 1993). Another report documented reduction in symptoms with levels of 93 and 110 µg/L (RachBeisel and Weintraub 1997). Concern has been raised over hepatotoxicity in patients with HIV taking valproic acid (Cozza et al. 2000). In cases of severe hepatic insufficiency, valproic acid probably should be avoided, but this has not been studied. Valproic acid also can affect hematopoietic function, so white blood cell and platelet counts must be monitored. In addition, sodium valproate has been reported to increase HIV replication in vitro (Jennings and Romanelli 1999; Moog et al. 1996; Simon et al. 1994; Witvrouw et al. 1997), as well as increase CMV replication (Jennings and Romanelli 1999).

Carbamazepine also may be effective, but concerns exist regarding the potential for synergistic bone marrow suppression in combination with antiviral medications and HIV itself. It also may lower serum levels of protease inhibitors (Ferrando and Wapenyi 2002).

There are anecdotal reports of effective treatment of psychosis in HIV-related mania with risperidone (Singh et al. 1997) and olanzapine (Ferrando and Wapenyi 2002). Atypical antipsychotics have the advantage of lower risk of tardive dyskinesia, but this is not an important issue for patients with end-stage AIDS. Reduction of the risk of EPS is a noteworthy consideration in selecting an antipsychotic, in addition to other factors including affordability. The common side effect of significant weight gain with some atypical antipsychotics is less problematic for patients with HIV who are cachectic. Clonazepam may also be useful in HIV-associated mania (Budman and Vandersall 1990).

Schizophrenia

In patients with severe chronic mental illnesses, primarily schizophrenia and bipolar disorder, HIV prevalence rates of between 2% and 20% have been found in both inpatient and outpatient samples (Ayuso-Mateos et al. 1997; Blank et al. 2002; Empfield et al. 1993; Meyer et al. 1993; Naber et al. 1994; Silberstein et al. 1994; Volavka et al. 1991; Walkup et al. 1999). Investigators have noted that clinicians working with patients with schizophrenia were often unaware of their increased risk for seropositivity (Cournos et al. 1991). However, many schizophrenic patients are sexually active (Cournos et al. 1994), often with higher-risk partners (Kalichman et al. 1994); seldom use condoms (Cournos et al. 1994); and do not otherwise practice safe sex. Substance abuse is very common in schizophrenic patients, including during sexual activity (Cournos et al. 1994). Patients with schizophrenia have significantly less knowledge about HIV infection and transmission than do persons without schizophrenia (Kalichman et al. 1994; J.A. Kelly et al. 1992). Suicidality is increased in patients with both schizophrenia and HIV infection. For all these reasons, clinicians should evaluate schizophrenic patients for risk behaviors and for their knowledge about HIV.

Treatment

Treatment of schizophrenia in patients infected with HIV follows the same basic principles as for other patients with schizophrenia—namely, control of symptoms with medications and psychosocial support and rehabilitation. Close collaboration with HIV providers is strongly suggested, so that HIV treatment can be coordinated and monitored. Schizophrenic patients are very likely to have difficulties accessing care, affording medication, and adhering to complex HAART regimens. Educational interventions have promoted safer sexual practices (Baer et al. 1988; Jacobs and Bobek 1991) and may decrease risk behaviors (Carmen and Brady 1990; Kalichman et al. 1995).

Haloperidol was found to be effective in treating psychotic symptoms of schizophrenia in patients with HIV (Mauri et al. 1997; Sewell et al. 1994a, 1994b). Patients with HIV may be highly sensitive to the EPS of antipsychotic medications. Treatment with thioridazine was reported to be efficacious without EPS (Sewell et al. 1994b). Molindone was reported to be of benefit for psychosis and agitation with few EPS in patients with HIV (Fernandez and Levy 1993). Clozapine also has shown efficacy in treating HIV-associated psychosis in patients with drug-induced parkinsonism (Lera and Zirulnik 1999). Risperidone also has been reported to be effective (Singh et al. 1997).

Substance Abuse and Addiction

Substance abuse is a primary vector for the spread of HIV for those who use intravenous drugs and their sexual partners and those who are disinhibited by intoxication or driven by addiction to unsafe sexual practices. In addition, intoxication and the behaviors necessary to obtain drugs interfere with access to, and effectiveness of, health care.

Triple diagnosis refers to a patient with a dual diagnosis (substance abuse and psychiatric disorder) who also has HIV. One study found that as many as 44% of the new entrants to the HIV medical clinic at the Johns Hopkins Hospital had an active substance use disorder. Of these patients, 24% had both a current substance use disorder and another nonsubstance-related Axis I diagnosis (Lyketsos et al. 1994).

In the United States at the end of 2001, the proportion of injection drug users with AIDS was 24% (Centers for Disease Control and Prevention 2001). Even among non–injection drug users, substance abuse plays a major, albeit more subtle, role in HIV transmission. Addiction and high-risk sexual behavior have been linked across a wide range of settings. For example, crack cocaine abusers are more likely to engage in prostitution to obtain money for drugs (Astemborski et al. 1994; Edlin et al. 1994). Men who use crack cocaine are more likely to engage in unprotected anal sex with casual male contacts (de Souza et al. 2002). Alcohol intoxication also can lead to risky sexual behaviors by way of cognitive impairment and disinhibition (Rees et al. 2001; Stein et al. 2000).

Neuropsychological testing of drug abusers with and without HIV indicates that substance use can contribute to the cognitive decline of HIV-associated dementia (Pakesch et al. 1992). Substance use may augment HIV replication in the CNS and increase HIV encephalopathy in early AIDS (Kibayashi et al. 1996).

One of the most extensively studied interventions in risk reduction is methadone maintenance, which resulted in sustained reductions in HIV risk and lower incidence of HIV infection (Metzger et al. 1991, 1998).

Substance Use Disorders and Interaction With HIV Treatment

The medical sequelae of chronic substance abuse accelerate the process of immunocompromise and amplify the burdens of HIV infection. Injection drug users are at higher risk for developing bacterial infections such as pneumonia, sepsis, and endocarditis. Tuberculosis, sexually transmitted diseases (STDs), viral hepatitis, coinfection with human CD4 cell lymphotrophic virus, and lymphomas also occur more commonly in injection drug users with HIV than in other patients with HIV. HIV-infected injection drug users are at higher risk for fungal or bacterial infections of the CNS. Alcohol abuse is immunosuppressive and increases risk for bacterial infections, tuberculosis, and dementia. Heroin may worsen HIV-associated nephropathy.

Important drug interactions occur between abused substances and antiretroviral and antibiotic drugs. Rifampin increases the elimination of methadone and may result in withdrawal symptoms. Decreased plasma levels of methadone also occur with concurrent administration of ritonavir, nelfinavir, efavirenz, and nevirapine (Gourevitch and Friedland 2000).

Posttraumatic Stress Disorder

Posttraumatic stress disorder (PTSD) and its symptoms occur at greatly increased rates in HIV-infected patients (Martinez et al. 2002). Of the HIV-infected women attending county medical clinics, 42% met diagnostic criteria for PTSD (Cottler et al. 2001). Male veterans with a diagnosis of PTSD are at increased risk for HIV infection, especially if they are substance abusers (Hoff et al. 1997). PTSD symptoms are associated with high-risk behaviors, including prostitution, choosing other high-risk sexual partners, injection drug use, and unsafe sexual practices (Stiffman et al. 1992). Among the HIV-infected female partners of male drug users, those who had a history of rape or being assaulted were more likely to engage in high-risk HIV behaviors (He et al. 1998). Finally, HIV infection itself may be the cause of PTSD. Rates of PTSD in response to HIV infection are higher than those in response to other debilitating illnesses (Fauerbach et al. 1997; Perez-Jimenez et al. 1994; van Driel and Op den Velde 1995). In one study, about 30% of persons recently diagnosed with HIV subsequently developed PTSD, with half of the cases appearing within 1 month of HIV diagnosis (B. Kelly et al. 1998).

PTSD has high rates of psychiatric comorbidity (up to 80%), most often depression (B. Kelly et al. 1998) and cocaine and opioid abuse (Kessler et al. 1995), which are also risks for HIV (Lyketsos and Federman 1995). PTSD symptoms in HIV-positive patients in one study predicted lower CD4 cell counts (Lutgendorf et al. 1997b).

Issues of Personality in Patients Infected With HIV

A disturbing trend in the HIV epidemic has been the persistence of modifiable risk factors among persons who are HIV infected. The fact that knowledge of HIV and its transmission is insufficient to deter these individuals from engaging in HIV risk behaviors suggests that certain personality characteristics may enhance a person's tendency to engage in such behaviors.

Traditional approaches in risk reduction counseling emphasize the avoidance of negative consequences in the future, such as condom use during sexual intercourse to prevent STDs. Such educational approaches have proved ineffective for individuals with certain personality characteristics (Kalichman et al. 1996; Trobst et al. 2000). In this section, we outline the role of personality characteristics and personality disorders in the risk of acquiring HIV and highlight specific interventions for individuals with these characteristics.

Implications for HIV Risk Behavior

Our clinical experience suggests that unstable extraverts are the most prone to engage in practices that place them at risk for HIV. These individuals are preoccupied by, and act on, their feelings, which are labile, leading to unpredictable and inconsistent behavior. Regardless of intellectual ability or knowledge of HIV, unstable extraverts can engage in extremely risky behavior. Past experience and future consequences have little importance in decision making for the individual who is ruled by feeling; the present is paramount. Their primary goal is to achieve immediate pleasure or removal of pain, regardless of circumstances. As part of their emotional instability, they experience intense fluctuations in mood. It is difficult for them to tolerate painful affects; they want to escape or avoid feelings as quickly as possible. They are motivated to pursue pleasurable experiences, however risky, to eliminate negative moods.

Unstable extraverts are more likely to engage in behavior that places them at risk for HIV infection and are more likely to pursue sex promiscuously. They are less likely to plan and carry condoms and more likely to have unprotected vaginal or anal sex. They are more fixed on the reward of sex and remarkably inattentive to the STD they may acquire if they do not use a condom. Unstable extraverts are also more likely to become injection drug users.

Personality Disorder in HIV

Prevalence rates of personality disorders among HIV-infected patients (19%–36%) and individuals at risk for HIV (15%–20%) (Jacobsberg et al. 1995; J.G. Johnson et al.

1995; Perkins et al. 1993) are high and significantly exceed rates found in the general population (10%) (J.G. Johnson et al. 1995). The most common personality disorders among HIV-infected patients are antisocial and borderline types (Golding and Perkins 1996). Antisocial personality disorder is the most common (Perkins et al. 1993) and is a risk factor for HIV infection (Weissman 1993). Individuals with personality disorder, particularly antisocial personality disorder, have high rates of substance abuse and are more likely to inject drugs and share needles compared with those without an Axis II diagnosis (Brooner et al. 1993; Dinwiddie et al. 1996; Golding and Perkins 1996). Approximately half of drug abusers may meet criteria for a diagnosis of antisocial personality disorder. Individuals with antisocial personality disorder are also more likely to have higher numbers of lifetime sexual partners, engage in unprotected anal sex, and contract STDs compared with individuals without antisocial personality disorder (Brooner et al. 1993; Hudgins et al. 1995; Kleinman et al. 1994).

In our AIDS clinic, patients are characterized along the dimensions of extraversion–introversion and emotional stability–instability rather than in the discrete categories provided by DSM's Axis II for several reasons. First, it is easier for staff to determine where a patient falls along two dimensions than to evaluate the many criteria for personality disorders. Second, it is simpler to design intervention strategies for two dimensions. Third, a diagnosis of antisocial or borderline personality disorder can be stigmatizing, particularly in a general medical clinic.

Implications for Medication Adherence

Adherence is especially challenging in HIV, which carries all of the components

of low adherence—long duration of treatment, preventive rather than curative treatment, asymptomatic periods, and frequent and complex medication dosing (Blackwell 1996; Haynes 1979; Kruse et al. 1991). Our clinical experience suggests that nonadherence is more common among our extraverted or unstable patients. The same personality characteristics that place them at risk for HIV also reduce their ability to adhere to demanding drug regimens. Specifically, their present-time orientation, combined with reward-seeking behavior, makes it more difficult to tolerate side effects from drugs whose benefits may not be immediately apparent. It is also difficult for feeling-driven individuals to maintain consistent, well-ordered routines, so following frequent, rigid dosing schedules is problematic.

Treatment Implications

We have found that a cognitive-behavioral approach is most effective in treating patients who present with extraverted and/or emotionally unstable personalities. Five principles guide our care:

1. *Focus on thoughts, not feelings.* Individuals with unstable, extraverted personalities often do not recognize the extent to which their actions are driven by feelings of the moment.
2. *Use a behavioral contract for all patients to build consistency.* The contract outlines goals for treatment and responsibilities and expectations of both the patient and the providers.
3. *Emphasize constructive rewards.* Positive outcomes, not adverse consequences, are salient to extraverts. Exhortations to use condoms to avoid STDs are unpersuasive. Eroticizing the use of condoms (Tanner and Pollack 1988) and incorporating novel techniques into sexual repertoires (Abramson and Pink-

erton 1995) have been successful. Similarly, the rewards of abstaining from drugs or alcohol are emphasized, such as having money to buy clothing, having a stable home, or maintaining positive relationships with children. Rewards of having an increased CD4 cell count and reduced viral load should be pursued.

4. *Use relapse prevention techniques.* The relapse prevention model, originally developed for treatment of substance abuse behavior, is an effective method for changing habitual ways of behaving.

5. *Develop a coordinated treatment plan.* The mental health professional coordinates with the medical care provider. Both professionals work in tandem to develop behavioral contracts to reduce HIV risk behaviors and build medication adherence.

Psychosocial Interventions to Prevent HIV Transmission

In intervention studies of men who have sex with other men (still the largest subgroup in terms of new HIV infections in the United States), many psychosocial interventions have shown a decrease in either risk behaviors or infection (Dilley et al. 2002; W.D. Johnson et al. 2002). A meta-analysis examining the effect of HIV prevention strategies found that psychosocial interventions can lead to sexual risk reduction among drug users (Semaan et al. 2002), as did a separate large study of cocaine-dependent patients (Woody et al. 2003). Studied interventions have included stress management and relaxation techniques, group counseling, education, cognitive training, negotiation skills training, psychotherapy directed at emotional distress reduction, education directed at eroticizing safer sex, assertiveness training,

and peer education in bars. All of these interventions showed a modest effect on either risk behavior or HIV infection.

Adherence Counseling

The single most important factor regarding outcome of HIV treatment is the patient's ability to adhere to a prescribed regimen. A recent study of HIV-infected prisoners reported that under directly observed therapy in a prison setting, 85% of the individuals developed undetectable viral loads with prisoners taking approximately 93% of doses (Kirkland et al. 2002). In contrast, antiretroviral adherence rates between 54% and 76% have been reported in other general clinic or community samples (Liu et al. 2001; McNabb et al. 2001; Paterson et al. 2000; Wagner and Ghosh-Dastidar 2002), including a group of patients with serious mental illness (Wagner et al. 2003).

The literature on adherence indicates that four groups of factors affect adherence: environmental factors, treatment factors, illness factors, and patient factors. Environmental factors include medication cost, work schedules, transportation, housing issues, and lack of supportive relationships (Lucas et al. 1999). Patient survey data indicate that the patient–provider relationship has a strong effect on adherence (Altice et al. 2001; Stone et al. 1998).

Treatment factors include the type of medication and amount of pill burden. Once-a-day medications are easier to remember to take regularly than twice-a-day medications, but both are markedly better for adherence than three- or four-times-a-day medications (Kleeberger et al. 2001). Perceived side effects also correlate with poor adherence and can prevent patients from taking all required doses in an attempt to prevent adverse consequences.

Illness chronicity, symptoms, and curability also affect adherence. Lifelong illnesses have the highest degree of nonadherence, as do illnesses that are asymptomatic, because the patient is unable to feel any benefit or effect from taking a medication. Similarly, illnesses that cause symptoms that are unrelieved by treatment are often associated with poor adherence.

Patient factors associated with nonadherence, including dementia, depression, psychosis, personality factors, and substance use, are detailed elsewhere in this chapter. Constant and consistent coaching of patients at each visit is imperative, including clarifying goals of treatment (both short-term and long-term) and anticipating misunderstandings.

More subtle factors affecting adherence include psychosocial support networks, individual coping skills, life structure, access to resources, and behavioral control. Interventions such as cognitive-behavioral psychotherapy, structured psychoeducational psychotherapy, supportive psychotherapy, and group interventions all have been used to improve patient adherence to medication regimens. The current literature on HIV medication adherence focuses on technical interventions, such as pillbox and timer reminders, less complex pharmacological interventions, and increased access to care.

Mental Health Care for Patients With HIV Infection

Patients with HIV infection are underserved with regard to mental health. Psychiatric disorders are underrecognized and undertreated in patients with many chronic medical conditions, but HIV-infected patients are especially likely to be impoverished, disenfranchised, vulnerable, and members of underserved minorities, all of which further decrease the likelihood that they will receive adequate treatment.

Integrated expert care by psychiatrists and other mental health professionals should be a high priority both to promote effective treatment of HIV infection and to stem the tide of an epidemic that spreads through modifiable behaviors.

Conclusion

The interrelationships between HIV/ AIDS and psychiatry are myriad and complex. In a sense, psychiatric disorders can be seen as vectors of HIV transmission, through associated high-risk behaviors. Comorbid psychopathology—including major depression, schizophrenia, addictions, personality vulnerabilities, and the effects of traumatic life experiences—is highly prevalent in patients with HIV/ AIDS. Each of these problems has the potential to sabotage treatment for HIV infection and its many complications. By developing a comprehensive diagnostic formulation on which to base treatment, even many of the most difficult patients can be successfully treated. At the heart of our work we try to impart hope for the future, therapeutic optimism, advocacy, sanctuary, and rehabilitation.

References

Abramson PR, Pinkerton SD: With Pleasure: Thought on the Nature of Human Sexuality. New York, Oxford University Press, 1995

Alfonso CA, Cohen MA: HIV-dementia and suicide. Gen Hosp Psychiatry 16:45–46, 1994

Altice FL, Mostashari F, Friedland GH: Trust and the acceptance of and adherence to antiretroviral therapy. J Acquir Immune Defic Syndr 28:47–58, 2001

American Psychiatric Association, Work Group on HIV/AIDS: Practice guideline for the treatment of patients with HIV/AIDS. Am J Psychiatry 157 (11 suppl):1–62, 2000

Anderson R, Grady C: Symptoms reported by "asymptomatic" HIV-infected subjects (abstract). Proceedings of the 7th Annual Association of Nurses in AIDS Care. Nashville, TN, November 10–12, 1994

Angelino AF, Treisman GJ: Management of psychiatric disorders in patients infected with human immunodeficiency virus. Clin Infect Dis 33:847–856, 2001

Antoni MH, Baggett L, Ironson G, et al: Cognitive-behavioral stress management buffers distress responses and immunologic changes following notification of HIV-1 seropositivity. J Consult Clin Psychol 59:906–915, 1991

Astemborski J, Vlahov D, Warren D, et al: The trading of sex for drugs or money and HIV seropositivity among female intravenous drug users. Am J Public Health 84:382–387, 1994

Atkinson JH Jr, Grant I, Kennedy CJ, et al: Prevalence of psychiatric disorders among men infected with human immunodeficiency virus: a controlled study. Arch Gen Psychiatry 45:859–864, 1988

Ayuso-Mateos JL, Montanes-Lastra L, De La Garza PJ, et al: HIV infection in psychiatric patients: an unlinked anonymous study. Br J Psychiatry 170:181–185, 1997

Baer JW, Dwyer PC, Lewitter-Koehler S: Knowledge about AIDS among psychiatric inpatients. Hosp Community Psychiatry 39:986–988, 1988

Batki SL, Manfredi LB, Murphy JM, et al: Randomized, placebo-controlled trial of paroxetine versus imipramine in depression in HIV-infected injection drug users (abstract PO-B16–1685). Berlin, Germany, International Conference on AIDS, June 1993

Berger D, Muurahainen N, Wittert H, et al: Hypogonadism and wasting in the era of HAART in HIV-infected patients (32174). Geneva, Switzerland, World AIDS Conference, June 1998

Bialer PA, Wallack JJ, Snyder SL: Psychiatric diagnosis in HIV-spectrum disorders. Psychiatr Med 9:361–375, 1991

Bialer PA, Wallack JJ, McDaniel S: Human immunodeficiency virus and AIDS, in Psychiatric Care of the Medical Patient, 2nd Edition. Edited by Stoudemire A, Fogel B, Greenberg D. New York, Oxford University Press, 2000, pp 871–887

Blackwell B: From compliance to alliance: a quarter century of research. Neth J Med 48:140–149, 1996

Blank MB, Mandell DS, Aiken L, et al: Co-occurrence of HIV and serious mental illness among Medicaid recipients. Psychiatr Serv 53:868–873, 2002

Boccellari A, Dilley JW, Shore MD: Neuropsychiatric aspects of AIDS dementia complex: a report on a clinical series. Neurotoxicology 9:381–390, 1988

Brechtl JR, Breitbart W, Galietta M, et al: The use of highly active antiretroviral therapy (HAART) in patients with advanced HIV infection: impact on medical, palliative care, and quality of life outcomes. J Pain Symptom Manage 21:41–51, 2001

Breitbart W, Marotta R, Platt M, et al: A double-blind trial of haloperidol, chlorpromazine and lorazepam in the treatment of delirium in hospitalized AIDS patients. Am J Psychiatry 153:231–237, 1996

Breitbart W, McDonald MV, Rosenfeld B, et al: Fatigue in ambulatory AIDS patients. J Pain Symptom Manage 15:159–167, 1998

Breitbart W, Rosenfeld B, Kaim M, et al: A randomized, double-blind, placebo-controlled trial of psychostimulants for the treatment of fatigue in ambulatory patients with human immunodeficiency virus disease. Arch Intern Med 161:411–420, 2001

Brew BJ, Brown SJ, Catalan J, et al: Phase III, randomized, double-blind, placebo-controlled, multicentre study to evaluate the safety and efficacy of abacavir (ABC, 1592) in HIV-1 infected subjects with AIDS dementia complex (CNA3001), in Abstracts of the 12th World AIDS Conference. Geneva, Switzerland, June 29–July 2, 1998

Brooner RK, Greenfield L, Schmidt CW, et al: Antisocial personality disorder and HIV infection among intravenous drug users. Am J Psychiatry 150:53–58, 1993

Brouillette M-J, Chouinard G, Lalonde R: Didanosine-induced mania in HIV infection (letter). Am J Psychiatry 151:1839–1840, 1994

Brown GR: The use of methylphenidate for cognitive decline associated with HIV disease. Int J Psychiatry 25:21–37, 1995

Budman CL, Vandersall TA: Clonazepam treatment of acute mania in an AIDS patient. J Clin Psychiatry 51:212, 1990

Buhrich N, Cooper DA: Requests for psychiatric consultation concerning 22 patients with AIDS and ARC. Aust N Z J Psychiatry 21:346–353, 1987

Carmen E, Brady SM: AIDS risk and prevention in the chronic mentally ill. Hosp Community Psychiatry 41:652–657, 1990

Centers for Disease Control and Prevention: HIV/AIDS Surveillance Report, 2001. Available at: http://www.cdc.gov. Accessed March 2004

Chang L, Speck O, Miller E, et al: Neural correlates of attention and working memory deficits in HIV patients. Neurology 57:1001–1007, 2001

Chesney MA, Folkman S, Chambers D: Coping effectiveness training for men living with HIV: preliminary findings. Int J STD AIDS 7:75–82, 1996

Chiesi A, Agresti MG, Dally LG, et al: Decrease in notifications of AIDS dementia complex in 1989–1990 in Italy: possible role of the early treatment with zidovudine. Medicina (Firenze) 10:415–416, 1990

Chiesi A, Vella S, Dally LG, et al: Epidemiology of AIDS dementia complex in Europe. AIDS in Europe Study Group. J Acquir Immune Defic Syndr Hum Retrovirol 11:39–44, 1996

Childs EA, Lyles RH, Selnes OA, et al: Plasma viral load and CD4 lymphocytes predict HIV-associated dementia and sensory neuropathy. Neurology 52:607–613, 1999

Ciesla JA, Roberts JE: Meta-analysis of the relationship between HIV infection and risk for depressive disorders. Am J Psychiatry 158:725–730, 2001

Clifford DB: Human immunodeficiency virus-associated dementia. Arch Neurol 57:321–324, 2000

Cottler LB, Nishith P, Compton WM III: Gender differences in risk factors for trauma exposure and post-traumatic stress disorder among inner-city drug abusers in and out of treatment. Compr Psychiatry 42:111–117, 2001

Cournos F, Empfield M, Horwath E, et al: HIV seroprevalence among patients admitted to two psychiatric hospitals. Am J Psychiatry 48:1225–1230, 1991

Cournos F, Guido JR, Coomaraswamy S, et al: Sexual activity and risk of HIV infection among patients with schizophrenia. Am J Psychiatry 151:228–232, 1994

Cozza KL, Swanton EJ, Humphreys CW: Hepatotoxicity with combination of valproic acid, ritonavir, and nevirapine: a case report. Psychosomatics 41:452–453, 2000

Crocker KS: Gastrointestinal manifestations of the acquired immunodeficiency syndrome. Nurs Clin North Am 24:395–406, 1989

Czub S, Koutsilieri E, Sopper S, et al: Enhancement of CNS pathology in early simian immunodeficiency virus infection by dopaminergic drugs. Acta Neuropathol 101:85–91, 2001

Dal Pan GJ, McArthur JH, Aylward E, et al: Patterns of cerebral atrophy in HIV-1-infected individuals: results of a quantitative MRI analysis. Neurology 42:2125–2130, 1992

Darko DF, McCutchan JA, Kripke DF, et al: Fatigue, sleep disturbance, disability and indices of progression of HIV infection. Am J Psychiatry 149:514–520, 1992

Davis HF, Skolasky RL Jr, Selnes OA, et al: Assessing HIV-associated dementia: modified HIV Dementia Scale versus the grooved pegboard. AIDS Reader 12:29–31, 38, 2002

de Souza CT, Diaz T, Sutmoller F, et al: The association of socioeconomic status and use of crack/cocaine with unprotected anal sex in a cohort of men who have sex with men in Rio de Janeiro, Brazil. J Acquir Immune Defic Syndr 29: 95–100, 2002

Dilley JW, Ochitill HN, Perl M, et al: Findings in psychiatric consultations with patients with acquired immune deficiency syndrome. Am J Psychiatry 142:82–86, 1985

Dilley JW, Woods WJ, Sabatino J, et al: Changing sexual behavior among gay male repeat testers for HIV: a randomized, controlled trial of a single-session intervention. J Acquir Immune Defic Syndr 30:177–186, 2002

Dinwiddie SH, Cottler L, Compton W, et al: Psychopathology and HIV risk behaviors among injection drug users in and out of treatment. Drug Alcohol Depend 43:1–11, 1996

Dobs A, Few W III, Blackman M, et al: Serum hormones in men with human immunodeficiency virus associated wasting. J Clin Endocrinol Metab 81:4108–4112, 1996

Dore GJ, Correll PK, Li Y, et al: Changes to AIDS dementia complex in the era of highly active antiretroviral therapy. AIDS 13:1249–1253, 1999

Duran S, Spire B, Raffi F, et al: Self-reported symptoms after initiation of a protease inhibitor in HIV-infected patients and their impact on adherence to HAART. HIV Clin Trials 2:38–45, 2001

Edelstein H, Knight RT: Severe parkinsonism in two AIDS patients taking prochlorperazine. Lancet 2(8554):341–342, 1987

Edlin BR, Irwin KL, Faruque S, et al: Multicenter Crack Cocaine and HIV Infection Study Team. Intersecting epidemics: crack cocaine use and HIV infection among inner-city young adults. N Engl J Med 331:1422–1427, 1994

Ellen SR, Judd FK, Mijch AM, et al: Secondary mania in patients with HIV infection. Aust N Z J Psychiatry 33:353–360, 1999

Elliott AJ, Roy-Byrne PP: Mirtazapine for depression in patients with human immunodeficiency virus (letter). J Clin Psychopharmacol 20:265–267, 2000

Elliott AJ, Uldall KK, Bergam K, et al: Randomized, placebo-controlled trial of paroxetine versus imipramine in depressed HIV-positive outpatients. Am J Psychiatry 155:367–372, 1998

Elliott AJ, Russo J, Bergam K, et al: Antidepressant efficacy in HIV-seropositive outpatients with major depressive disorder: an open trial of nefazodone. J Clin Psychiatry 60:226–231, 1999

Empfield M, Cournos F, Meyer I, et al: HIV seroprevalence among homeless patients admitted to a psychiatric inpatient unit. Am J Psychiatry 150:47–52, 1993

Ernst T, Chang L, Jovicich J, et al: Abnormal brain activation on functional MRI in cognitively asymptomatic HIV patients. Neurology 59:1343–1349, 2002

Fauerbach JA, Lawrence J, Haythornthwaite J, et al: Preburn psychiatric history affects post-trauma morbidity. Psychosomatics 38:374–385, 1997

Fawcett J: Suicide risk factors in depressive disorders and in panic disorder. J Clin Psychiatry 53 (suppl):93–95, 1992

Fernandez F, Levy JK: The use of molindone in the treatment of psychotic and delirious patients infected with the human immunodeficiency virus: case reports. Gen Hosp Psychiatry 15:31–35, 1993

Fernandez F, Levy J: Efficacy of venlafaxine in HIV-depressive disorders. Psychosomatics 38:173–174, 1997

Fernandez F, Levy JK, Mansell PW: Management of delirium in terminally ill AIDS patients. Int J Psychiatry Med 19:165–172, 1989

Fernandez F, Levy JK, Samley HR, et al: Effects of methylphenidate in HIV-related depression: a comparative trial with desipramine. Int J Psychiatry Med 25:53–67, 1995

Ferrando S, Wapenyi K: Psychopharmacological treatment of patients with HIV and AIDS. Psychiatr Q 73:33–49, 2002

Ferrando SJ, Goldman JG, Charness W: SSRI treatment of depression in symptomatic HIV infection and AIDS: improvements in affective and somatic symptoms. Gen Hosp Psychiatry 19:89–97, 1997

Ferrando S, Evans S, Goggin K, et al: Fatigue in HIV illness: relationship to depression, physical limitations, and disability. Psychosom Med 60:759–764, 1998a

Ferrando S, van Gorp W, McElhiney M, et al: Highly active antiretroviral treatment in HIV infection: benefits for neuropsychological function. AIDS 12 (suppl):F65–F70, 1998b

Ferrando SJ, Rabkin JG, de Moore G, et al: Antidepressant treatment of depression in HIV+ women. J Clin Psychiatry 60:741–746, 1999

Fichtner CG, Braun BG: Bupropion-associated mania in a patient with HIV infection (letter). J Clin Psychopharmacol 12:366–367, 1992

Gabel RM, Barnard M, Norko M, et al: AIDS presenting as mania. Compr Psychiatry 27:251–254, 1986

Giesen HJV, Hefter H, Jablonowski H, et al: HAART is neuroprophylactic in HIV-1 infection. J Acquir Immune Defic Syndr 23:380–385, 2000

Golding M, Perkins DO: Personality disorder in HIV infection. Int Rev Psychiatry 8:253–258, 1996

Gourevitch MN, Friedland GH: Interactions between methadone and medications used to treat HIV infection: a review. Mt Sinai J Med 67:429–436, 2000

Grassi L: Risk of HIV infection in psychiatrically ill patients. AIDS Care 8:103–116, 1996

Grinspoon S, Anderson C, Schoenfeld D, et al: Long-term effects of androgen administration in men with AIDS wasting (32176). Geneva, Switzerland, World AIDS Conference, June 1998

Halman M, Rourke SB: HAART and neuropsychological impairment: neuroscience in HIV infection, Edinburgh 22–24 June 2000 (abstract 03). J Neurovirol 6:246, 2000

Halman MM, Worth JL, Sanders KM, et al: Anticonvulsant use in the treatment of manic syndromes in patients with HIV-1 infection. J Clin Neuropsychiatry Clin Neurosci 5:430–434, 1993

Handelsman L, Aronson M, Maurer G, et al: Neuropsychological and neurological manifestations of HIV-1 dementia in drug users. J Neuropsychiatry Clin Neurosci 4:21–28, 1992

Hartgers C, Van Den Hoek JAR, Coutinho RA, et al: Psychopathology, stress and HIV-risk injecting behaviour among drug users. Br J Addict 87:857–865, 1992

Haynes RB: Determinants of compliance: the disease and the mechanics of treatment, in Compliance in Health Care. Edited by Haynes RB, Taylor DW, Sackett DL. Baltimore, MD, Johns Hopkins University Press, 1979, pp 46–62

He H, McCoy HV, Stevens SJ, et al: Violence and HIV sexual risk behaviors among female sex partners of male drug users. Women Health 27:161–175, 1998

Hinkin CH, Castellon SA, Hardy DJ, et al: Methylphenidate improves HIV-1-associated cognitive slowing. J Neuropsychiatry Clin Neurosci 13:248–254, 2001

Hoff RA, Beam-Goulet J, Rosenheck RA: Mental disorder as a risk factor for human immunodeficiency virus infection in a sample of veterans. J Nerv Ment Dis 185:556–560, 1997

Hoffman RS: Neuropsychiatric complications of AIDS. Psychosomatics 25:393–400, 1984

Holland NR, Power C, Mathews VP, et al: Cytomegalovirus encephalitis in acquired immunodeficiency syndrome (AIDS). Neurology 44:507–514, 1994

Hollander H, Golden J, Mendelson T, et al: Extrapyramidal symptoms in AIDS patients given low-dose metoclopramide or chlorpromazine (letter). Lancet 2(8465):1186, 1985

Holmes VF, Ficchione GL: Hypomania in an AIDS patient receiving amitriptyline for neuropathic pain. Neurology 39:305, 1989

Holmes VF, Ficchione GL: Hypomania in an AIDS patient receiving amitriptyline for neuropathic pain. Neurology 39:305, 1989

Holmes VF, Fernandez F, Levy JK: Psychostimulant response in AIDS-related complex patients. J Clin Psychiatry 50:5–8, 1989

Hoover DR, Saah AJ, Bacellar H, et al: Signs and symptoms of "asymptomatic" HIV-1 infection in homosexual men. J Acquir Immune Defic Syndr 6:66–71, 1993

Hriso E, Kuhn T, Masdeu JC, et al: Extrapyramidal symptoms due to dopamine-blocking agents in patients with AIDS encephalopathy. Am J Psychiatry 148:1558–1561, 1991

Hudgins R, McCusker J, Stoddard A: Cocaine use and risky injection and sexual behaviors. Drug Alcohol Depend 37:7–14, 1995

Ickovics JR, Hamburger ME, Vlahov D, et al: Mortality, CD4 cell count decline, and depressive symptoms among HIV-seropositive women: longitudinal analysis from the HIV epidemiology research study. JAMA 285:1466–1474, 2001

Jacobs P, Bobek SC: Sexual needs of the schizophrenic client. Perspect Psychiatr Care 27:15–20, 1991

Jacobsberg L, Frances A, Perry S: Axis II diagnoses among volunteers for HIV testing and counseling. Am J Psychiatry 152:1222–1224, 1995

Jarvik JG, Hesselink JR, Kennedy C, et al: Acquired immunodeficiency syndrome: magnetic resonance patterns of brain involvement with pathologic correlation. Arch Neurol 45: 731–736, 1988

Jennings HR, Romanelli F: The use of valproic acid in HIV-positive patients. Ann Pharmacol 33:1113–1116, 1999

Johannessen DJ, Wilson LG: Mania with cryptococcal meningitis in two AIDS patients. J Clin Psychiatry 49:200–201, 1988

Johnson JG, Williams JBW, Rabkin JG, et al: Axis I psychiatric symptomatology associated with HIV infection and personality disorder. Am J Psychiatry 152:551–554, 1995

Johnson WD, Hedges LV, Ramirez G, et al: HIV prevention research for men who have sex with men: a systematic review and meta-analysis. J Acquir Immune Defic Syndr 30 (suppl 1): S118–S129, 2002

Kalayjian RC, Cohen ML, Bonomo RA, et al: Cytomegalovirus ventriculoencephalitis in AIDS: a syndrome with distinct clinical and pathologic features. Medicine (Baltimore) 72:67–77, 1993

Kalichman SC, Sikkema KJ, Kelly JA, et al: Factors associated with risk for HIV infection among chronic mentally ill adults. Am J Psychiatry 15:221–227, 1994

Kalichman SC, Sikkema KJ, Kelly JA, et al: Use of a brief behavioral skills intervention to prevent HIV infection among chronic mentally ill adults. Psychiatr Serv 46:275–280, 1995

Kalichman SC, Heckkman T, Kelly JA: Sensation-seeking as an explanation for the association between substance use and HIV-related risky sexual behavior. Arch Sex Behav 25:141–154, 1996

Kelly B, Raphael B, Judd F, et al: Posttraumatic stress disorder in response to HIV infection. Gen Hosp Psychiatry 20:345–352, 1998

Kelly JA, Murphy DA, Bahn GR, et al: AIDS/HIV risk behaviour among the chronic mentally ill. Am J Psychiatry 149: 886–889, 1992

Kelly J: Group psychotherapy for persons with HIV and AIDS-related illnesses. Int J Group Psychother 98:143–162, 1998

Kermani EJ, Borod JC, Brown PH, et al: New psychopathologic findings in AIDS: case report. J Clin Psychiatry 46:240–241, 1985

Kessler RC, Sonega A, Bromer E: Posttraumatic stress disorder in the national comorbidity survey. Arch Gen Psychiatry 52:1048–1060, 1995

Kibayashi K, Mastri AR, Hirsch CS: Neuropathology of human immunodeficiency virus infection at different disease stages. Hum Pathol 27:637–642, 1996

Kieburtz KD, Epstein LG, Gelbard HA, et al: Excitotoxicity and dopaminergic dysfunction in the acquired immunodeficiency syndrome dementia complex: therapeutic implications. Arch Neurol 48:1281–1284, 1991a

Kieburtz K, Zettelmaier AE, Ketonen L, et al: Manic syndromes in AIDS. Am J Psychiatry 148:1068–1070, 1991b

Kirkland LR, Fischl MA, Tashima KT, et al: Response to lamivudine-zidovudine plus abacavir twice daily in antiretroviral-naive, incarcerated patients with HIV infection taking directly observed treatment. Clin Infect Dis 34:511–518, 2002

Kleeberger CA, Phair JP, Strathdee SA, et al: Determinants of heterogeneous adherence to HIV-antiretroviral therapies in the Multicenter AIDS Cohort Study. J Acquir Immune Defic Syndr 26:82–92, 2001

Kleinman PH, Millman RB, Robinson H, et al: Lifetime needle sharing: a predictive analysis. J Subst Abuse Treat 11:449–455, 1994

Kopicko JJ, Momodu I, Adedokun A, et al: Characteristics of HIV-infected men with low serum testosterone levels. Int J STD AIDS 10:817–820, 1999

Koutsilieri E, Sopper S, Scheller C, et al: Parkinsonism in HIV dementia. J Neural Transm 109:767–775, 2002

Krauthammer C, Klerman GL: Secondary mania: manic syndromes associated with antecedent physical illness or drugs. Arch Gen Psychiatry 35:1333–1339, 1978

Krikorian R, Wrobel AJ, Meinecke C, et al: Cognitive deficits associated with human immunodeficiency virus encephalopathy. J Neuropsychiatry Clin Neurosci 2:256–260, 1990

Kruse W, Eggert-Kruse W, Rampmaier J, et al: Dosage frequency and drug-compliance behavior: a comparative study on compliance with a medication to be taken twice or four times daily. Eur J Clin Pharmacol 41:589–592, 1991

Laudat A, Blum L, Guechot J, et al: Changes in systemic gonadal and adrenal steroids in symptomatic human immunodeficiency virus infected men: relationship with CD4 cell counts. Eur J Endocrinol 133:418–424, 1995

Lera G, Zirulnik J: Pilot study with clozapine in patients with HIV-associated psychosis and drug-induced parkinsonism. Mov Disord 14:128–131, 1999

Letendre S, Ellis R, Rippeth J, et al: Reduction of HIV RNA levels correlates with reversal of HIV-induced cognitive dysfunction: neuroscience in HIV infection. Edinburgh 22–24 June 2000 (abstract 04). J Neurovirol 6:246, 2000

Liu H, Golin CE, Miller LG, et al: A comparison study of multiple measures of adherence to HIV protease inhibitors. Ann Intern Med 134:968–977, 2001

Longo MB, Spross JA, Locke AM: Identifying major concerns of persons with acquired immunodeficiency syndrome: a replication. Clin Nurse Spec 4:21–26, 1990

Lopez OL, Smith G, Meltzer CC, et al: Dopamine systems in human immunodeficiency virus-associated dementia. Neuropsychiatry Neuropsychol Behav Neurol 12:184–192, 1999

Louhivuori KA, Hakama M: Risk of suicide among cancer patients. Am J Epidemiol 109:50–65, 1979

Lucas GM, Chaisson RE, Moore RD: Highly active antiretroviral therapy in a large urban clinic: risk factors for virologic failure and adverse drug reactions. Ann Intern Med 131:81–87, 1999

Lutgendorf S, Antoni MH, Ironson G, et al: Cognitive-behavioral stress management decreases dysphoric mood and herpes simplex virus-type 2 antibody titers in symptomatic HIV-seropositive gay men. J Consult Clin Psychol 65:31–43, 1997a

Lutgendorf SK, Antoni MH, Ironson G, et al: Cognitive processing style, mood, and immune function following HIV seropositivity notification. Cognit Ther Res 21:157–184, 1997b

Lyketsos CG, Federman EB: Psychiatric disorders and HIV infection: impact on one another. Epidemiol Rev 17:152–164, 1995

Lyketsos CG, Hoover DR, Guccione M, et al: Depressive symptoms as predictors of medical outcomes in HIV infection. Multicenter AIDS Cohort Study. JAMA 270:2563–2567, 1993a

Lyketsos CG, Hanson AL, Fishman M, et al: Manic syndrome early and late in the course of HIV. Am J Psychiatry 150:326–327, 1993b

Lyketsos CG, Hanson A, Fishman M, et al: Screening for psychiatric morbidity in a medical outpatient clinic for HIV infection: the need for a psychiatric presence. Int J Psychiatry Med 24:103–113, 1994

Lyketsos CG, Hoover DR, Guccione M, et al: Changes in depressive symptoms as AIDS develops. Am J Psychiatry 153: 1430–1437, 1996a

Lyketsos CG, Hutton H, Fishman M, et al: Psychiatric morbidity on entry to an HIV primary care clinic. AIDS 10:1033–1039, 1996b

Lyketsos CG, Schwartz J, Fishman M, et al: AIDS mania. J Neuropsychiatry Clin Neurosci 9:277–279, 1997

Maj M: Psychiatric aspects of HIV-1 infection and AIDS. Psychol Med 20:547–563, 1990

Maj M, Satz P, Janssen R, et al: WHO Neuropsychiatric AIDS Study, cross-sectional phase II: neuropsychological and neurological findings. Arch Gen Psychiatry 51:51–61, 1994

Manning D, Jacobsberg L, Erhart S, et al: The efficacy of imipramine in the treatment of HIV-related depression (abstract no. Th.B.32). International Conference on AIDS, San Francisco, CA, June 20–23, 1990

Markowitz JC, Kocsis JH, Fishman B, et al: Treatment of depressive symptoms in human immunodeficiency virus-positive patients. Arch Gen Psychiatry 55:452–457, 1998

Martinez A, Israelski D, Walker C, et al: Post-traumatic stress disorder in women attending human immunodeficiency virus outpatient clinics. AIDS Patient Care STDS 16:283–291, 2002

Masand PS, Tesar GE: Use of stimulants in the medically ill. Psychiatr Clin North Am 19:515–547, 1996

Mauri MC, Fabiano L, Bravin S, et al: Schizophrenic patients before and after HIV infection: a case-control study. Encephale 23:437–441, 1997

Maxwell S, Scheftner WA, Kessler MA, et al: Manic syndromes associated with zidovudine therapy (letter). JAMA 259:3406–3407, 1988

McArthur JC, Hoover DR, Bacellar H, et al: Dementia in AIDS patients: incidence and risk factors. Multicenter AIDS Cohort Study. Neurology 43:2245–2252, 1993

McArthur JC, McClernon DR, Cronin MR, et al: Relationship between human immunodeficiency virus-associated dementia and viral load in cerebrospinal fluid and brain. Ann Neurol 42:689–698, 1997

McDermott BE, Sautter FJ, Winstead DK, et al: Diagnosis, health beliefs, and risk of HIV infection in psychiatric patients. Hosp Community Psychiatry 45:580–585, 1994

McKegney FP, O'Dowd MA, Feiner C, et al: A prospective comparison of neuropsychologic function in HIV-seropositive and seronegative methadone-maintained patients. AIDS 4:565–569, 1990

McNabb J, Ross JW, Abriola K, et al: Adherence to highly active antiretroviral therapy predicts outcome at an inner-city human immunodeficiency virus clinic. Clin Infect Dis 33: 700–705, 2001

Metzger DS, Woody GE, DePhillipis D, et al: Risk factors for needle sharing among methadone patients. Am J Psychiatry 148:636–640, 1991

Metzger DS, Navaline H, Woody GE: Drug abuse treatment as AIDS prevention. Public Health Rep 113 (suppl 1):97–106, 1998

Meyer I, McKinnon K, Cournos F, et al: HIV seroprevalence among long-stay patients in a state psychiatric hospital. Hosp Community Psychiatry 44:282–284, 1993

Miller RG, Carson PJ, Moussavi RS, et al: Fatigue and myalgia in AIDS patients. Neurology 41:1603–1607, 1991

Mintz M, Tardieu M, Hoyt L, et al: Levodopa therapy improves motor function in HIV-infected children with extrapyramidal syndromes. Neurology 47:1583–1585, 1996

Mirsattari SM, Power C, Nath A: Parkinsonism with HIV infection. Mov Disord 13:684–689, 1998

Moog C, Kuntz-Simon G, Caussin-Schwemling C, et al: Sodium valproate, an anticonvulsant drug, stimulates human immunodeficiency virus type 1 replication independently of glutathione levels. J Gen Virol 77:1993–1999, 1996

Morrill AC, Ickovics JR, Golubchikov VV, et al: Safer sex: social and psychological predictors of behavioral maintenance and change among heterosexual women. J Consult Clin Psychol 64:819–828, 1996

Murphy GE: Suicide and attempted suicide. Hosp Pract 12:78–81, 1977

Muurahainen N, Mulligan K: Clinical trial updates in human immunodeficiency virus wasting. Semin Oncol 25:104–111, 1998

Naber D, Pajonk FG, Perro C, et al: Human immunodeficiency virus antibody test and seroprevalence in psychiatric patients. Acta Psychiatr Scand 89:358–361, 1994

Nath A, Maragos WF, Avison MJ, et al: Acceleration of HIV dementia with methamphetamine and cocaine. J Neurovirol 7:66–71, 2001

Navia BA, Jordan BD, Price RW: The AIDS dementia complex, I: clinical features. Ann Neurol 19:517–524, 1986

Navia BA, Jordan BD, Price RW: The AIDS dementia complex, I: clinical features. Ann Neurol 19:517–524, 1986

Navia BA, Dafni U, Simpson D, et al (for the AIDS Clinical Trials Group): A phase I/II trial of nimodipine for HIV-related neurologic complications. Neurology 51:221–228, 1998

Nightingale SD, Kosto FT, Mertz CJ, et al: Clarithromycin-induced mania in two patients with AIDS. Clin Infect Dis 20:1563–1564, 1995

Nyamathi A: Comparative study of factors relating to HIV risk level of black homeless women. J Acquir Immune Defic Syndr 5:222–228, 1992

O'Dowd MA, McKegney FP: Manic syndrome associated with zidovudine (letter). JAMA 260:3587, 1988

Orr S, Celentano DD, Santelli J, et al: Depressive symptoms and risk factors for HIV acquisition among black women attending urban health centers in Baltimore. AIDS Educ Prev 6:230–236, 1994

Pakesch G, Loimer N, Grunberger J, et al: Neuropsychological findings and psychiatric symptoms in HIV-1 infected and non-infected drug users. Psychiatry Res 41:163–177, 1992

Paterson DL, Swindells S, Mohn J, et al: Adherence to protease inhibitor therapy and outcomes in patients with HIV infection. Ann Intern Med 133:21–30, 2000

Perez-Jimenez JP, Gomez-Bajo GJ, Lopez-Castillo JJ, et al: Psychiatric consultation and post-traumatic stress disorder in burned patients. Burns 20:532–536, 1994

Perkins DO, Davidson EJ, Leserman J, et al: Personality disorder in patients infected with HIV: a controlled study with implications for clinical care. Am J Psychiatry 150:309–315, 1993

Perkins DO, Stern RA, Golden RN, et al: Mood disorders in HIV infection: prevalence and risk factors in a nonepicenter of the AIDS epidemic. Am J Psychiatry 151:233–236, 1994

Perkins DO, Leserman J, Stern RA, et al: Somatic symptoms and HIV infection: relationship to depressive symptoms and indicators of HIV disease. Am J Psychiatry 152:1776–1781, 1995

Perry S, Jacobsen P: Neuropsychiatric manifestations of AIDS-spectrum disorders. Hosp Community Psychiatry 37:135–142, 1986

Pickles RW, Spelman DW: Suspected ethambutol-induced mania. Med J Aust 164:445–446, 1996

Portegies P, De Gans J, Lange JM, et al: Declining incidence of AIDS dementia complex after introduction of zidovudine treatment. BMJ 299:819–821, 1989 (published erratum appears in BMJ 299:1141, 1989)

Price RW, Brew BJ: The AIDS dementia complex. J Infect Dis 158:1079–1083, 1988

Price RW, Yiannoutsos CT, Cliffort DB, et al: Neurological outcomes in late HIV infection: adverse impact of neurological impairment on survival and protective effect of antiviral therapy. AIDS 13:1677–1685, 1999

Pugh K, O'Donnell I, Catalan J: Suicide and HIV disease. AIDS Care 4:391–400, 1993

Rabkin JG, Remien R, Katoff L, et al: Suicidality in AIDS long-term survivors: what is the evidence? AIDS Care 5:401–411, 1993

Rabkin JG, Rabkin R, Harrison W, et al: Effect of imipramine on mood and enumerative measures of immune status in depressed patients with HIV illness. Am J Psychiatry 151:516–523, 1994a

Rabkin JG, Rabkin R, Wagner G: Effects of fluoxetine on mood and immune status in depressed patients with HIV illness. J Clin Psychiatry 55:92–97, 1994b

Rabkin JG, Wagner GJ, Rabkin R: Fluoxetine treatment for depression in patients with HIV and AIDS: a randomized, placebo-controlled trial. Am J Psychiatry 156:101–107, 1999a

Rabkin JG, Wagner GJ, Rabkin R: Testosterone therapy for human immunodeficiency virus-positive men with and without hypogonadism. J Clin Psychopharmacol 19:19–27, 1999b

Rabkin JG, Ferrando SJ, Wagner G, et al: DHEA treatment of men and women with HIV infection. Psychoneuroendocrinology 25:53–68, 2000a

Rabkin JG, Wagner GJ, Rabkin R: A double-blind, placebo-controlled trial of testosterone therapy for HIV-positive men with hypogonadal symptoms. Arch Gen Psychiatry 57:141–147, 2000b

RachBeisel JA, Weintraub E: Valproic acid treatment of AIDS-related mania. J Clin Psychiatry 58:406–407, 1997

Rees V, Saitz R, Horton NJ, et al: Association of alcohol consumption with HIV sex- and drug-risk behaviors among drug users. J Subst Abuse Treat 21:129–134, 2001

Regier DA, Farmer ME, Rae DS, et al: Comorbidity of mental disorders with alcohol and other drug abuse. JAMA 264:2511–2518, 1990

Revicki DA, Brown RE, Henry DH, et al: Recombinant human erythropoietin and health-related quality of life of AIDS patients with anemia. J Acquir Immune Defic Syndr 7:474–484, 1994

Richman DD, Fischl MA, Grieco MH, et al: The toxicity of azidothymidine (AZT) in the treatment of patients with AIDS and AIDS-related complex. N Engl J Med 317:192–197, 1987

Sacks M, Dermatis H, Looser-Ott S, et al: Undetected HIV infection among acutely ill psychiatric inpatients. Am J Psychiatry 149:544–545, 1992

Sacktor NC, Lyles RH, McFarlane G, et al (for the Multicenter AIDS Cohort Study): The changing incidence of HIV-1 related neurologic diseases (abstract 145), in Abstracts of the 6th Conference on Retroviruses and Opportunistic Infections. Chicago, IL, January 31–February 4, 1999a

Sacktor NC, Lyles RH, McFarlane G, et al: HIV-1-related neurological disease incidence changes in the era of highly active antiretroviral therapy. Neurology 52:A252–A253, 1999b

Sacktor N, Lyles RH, Skolasky R, et al: HIV-associated neurologic disease incidence changes: Multicenter AIDS Cohort Study, 1990–1998. Neurology 56:257–260, 2001

Schmidt U, Miller D: Two cases of hypomania in AIDS. Br J Psychiatry 152:839–842, 1988

Schwartz JAJ, McDaniel JS: Double-blind comparison of fluoxetine and desipramine in the treatment of depressed women with advanced HIV disease: a pilot study. Depress Anxiety 9:70–74, 1999

Semaan S, Des Jarlais DC, Sogolow E, et al: A meta-analysis of the effect of HIV prevention interventions on the sex behaviors of drug users in the United States. J Acquir Immune Defic Syndr 30 (suppl 1):S73–S93, 2002

Sewell D, Jeste D, Atkinson J, et al: HIV-associated psychosis: a study of 20 cases. Am J Psychiatry 151:237–242, 1994a

Sewell DD, Jeste DV, McAdams LA, et al: Neuroleptic treatment of HIV-associated psychosis. HNRC group. Neuropsychopharmacology 10:223–229, 1994b

Sidtis JJ, Gatsonis C, Price RW, et al (for the AIDS Clinical Trials Group): Zidovudine treatment of the AIDS dementia complex: results of a placebo-controlled trial. Ann Neurol 33:343–349, 1993

Silberstein C, Galanter M, Marmor M, et al: HIV-1 among inner city dually diagnosed inpatients. Am J Drug Alcohol Abuse 20:201–213, 1994

Simon G, Moog C, Obert G: Valproic acid reduces the intracellular level of glutathione and stimulates human immunodeficiency virus. Chem Biol Interact 91:111–121, 1994

Singh A, Golledge H, Catalan J: Treatment of HIV-related psychotic disorders with risperidone: a series of 21 cases. J Psychosom Res 42:489–493, 1997

St. John's wort and HAART. AIDS Patient Care STDS 14:281–283, 2000

Steer RA, Iguchi MY, Platt JJ: Hopelessness in IV drug users not in treatment and seeking HIV testing and counseling. Drug Alcohol Depend 34:99–103, 1994

Stein MD, Hanna L, Natarajan R, et al: Alcohol use patterns predict high-risk HIV behaviors among active injection drug users. J Subst Abuse Treat 18:359–363, 2000

Stiffman AR, Dore P, Earls F, et al: The influence of mental health problems on AIDS-related risk behaviors in young adults. J Nerv Ment Dis 180:314–320, 1992

Stone VE, Clarke J, Lovell J, et al: HIV/AIDS patients' perspectives on adhering to regimens containing protease inhibitors. J Gen Intern Med 13:586–593, 1998

Stout JC, Ellis RJ, Jernigan TL, et al: Progressive cerebral volume loss in human immunodeficiency virus infection: a longitudinal volumetric magnetic resonance imaging study. HIV Neurobehavioral Research Center Group. Arch Neurol 55:161–168, 1998

Tanner WM, Pollack RH: The effect of condom use and erotic instructions on attitudes towards condoms. J Sex Res 25:537–541, 1988

Thurnher MM, Schindler EG, Thurnher SA, et al: Highly active antiretroviral therapy for patients with AIDS dementia complex: effect on MR imaging findings and clinical course. Am J Neuroradiol 21:670–678, 2000

Tozzi V, Balestra P, Galgani S, et al: Positive and sustained effects of highly active anti-retroviral therapy on HIV associated neurocognitive impairment. AIDS 13:1889–1897, 1999

Tozzi V, Balestra P, Galgani S, et al: Changes in neurocognitive performance in a cohort of patients treated with HAART for 3 years. J Acquir Immune Defic Syndr Hum Retrovirol 28:19–27, 2001

Treisman GJ, Fishman M, Schwartz J, et al: Mood disorders in HIV infection. Depress Anxiety 7:178–187, 1998

Trobst KK, Wiggins JS, Costa PT Jr, et al: Personality psychology and problem behaviors: HIV risk and the five-factor model. J Pers 68:1232–1252, 2000

Uldall KK, Berghuis JP: Delirium in AIDS patients: recognition and medication factors. AIDS Patient Care STDS 11:435–441, 1997

Uldall KK, Harris VL, Lalonde B: Outcomes associated with delirium in acutely hospitalized acquired immune deficiency syndrome patients. Compr Psychiatry 41:88–91, 2000a

Uldall KK, Ryan R, Berghuis JP, et al: Association between delirium and death in AIDS patients. AIDS Patient Care STDS 14:95–100, 2000b

UNAIDS Joint United Nations Programme on HIV/AIDS. AIDS Epidemic Update: December 2000. Available at: http://www.thebody.com/unaids/update/contents.html. Accessed March 2004.

van Driel RC, Op den Velde W: Myocardial infarction and posttraumatic stress disorder. J Trauma Stress 8:151–159, 1995

van Servellen G, Chang B, Garcia L, et al: Individual and system level factors associated with treatment nonadherence in human immunodeficiency virus-infected men and women. AIDS Patient Care STDS 16:269–281, 2002

Vlahov D, Munow A, Solomon L, et al: Comparison of clinical manifestations of HIV infection between male and female injecting drug users. AIDS 8:819–823, 1994

Volavka J, Convit A, Czobor P, et al: HIV seroprevalence and risk behaviours in psychiatric inpatients. Psychiatry Res 39: 109–114, 1991

Wagner GJ, Ghosh-Dastidar B: Electronic monitoring: adherence assessment or intervention? HIV Clin Trials 3:45–51, 2002

Wagner GJ, Rabkin R: Effects of dextroamphetamine on depression and fatigue in men with HIV: a double-blind, placebo-controlled trial. J Clin Psychiatry 61:436–440, 2000

Wagner G, Rabkin J, Rabkin R: Illness stage, concurrent medications, and other correlates of low testosterone in men with HIV illness. J Acquir Immune Defic Syndr Hum Retrovirol 8:204–207, 1995

Wagner GJ, Rabkin JG, Rabkin R: A comparative analysis of standard and alternative antidepressants in the treatment of human immunodeficiency virus patients. Compr Psychiatry 37:402–408, 1996

Wagner GJ, Rabkin JG, Rabkin R: Dextroamphetamine as a treatment for depression and low energy in AIDS patients: a pilot study. J Psychosom Res 42:407–411, 1997

Wagner GJ, Rabkin JG, Rabkin R: Testosterone as a treatment for fatigue in HIV+ men. Gen Hosp Psychiatry 20:209–213, 1998

Wagner GJ, Kanouse DE, Koegel P, et al: Adherence to HIV antiretrovirals among persons with serious mental illness. AIDS Patient Care STDS 17:179–186, 2003

Walkup J, Crystal S, Sambamoorthri U: Schizophrenia and major affective disorder among Medicaid recipients with HIV/AIDS in New Jersey. Am J Public Health 89:1101–1103, 1999

Weinhardt LS, Carey KB: Prevalence of infection with HIV among the seriously mentally ill: review of research and implications for practice. Prof Psychol 26:262–268, 1995

Weissman MM: The epidemiology of personality disorders: a 1990 update. J Personal Disord 7 (suppl):44–62, 1993

White JC, Christensen JF, Singer CM: Methylphenidate as a treatment for depression in acquired immunodeficiency syndrome: an n-of-1 trial. J Clin Psychiatry 53:153–156, 1992

Wilkie FL, Eisdorfer C, Morgan R, et al: Cognition in early human immunodeficiency virus infection. Arch Neurol 41: 433–440, 1990

Witvrouw M, Schmit JC, Van Remoortel B, et al: Cell type-dependent effect of sodium valproate on human immunodeficiency virus type 1 replication in vitro. AIDS Res Hum Retroviruses 13:87–92, 1997

Woody GE, Gallop R, Luborsky L, et al: HIV risk reduction in the National Institute on Drug Abuse Cocaine Collaborative Treatment Study. J Acquir Immune Defic Syndr 33:82–87, 2003

Wright JM, Sachder PS, Perkins RJ, et al: Zidovudine-related mania. Med J Aust 150:334–341, 1989

Zisook S, Peterkin J, Goggin KJ, et al: Treatment of major depression in HIV-seropositive men. J Clin Psychiatry 59:217–224, 1998

Self-Assessment Questions

Select the single best response for each question.

1. The most common neoplasm seen in AIDS patients is

    A. Sarcoma.
    B. Lung cancer.
    C. Pancreatic cancer.
    D. Colon cancer.
    E. Lymphoma.

2. The addition of zidovudine to antiviral treatment regimens for HIV infection has resulted in

    A. Worsening of cognitive functioning.
    B. Improvement in cognitive functioning.
    C. Onset of parkinsonian symptoms.
    D. Increased risk for psychosis.
    E. Increased delirium.

3. HIV is believed to increase the risk of developing major depression through which of the following mechanisms?

    A. Chronic stress.
    B. Worsening social isolation.
    C. Demoralization.
    D. Direct injury to subcortical brain areas.
    E. All of the above.

4. AIDS mania often has a clinical profile different from that of primary mania. All of the following are characteristics of AIDS mania *except*

    A. Irritable mood.
    B. Infrequent spontaneous remissions.
    C. Psychomotor agitation.
    D. More chronic than episodic course.
    E. None of the above.

5. Which of the following personality characteristics *best* describes the majority of patients who would be seen in an AIDS clinic in a metropolitan area?

    A. Unstable extravert.
    B. Stable extravert.
    C. Unstable introvert.
    D. Stable introvert.
    E. None of the above.

12 Dermatology

Lesley M. Arnold, M.D.

PSYCHOCUTANEOUS DISORDERS include dermatological diseases that are affected by psychological factors and psychiatric illnesses in which the skin is the target of disordered thinking, behavior, or perception. Emerging evidence of the role of the nervous system in skin pathophysiology provides clues into possible links between stress and dermatological diseases. In this chapter, I review the pathophysiology of these dermatological diseases, emphasizing the involvement of the central nervous system (CNS), and examine recent developments in the management of psychocutaneous disorders.

Classification

Table 12–1 shows the classification of psychocutaneous disorders in DSM-IV-TR (American Psychiatric Association 2000) categories. Psychological factors affecting medical condition includes dermatological diseases that are commonly affected by psychiatric factors. Somatoform disorders include disorders of the skin that are not fully explained by a known dermatological disease. Delusional disorder, somatic type, is the most common diagnosis in patients with delusional parasitosis, but the differential diagnosis of delusions of parasitosis includes major depressive disorder, bipolar disorder, schizophrenia, psychotic disorder due to a general medical condition, and substance-induced psychotic disorder. A preoccupation with a defect in appearance (body dysmorphic disorder) has a delusional variant, classified as a delusional disorder, somatic type. Trichotillomania is classified under the impulse-control disorders. Psychogenic excoriation and onychophagia are not currently included in DSM-IV-TR but could probably be classified under the category of impulse-control disorder not otherwise specified. Trichotillomania, psychogenic excoriation, and onychophagia frequently have symptoms that overlap with obsessive-compulsive disorder. Factitious disorders include factitious dermatitis (also called dermatitis artefacta) and psychogenic purpura.

TABLE 12–1. Classification of psychocutaneous disorders by DSM-IV-TR categories

I. Psychological factors affecting medical condition
    Atopic dermatitis
    Psoriasis
    Alopecia areata
    Urticaria and angioedema
    Acne vulgaris

II. Somatoform disorders
    Chronic idiopathic pruritus
    Idiopathic pruritus ani, vulvae, and scroti
    Body dysmorphic disorder

III. Delusional disorder, somatic type
    Delusional parasitosis
    Delusions of a defect in appearance
    Delusions of a foul body odor

IV. Impulse-control disorders
    Psychogenic excoriation
    Trichotillomania
    Onychophagia

V. Factitious disorders
    Factitious dermatitis (dermatitis artefacta)
    Psychogenic purpura

Psychological Factors Affecting Medical Condition

Atopic Dermatitis

Atopic dermatitis, a chronic skin disorder characterized by pruritus and inflammation (eczema), often begins as an erythematous, pruritic, maculopapular eruption (Ehlers et al. 1995; Gil et al. 1987; Lammintausta et al. 1991). Lichenification, excoriations, and infections frequently occur in response to excessive scratching (Gil et al. 1987). Atopic dermatitis typically begins in early infancy, childhood, or adolescence and is frequently associated with a personal or family history of atopic dermatitis, allergic rhinitis, or asthma (Ginsburg et al. 1993). Atopic dermatitis is a common disorder,

with a female-to-male ratio of 1.2:1.0 (M.L. Johnson 1977; Rajka 1989). The prevalence of atopic dermatitis has increased to greater than 10% in the past decade, possibly as a result of greater exposure to provocative factors (Leung et al. 1999; Rothe and Grant-Kels 1996; Williams 1992, 1995). Mild cases of atopic dermatitis may spontaneously resolve, but most patients experience persistent or relapsing symptoms (Kissling and Wuthrich 1994; Lammintausta et al. 1991).

Although genetic factors are probably involved in the pathophysiology of atopic dermatitis (Schultz Larson 1993; Uehara and Kimura 1993), environmental factors frequently trigger or exacerbate the disease (Ehlers et al. 1995; Morren et al. 1994). A vicious cycle of itching, scratching, and lesion aggravation frequently develops and contributes to symptom chronicity (Gil et al. 1987; Gupta and Gupta 1996; Morren et al. 1994). Stressful life events often precede the onset or exacerbation of atopic dermatitis (Kodama et al. 1999; Morren et al. 1994; Picardi and Abeni 2001). Stress may have an effect on atopic dermatitis through an interaction between the CNS and the immune system (Buske-Kirshbaum et al. 2001).

Controlled studies have found that adult patients with atopic dermatitis are more anxious and depressed compared with clinical and disease-free control groups (Ehlers et al. 1995; Gupta and Gupta 2003; Hashiro and Okumura 1997). Distress appears to perturb the epidermal permeability barrier homeostasis, resulting in inflammation and pruritus. The stress-induced deterioration of the barrier function may be mediated by glucocorticoids or by neuropeptides released within the epidermis (Garg et al. 2001).

In a study of children with atopic dermatitis, about a third of the children with severe atopic dermatitis symptoms had significantly higher morbidity levels on behavioral screening questionnaires (Daud et al. 1993). In another study, children with moderate to severe atopic dermatitis were significantly more likely to be distressed than a control group with minor skin problems (Absolon et al. 1997). Certain dimensions of family environment, such as independence and organization, correlated with less severe symptoms of atopic dermatitis, whereas parental responses of attention or physical contact reinforced scratching (Gil and Sampson 1989).

Treatment of atopic dermatitis strives to interrupt the vicious cycle of itching and scratching. Psychiatric treatment modalities include psychological or behavioral therapies and psychotropic medications. In controlled studies, relaxation training, habit reversal training, cognitive-behavioral techniques, and stress management training resulted in significant and stable adjunctive treatment responses to standard medical care and reduction in anxiety and depression (Ehlers et al. 1995). Topical 5% doxepin cream, which has potent histamine antagonism, was effective in reducing pruritus in patients with atopic dermatitis in controlled trials (Drake and Millikan 1995; Drake et al. 1994). Another antidepressant with histamine receptor antagonism, trimipramine (50 mg/day), decreased the fragmentation of sleep and reduced the time spent in Stage I sleep, which reduced the amount of scratching during the night in atopic dermatitis patients (Savin et al. 1979).

Psoriasis

Psoriasis is a chronic, relapsing disease of the skin with characteristic lesions that involve both the vasculature and the epidermis and have clear-cut borders and noncoherent silvery scales over a glossy, homogeneous erythema. Lesions vary from pinpoint plaques to extensive (erythrodermic) skin involvement, nail dystrophy, and

arthritis (Christophers and Mrowietz 1999). Psoriasis affects about 2% of the U.S. general population and is equally common in women and men. Most develop initial lesions in the third decade of life (Christophers and Mrowietz 1999). Although spontaneous remissions have been reported and have lasted between 1 and 54 years (Farber and Nall 1974), most patients with psoriasis experience unpredictable exacerbations throughout life.

The pathogenesis of psoriasis appears to involve skin repair systems, inflammatory defense mechanisms, and immunity. Both genetic (Christophers and Mrowietz 1999) and environmental factors probably contribute to the liability to psoriasis (Christophers and Mrowietz 1999). Lithium-induced psoriasis typically occurs within the first few years of treatment, is resistant to treatment, and resolves after discontinuation of lithium (Krahn and Goldberg 1994).

Psoriasis is associated with substantial impairment of health-related quality of life, with a negative effect on psychological, vocational, social, and physical function (Fortune et al. 1997b; Gupta et al. 1990b; McKenna and Stern 1997; Rapp et al. 1999). Studies have found that psychological factors, including perceived health, perceptions of stigmatization, and depression, are stronger determinants of disability in patients with psoriasis than are disease severity, location, and duration (Rapp et al. 1997; Richards et al. 2001).

Stress has been reported to trigger psoriasis (Al'Abadie et al. 1994; Farber and Nall 1993; Gaston et al. 1987). Most patients who report episodes of psoriasis triggered by stress describe disease-related stress, resulting from the cosmetic disfigurement and social stigma of psoriasis, rather than stressful major life events or general levels of distress (Fortune et al. 1997a; Ginsburg 1995; Gupta et al. 1989, 1990b; Richards et al. 2001). The mechanism of stress-induced exacerbations may involve the nervous, endocrine, and immune systems (Farber 1995; Harvima et al. 1993; Raychaudhuri et al. 1995).

In controlled studies, patients with psoriasis had high levels of anxiety and depression and significant comorbidity with several personality disorders, including schizoid, avoidant, passive-aggressive, and compulsive personality disorders (Devrimci-Ozguven et al. 2000; Fried et al. 1995; Gupta and Gupta 1998; Richards et al. 2001; Rubino et al. 1995). A direct correlation was found between patients' self-report of psoriasis severity and depression and suicidal ideation. Furthermore, comorbid depression reduced the threshold for pruritus in psoriatic patients (Gupta et al. 1993b, 1994).

Evidence of psychological morbidity associated with psoriasis has led to the development of psychosocial interventions as part of its treatment. Meditation, hypnosis, relaxation training, cognitive-behavioral stress management, and symptom control imagery training were effective in reducing psoriasis activity in controlled studies (Fortune et al. 2002; Gaston et al. 1991; Kabat-Zinn et al. 1998; Zachariae et al. 1996).

Alopecia Areata

Alopecia areata is characterized by non-scarring hair loss in patches of typically well-demarcated smooth skin. Breakage of the hair shaft results in characteristic "exclamation-mark hairs." Hair loss often occurs on the scalp but also can affect the eyebrows, eyelashes, beard, and body hair and varies from a single patch to multiple patches or total hair loss (Koblenzer 1987). Alopecia areata accounts for about 2% of new dermatological outpatient visits in the United States. An estimated 1% of the U.S. population will have at least one episode by age 50 years (Price 1991).

The incidence is equal in men and women and peaks during the third to fifth decade (Olsen 1999). Of the patients with alopecia areata, 30% completely recover, but 20%–30% never recover from the first episode (Koblenzer 1987; Olsen 1999). The pathogenesis of alopecia areata probably involves immunological and genetic factors (Olsen 1999).

Debate continues about the role of psychiatric factors in the development of alopecia areata (Picardi and Abeni 2001). In one controlled study, patients with alopecia areata reported significantly more life events with a substantial effect, including exits from social fields (e.g., death, divorce), uncontrolled events, and socially desirable and undesirable events in the 6 months preceding the onset of symptoms than did control subjects (Perini et al. 1984). In uncontrolled studies of lifetime comorbid psychiatric disorders in adults with alopecia areata, many patients reported lifetime psychiatric diagnoses, particularly major depression, generalized anxiety disorder, and paranoid disorder (Colón et al. 1991; Koo et al. 1994). Patients with highly stress-reactive alopecia areata reported more depressive symptoms than did patients without stress-reactive alopecia areata (Gupta et al. 1997). Finally, children with alopecia areata reported more symptoms of depression and anxiety than did control subjects (Liakopoulou et al. 1997).

Locally released corticotropin-releasing hormone or other neuropeptides in the skin from dorsal root ganglia or immune cells in response to stress might contribute to the intense local inflammation around hair follicles and symptoms of alopecia areata (Katsarou-Katsari et al. 2001; Toyoda et al. 2001).

In a double-blind, placebo-controlled trial, patients taking imipramine (75 mg/day) had significantly more hair regrowth than did control subjects, an effect that was independent of a reduction in anxiety or depression (Perini et al. 1994). Patients with alopecia areata and comorbid depressive and anxiety disorders who received selective serotonin reuptake inhibitors (SSRIs) in open trials and a small controlled study also experienced improvement in the symptoms of alopecia areata (Cipriani et al. 2001; Ruiz-Doblado et al. 1999). Uncontrolled studies of psychotherapy and relaxation training have been promising in the treatment of alopecia areata, but more study is needed (García-Hernández et al. 1999).

Urticaria and Angioedema

Urticaria (hives) is characterized by circumscribed, raised, erythematous, usually pruritic areas of edema that involve the superficial dermis. Angioedema occurs when the edema extends into the deep dermis, subcutaneous, or submucosal layers (Soter 1999). About 15%–20% of the general population develops urticaria, with a peak incidence between ages 20 and 40 (Koblenzer 1987). The male-to-female ratio is equal in children, but more women than men develop urticaria in adulthood (Koblenzer 1987). Most patients with acute urticaria (duration of less than 6 weeks) readily respond to treatment of the underlying cause, usually infection or intolerance to specific drugs or food. However, the cause of chronic urticaria or angioedema (duration of greater than 6 weeks) in about 70% of patients is unknown. Chronic idiopathic urticaria often responds poorly to usual dermatological treatment. About 20% of the patients with chronic idiopathic urticaria have persistent symptoms after 10 years (Champion et al. 1969).

The manifestations of urticaria are a result of the release of vasoactive mediators in the skin, primarily histamine from mast cells or basophils (Soter 1999). The etiology of chronic idiopathic urticaria is unknown, but studies suggest an autoimmune pathogenesis in some patients (Demera et al. 2001).

The relation between chronic idiopathic urticaria or angioedema and psychiatric factors is unclear. Controlled studies have found that patients, particularly females, with chronic idiopathic urticaria are frequently depressed and anxious (Badoux and Levy 1994; Hashiro and Okumura 1994; Sheehan-Dare et al. 1990; Sperber et al. 1989). Controlled studies also demonstrated an association between stressful life events and the onset of urticaria (Fava et al. 1980; Lyketsos et al. 1985). Stress may lead to the secretion of neuropeptides, such as vasoactive intestinal peptide and substance P, that can cause vasodilation and contribute to the development of urticarial wheals (see Koblenzer 1987).

In a controlled study of psychological treatment of chronic idiopathic urticaria, hypnosis with relaxation reduced pruritus but not the number of hives (Shertzer and Lookingbill 1987). Controlled trials indicated that antidepressant medications were effective in the management of chronic idiopathic urticaria. Doxepin (10 mg three times a day) was more effective than diphenhydramine (25 mg three times a day) for the control of chronic idiopathic urticaria (Greene et al. 1985), and nortriptyline (25 mg three times a day) was significantly better than placebo in the treatment of pruritus and wheals (Morley 1969). In two case reports, both comorbid panic disorder and urticaria responded to treatment with the SSRI fluoxetine (40 mg/day) or sertraline (100 mg/day), suggesting a possible role for serotonergic mechanisms (Gupta and Gupta 1995).

Acne Vulgaris

Acne vulgaris, a common sebaceous gland disease, is characterized by a variety of lesions, including comedones, papules, pustules, and nodules. Possible complications from the lesions include development of pitted or hypertrophic scars. Most cases of acne vulgaris develop between the middle and late teenage years. The course of acne vulgaris is usually self-limited, with spontaneous remission after several years, but it may persist through the third decade and later. Although women are more likely than men to have persistent acne, it tends to be more severe in men (Strauss and Thiboutot 1999).

Although the cause of acne vulgaris is unknown, many factors are probably involved in its pathogenesis, including stress. Stress-induced aggravation of acne might be caused by the release of adrenal steroids, which affect the sebaceous glands (Koo and Smith 1991; Strauss and Thiboutot 1999).

Severe acne is associated with increased anxiety and poor self-image (Koo and Smith 1991). Acne can substantially interfere with social and occupational functioning (Gupta et al. 1990a). Successful treatment of acne with isotretinoin led to a reduction in both anxiety and depressive symptoms and a significant improvement in self-image (Kellett and Gawkrodger 1999; Rubinow et al. 1987). Also, case reports have shown improvement in acne after treatment of depression with paroxetine (Moussavian 2001). In another study, biofeedback-assisted relaxation and cognitive imagery added to usual dermatological treatment resulted in significant reduction in acne severity compared with medical control groups (Hughes et al. 1983).

The use of isotretinoin for treatment of acne vulgaris has been associated with depression, suicidal ideation, suicide attempts, and suicide in anecdotal reports that received extensive media attention (Jick et al. 2000). The U.S. Food and Drug Administration (FDA) MedWatch system reports of psychiatric disorders linked to use of isotretinoin led to additional label warnings in 1998. Recently, the FDA and isotretinoin's manufacturer added the possible development of aggressive and/or violent behavior to the psychiatric disorder warning section of the package insert (Enders and Enders 2003). Therefore, it is important to educate patients about the risk of major depressive disorder, suicide, and other psychiatric disorders and to monitor each patient carefully (Gupta and Gupta 2001).

Somatoform Disorders

Chronic Idiopathic Pruritus

Pruritus, or itchiness, is a common symptom of dermatological diseases, of several systemic diseases, and of advanced age (Gilchrest 1982). The pathophysiology of pruritus is not completely understood (Greaves and Wall 1996).

In a study of histamine-induced pruritus, psychic trauma lowered itch threshold, aggravated itch intensity, and prolonged itch duration. Furthermore, the duration of the pruritus was more pronounced in subjects reporting "moodiness" during stressor exposure (Fjellner and Arnetz 1985; Fjellner et al. 1985). Recent stressful life events also have been correlated with an increased ability to detect itch. A study of pruritus in psoriasis, atopic dermatitis, and chronic idiopathic urticaria found a direct correlation between pruritus severity and the degree of depressive symptoms, possibly a result of a reduced itch threshold (Gupta et al. 1994).

Antidepressant medications, particularly the tricyclic antidepressants, can relieve chronic idiopathic pruritus. Behavioral treatment, such as habit reversal training and cognitive-behavioral therapy (Rosenbaum and Ayllon 1981; Welkowitz et al. 1989), aimed at interrupting the itch-scratch cycle may help to prevent complications of long-term scratching, such as lichen simplex chronicus, a condition of prominent skin markings and thickening of the tissue.

Body Dysmorphic Disorder

Body dysmorphic disorder is a preoccupation with an imagined defect in appearance (Phillips et al. 1993). Body dysmorphic disorder is common in dermatology practice. Approximately 12% of the patients seeking dermatological treatment for concerns about the skin or hair had positive screening test results for body dysmorphic disorder, and it was equally common in men and women (Phillips et al. 2000). Although body dysmorphic disorder is classified as a somatoform disorder, it has phenomenological similarities to obsessive-compulsive disorder (Phillips et al. 1995). Dermatological treatment alone is not effective for body dysmorphic disorder, which often responds to treatment with SSRIs and cognitive-behavioral therapy (Phillips et al. 2002).

Delusional Disorder, Somatic Type

Delusional Parasitosis

Delusional parasitosis is characterized by a fixed, false conviction that one is infested with living organisms (G.C. Johnson and Anton 1985). Patients with delusional parasitosis seek treatment from dermatologists because the delusions often involve a cutaneous invasion. There are also cases of delusional oral, ocular, and intestinal parasitosis (Ford et al. 2001; Maeda et al. 1998; Sherman et al. 1998). Delusional parasitosis typically occurs as a single somatic delusion with no other impairment of thought or thought process (Munro 1978). Occasionally, patients describe tactile sensations of crawling, biting, or stinging and other perceptual abnormalities such as

buzzing or other sounds. Delusional parasitosis appears to be uncommon, with an equal sex distribution in patients younger than 50 years and a female-to-male ratio of 3:1 in patients ages 50 years and older (Lyell 1983).

The differential diagnosis of delusions of parasitosis includes numerous medical and neurological disorders (G.C. Johnson and Anton 1985; Morris 1991; Wykoff 1987). Patients with other psychiatric disorders, including major depressive disorder, bipolar disorder, and schizophrenia, also may have delusions of parasitosis (Freinhar 1984; G.C. Johnson and Anton 1985). Finally, delusions of parasitosis are associated with long-term use of amphetamines, methylphenidate, cocaine, alcohol, phenelzine, pargyline, or corticosteroids. The delusions usually resolve with discontinuation of the drug (G.C. Johnson and Anton 1985; Morris 1991; Wykoff 1987).

Characteristic features of delusional parasitosis include a specific precipitant, a history of potential or actual exposure to contagious organisms or actual infestation, and a history of multiple consultations with physicians and other professionals such as entomologists and exterminators (Lyell 1983). Patients make multiple attempts at treatment, including repetitive washing, checking, and cleaning; excoriation of the skin with needles, knives, or fingernails; discarding or destroying possessions; and excessive use of insect repellents and insecticides (Lyell 1983; Wykoff 1987). Other individuals may share the delusion (folie à deux), and the fear of contaminating others is often present (Lyell 1983; Morris 1991). Also, cases of delusional parasitosis by proxy involve children or pets (Nel et al. 2001). Descriptions of the offending parasite vary from the imprecise "things" or "bugs" to detailed explanations of the organism's (usually insects, spiders, or worms) appearance, behavior, and life cycle (Lyell 1983; Morris 1991; Wykoff 1987). The mistaken worries about infestation span a spectrum from nondelusional to delusional thinking (Wykoff 1987). Sometimes the preoccupation with infestation resembles obsessions in that it is distressing, anxiety-provoking, persistent, recurrent, and difficult to resist or control. The repetitive behaviors accompanying the preoccupation are often compulsive in nature. Patients frequently report social isolation and loss of employment as a result of the delusions (Wykoff 1987).

Patients with delusional parasitosis respond to treatment with the potent neuroleptic pimozide. Only one controlled study of the treatment of delusional parasitosis with pimozide has been done, in which 10 of 11 patients improved after 6 weeks of 1–5 mg/day (Hamann and Avnstorp 1982). A follow-up study indicated that many patients taking pimozide could discontinue the medication after a mean treatment duration of 5 months without recurrence of the delusions (Lindskov and Baadsgaard 1985). In other anecdotal reports, pimozide dosages of up to 12 mg/day have been used in delusional parasitosis (G.C. Johnson and Anton 1985). Full remission of delusional parasitosis has been reported in 50% of the patients receiving pimozide (Trabert 1995). There are uncontrolled reports of efficacy with other antipsychotic medications, including chlorpromazine, trifluoperazine, haloperidol, risperidone, and fluphenazine decanoate (De Leon et al. 1997; Freinhar 1984; Gallucci and Beard 1995; Kitamura 1997; Morris 1991; Songer and Roman 1996). Although pimozide is most commonly advocated for the treatment of delusional parasitosis, no conclusive evidence indicates that pimozide is superior to other antipsychotics. However, pimozide is the only neuroleptic used in the treatment of delusional parasitosis that is a potent opiate antagonist (Creese et al.

1976). Pimozide may be antipruritic as a result of its opiate antagonism, and the relief of pruritus or paresthesias could contribute to improvement in delusional parasitosis (G.C. Johnson and Anton 1983; Krishnan and Koo 2005).

Case reports show successful treatment of delusional parasitosis with tricyclic antidepressants, SSRIs, and electroconvulsive therapy (Bhatia et al. 2000; Morris 1991; Pylko and Sicignan 1985; Slaughter et al. 1998). Because of the obsessive-compulsive symptoms in many patients with delusional parasitosis, controlled studies with the SSRIs are needed. Psychotherapy has minimal efficacy in the treatment of delusional parasitosis (Freinhar 1984).

Other Delusional Disorders, Somatic Type

In the delusional variant of body dysmorphic disorder, the preoccupations with a defect in appearance are of delusional intensity, although the distinction between an obsessive concern and delusions is not always clear (see McElroy et al. 1993; Phillips et al. 1994). Delusional body dysmorphic disorder may respond preferentially to SSRIs, and if a patient's symptoms do not completely respond to an SSRI, the addition of an antipsychotic, such as pimozide, may be helpful (Phillips 1996; Phillips et al. 2002).

The delusion of a foul body odor is another encapsulated somatic delusion that a dermatologist may encounter in patients. Treatment data are limited, but pimozide and other antipsychotic medications may be effective (Manschreck 1996).

Impulse-Control Disorders

Psychogenic Excoriation

Psychogenic excoriation (neurotic excoriation, acne excoriée, pathological or compulsive skin picking, or dermatotillomania) is a disorder characterized by self-induced skin lesions from excoriating the skin in response to skin sensations or an urge to remove an irregularity on the skin (Gupta et al. 1987). Lesions are found in areas that the patient can easily reach, such as the face, upper back, and upper and lower extremities. Psychogenic excoriation occurs in about 2% of dermatology outpatients and is more common in women (Gupta et al. 1986). Most studies report a mean age at onset between 30 and 45 years, although the disorder can begin in adolescence. The mean duration of symptoms is 5 years, with a better prognosis for patients who have had the symptoms for less than 1 year (Gupta et al. 1986).

The behavior associated with psychogenic excoriation is heterogeneous. Some patients exhibit behavior that resembles obsessive-compulsive disorder in that it is repetitive, ritualistic, and tension reducing, and patients attempt, often unsuccessfully, to resist excoriating, a behavior they find ego-dystonic (Stein and Hollander 1992a). Patients sometimes describe obsessions about an irregularity on the skin or preoccupations with having smooth skin and may excoriate in response to such thoughts (Phillips and Taub 1995). Patients also may describe symptoms of impulse-control disorders, such as an increase in tension before the behavior and transient pleasure or relief immediately afterward (Arnold et al. 1998). As in other impulse-control disorders, patients with psychogenic excoriation often find themselves acting automatically. Behaviors thus can span a "compulsivity–impulsivity" continuum from purely obsessive-compulsive to purely impulsive, with mixed symptoms between these poles (Arnold et al. 2001; McElroy et al. 1994).

Depressive and anxiety disorders are common in patients with psychogenic excoriation (Arnold et al. 1998; Gupta et al. 1987; Simeon et al. 1997).

Case reports and open trials suggest that psychogenic excoriation responds to treatment with oral doxepin (Harris et al. 1987) and the serotonin reuptake inhibitors fluoxetine (Gupta and Gupta 1993; Phillips and Taub 1995; Stein et al. 1993; Stout 1990; Vittorio and Phillips 1997), sertraline (Kalivas et al. 1996), paroxetine (Biondi et al. 2000; Ravindran et al. 1999), and fluvoxamine (Arnold et al. 1999) and the tricyclic antidepressant clomipramine (Gupta et al. 1986). There are also case reports of successful treatment of psychogenic excoriation with olanzapine (Blanch et al. 2004; Garnis-Jones et al. 2000; Gupta and Gupta 2000), pimozide (Duke 1983), and naltrexone (Lienemann and Walker 1989). A 10-week double-blind, placebo-controlled trial found that fluoxetine, at a mean dosage of 55 mg/day, was significantly better than placebo in reducing psychogenic excoriation (Simeon et al. 1997). A study of open-label fluoxetine, at a mean dosage of 41 mg/day for 6 weeks followed by a 6-week double-blind, placebo-controlled phase, also reported that fluoxetine significantly reduced skin excoriation (Block et al. 2000). Studies of the behavioral treatment of psychogenic excoriation are limited to case reports, which showed promising results (Deckersbach et al. 2002; Kent and Drummond 1988; Welkowitz et al. 1989).

Trichotillomania

Trichotillomania is a disorder of chronic pulling out of one's hair. Trichotillomania is classified as an impulse-control disorder in DSM-IV-TR but, like psychogenic excoriation, has both impulsive and compulsive features (Stein et al. 1995a, 1995b). Trichotillomania causes substantial distress and impairment in functioning and leads to alopecia, most commonly involving the scalp hair but also eyelashes, eyebrows, pubic hair, and other body hair (Christenson et al. 1991a). The extracted hair is sometimes chewed or swallowed, resulting in the development of trichobezoars (Christenson and Crow 1996). Patients may develop infections at the site of hair pulling, change in texture or color of the hair, or carpal tunnel syndrome from pulling (Christenson and Crow 1996).

In a survey of college freshmen, the lifetime prevalence of trichotillomania (by strict criteria) was 0.6% for both men and women but rose to 3.4% for women and 1.5% for men if all hair pulling with noticeable hair loss was included (Christenson et al. 1991b). The condition typically persists for years, with a mean age at onset of 13 years (Christenson et al. 1991a).

There are two types of hair pulling (Christenson and Crow 1996). In the "focused style," patients focus solely on the pulling without attention to other thoughts and activities. Symptoms resemble obsessive-compulsive disorder in that the patient resists the pulling and feels relief with pulling. However, most patients engage in an "automatic style" of pulling that occurs during situations described as sedentary or contemplative, such as reading or watching television, which is consistent with impulse-control disorders. Many patients have a combination of these two styles (Christenson et al. 1993).

Comorbid psychiatric disorders in patients with trichotillomania include anxiety, mood, substance abuse/dependence, eating, and personality disorders (Christenson et al. 1991a; Cohen et al. 1995; Schlosser et al. 1994; Swedo and Leonard 1992).

In a double-blind crossover study, trichotillomania responded preferentially to the antiobsessional agent clomipramine, at a mean dose of 180 mg/day, over desipramine, at a mean dose of 173 mg/day (Swedo et al. 1989). Open studies of the SSRI fluoxetine reported positive short- and long-term results (Koran et al. 1992; Winchel et al. 1992); however, controlled studies have yielded mixed findings. Two placebo-controlled studies found that fluoxetine was not superior to placebo in the treatment of trichotillomania (Christenson et al. 1991c; Streichenwein and Thornby 1995), but in a double-blind crossover study of clomipramine and fluoxetine, both medications had positive treatment effects on trichotillomania (Pigott et al. 1992). Case reports and open trials reported positive responses to treatment with other drugs, including fluvoxamine (Christenson et al. 1998; Stanley et al. 1997), paroxetine (Reid 1994), sertraline (Bradford and Gratzer 1995; Rahman and Gregory 1995), citalopram (Stein et al. 1997), venlafaxine (Ninan et al. 1998), other antidepressants (Christenson and Crow 1996), lithium (Christenson et al. 1991d), and buspirone (Reid 1992). Pimozide augmentation of clomipramine or fluoxetine also has proved useful in a small case series (Stein and Hollander 1992b). A case series of olanzapine augmentation of citalopram was effective in three of four patients (Ashton 2001). Finally, there are case reports of successful treatment of resistant trichotillomania with a combination of risperidone and fluvoxamine (Gabriel 2001) and with risperidone alone (Sentürk and Tanrtverdi 2002).

The behavioral treatment of habit reversal has been reported to be effective in trichotillomania and involves increasing awareness of situations or stressors associated with hair pulling, relaxation training, and competing response training (Azrin et al. 1980). A small 9-week controlled study examining efficacy of cognitive-behavioral therapy and clomipramine compared with placebo found that cognitive-behavioral therapy substantially reduced the symptoms of trichotillomania and was significantly more effective than clomipramine or placebo (Ninan et al. 2000). A 12-week controlled study compared fluoxetine with behavioral treatment that consisted of six individual 45-minute sessions aimed at self-control, which relied on self-report and self-monitoring. The behavioral treatment resulted in significantly greater reduction in trichotillomania symptoms compared with the fluoxetine or a waiting-list control condition (van Minnen et al. 2003). Hypnosis and other behavioral treatments also have been useful according to case reports (Peterson et al. 1994). Preliminary evidence suggests that concurrent use of behavioral therapies and medication treatment for trichotillomania may be more effective than either treatment alone, but more study is needed (Keuthen et al. 1998; Walsh and McDougle 2005).

Onychophagia

Onychophagia, or repetitive nail biting, is a common behavior that can begin as early as age 4 years, with a peak between ages 10 and 18 years, and that appears to be familial (Leonard et al. 1991). Severe onychophagia can lead to significant medical and dental problems, such as hand infection (Zook 1986) and craniomandibular disorders (Westling 1988). Onychotillomania, the picking or tearing of the nail, may be a variant of the behavior. Like trichotillomania and psychogenic excoriation, onychophagia has the phenomenological features of repetition, resistance, and relief (Leonard et al. 1991).

A double-blind crossover study reported that onychophagia responded preferentially to clomipramine, at a mean dosage of 120 mg/day, over desipramine, at a mean dosage of 135 mg/day (Leonard et al. 1991). Many forms of behavior therapy, including habit reversal, have been efficacious (Peterson et al. 1994). In a recent controlled study of chronic nail biting, habit reversal training (a total of 2 hours spread over three sessions) was compared with a placebo treatment in which patients simply discussed their nail biting. The habit reversal intervention produced a greater increase in nail length compared with the placebo (Twohig et al. 2003).

Factitious Disorders

Factitious Dermatitis

Factitious dermatitis (dermatitis artefacta) is a disorder in which patients intentionally produce skin lesions in order to assume the sick role. Patients typically deny the self-inflicted nature of the disorder (Gupta et al. 1987).

Factitious dermatitis can present with a wide variety of lesions depending on the methods used by the patient. Patients may either simulate actual medical dermatoses or aggravate a preexisting dermatological condition (Koblenzer 1987). Lesions include excoriations, blisters, purpura, ulcers, erythema, edema, sinuses, and nodules (Gupta et al. 1987). Methods used by patients include rubbing; scratching; picking; cutting; puncturing; sucking; biting; applying suction cups; occluding; applying dye, heat, or caustic substances onto the skin; or injecting caustics, infected material, blood, feces, or other substances into the skin (Gupta et al. 1987; Koblenzer 1987; Lyell 1979; Spraker 1983).

Skin damage can be extensive, with full-thickness skin loss and severe scarring requiring plastic surgery or even amputation (Hollender and Abram 1973). Affected sites tend to be easily accessible to the patient and are more prominent on one side of the body, depending on the handedness of the patient (Hollender and Abram 1973). Excoriated lesions frequently have sharp geometric borders with normal surrounding skin or lines at the margin if a caustic was used and some liquid dripped out of the site (Hollender and Abram 1973; Spraker 1983). The natural progression of the lesions through the different stages of development is not evident (Spraker 1983).

The history is often vague and "hollow" (Lyell 1979), and patients are often very suggestible as to the site of the next lesion (Hollender and Abram 1973). The use of an occlusive dressing such as an Unna's paste boot (a dressing that hardens to form a protective covering) can help make the diagnosis because the lesions heal when the patients are unable to reach them (Hollender and Abram 1973; Koblenzer 1987).

Factitious dermatitis occurs in about 0.3% of dermatology patients (Gupta et al. 1987), with a female-to-male ratio between 3:1 and 8:1 and the greatest frequency in adolescents and young adults (Koblenzer 1987). It reportedly begins after severe psychosocial stress, usually involving loss, threatened loss, or isolation (Stein and Hollander 1992a). As in other factitious disorders, the patient often has experience in medicine as a result of either prior exposure to illness or employment in a health care field. The prognosis varies; some cases resolve after a brief episode, whereas others become lifelong problems (Lyell 1979). In a classic long-term study, 30% of the patients continued to produce lesions more than 12 years after the onset of their symptoms (Sneddon and Sneddon 1975).

No controlled trials of the treatment of factitious dermatitis have been published, and treatment recommendations are based on anecdotal experience (Koblenzer 1987; Spraker 1983).

Psychogenic Purpura

The spontaneous appearance of recurrent bruising (purpura) is a rare dermatological disorder that often follows an injury or a surgical procedure and typically is initiated by pain, burning, or stinging, followed by warmth, erythema, swelling, and sometimes pruritus and, after hours or days, by ecchymosis (Gardner and Diamond 1955). Blood coagulation and hemostatic tests, however, have normal results (Koblenzer 1987;

Stocker and McIntyre 1977). The incidence is unknown, but it affects women more frequently than men, with a female-to-male ratio of 20:1. The age at onset varies from 9 to 53 years, with most cases occurring between ages 14 and 40 (Koblenzer 1987).

In support of a psychogenic cause of the purpura, studies have found that it often begins after significant psychosocial stressors. Most patients present with several other unexplained somatic symptoms and have significant comorbid psychiatric symptoms, including depression, anxiety, and personality disorders, particularly borderline and histrionic personality disorders (Ratnoff 1989). The differentiation between conversion and factitious purpura is unclear because patients thought to have conversion symptoms and those found to have factitious disorder share many common features (Stocker and McIntyre 1977). In addition, physicians can identify no mechanism for a conversion reaction or convincingly disprove factitious causation in many cases (Stocker and McIntyre 1977). Although more study is needed, it appears that factitious disorder is the most likely cause of psychogenic purpura.

Conclusion

Patients with psychocutaneous disorders are a diverse group who frequently present to dermatologists for evaluation and treatment. Included in this group are patients who have dermatological diseases (e.g., psoriasis), in which the course may be affected by psychological factors, such as stress or comorbid mood and anxiety disorders. Patients who have primary psychiatric disorders with skin-related symptoms (e.g., delusional parasitosis) are also included under the broad category of psychocutaneous disorders. Psychocutaneous disorders can be particularly challenging for dermatologists because patients with these disorders are often reluctant to seek psychiatric treatment. Furthermore, the understanding of the pathophysiology of these disorders is limited, and relatively few treatment studies are available to guide the management of these disorders.

Patients may be more willing to accept a psychiatric evaluation if a psychiatrist is working within the dermatology clinic. In a study of a dermatology liaison clinic, most of the psychiatric workload involved the treatment of comorbid depressive and anxiety disorders. Furthermore, most of the patients who were seen in the liaison clinic responded well to psychiatric treatment (Woodruff et al. 1997). However, many communities do not have psychiatrists available to perform a liaison function within dermatology settings. As an alternative, psychiatrists with an interest in psychocutaneous disorders could develop working relationships with dermatologists to improve the access to psychiatric evaluation and treatment. Collaboration between the psychiatrist and dermatologist is likely to positively affect the treatment outcome of patients with psychocutaneous disorders.

References

Absolon CM, Cottrell D, Eldridge SM, et al: Psychological disturbance in atopic eczema: the extent of the problem in school aged children. Br J Dermatol 137:241–245, 1997

Al'Abadie MS, Kent GG, Gawkrodger DJ: The relationship between stress and the onset and exacerbation of psoriasis and other skin conditions. Br J Dermatol 130:199–203, 1994

American Psychiatric Association: Diagnostic and Statistical Manual of Mental Disorders, 4th Edition, Text Revision. Washington, DC, American Psychiatric Association, 2000

Arnold LM, McElroy SL, Mutasim DF, et al: Characteristics of 34 adults with psychogenic excoriation. J Clin Psychiatry 59:509–514, 1998

Arnold LM, Mutasim DF, Dwight MM, et al: An open clinical trial of fluvoxamine treatment of psychogenic excoriation. J Clin Psychopharmacol 19:15–18, 1999

Arnold LM, Auchenbach MB, McElroy SL: Psychogenic excoriation: clinical features, proposed diagnostic criteria, epidemiology and approaches to treatment. CNS Drugs 15: 351–359, 2001

Ashton AK: Olanzapine augmentation for trichotillomania. Am J Psychiatry 158:1929–1930, 2001

Azrin NH, Nunn RG, Frantz SE: Treatment of hairpulling (trichotillomania): a comparative study of habit reversal and negative practice training. J Behav Ther Exp Psychiatry 11: 13–20, 1980

Badoux A, Levy DA: Psychologic symptoms in asthma and chronic urticaria. Ann Allergy 72:229–234, 1994

Bhatia MS, Jagawat T, Choudhary S: Delusional parasitosis: a clinical profile. Int J Psychiatry Med 30:83–91, 2000

Biondi M, Arcangeli T, Petrucci RM: Paroxetine in a case of psychogenic pruritus and neurotic excoriations. Psychother Psychosom 69:165–166, 2000

Blanch J, Grimalt F, Massana G, et al: Efficacy of olanzapine in the treatment of psychogenic excoriation. Br J Dermatol 151: 714–716, 2004

Block MR, Elliott MA, Thompson H, et al: Fluoxetine for skin picking. Abstracts of the New Clinical Drug Evaluation Unit Annual Meeting. Boca Raton, FL, May 30–June 2, 2000

Bradford JMW, Gratzer TG: A treatment for impulse control disorders and paraphilia: a case report. Can J Psychiatry 40: 4–5, 1995

Buske-Kirschbaum A, Geiben A, Hellhammer D: Psychobiological aspects of atopic dermatitis: an overview. Psychother Psychosom 70:6–16, 2001

Champion RH, Roberts SOB, Carpenter RG, et al: Urticaria and angio-oedema: a review of 554 patients. Br J Dermatol 81:588–597, 1969

Christenson GA, Crow SJ: The characterization and treatment of trichotillomania. J Clin Psychiatry 57:42–49, 1996

Christenson GA, Mackenzie TB, Mitchell JE: Characteristics of 60 adult chronic hair pullers. Am J Psychiatry 148:365–370, 1991a

Christenson GA, Pyle RL, Mitchell JE: Estimated lifetime prevalence of trichotillomania in college students. J Clin Psychiatry 52:415–417, 1991b

Christenson GA, Mackenzie TB, Mitchell JE, et al: A placebo-controlled, double-blind crossover study of fluoxetine in trichotillomania. Am J Psychiatry 148:1566–1571, 1991c

Christenson GA, Popkin MK, Mackenzie TB, et al: Lithium treatment of chronic hair pulling. J Clin Psychiatry 52:116–120, 1991d

Christenson GA, Ristvedt SL, Mackenzie TB: Identification of trichotillomania cue profiles. Behav Res Ther 31:315–320, 1993

Christenson GA, Crow SJ, Mitchell JE, et al: Fluvoxamine in the treatment of trichotillomania: an 8-week, open-label study. CNS Spectr 3:64–71, 1998

Christophers E, Mrowietz U: Epidermis: disorders of persistent inflammation, cell kinetics and differentiation, in Fitzpatrick's Dermatology in General Medicine, 5th Edition. Edited by Freedberg IM, Eisen AZ, Wolff K, et al. New York, McGraw-Hill, 1999, pp 495–521

Cipriani R, Perini GI, Rampinelli S: Paroxetine in alopecia areata. Int J Dermatol 40:600–601, 2001

Cohen LJ, Stein DJ, Simeon D, et al: Clinical profile, comorbidity, and treatment history in 123 hair pullers: a survey study. J Clin Psychiatry 56:319–326, 1995

Colón EA, Popkin MK, Callies AL, et al: Lifetime prevalence of psychiatric disorders in patients with alopecia areata. Compr Psychiatry 32:245–251, 1991

Creese I, Feinberg AP, Snyder SH: Butyrophenone influences on the opiate receptor. Eur J Pharmacol 36:231–235, 1976

Daud IR, Garralda ME, David TJ: Psychosocial adjustment in preschool children with atopic eczema. Arch Dis Child 69:670–676, 1993

Deckersbach T, Wilhelm S, Keuthen NJ, et al: Cognitive-behavior therapy for self-injurious skin picking. Behav Modif 26:361–377, 2002

De Leon OA, Furmaga KM, Canterbury AL, et al: Risperidone in the treatment of delusions of infestation. Int J Psychiatry Med 27:403–409, 1997

Demera RS, Ryhal B, Gershwin ME: Chronic idiopathic urticaria. Compr Ther 27:213–217, 2001

Devrimci-Ozguven H, Kundakci N, Kumbasar H, et al: The depression, anxiety, life satisfaction and affective expression levels in psoriasis patients. J Eur Acad Dermatol Venereol 14:267–271, 2000

Drake LA, Millikan LE: The Doxepin Study Group: the antipruritic effect of 5% doxepin cream in patients with eczematous dermatitis. Arch Dermatol 131:1403–1408, 1995

Drake LA, Fallon JD, Sober A, et al: Relief of pruritus in patients with atopic dermatitis after treatment with topical doxepin cream. J Am Acad Dermatol 31:613–616, 1994

Duke EE: Clinical experience with pimozide: emphasis on its use in postherpetic neuralgia. J Am Acad Dermatol 8:845–850, 1983

Ehlers A, Stangier U, Gieler U: Treatment of atopic dermatitis: a comparison of psychological and dermatological approaches to relapse prevention. J Consult Clin Psychol 63:624–635, 1995

Enders SJ, Enders JM: Isotretinoin and psychiatric illness in adolescents and young adults. Ann Pharmacother 37:1124–1127, 2003

Farber EM: Therapeutic perspectives in psoriasis. Int J Dermatol 34:456–460, 1995

Farber EM, Nall ML: The natural history of psoriasis in 5600 patients. Dermatologica 148:1–18, 1974

Farber EM, Nall L: Psoriasis: a stress-related disease. Cutis 51: 322–326, 1993

Fava GA, Perini GI, Santonastaso P, et al: Life events and psychological distress in dermatologic disorders: psoriasis, chronic urticaria and fungal infections. Br J Med Psychol 53:277–282, 1980

Fjellner B, Arnetz BB: Psychological predictors of pruritus during mental stress. Acta Derm Venereol 65:504–508, 1985

Fjellner B, Arnetz BB, Eneroth P, et al: Pruritus during standardized mental stress: relationship to psychoneuroendocrine and metabolic parameters. Acta Derm Venereol 65:199–205, 1985

Ford EB, Calfee DP, Pearson RD: Delusions of intestinal parasitosis. South Med J 94:545–547, 2001

Fortune DG, Main CJ, O'Sullivan TM, et al: Assessing illness-related stress in psoriasis: the psychometric properties of the psoriasis life stress inventory. J Psychosom Res 42:467–475, 1997a

Fortune DG, Main CJ, O'Sullivan TM, et al: Quality of life in patients with psoriasis: the contribution of clinical variables and psoriasis-specific stress. Br J Dermatol 137:755–760, 1997b

Fortune DG, Richards HL, Kirby B, et al: A cognitive-behavioural symptom management programme as an adjunct in psoriasis therapy. Br J Dermatol 146:458–465, 2002

Freinhar JP: Delusions of parasitosis. Psychosomatics 25:47–53, 1984

Fried RG, Friedman S, Paradis C, et al: Trivial or terrible? The psychosocial impact of psoriasis. Int J Dermatol 34:101–105, 1995

Gabriel A: A case of resistant trichotillomania treated with risperidone-augmented fluvoxamine (letter). Can J Psychiatry 46:285–286, 2001

Gallucci G, Beard G: Risperidone and the treatment of delusions of parasitosis in an elderly patient. Psychosomatics 36:578–580, 1995

García-Hernández MJ, Ruiz-Doblado S, Rodriguez-Pichardo A, et al: Alopecia areata, stress and psychiatric disorders: a review. J Dermatol 26:625–632, 1999

Gardner FH, Diamond LK: Autoerythrocyte sensitization: a form of purpura, producing painful bruising following autosensitization to red blood cells in certain women. Blood 10: 675–690, 1955

Garg A, Chren MM, Sands LP, et al: Psychological stress perturbs epidermal permeability barrier homeostasis. Arch Dermatol 137:53–59, 2001

Garnis-Jones S, Collins S, Rosenthal D: Treatment of self-mutilation with olanzapine. J Cutan Med Surg 4:161–163, 2000

Gaston L, Lassonde M, Bernier-Buzzanga J, et al: Psoriasis and stress: a prospective study. J Am Acad Dermatol 17:82–86, 1987

Gaston L, Crombez J, Lassonde M, et al: Psychological stress and psoriasis: experimental and prospective correlational studies. Acta Derm Venereol 156:37–43, 1991

Gil KM, Sampson HA: Psychological and social factors of atopic dermatitis. Allergy 44:84–89, 1989

Gil KM, Keefe FJ, Sampson HA, et al: The relation of stress and family environment to atopic dermatitis symptoms in children. J Psychosom Res 31:673–684, 1987

Gilchrest BA: Pruritus: pathogenesis, therapy, and significance in systemic disease states. Arch Intern Med 142:101–105, 1982

Ginsburg IH: Psychological and psychophysiological aspects of psoriasis. Dermatol Clin 13:793–804, 1995

Ginsburg IH, Prystowsky JH, Kornfeld DS, et al: Role of emotional factors in adults with atopic dermatitis. Int J Dermatol 32:656–660, 1993

Greaves MW, Wall PD: Pathophysiology of itching. Lancet 348:938–940, 1996

Greene SL, Reed CE, Schroeter AL: Double-blind crossover study comparing doxepin with diphenhydramine for the treatment of chronic urticaria. J Am Acad Dermatol 12:669–675, 1985

Gupta MA, Gupta AK: Fluoxetine is an effective treatment for neurotic excoriations: case report. Cutis 51:386–387, 1993

Gupta MA, Gupta AK: Chronic idiopathic urticaria associated with panic disorder: a syndrome responsive to selective serotonin reuptake inhibitor antidepressants? Cutis 56:53–54, 1995

Gupta MA, Gupta AK: Psychodermatology: an update. J Am Acad Dermatol 34:1030–1046, 1996

Gupta MA, Gupta AK: Depression and suicidal ideation in dermatology patients with acne, alopecia areata, atopic dermatitis and psoriasis. Br J Dermatol 139:846–850, 1998

Gupta MA, Gupta AK: Olanzapine is effective in the management of some self-induced dermatoses: three case reports. Cutis 66:143–146, 2000

Gupta MA, Gupta AK: The psychological co-morbidity in acne. Clin Dermatol 19:360-363, 2001

Gupta MA, Gupta AK: Psychiatric and psychological co-morbidity in patients with dermatologic disorders. Am J Clin Dermatol 4:833–842, 2003

Gupta MA, Gupta AK, Haberman HF: Neurotic excoriations: a review and some new perspectives. Compr Psychiatry 27:381–386, 1986

Gupta MA, Gupta AK, Haberman HF: The self-inflicted dermatoses: a critical review. Gen Hosp Psychiatry 9:45–52, 1987

Gupta MA, Gupta AK, Kirkby S, et al: A psycho-cutaneous profile of psoriasis patients who are stress reactors: a study of 127 patients. Gen Hosp Psychiatry 11:166–173, 1989

Gupta MA, Gupta AK, Schork NJ, et al: Psychiatric aspects of the treatment of mild to moderate facial acne; some preliminary observations. Int J Dermatol 29:719–721, 1990a

Gupta MA, Gupta AK, Ellis CN, et al: Some psychosomatic aspects of psoriasis. Adv Dermatol 5:21–32, 1990b

Gupta MA, Schork NJ, Gupta AK, et al: Suicidal ideation in psoriasis. Int J Dermatol 32:188–190, 1993b

Gupta MA, Gupta AK, Schork NJ, et al: Depression modulates pruritus perception: a study of pruritus in psoriasis, atopic dermatitis, and chronic idiopathic urticaria. Psychosom Med 56:36–40, 1994

Gupta MA, Gupta AK, Watteel GN: Stress and alopecia areata: a psychodermatologic study. Acta Derm Venereol 77:296–298, 1997

Hamann K, Avnstorp C: Delusions of infestation treated by pimozide: a double-blind crossover clinical study. Acta Derm Venereol 62:55–58, 1982

Harris BA, Sherertz EF, Flowers FP: Improvement of chronic neurotic excoriations with oral doxepin therapy. Int J Dermatol 26:541–543, 1987

Harvima IT, Viinamäki H, Naukkarinen A, et al: Association of cutaneous mast cells and sensory nerves with psychic stress in psoriasis. Psychother Psychosom 60:168–176, 1993

Hashiro M, Okumura M: Anxiety, depression, psychosomatic symptoms and autonomic nervous function in patients with chronic urticaria. J Dermatol Sci 8:129–135, 1994

Hashiro M, Okumura M: Anxiety, depression and psychosomatic symptoms in patients with atopic dermatitis: comparison with normal controls and among groups of different degrees of severity. J Dermatol Sci 14:63–67, 1997

Hollender MH, Abram HS: Dermatitis factitia. South Med J 66:1279–1285, 1973

Hughes H, Brown BW, Lawlis GF, et al: Treatment of acne vulgaris by biofeedback relaxation and cognitive imagery. J Psychosom Res 27:185–191, 1983

Jick SS, Kremers HM, Vasilakis-Scaramozza C: Isotretinoin use and risk of depression, psychotic symptoms, suicide, and attempted suicide. Arch Dermatol 136:1231–1236, 2000

Johnson GC, Anton RF: Pimozide in delusions of parasitosis (letter). J Clin Psychiatry 44:233, 1983

Johnson GC, Anton RF: Delusions of parasitosis: differential diagnosis and treatment. South Med J 78:914–918, 1985

Johnson ML: Prevalence of dermatologic disease among persons 1–74 years of age: United States, in Advance Data from Vital and Health Statistics of the National Center for Health Statistics, no 4. Washington, DC, U.S. Department of Health, Education, and Welfare, U.S. Government Printing Office, January 26, 1977

Kabat-Zinn J, Wheeler E, Light T, et al: Influence of a mindfulness meditation-based stress reduction intervention on rates of skin clearing in patients with moderate to severe psoriasis undergoing phototherapy (UVB) and photochemotherapy (PUVA). Psychosom Med 60:625–632, 1998

Kalivas J, Kalivas L, Gilman D, et al: Sertraline in the treatment of neurotic excoriations and related disorders. Arch Dermatol 132:589–590, 1996

Katsarou-Katsari A, Singh LK, Theoharides TC: Alopecia areata and affected skin CRH receptor upregulation induced by acute emotional stress. Dermatology 203: 157–161, 2001

Kellett SC, Gawkrodger DJ: The psychological and emotional impact of acne and the effect of treatment with isotretinoin. Br J Dermatol 140:273–282, 1999

Kent A, Drummond LM: Acne excoriée—a case report of treatment using habit reversal. Clin Exp Dermatol 14:163–164, 1988

Keuthen NJ, O'Sullivan RI, Goodchild P, et al: Behavior therapy and pharmacotherapy for trichotillomania: choice of treatment, patient acceptance, and long-term outcome. CNS Spectr 3:72–78, 1998

Kissling S, Wuthrich B: Dermatitis in young adults: personal follow-up 20 years after diagnosis in childhood. Hautarzt 45:368–371, 1994

Kitamura H: A case of somatic delusional disorder that responded to treatment with risperidone (letter). Psychiatry Clin Neurosci 51:337, 1997

Koblenzer CS: Psychocutaneous Disease. Orlando, FL, Grune & Stratton, 1987

Kodama A, Horikawa T, Suzuki T, et al: Effect of stress on atopic dermatitis: investigation in patients after the Great Hanshin Earthquake. J Allergy Clin Immunol 104:173–176, 1999

Koo JYM, Smith LL: Psychologic aspects of acne. Pediatr Dermatol 8:185–188, 1991

Koo JYM, Shellow WVR, Hallman CP, et al: Alopecia areata and increased prevalence of psychiatric disorders. Int J Dermatol 33:849–850, 1994

Koran LM, Ringold A, Hewlett W: Fluoxetine for trichotillomania: an open clinical trial. Psychopharmacol Bull 28: 145–149, 1992

Krahn LE, Goldberg RL: Psychotropic medications and the skin, in Psychotropic Drug Use in the Medically Ill. Edited by Silver PA. Basel, Switzerland, S Karger AG, 1994, pp 90–106

Krishnan A, Koo J: Psyche, opioids, and itch: therapeutic consequences. Dermatol Ther 18;314–322, 2005

Lammintausta K, Kalimo K, Raitala R, et al: Prognosis of atopic dermatitis, a prospective study in early adulthood. Int J Dermatol 30:563–568, 1991

Leonard HL, Lenane MC, Swedo SE, et al: A double-blind comparison of clomipramine and desipramine treatment of severe onychophagia (nail biting). Arch Gen Psychiatry 48: 821–827, 1991

Leung DYM, Tharp M, Boguniewicz M: Atopic dermatitis, in Fitzpatrick's Dermatology in General Medicine, 5th Edition. Edited by Freedberg IM, Eisen AZ, Wolff K, et al. New York, McGraw-Hill, 1999, pp 1464–1480

Liakopoulou M, Alifieraki T, Katideniou A, et al: Children with alopecia areata: psychiatric symptomatology and life events. J Am Acad Child Adolesc Psychiatry 36:678–684, 1997

Lienemann J, Walker FD: Reversal of self-abusive behavior with naltrexone (letter). J Clin Psychopharmacol 9:448–449, 1989

Lindskov R, Baadsgaard O: Delusions of infestation treated with pimozide: a follow-up study. Acta Derm Venereol 65:267–270, 1985

Lyell A: Cutaneous artifactual disease: a review amplified by personal experience. J Am Acad Child Adolesc Psychiatry 1:391–407, 1979

Lyell A: Delusions of parasitosis. Br J Dermatol 108:485–499, 1983

Lyketsos GC, Stratigos J, Tawil G, et al: Hostile personality characteristics, dysthymic states and neurotic symptoms in urticaria, psoriasis and alopecia. Psychother Psychosom 44:122–131, 1985

Maeda K, Yamamoto Y, Yasuda M, et al: Delusions of oral parasitosis. Prog Neuropsychopharmacol Biol Psychiatry 22:243–248, 1998

Manschreck TC: Delusional disorder: the recognition and management of paranoia. J Clin Psychiatry 57:32–38, 1996

McElroy SL, Phillips KA, Keck PE, et al: Body dysmorphic disorder: does it have a psychotic subtype? J Clin Psychiatry 54:389–395, 1993

McElroy SL, Phillips KA, Keck PE: Obsessive compulsive spectrum disorder. J Clin Psychiatry 55:33–51, 1994

McKenna KE, Stern RS: The impact of psoriasis on the quality of life of patients from the 16-center PUVA follow-up cohort. J Am Acad Dermatol 36:388–394, 1997

Morley WN: Nortriptyline in the treatment of chronic urticaria. Br J Clin Pract 23:305–306, 1969

Morren MA, Przybilla B, Bamelis M, et al: Atopic dermatitis: triggering factors. J Am Acad Dermatol 31:467–473, 1994

Morris M: Delusional infestation. Br J Psychiatry 159:83–87, 1991

Moussavian H: Improvement of acne in depressed patients treated with paroxetine. J Am Acad Child Adolesc Psychiatry 40:505–506, 2001

Munro A: Monosymptomatic hypochondriacal psychosis manifesting as delusions of parasitosis: a description of four cases treated with pimozide. Arch Dermatol 114:940–943, 1978

Nel M, Schoeman JP, Lobetti RG: Delusions of parasitosis in clients presenting pets for veterinary care. J S Afr Vet Assoc 72:167–169, 2001

Ninan PT, Knight B, Kirk L, et al: A controlled trial of venlafaxine in trichotillomania: interim phase I results. Psychopharmacol Bull 34:221–224, 1998

Ninan PT, Rothbaum BO, Marsteller FA, et al: A placebo-controlled trial of cognitive-behavioral therapy and clomipramine in trichotillomania. J Clin Psychiatry 61:47–50, 2000

Olsen EA: Disorders of epidermal appendages and related disorders, in Fitzpatrick's Dermatology in General Medicine, 5th Edition. Edited by Freedberg IM, Eisen AZ, Wolff K, et al. New York, McGraw-Hill, 1999, pp 729–751

Perini GI, Fornasa CV, Cipriani R, et al: Life events and alopecia areata. Psychother Psychosom 41:48–52, 1984

Perini G, Zara M, Cipriani R, et al: Imipramine in alopecia areata: a double-blind, placebo-controlled study. Psychother Psychosom 61:195–198, 1994

Peterson AL, Campise RL, Azrin NH: Behavioral and pharmacological treatments for tic and habit disorders: a review. J Dev Behav Pediatr 15:430–441, 1994

Phillips KA: Body dysmorphic disorder: diagnosis and treatment of imagined ugliness. J Clin Psychiatry 57:61–65, 1996

Phillips KA, Taub SL: Skin picking as a symptom of body dysmorphic disorder. Psychopharmacol Bull 31:279–288, 1995

Phillips KA, McElroy SL, Keck PE, et al: Body dysmorphic disorder: 30 cases of imagined ugliness. Am J Psychiatry 150:302–308, 1993

Phillips KA, McElroy SL, Keck PE, et al: A comparison of delusional and nondelusional body dysmorphic disorder in 100 cases. Psychopharmacol Bull 30:179–186, 1994

Phillips KA, McElroy SL, Hudson JI, et al: Body dysmorphic disorder: an obsessive-compulsive spectrum disorder, a form of affective spectrum disorder, or both? J Clin Psychiatry 56:41–51, 1995

Phillips KA, Dufresne RG, Wilkel CS, et al: Rate of body dysmorphic disorder in dermatology patients. J Am Acad Dermatol 42:436–441, 2000

Phillips KA, Albertini RS, Rasmussen SA: A randomized placebo-controlled trial of fluoxetine in body dysmorphic disorder. Arch Gen Psychiatry 59:381–388, 2002

Picardi A, Abeni D: Stressful life events and skin diseases: disentangling evidence from myth. Psychother Psychosom 70: 118–136, 2001

Pigott TA, L'Heueux F, Grady TA, et al: Controlled comparison of clomipramine and fluoxetine in trichotillomania, in Abstracts of Panels and Posters of the 31st Annual Meeting of the American College of Neuropsychopharmacology, San Juan, Puerto Rico, December 1992

Price V: Alopecia areata: clinical aspects. J Invest Dermatol 96: 68, 1991

Pylko T, Sicignan J: Nortriptyline in the treatment of a monosymptomatic delusion (letter). Am J Psychiatry 142:1223, 1985

Rahman MA, Gregory R: Trichotillomania associated with HIV infection and response to sertraline (letter). Psychosomatics 36:417–418, 1995

Rajka G: Essential Aspects of Atopic Dermatitis. Berlin, Germany, Springer, 1989

Rapp SR, Lyn Exum M, Reboussin DM, et al: The physical, psychological and social impact of psoriasis. Br J Health Psychol 2:525–537, 1997

Rapp SR, Feldman SR, Exum ML, et al: Psoriasis causes as much disability as other major medical diseases. Am Acad Dermatol 41:401–407, 1999

Ratnoff OD: Psychogenic purpura (autoerythrocyte sensitization): an unsolved dilemma. Am J Med 87:16–21, 1989

Ravindran AV, Lapierre YD, Anisman H: Obsessive-compulsive spectrum disorders: effective treatment with paroxetine. Can J Psychiatry 44:805–807, 1999

Raychaudhuri SP, Rein G, Farber EM: Neuropathogenesis and neuropharmacology of psoriasis. Int J Dermatol 34:685–693, 1995

Reid TL: Treatment of generalized anxiety disorder and trichotillomania with buspirone (letter). Am J Psychiatry 149:573–574, 1992

Reid TL: Treatment of resistant trichotillomania with paroxetine (letter). Am J Psychiatry 151:290, 1994

Richards HL, Fortune DG, Griffiths CEM, et al: The contribution of perceptions of stigmatization to disability in patients with psoriasis. J Psychsom Res 50:11–15, 2001

Rosenbaum MS, Ayllon T: The behavioral treatment of neurodermatitis through habit-reversal. Behav Res Ther 19:313–318, 1981

Rothe MJ, Grant-Kels JM: Atopic dermatitis: an update. J Am Acad Dermatol 35:1–13, 1996

Rubino IA, Sonnino A, Pezzarossa B, et al: Personality disorders and psychiatric symptoms in psoriasis. Psychol Rep 77:547–553, 1995

Rubinow DR, Peck GL, Squillace KM, et al: Reduced anxiety and depression in cystic acne patients after successful treatment with oral isotretinoin. J Am Acad Dermatol 17:25–32, 1987

Ruiz-Doblado S, Carrizosa A, Garcia-Hernandez MJ, et al: Selective serotonin reuptake inhibitors (SSRIs) and alopecia areata. Int J Dermatol 10:798–799, 1999

Savin JA, Paterson WD, Adam K, et al: Effects of trimeprazine and trimipramine on nocturnal scratching in patients with atopic eczema. Arch Dermatol 115:313–315, 1979

Schlosser S, Black DW, Blum N, et al: The demography, phenomenology, and family history of 22 persons with compulsive hair pulling. Ann Clin Psychiatry 6:147–152, 1994

Schultz Larson F: Atopic dermatitis: a genetic-epidemiologic study in a population-based twin sample. J Am Acad Dermatol 28:719–723, 1993

Sentürk V, Tanrtverdi N: Resistant trichotillomania and risperidone (letter). Psychosomatics 43:429–430, 2002

Sheehan-Dare RA, Henderson MJ, Cotterill JA: Anxiety and depression in patients with chronic urticaria and generalized pruritus. Br J Dermatol 123:769–774, 1990

Sherman MD, Holland GN, Holsclaw DS, et al: Delusions of ocular parasitosis. Am J Ophthalmol 125:852–856, 1998

Shertzer CL, Lookingbill DP: Effects of relaxation therapy and hypnotizability in chronic urticaria. Arch Dermatol 123:913–916, 1987

Simeon D, Stein DJ, Gross S, et al: A double-blind trial of fluoxetine in pathologic skin picking. J Clin Psychiatry 58:341–347, 1997

Slaughter JR, Zanol K, Rezvani H, et al: Psychogenic parasitosis. Psychosomatics 39:491–500, 1998

Sneddon I, Sneddon J: Self-inflicted injury: a follow-up study of 43 patients. BMJ 2:527–530, 1975

Songer DA, Roman B: Treatment of somatic delusional disorder with atypical antipsychotic agents. Am J Psychiatry 153:578–579, 1996

Soter NA: Urticaria and angioedema, in Fitzpatrick's Dermatology in General Medicine, 5th Edition. Edited by Freedberg IM, Eisen AZ, Wolff K, et al. New York, McGraw-Hill, 1999, pp 1409–1418

Sperber J, Shaw J, Bruce S: Psychological components and the role of adjunct interventions in chronic idiopathic urticaria. Psychother Psychosom 51:135–141, 1989

Spraker MK: Cutaneous artifactual disease: an appeal for help. Pediatr Clin North Am 30:659–668, 1983

Stanley MA, Breckenridge JK, Swann AC, et al: Fluvoxamine treatment of trichotillomania. J Clin Psychopharmacol 17: 278–283, 1997

Stein DJ, Hollander E: Dermatology and conditions related to obsessive-compulsive disorder. J Am Acad Dermatol 26:237–242, 1992a

Stein DJ, Hollander E: Low-dose pimozide augmentation of serotonin reuptake blockers in the treatment of trichotillomania. J Clin Psychiatry 53:123–126, 1992b

Stein DJ, Hutt CS, Spitz JL, et al: Compulsive picking and obsessive-compulsive disorder. Psychosomatics 34:177–181, 1993

Stein DJ, Mullen L, Islam MN, et al: Compulsive and impulsive symptomatology in trichotillomania. Psychopathology 28:208–213, 1995a

Stein DJ, Simeon D, Cohen LJ, et al: Trichotillomania and obsessive-compulsive disorder. J Clin Psychiatry 56:28–34, 1995b

Stein DJ, Bouwer C, Maud CM: Use of the selective serotonin reuptake inhibitor citalopram in treatment of trichotillomania. Eur Arch Psychiatry Clin Neurosci 247:234–236, 1997

Stocker WW, McIntyre OR, Clendenning WE: Psychogenic purpura. Arch Dermatol 113:606–609, 1977

Stout RJ: Fluoxetine for the treatment of compulsive facial picking (letter). Am J Psychiatry 147:370, 1990

Strauss JS, Thiboutot DM: Diseases of the sebaceous glands, in Fitzpatrick's Dermatology in General Medicine, 5th Edition. Edited by Freedberg IM, Eisen AZ, Wolff K, et al. New York, McGraw-Hill, 1999, pp 769–784

Streichenwein SM, Thornby JI: A long-term, double-blind, placebo-controlled crossover trial of the efficacy of fluoxetine for trichotillomania. Am J Psychiatry 152:1192–1196, 1995

Swedo SE, Leonard HL: Trichotillomania: an obsessive compulsive spectrum disorder? Psychiatr Clin North Am 15:777–790, 1992

Swedo SE, Leonard HL, Rapoport JL, et al: A double-blind comparison of clomipramine and desipramine in the treatment of trichotillomania (hair pulling). N Engl J Med 321:497–501, 1989

Toyoda M, Makino T, Kagoura M, et al: Expression of neuropeptide-degrading enzymes in alopecia areata: an immunohistochemical study. Br J Dermatol 144:46–54, 2001

Trabert W: 100 years of delusional parasitosis: meta-analysis of 1,223 case reports. Psychopathology 28:238–246, 1995

Twohig MP, Woods DW, Marcks BA, et al: Evaluating the efficacy of habit reversal: comparison with a placebo control. J Clin Psychiatry 64:40–48, 2003

Uehara M, Kimura C: Descendant family history of atopic dermatitis. Acta Derm Venereol 73:62–63, 1993

van Minnen A, Hoogduin KAL, Keijsers GPJ, et al: Treatment of trichotillomania with behavioral therapy or fluoxetine. Arch Gen Psychiatry 60:517–522, 2003

Vittorio CC, Phillips KA: Treatment of habit-tic deformity with fluoxetine. Arch Dermatol 133:1203–1204, 1997

Walsh KH, McDougle CJ: Pharmacological strategies for trichotillomania. Expert Opin Pharmacother 6:975–984, 2005

Welkowitz LA, Held JL, Held AL: Management of neurotic scratching with behavioral therapy. J Am Acad Dermatol 21: 802–804, 1989

Westling L: Fingernail biting. Cranio 6:182–187, 1988

Williams HC: Is the prevalence of atopic dermatitis increasing? Clin Exp Dermatol 17:385–391, 1992

Williams HC: On the definition and epidemiology of atopic dermatitis. Dermatol Clin 13:649–657, 1995

Winchel RM, Jones JS, Stanley B, et al: Clinical characteristics of trichotillomania and its response to fluoxetine. J Clin Psychiatry 53:304–308, 1992

Woodruff PWR, Higgins EM, du Vivier AWP, et al: Psychiatric illness in patients referred to a dermatology-psychiatry clinic. Gen Hosp Psychiatry 19:29–35, 1997

Wykoff RF: Delusions of parasitosis: a review. Rev Infect Dis 9:433–437, 1987

Zachariae R, Øster H, Bjerring P, et al: Effects of psychologic intervention on psoriasis: a preliminary report. J Am Acad Dermatol 34:1008–1015, 1996

Zook F: Complications of the perionychium. Hand Clin 2:407–442, 1986

Self-Assessment Questions

Select the single best response for each question.

1. Atopic dermatitis is an often-chronic clinical problem with meaningful psychiatric co-morbidity. Which of the following statements is *not* true?
   A. Stressful life events often precede the onset or exacerbation of atopic dermatitis.
   B. Stress may have an effect on atopic dermatitis through an interaction between the central nervous system (CNS) and the immune system.
   C. Various behavioral therapy models have been shown to reduce anxiety and depression in patients with atopic dermatitis.
   D. Topical doxepin cream has been shown to decrease itching in atopic dermatitis.
   E. Trimipramine has been shown to reduce nighttime scratching by increasing the time spent in Stage I sleep.

2. Psoriasis is a chronic and relapsing dermatological disease of major importance to the psychiatrist, both because the disease is associated with significant psychiatric comor-bidity and because it can occur as a side effect of psychiatric treatment. Which of the following statements is *true?*
   A. Lithium-induced psoriasis typically persists after lithium is discontinued.
   B. Lithium-induced psoriasis typically occurs after several years of lithium treat-ment and rarely during the first few years of treatment.
   C. Psoriasis patients have been shown to be at high risk for comorbid personality dis-orders, including schizoid and avoidant personality disorders.
   D. Disability from psoriasis is more strongly correlated with disease severity and location than with psychosocial variables.
   E. Psoriasis is much more common in men (2:1) than in women.

3. Delusional parasitosis is an unusual syndrome in which the patient believes that he or she is infested with living organisms. Which of the following is *not* true?
   A. Patients typically have experienced a specific precipitating event.
   B. Patients typically have had actual exposure to parasites.
   C. Delusional parasitosis typically occurs with other delusions and with other im-pairment of thought or thought processes.
   D. Affected patients often respond to treatment with pimozide.
   E. Delusional parasitosis has a female-to-male ratio of 3:1 in patients age 50 years and older.

4. Psychogenic excoriation may lead to substantial dermatological problems. Depressive and anxiety disorders are common in patients with this condition. Case reports and small open trials have shown some efficacy for psychotropic medications in psy-chogenic excoriation. Which two tricyclic antidepressants (TCAs) have been shown to be effective?
   A. Nortriptyline and doxepin.
   B. Doxepin and clomipramine.
   C. Nortriptyline and desipramine.

    D. Imipramine and doxepin.

    E. Imipramine and desipramine.

5. Which of the following is *not* true of trichotillomania or its psychiatric comorbidity?

    A. The mean age at onset of trichotillomania is after age 15 years.

    B. Anxiety, mood, and substance use disorders are commonly comorbid with trichotillomania.

    C. The lifetime prevalence of trichotillomania is 0.6% for both men and women.

    D. The behavioral treatment of habit reversal has been reported to be effective in trichotillomania.

    E. Clomipramine has been shown to be superior to desipramine for treatment, supporting an "obsessive-compulsive spectrum" construct for trichotillomania.

13 Surgery

Pauline S. Powers, M.D.
Carlos A. Santana, M.D.

SURGICAL PATIENTS OFTEN have preexisting psychiatric disorders, and a range of psychosocial problems may become evident after surgery. Estimates of the prevalence of psychiatric problems in surgical patients range from 15% to 50% (Kain et al. 2002; Strain 1982). Surgeons are less likely to refer patients to psychiatrists than are other physicians, who themselves generally underestimate the prevalence of psychiatric disorders among their patients. Thus, a large proportion of psychopathology in surgical patients is either undiagnosed or misdiagnosed.

In the hospital, psychiatrists provide consultations for patients on general surgical floors, but they are more likely to provide liaison services to specialized surgical units such as burn units or organ transplant units. Consultations for general surgical patients often involve preoperative issues such as consent for surgery, fear of anesthesia or surgery, or management of preexisting psychiatric disorders during hospitalization. Postoperative hospital consultations are often initiated for assessment and treatment of delirium or behavioral problems.

General Conceptual Model

To conceptualize the problems requiring psychiatric intervention, the perioperative period can be divided into preoperative and postoperative periods. Although these periods are considered separately because special strategies and different personnel may be required in each, the connection between preoperatively identified psychiatric problems and outcome of surgery has been a topic widely studied. For example, in a study of patients with severe low back pain who underwent surgery, low presurgical neuroticism scores were associated with better postoperative functional improvement (Hagg et al. 2003). In another study of patients with gastroesophageal reflux disorder undergoing laparoscopic antireflux surgery (Kamolz et al. 2003), all the patients had normalized physiological findings after surgery, but patients with comorbid major depression had significantly more symptoms of postoperative dysphagia and had less improvement in quality of life than did the patients without depression.

Psychiatry is often consulted in the preoperative period around the issues of consent for treatment or refusal of surgery and may be consulted at any time when the patient threatens to sign out against medical advice. Preexisting psychiatric disorders and their management often are also the reason for a psychiatric consultation. Fear of surgery, anesthesia, needles, or machines may result in preoperative panic and necessitate psychiatric intervention.

With the emergence of outpatient surgery and use of drugs that induce a lighter stage of anesthesia, some patients may recall events from the intraoperative period. Psychiatric consultation may be needed to assist the patient in coping with these memories.

In the postoperative period, delirium (including withdrawal from various substances) is a very common cause for consultation. Agitation and management problems are also common. Patients who were admitted because of trauma (including burns) may begin to develop symptoms of posttraumatic stress disorder (PTSD). Other issues in this time period include ventilator weaning and the "intensive care unit (ICU) syndrome."

General Preoperative Issues

Capacity and Consent

The ethical practice of surgery requires a patient's voluntary informed consent. In some instances, however, direct consent is impossible, and surgeons seek permission from surrogates or guidance from written advance directives. Informed consent and decision making are at the core of the preoperative period. The communication of factual information understandable to the patient is the responsibility of the surgeon. It should include diagnosis, reasons that the operation is thought to be the treat-

ment of choice, and expected risks and benefits and their probabilities. Alternatives and their consequences, as well as financial costs, also should be discussed. Competent patients have a right to decide whether to accept or reject proposed surgery. A psychiatric consultant cannot legally declare a patient incompetent, but the consultant can evaluate the decision-making capacity of the patient. Examiners must be aware of the legal standards governing determination of competence in their jurisdiction. The assessment also includes a determinations of the cause of the patient's limitations (i.e., the nature of the mental disorder) and recommendations for treatment, if treatment is possible.

Preoperative Psychiatric Evaluation

The preoperative period is the time to obtain a psychiatric history. Patients with a history of anxiety disorder, depression, bipolar disorder, or psychosis are at risk for experiencing symptoms of these disorders during the postoperative period. Knowing what medications have been effective or not tolerated in the past is obviously valuable. Certain personality disorders and traits are known to predispose to behavioral problems during the postoperative period.

When a surgeon requests a psychiatric consultation, the consultant should establish the urgency. Surgical patients seldom initiate or request a psychiatric consultation and may even assume an adversarial attitude toward the consultant. However, one reason for the under-referral of surgical inpatients is under-recognition (or dismissal) of psychological distress by the surgical team. In some cases, surgical inpatients have felt the need to refer themselves for psychiatric evaluation of anxiety, although the surgical staff did not consider their anxiety sufficient to warrant a consultation (Fulop and Strain 1985). On the other hand, inappropriate or premature psychiatric consultation sometimes occurs when a patient expresses normal feelings (e.g., starts to cry) that the surgeon finds uncomfortable. One of the psychiatrist's major tasks is establishing a relationship with the referring surgeon, who may or may not be knowledgeable about psychiatric issues.

Psychiatric Disorders in the Perioperative Period

Depression
The proportion of patients taking antidepressants who undergo surgery is reported to be 35% (Scher and Anwar 1999). In the past, when monoamine oxidase inhibitors were more frequently prescribed, it was common to discontinue antidepressants prior to general anesthesia. This is no longer the case. In their study of 80 depressed patients who were scheduled to undergo orthopedic surgery under general anesthesia, Kudoh and colleagues (2002) determined that antidepressants administered to depressed patients should be continued. They concluded that discontinuation of antidepressants did not increase the incidence of hypotension or arrhythmias during anesthesia, but discontinuation increased the symptoms of depression and delirium.

Schizophrenia
The management of the schizophrenic patient requiring surgery can be difficult. Bizarre behavior and expression by schizophrenic patients can confuse and upset surgeons, nurses, and other patients, eliciting fear, anger, and nontherapeutic responses. Patients with paranoid delusions may refuse surgery because of psychotic misperception of the surgeon's intentions. Schizophrenic patients may also have deficits in the processing of cognitive or sensory information and concrete reasoning. These deficits may complicate the consent

process and the patient's ability to cooperate with treatment, and the staff may need to make changes in management (Adler and Griffith 1991).

Bipolar Disorder
The stress of surgery may psychologically and physiologically destabilize bipolar disorder, and acute relapse into mania in the postoperative period can be extremely disruptive to care, even life-threatening. Periods without oral intake in the perioperative period preclude the use of lithium, antidepressants, most antipsychotics, and anticonvulsants. During this time parenteral antipsychotics serve as the primary substitute for mood stabilization. Lithium is difficult to use safely during periods of rapid fluid shifts (e.g., after cardiac surgery and acute burns).

Preoperative Anxiety

Fear of Surgery and Anesthesia
Nearly 20 years ago, Regal and colleagues (1985) systematically assessed 150 patients before surgery and found that 54% were anxious. Many were anxious about the anesthesia: patients often feared that the anesthetic would prematurely wear off or that they would not wake up from the anesthesia. Nearly one-third of patients are afraid of anesthesia, as distinct from the operation itself (van Wijk and Smalhout 1990).

It has been consistently shown that appropriate provision of information in an empathic relationship can reduce preoperative anxiety, postoperative pain, and length of hospital stay (Klafta and Roizen 1996; Koivula et al. 2002; Nelson 1996). Timing the delivery of information is important and may vary depending on the surgery. For example, among patients undergoing elective coronary artery bypass grafting, fear is highest during the waiting period prior to hospital admission. Providing support and information during this period produces the greatest benefit. Nurses have been in the forefront of devising methods for delivering these services, and the results of their investigations can also inform psychiatric practice.

Treatment of Preoperative Anxiety

Preoperative anxiety has been treated with antianxiety medications, particularly benzodiazepines. Although the Cochrane Database reviewers concluded that the use of benzodiazepines does not delay discharge from adult outpatient surgery, less is known about the actual clinical benefit of these medications for preoperative anxiety (Smith and Pittaway 2003). For example, in an outpatient surgery program, preoperative benzodiazepines were shown to decrease levels of stress hormones, but the actual effect on clinical anxiety was equivocal (Duggan et al. 2002). However, pediatric dental and oral surgery patients have been the most thoroughly studied, and most of these patients seem to benefit from use of benzodiazepines (see Erlandsson et al. 2001; Marshall et al. 1999).

Although providing information and social support is more time-consuming than prescribing an antianxiety agent, it may be more effective than medication in reducing preoperative anxiety and is likely to have postoperative benefits as well.

Fear of Needles, Blood, and Medical Equipment

Fear of needles is common and may first become evident in the preoperative period. Estimates of the prevalence of needle phobia have ranged from 10% to 21% (Hamilton 1995; Nir et al. 2003), but probably about 8%–10% of adults have unreasonable fears of needles that interfere with treatment. Needle phobia appears to be partly inherited (especially the vasovagal response that may result in fainting) and partly learned from conditioned responses, including past fainting

spells when injected or after watching others be vaccinated (Hamilton 1995; Neale et al. 1994; Nir et al. 2003). Individuals who experience disgust in response to needles may be more likely to faint (Page 2003). Treatments for needle phobia have been primarily described in case reports and include behavioral strategies (exposure techniques and participant modeling) and empathy from treating professionals.

Fear of blood is closely related to fear of needles. Some patients are fearful of contracting HIV or hepatitis virus from blood transfusions (now a very rare occurrence) or from needles contaminated with blood (although this should never occur, except in very poor countries). Correcting misconceptions and providing accurate information can be reassuring.

Blood transfusion refusal is common and is usually related to religious beliefs or fear of bloodborne infections. Because Jehovah's Witnesses and others have refused blood transfusions, there has been a rigorous pursuit of alternatives. Many surgeries previously thought to require transfusions are now routinely done without them. If the patient refuses blood, a careful psychiatric assessment may be needed to determine why the patient is refusing and whether the patient is competent to refuse treatment. For anxious patients, cognitive-behavioral interventions and benzodiazepines are helpful. If the patient is a child and the parents refuse transfusion on the basis of the parents' beliefs, legal and ethical consultation should be obtained, but the decision is usually to transfuse the child.

General Postoperative Issues

Alcohol Dependence

Chronic alcohol misuse is more common in surgical patients than in psychiatric or neurological patients. More than 50% of patients with carcinoma of the gastrointestinal tract have alcohol dependence (Seitz and Simanowski 1986). Almost half of all trauma beds are occupied by patients who were injured while under the influence of alcohol (Gentilello et al. 1995; Spies et al. 1996). In addition to the life-threatening complications of the alcohol withdrawal syndrome, the rates of morbidity and mortality resulting from infections, cardiopulmonary insufficiency, and bleeding disorders are two to four times greater in patients with chronic alcoholism (Spies et al. 1997). The development of an alcohol withdrawal syndrome can change a routine postoperative course into a life-threatening situation in which the patient requires ICU treatment.

An alcohol-related history is frequently unobtainable in trauma patients because of their injuries (which may include closed head injury) and subsequent endotracheal intubation. Laboratory tests with sufficient sensitivity and specificity may assist in the diagnosis and possible prevention of complications (Sillanaukee 1996). If an ordinary alcohol history is not obtainable, the biological marker known as carbohydrate-deficient transferrin is a useful alternative and correlates with alcohol consumption in surgical patients (Tønnesen et al. 1999).

Chronic alcohol intake may produce either enhanced or reduced sensitivity to anesthetics. The net effect varies with the amount of alcohol used, the relative affinity of alcohol and the other drugs for microsomal enzymes, and the severity of any underlying liver disease (Lieber 1995).

Alcohol dependence is often complicated by disorders such as cirrhosis, seizures, pancreatitis, polyneuropathy, or cardiomyopathy. It seems obvious that surgical interventions in an alcoholic patient with one or more of these disorders may be associated with increased morbidity and mortality. Increased risk of complications is seen after both minor and major surgery,

as well as after elective and emergency procedures. In general, the risk of postoperative infections is related to decreased immune function and enhanced stress response to surgical trauma. This enhanced stress response is characterized by a greater release of stress hormones and catecholamines in patients with alcoholism compared with control subjects (Moesgaard and Lykkegaard-Nielsen 1989; Tønnesen et al. 1992). Alcoholic patients are at risk for excessive surgical blood loss secondary to coagulopathy from liver disease and platelet dysfunction. Many alcoholic patients are chronically malnourished, which retards wound healing.

Opioid Dependence

No evidence indicates that provision of appropriate doses of opioids for postoperative pain in the hospital creates addiction, yet some patients who fear becoming dependent decline or underuse postoperative opioids. If a surgical patient is receiving methadone maintenance, the dose used for maintenance should be continued throughout the surgical hospitalization. If the opioid-dependent patient does not have an established maintenance regimen, control of opioid withdrawal can, in most cases, be achieved with methadone dosages of 10–30 mg/day. Once-daily dosing is usually sufficient to prevent withdrawal, but the total daily dose can be split into two or three doses to prevent breakthrough symptoms. If anesthesia is necessary, the anesthesiologist obviously should be provided with the history of the patient's opioid dependence.

Postoperative opioid-dependent patients require higher doses of opioids to control surgical pain because of tolerance. When such patients are given only "normal" doses, they complain of not receiving enough and often are considered to be inappropriately "drug-seeking" when in fact they are being undermedicated.

Postoperative Delirium

Postoperative delirium is very common, particularly in elderly patients undergoing certain operations such as emergency repair of hip fractures, major gastrointestinal surgery, or cardiac surgery. Elderly orthopedic surgery patients have been the best studied, with rates of delirium higher than 40% documented (Galanakis et al. 2001). Estimates of prevalence among post–cardiac surgery patients range from 2% to more than 30%, depending on several factors, including age, the type of surgery, and whether the patient was on heart-lung bypass (Bayindir et al. 2000; Segatore et al. 1998). Delirium may be even more common and severe after certain procedures such as lung transplant (Craven 1990).

Risk Factors and Diagnosis

Multiple preoperative risk factors for postoperative delirium have been identified and include older age, alcohol use, cognitive impairment (especially dementia), chronic comorbid illnesses and medications used to treat these illnesses, and the severity of the acute illness, in addition to anesthesia and the type of surgery (Flacker and Marcantonio 1998; Williams-Russo et al. 1992). Postoperative changes in the sleep–wake cycle (Kaneko et al. 1997), inadequately treated pain, and use of medications such as benzodiazepines increase the likelihood of delirium.

Postoperative delirium usually is identified 2–5 days after surgery and typically, although certainly not always, resolves in about a week. Despite reliable methods for detecting delirium, it is often not diagnosed, or is misdiagnosed as another psychiatric disorder, particularly in the postoperative period.

Treatment

Psychiatrists are often consulted on an emergency basis for patients with postoperative delirium. Management is the same as that for other deliria, starting with an attempt to identify a remediable cause.

Several controlled trials have examined interventions that might prevent postoperative delirium. In one study (Aizawa et al. 2002), half the patients were given diazepam for 3 days immediately following surgery to try to prevent disruption of their sleep–wake cycle; only 5% of the treated patients developed delirium compared with 35% of the nontreated group. This study contradicts the usual wisdom that benzodiazepines are contraindicated in delirium, but the diazepam was given at a particular time with the specific goal of maintaining a normal sleep–wake pattern after surgery. Tokita et al. (2001) found that better pain control through patient-controlled analgesia (compared with a fixed continuous regimen) reduced the incidence of delirium following hepatectomy. Procholinergic drugs for prevention of delirium have not been found beneficial (Diaz et al. 2001).

Controlled trials of nonpharmacological interventions also have been conducted. Geriatric consults for elderly patients admitted for hip fracture surgery were associated with less postoperative delirium (32% vs. 50%) and even greater improvement in cases of severe delirium (12% vs. 29%) (Marcantonio et al. 2001). Compared with usual care, a nurse-led interdisciplinary psychosocial intervention program for delirium in elderly patients with hip fractures reduced the length and severity, but not the incidence, of postoperative delirium (Milisen et al. 2001).

Intensive Care Unit Psychosis

The concept of ICU psychosis emerged after Kornfeld and colleagues (1965) described a delirium that occurred in 38% of the patients in the recovery room after open-heart surgery. Their report noted several organic factors that they thought contributed to the delirium. Patients also were interviewed soon after they left the recovery room. They complained of lack of sleep and "the frightening environment, unusual sounds and sense of being chained" (p. 287). This article was very influential and resulted in many positive changes in the ICU environment, including adding windows (so that patients could determine whether it was day or night) and clocks within sight of the patients. It also became standard practice for the ICU staff to reorient patients and help them to understand ongoing procedures.

Despite the fact that the original authors emphasized that this was an acute organic psychosis influenced by environmental factors, the term *ICU psychosis* has come to imply that environmental factors are capable of inducing psychosis. It seems likely that environmental factors can worsen delirium caused by any of a variety of physiological factors, but psychosis resulting from solely a frightening environment occurs rarely, if ever. The danger of invoking the term *ICU psychosis* is that the underlying physiological cause of postoperative delirium will be unrecognized and untreated. Clarifying the diagnosis and treatment of postoperative delirium is an important role for the psychiatric consultant.

Posttraumatic Stress Disorder in the Postoperative Period

In the surgical arena, PTSD has been best studied in trauma patients (especially burn patients and motor vehicle accident victims) (Klein et al. 2003), but a significant percentage of patients also develop PTSD following cardiac surgery or neurosurgery (Powell et al. 2002; Stoll et al. 2000). Full syndromal PTSD may develop in 18%–40% of adult patients after trauma, but many more develop some of the symptoms of PTSD. Children who experience traumatic disfiguring injuries seem to be at

particular risk, with up to 82% having some symptoms of PTSD 1 month after the trauma (Rusch et al. 2002). Quality of life is significantly impaired in patients who develop PTSD posttrauma or postsurgery, compared with patients who do not develop PTSD (Zatzick et al. 2002).

Several studies have tried to identify factors that predict the emergence of PTSD (for review, see Tedstone and Tarrier 2003). As expected, better prior emotional adjustment and social support are relatively protective. However, contrary to expectation, the severity of the injury, or the severity of the illness requiring surgery, is not clearly correlated with the emergence of PTSD. Some patients with no apparent predisposing factors develop PTSD. Alcohol intoxication or concussion at the time of the trauma seems to decrease the likelihood of PTSD (perhaps because memory for the event is impaired). Symptoms usually appear within the first week after a trauma and increase in intensity over the next 3 months. Perhaps the best predictor of PTSD at 1 year is the presence of acute stress symptoms during the acute hospitalization after a trauma (Zatzick et al. 2002). Although most studies show that symptoms decrease by 1 year, some patients continue to meet full criteria, and many more still have symptoms.

Diagnosis of acute stress disorder, PTSD's predecessor, can be difficult in surgical trauma or postoperative patients who manifest symptoms of delirium. For the diagnosis of PTSD, the duration criterion is often not met in hospitalized patients because of relatively brief hospital stays. Almost all patients who meet full criteria will have nightmares, but among patients with only some symptoms, the cluster of symptoms varies. For example, female burn victims with facial burns have been reported to have predominantly avoidance and emotional numbness symptoms (Fukunishi 1999), whereas reexperiencing and startle symptoms are more likely in other burn patients (Ehde et al. 1999).

Few studies of treatment of PTSD have been done specifically in surgical patients, but general principles appear applicable. Cognitive-behavioral therapy has been shown to be more effective than a waiting-list control condition or supportive psychotherapy for PTSD among motor vehicle accident survivors (Blanchard et al. 2003). There is general agreement (although not much evidence) that psychotherapy should be the primary treatment of trauma-related PTSD in children and that the selective serotonin reuptake inhibitors should be adjunctive (Putnam and Hulsmann 2002).

Postoperative Pain

Unrelieved postoperative pain is still reported to be common, partly related to inadequate pain assessment (Sjostrom et al. 1997). Postoperative pain management remains suboptimal on many surgical wards despite the availability of effective analgesics. New technologies for drug administration and clinical practice guidelines for pain management are now available (Stomberg et al. 2003). The appropriate and optimal use of analgesics is essential for the adequate management of postoperative pain. Greer and colleagues (2001) concluded that fear of addiction is not prevalent among postoperative patients, but better communication by clinicians can further decrease the proportion of surgical patients who fear addiction to pain medication.

During the 1990s, the Joint Commission on Accreditation of Health Care Organizations (JCAHO) studied patterns of pain assessment and management and found that pain was underrecognized and inadequately treated when diagnosed. Multiple reasons were identified, including an inappropriate fear of addiction. It was repeatedly documented that many doctors and nurses based clinical practice on myths and misconceptions about pain medications rather than on evidence-based research (Curtiss 2001; Summers 2001).

Body Image and Surgery

In three important surgical areas, body image is key to patient outcome: 1) amputation and the phenomenon of phantom limb pain; 2) change in body image that may occur after trauma or surgery, including cosmetic surgery; and 3) body image concerns in bariatric surgery patients.

Phantom limb is the experience of feeling as if an amputated part is still present, first described by surgeon Ambrose Paré in 1649. In the United States, more than 200,000 surgical amputations occur each year. Up to 70% of these patients experience phantom limb pain immediately after the amputation, and 50% still experience it 5 years later (Bloomquist 2001). The occurrence of phantom limb pain has been shown to be associated with poorer health-related quality of life (van der Schans et al. 2002). There is general agreement that avoiding as much pain as possible prior to amputation decreases the likelihood of phantom limb pain, but other factors contribute as well. For example, phantom limb pain in burned children is more common after electrical injuries than after thermal injuries (Thomas et al. 2003). The exact etiology of both phantom limb and the paresthesias that often accompany it is complex and poorly understood.

Body image can change after trauma or surgery. Trauma, as in the case of burn injures, may cause dramatic changes in the body that require significant adaptation and integration of the changes into a new body image. However, the ease with which this integration occurs is influenced more by premorbid adjustment and stage of development than by the actual total body surface area burned. The type of surgery may influence body image outcome; for example, total abdominal hysterectomy is associated with greater body image dissatisfaction than is vaginal hysterectomy because of the abdominal scar (Gutl et al. 2002).

General Determinants of Functional Outcome

Notably, the actual severity of the underlying trauma or surgery does not necessarily determine quality of life. For example, the total body surface area burned does not directly correlate with the likelihood of PTSD, nor does the size of a scar necessarily correlate with posttrauma adjustment.

A confluence of factors determines functional outcome. These factors include the condition requiring surgical intervention, presurgical psychiatric status, and surgical strategy. It has been repeatedly demonstrated that an adequate social support system is positively correlated with postsurgical and posttrauma adaptation. Other factors that may improve outcome include preparation of the patient and family for surgery, detection and management of preoperative fears, respectful attitude of the surgeon and operating room personnel during surgery, detection and appropriate treatment of pain, and detection and management of various psychiatric problems following surgery, including delirium and PTSD.

Specific Topics in Surgery

Burn Trauma

The experience of being seriously burned and the treatment that follows for the survivors is one of the most frightening and painful known to humanity. Perhaps because of this, several important concepts

in psychiatry and medicine have been learned from the study of burn victims. For example, Erich Lindemann (1944/1994) described the evaluation and treatment of survivors, friends, and relatives of people who died in the Coconut Grove fire. He identified five major symptoms of normal grief: somatic distress, preoccupation with the image of the deceased, guilt, hostile reactions, and loss of patterns of conduct. These concepts continue to guide the detection and management of normal and pathological acute grief in burn units and elsewhere.

Imbus and Zawacki (1977) opened an ethical debate over prolongation of life that continues today. An unusual aspect of burns is that even mortally burned patients often have a lucid period that lasts for a few hours during which patients can participate in making decisions about their own care. For every severely burned patient, these investigators searched the literature to determine whether cases of survival had been reported, and, if not, they offered the patients a choice between a full therapeutic regimen and palliative care. They concluded that the mortality rate did not change but that this strategy increased the autonomy of patients and increased the empathy that they received. This report ignited a controversy that has grown to encompass all critical care: when is treatment futile, and who should decide?

In the United States, annually, thermal burns result in 1 million injuries, 4,500 deaths, 700,000 emergency department visits, and 45,000 general hospital admissions, half of which are to specialized burn centers. During the past 40 years, interdisciplinary burn centers have emerged, staffed by physicians, nurses, physical and occupational therapists, pain specialists, mental health professionals, social workers, and chaplains (American Burn Association 2004).

Psychiatric Disorders Among Burn Patients

Many burn patients have preexisting psychiatric disorders, the most common of which are substance use and mood disorders. The classic studies of adults by Andreasen and colleagues (1972) and of children by N.R. Bernstein (1976) led to the recognition that psychiatric problems are very common among burn patients. It is now known that about 35% of patients have an Axis I psychiatric disorder prior to the burn injury (Powers et al. 2000) and that 20%–30% of patients (many of whom do not have preexisting psychiatric disorders) develop full syndromal PTSD while in the hospital or after discharge (Powers et al. 1994a; Yu et al. 1999). In addition, many patients have preexisting maladaptive coping mechanisms or dysfunctional families, and these factors are known to contribute to poor functional outcomes.

The best-studied psychiatric topics in burn care include substance use disorders (particularly alcohol use), self-immolation, and PTSD. The neuropsychiatric consequences of electrical burn injuries also have been studied (Kelley et al. 1999). There are a few reports on the long-term psychiatric and functional consequences of burns in both children and adults. Several studies have tried to compare preburn adjustment and/or immediate postburn psychiatric status with outcome. The meaning and psychological importance of burn scars (particularly of the face, hands, and genital area) have been studied as well. Equally important in burn care is the delirium that frequently occurs during the acute-care phase. Psychiatric consultants also have described effective methods for the management of pain in burn patients (N.R. Bernstein 1976; Watkins et al. 1992).

Burns and substance use disorders. Preinjury substance use disorders are common among burn victims. Reports of alcohol abuse or dependence in burn patients have ranged from 6% to 29% (Barillo and Goode 1996; Jones et al. 1991; Powers et al. 1994b; Tabares and Peck 1997), based on blood alcohol assay or physician report. However, much higher rates (over 50%) have been identified with screening instruments like the CAGE (L. Bernstein et al. 1992) or Michigan Alcoholism Screening Test (Steenkamp et al. 1994). Concomitant abuse of other drugs is also very common (Barillo and Goode 1996). Alcohol use has been found to be associated with increased total body surface area burned, an increased likelihood of death, longer length of hospital stay, and, consequently, increased medical costs (Jones et al. 1991; Powers et al. 1994a).

Withdrawal symptoms from alcohol dependence are common during the acute-care phase but may be difficult to distinguish from other causes of delirium. The best approach in a burn unit may be a standard withdrawal protocol with a relatively long-acting benzodiazepine (e.g., chlordiazepoxide). Because the development of alcohol withdrawal can be particularly dangerous in a burn patient, a liberal approach to prescribing the withdrawal regimen among patients suspected of alcohol dependence is probably the safest course of treatment. Haloperidol is frequently added to the regimen for psychotic symptoms during withdrawal but should not be used alone.

Even though burn patients have a high rate of preexisting drug abuse, withdrawal from narcotics is less likely because most patients require narcotic treatment for pain. However, it is important to remember that opioid-dependent patients may require a larger dose of narcotics for pain, and this larger dose should be provided.

Self-inflicted burn injuries. The frequency of self-immolation varies widely from nation to nation. In India, ritual self-immolation is common; 32% of married women with lethal burn injuries have self-inflicted the burn (Kumar 2003). In Zimbabwe, 22% of the adult burn patients have been reported to have self-immolated; most are married women, and the most common reason for self-immolation is conflict in a love relationship (Mzezewa et al. 2000).

In the United States, the frequency of self-inflicted injuries among patients who are admitted to a burn center ranges from 0.067% to 9% (Daniels et al. 1991; Scully and Hutcherson 1983). Although political and cultural motivations for self-immolation may predominate in some cultures, in the United States, most patients have a preexisting Axis I psychiatric disorder, including major depression, schizophrenia, and substance abuse. Not all of these patients are actually suicidal: psychotic patients may be responding to command hallucinations.

Patients who have self-inflicted their burn injuries often elicit intense countertransference reactions from the entire staff, including the psychiatric team. Burn center teams understand chronic medical illness and the need for expert treatment, and this "medical model" analogy may help them better understand and empathize with a patient who has chronic mental illness and who has self-inflicted a burn injury.

PTSD in burn patients. PTSD occurs in a significant minority of patients who have been burned. Estimates range from 21% to 43% (Ehde et al. 2000; Powers et al. 1994a). The difficulties in estimating frequency include the confounding effects of delirium and the duration criterion requirement of 1 month. Many patients have been discharged from the hospital before a month elapses, and less severely injured patients may not be seen again; thus, a diagnosis is not made. Nonetheless, many patients do develop the full syndrome of PTSD, and many more have symptoms in the reexperiencing cluster even though they do not meet the other criteria. Some

patients also have PTSD symptoms related to their treatment, especially the extreme pain inflicted during debridement and dressing changes. Some patients also have traumatic memories of psychotic experiences they suffered during the delirium that often occurs during the acute phase of treatment.

Treatment of PTSD in burn patients is similar to treatment of PTSD in others and includes psychotherapeutic techniques and medication. Increasing a sense of control and alleviating pain in patients when they are being treated at the burn center also may prevent some PTSD symptoms.

Delirium and psychosis in burn patients. Delirium during the acute care of severely burned patients is very common, related to sepsis, pain medication, or other organic factors. Other causes of delirium in burn patients include hypoxia from smoke inhalation and massive fluid shifts and electrolyte imbalance, especially hyponatremia and hypophosphatemia. The psychotic symptoms that occur most often include hallucinations (often visual and not always distressing) and delusions. The delusions are often paranoid, as the delirious patient may misinterpret care interventions and then suspect nurses and other providers of malevolent intent. It is often difficult to distinguish between pain, agitation, anxiety, and confusion in the ICU, and the psychiatric consultant is invaluable in this differentiation. The principles of treatment of delirium in the burn unit are the same as described earlier for postoperative delirium.

Burn Pain Management

Pain in burn care arises from both the pain from various procedures, including dressing changes and burn wound debridement, and the background pain of the injury itself. The key concept in managing pain on the burn unit is to recognize that it is often undertreated, and this can result in worsening delirium, anxiety, and other management problems. Pain is undertreated for many reasons, but the most important reasons are an unrealistic fear of addiction (both by the patient and by the physician) and fear of respiratory compromise. Burn wound debridement (in which the eschar is removed) is an excruciatingly painful procedure, but various techniques are now available to alleviate much of the pain. When sharp debridement (involving use of a scalpel) is needed, general anesthesia offers the greatest relief of pain and also may facilitate a more thorough debridement (Powers et al. 1993). Parenteral use of narcotics, especially intravenous morphine, is often preferable for blunt debridement (in which scalpels are not used) and dressing changes. A common error is not waiting the 10–15 minutes required for adequate distribution after intravenous injection before beginning blunt debridement. Intramuscular injections are often contraindicated because they may add to the pain, and sufficient injection sites may not be available.

The background pain of burn injuries is best managed with oral narcotics whenever possible. Fentanyl is often helpful for intermittent pain because it is short acting and will allow the patient to be awake to participate in various rehabilitation activities. Meperidine is usually contraindicated because it is relatively ineffective orally and may aggravate delirium. Benzodiazepines are often used to promote sedation and reduce anxiety but are often inappropriate to treat pain. If pain is adequately managed and the patient has anxiety in anticipation of debridement, use of benzodiazepines is then very helpful.

Treatment of Burns in Children

Consideration of the developmental stage of the burned child and careful, age-appropriate assessment and treatment of pain and anxiety are important in the treatment of burned children (Martin-Herz et al. 2003; Stoddard et al. 2002). Appropriate management of pain partially predicts the long-term outcome for the child. For example, higher level of morphine in the hospital was associated with fewer PTSD symptoms in children at follow-up 6 months later (Saxe et al. 2001). Guidelines are available for the management of pain and anxiety in burned children (Stoddard et al. 2002). Although many psychological treatments may ultimately prove to be effective for children with burns, several are not. For example, imagery-based interventions do not seem to help, and having a parent in the room during procedures seems to make the experience worse for the child (and probably for the parent) (Foertsch et al. 1998).

Brief small follow-up studies of burned children have sometimes seemed to indicate that children do not develop significant long-term psychological or behavioral problems (e.g., Kent et al. 2000). However, Stoddard et al. (1992) found the rate of long-term depression in children to be high. One important confounding factor is that many children who are burned have preexisting psychosocial problems that influence long-term outcome.

Psychiatric Practice Guideline for Adults With Acute Burns

Although the evidence base is sparse, a practice guideline has been proposed for the management of adult psychiatric disorders in burn patients during their initial hospitalization (Powers and Santana 2005).

Facial Disfigurement and Scars

The adaptation to facial disfigurement depends, in part, on the age at which the disfigurement occurs. Children with congenital disfigurement often encounter significant developmental difficulties and are frequently stigmatized by peers, adults, and even health care personnel. These problems may be incorporated into an enduring negative sense of self. If the child has a strong social support system and receives well-informed medical and psychological care, these problems can be mitigated.

The adjustment to facial disfigurement also depends on the patient's preexisting personality and mental defense mechanisms. In his classic book, N.R. Bernstein (1976) described variables critical to adaptation, including the following: adaptive versus maladaptive defenses; active coping versus passive surrender; loving exchange versus rage; leading and co-managing treatment versus resisting treatment; and denial versus overawareness. For example, a patient who participates in managing his or her own care; who has a flexible, extensive repertoire of mental defense mechanisms; and who has loving exchanges with friends and family is likely to make a successful adjustment to a facial disfigurement.

Irrespective of the cause of the facial disfigurement, the objective nature of the disfigurement usually is not correlated with the patient's self-perception. For example, among 50 patients who received extensive multidisciplinary treatment from birth to age 18 years for cleft palate, no correlation was found between the objective measure of the residual deformities and the patient's subjective judgment of the remaining deformity (Vegter and Hage 2001). Thus, the subjective assessment of the deformity is probably more important than its actual nature in determining quality of life. Other factors that are important include proneness to shame, body image, and self-esteem (Van Loey and Van Son 2003).

Despite the recognition that the *emotional* experience of the facial disfigurement is one of the primary determinants of quality of life, little research is available on possible interventions. In addition to self-help interventions for patients, improving health care professionals' ability to cope with patients' facial disfigurement enhances psychosocial rehabilitation (Clarke and Cooper 2001).

Trauma Victims of Terrorist Attacks

The psychological consequences of trauma or disaster may include a variety of clinical symptoms, including a disruption of homeostasis, a shattering of ego integrity, and a feeling of fright and being overwhelmed (Figley 1978; Wilkinson 1983). The federal disaster mental health approach in the United States was developed largely out of experiences with natural disasters. The 1995 Oklahoma City bombing and the events of September 11, 2001, highlighted how little we know about the provision of services in the aftermath of mass trauma caused by humans.

The U.S. federal approach emphasizes crisis intervention, support services, triage, referral, outreach, and public education for affected individuals (Center for Mental Health Services 1994; Myers 1994). The federal program concluded that although many individuals may have psychological reactions to a natural disaster, few actually develop diagnosable mental disorders significant enough to warrant more than crisis intervention, brief treatment, or supportive therapy (Flynn and Nelson 1998; Myers 1994). However, in the Oklahoma City bombing, 6 months after the incident, 45% of the sample had an active psychiatric disorder, and one-third had PTSD (North et al. 1999). Experiences in Oklahoma City suggest that large-scale disasters caused by humans may result in greater psychiatric impairment of direct victims than do natural disasters (North et al. 1999). In a developing field like disaster mental health, in which experience is expanding faster than research and in which we are faced with events for which models were not designed, the learning curve is both steep and incomplete.

Bariatric Surgery

The National Heart, Lung, and Blood Institute (1998) clinical guidelines define *extreme obesity* as a body mass index (BMI) greater than 40 kg/m^2. BMI is a calculated number attained by dividing weight in kilograms by height in meters squared. Extreme obesity is also called *morbid obesity* because it is associated with high premature morbidity and mortality, most commonly as a result of complications of type 2 diabetes mellitus, hypertension, hyperlipidemia, or sleep apnea. Multiple treatments have been tried for morbid obesity, but clearly the most effective is bariatric surgery (Fisher and Schauer 2002). The current weight criterion for bariatric (or obesity) surgery is a BMI greater than 40 or a BMI greater than 35 with life-threatening comorbidities. Fifteen million people in the United States, or 1 out of 20 people, have a BMI of 35 kg/m^2 or greater (Buchwald and Buchwald 2002).

Bariatric surgery works in one of two ways: 1) by restricting a patient's ability to eat (restrictive procedures) and 2) by interfering with absorption of ingested food (malabsorptive procedures). Although more than five bariatric procedures are currently performed, the Roux-en-Y gastric bypass (RYGBP) and the laparoscopic adjustable gastric banding (LAGB) are the most widely used. The RYGBP combines restriction and malabsorption principles and results in greater weight loss than the previously popular vertical banded gastroplasty (so-called stomach stapling) that was purely a restrictive procedure. The restrictive element of the RYGBP involves creation of a small gastric pouch with a small outlet; the malabsorptive element involves bypass of the distal stomach, the entire duodenum, and about 20–40 cm of the proximal jejunum. The LAGB is a purely restrictive procedure and involves placement of a silicone band around the upper stomach.

In the bariatric surgery field, there has been a strong effort to standardize reports of weight loss following surgery by using either percent initial excess weight loss or percent initial BMI loss. Both the RYGBP and the LAGB result in approximately 33% initial BMI loss at 1 year (Buchwald 2002; Fox et al. 2003). Weight loss continues during the next year, but not all weight loss is maintained during the next 5–10 years. These results mean that the average patient has a meaningful weight loss but does not achieve ideal body weight; that is, morbid obesity is exchanged for moderate obesity. Perhaps the most important question is whether bariatric surgery results in improvement in the usual physiological complications of morbid obesity. The evidence for significant and sustained improvement in type 2 diabetes mellitus is strong (Greenway et al. 2002), and, although less impressive, reduction in hypertension and improvement in lipid metabolism usually occur.

Psychosocial Aspects

Multiple studies have attempted to identify psychosocial predictors of outcome after bariatric surgery. Early studies of the vertical banded gastroplasty procedure found no relation between presurgical psychiatric diagnoses or presurgical eating pathology and degree of weight loss at follow-up (Powers et al. 1997, 1999). This does not allow one to conclude that psychopathology will have no influence on postoperative adherence and outcome because 1) published studies are not large enough to examine the effect of each specific psychiatric disorder, and 2) patients with severe psychiatric disorders tend not to be referred by their physicians to bariatric surgeons.

More recent studies have looked at the question another way and have convincingly shown that many measures of psychopathology and quality of life improve after bariatric surgery (Bocchieri et al.

2002; Guisado et al. 2002). In addition, one study showed that patients who received preoperative brief strategic therapy (average six sessions) had a greater weight loss at 1 year after LAGB than did patients who did not receive this therapy (Caniato and Skorjanec 2002).

It is worth remembering that some patients who might benefit substantially from the surgery (in terms of both weight loss and quality of life) do not receive it. Examples include patients with schizophrenia or bipolar disorder, whose obesity may have been caused by psychotropic medications. Many surgeons exclude these patients because of early reports in the literature of negative outcomes and concerns about whether they would comply with postoperative requirements. Finally, some health insurers refuse to cover, or make access difficult to, bariatric surgery.

Eating Disorders and Bariatric Surgery

Presurgical binge-eating disorder occurs among 16%–33% of patients who have bariatric surgery, and an even greater percentage have subsyndromal binge-eating disorder (Powers et al. 1999; Saunders 1999). These figures are significantly higher than those reported in the general population. Presurgical night-eating syndrome also appears to be more common among bariatric surgery patients than in the general population (Kuldau and Rand 1986). Although binge eating is usually absent after surgery, vomiting is frequent after vertical banded gastroplasty, sometimes resulting from failed attempts to binge (Powers et al. 1999). In other cases, such vomiting may represent a continuation of conditioned vomiting in patients who had frequently purged before surgery. However, before postgastroplasty vomiting is attributed to a behavior, a mechanical cause (i.e., overly restrictive anatomy) should be ruled out.

Ophthalmological Surgery

Cataract Surgery

Early on, there were reports by psychiatric consultants of "black patch" psychosis following cataract surgery (Weisman and Hackett 1958). They focused on the sensory deprivation that occurred after bilateral cataract removal and led to the recommendation that only one eye be operated on at a time. Subsequently, "black patch" psychosis was identified as a postoperative delirium that was relatively uncommon. Milstein and colleagues (2002) found that following cataract surgery, 4.4% of 296 patients had an immediate postoperative delirium according to the Confusion Assessment Method (Inouye 1998), a standardized measure of delirium. Factors found to be statistically associated with postoperative delirium included very old age (82 years compared with 73 years) and frequent preoperative use of benzodiazepines.

Cataract surgery usually is performed in an outpatient setting, and typically either topical or regional anesthesia is used. These anesthetic approaches usually result in the patient being aware during the surgery, and patients often have visual experiences: most patients see light; some see various colors (especially red and yellow); and a minority see vague movements, instruments, and the surgeon's hands (Au Eong et al. 1999). Almost all patients (93%) find these visual experiences acceptable, but 4% find them unpleasant, and 3% are frightened by the experiences (Prasad et al. 2003). Preoperative counseling and inclusion of the possibility of these experiences in the informed consent process for surgery have been recommended. A controlled study (Moon and Cho 2001) found that handholding during cataract surgery decreased both anxiety and epinephrine levels.

Cosmetic Surgery

In an age and a culture in which people have an increased interest in physical attractiveness, cosmetic surgery has dramatically increased. In 1998, more than 132,000 women had breast augmentation procedures in the United States (Sarwer et al. 2000). Early studies found that psychopathology was common among cosmetic surgery candidates. Findings from more recent studies suggest that because more people consider cosmetic surgery a reasonable choice, the percentage of applicants with psychiatric disorders may be relatively lower. Most patients do well with cosmetic surgery, although it is thought that so-called type changes (e.g., rhinoplasty) require more extensive psychological adjustment than do restorative changes such as face-lifts (Castle et al. 2002).

Age at the time of cosmetic surgery is also important because it may be easier to incorporate changes into body image during childhood or adolescence. Cosmetic surgery is usually helpful in adolescents with a true defect if they are selected carefully and if genuine informed consent is obtained before surgery (McGrath and Mukerji 2000).

Because quality of life is significantly influenced by body image, a philosophical question is whether or which cosmetic surgery should be considered medically necessary. The focus on possible negative body image changes after lifesaving surgeries for illnesses such as breast cancer has resulted in trials comparing the effectiveness (in terms of survival) of less disfiguring surgeries with that of more radical approaches. A persuasive argument can be made that improvements in body image and self-esteem may dramatically improve quality of life, but this issue remains controversial.

Preoperative Assessment

Even though the percentage of patients with psychiatric disorders may be lower among patients seeking aesthetic surgery than in previous decades, it is probably still higher than among most other surgical candidates. Most patients with body dysmorphic disorder are primarily encountered by plastic surgeons, not by psychiatrists. Several research groups have attempted to determine which patients should not have cosmetic surgery at all and which patients should have psychiatric treatment before aesthetic surgery. A series of questions designed to detect psychiatric problems has been proposed (Grossbart and Sarwer 1999). One problem in determining who is likely to benefit from cosmetic surgery is that there is no widely accepted method for determining patient satisfaction with the surgical results. Ching and colleagues (2003) have reviewed the literature and suggested specific measures of body image and quality of life likely to provide valid evidence concerning the question of who should receive surgery.

References

Adler LE, Griffith JM: Concurrent medical illness in the schizophrenic patient: epidemiology, diagnosis, and management. Schizophr Res 4:91–107, 1991

Aizawa KI, Kanai T, Saikawa Y, et al: A novel approach to the prevention of postoperative delirium in the elderly after gastrointestinal surgery. Surgery Today 32:310–314, 2002

American Burn Association: Burn Incidence Fact Sheet. Available at: http://www.ameriburn.org. Accessed July 2, 2004.

Andreasen NJ, Noyes R Jr, Hartford CE, et al: Management of emotional reactions in seriously burned adults. N Engl J Med 286:65–69, 1972

Au Eong KG, Lee HM, Lim AT, et al: Subjective visual experience during extracapsular cataract extraction and intraocular lens implantation under retrobulbar anaesthesia. Eye 13(Pt 3a):325–328, 1999

Barillo DJ, Goode R: Substance abuse in victims of fire. J Burn Care Rehabil 17:71–76, 1996

Bayindir O, Akpinar B, Can E, et al: The use of the 5-HT$_3$-receptor antagonist ondansetron for the treatment of postcardiotomy delirium. J Cardiothorac Vasc Anesth 14:288–292, 2000

Bernstein L, Jacobsberg L, Ashman T, et al: Detection of alcoholism among burn patients. Hosp Community Psychiatry 43:255–256, 1992

Bernstein NR: Emotional Care of the Facially Burned and Disfigured. Boston, MA, Little, Brown, 1976

Blanchard EB, Hickling EJ, Devineni T, et al: A controlled evaluation of cognitive behavioural therapy for posttraumatic stress in motor vehicle accident survivors. Behav Res Ther 41:79–96, 2003

Bloomquist T: Amputation and phantom limb pain: a pain-prevention model. AANA J 69:211–217, 2001

Bocchieri LE, Meana M, Fisher BL: A review of psychosocial outcomes of surgery for morbid obesity. J Psychosom Res 52:155–165, 2002

Buchwald H: A bariatric surgery algorithm. Obes Surg 12:733–746, 2002

Buchwald H, Buchwald JN: Evolution of operative procedures for the management of morbid obesity 1950–2000. Obes Surg 12:705–717, 2002

Caniato D, Skorjanec B: The role of brief strategic therapy on the outcome of gastric banding. Obes Surg 12:666–671, 2002

Castle DJ, Honigman RJ, Phillips KA: Does cosmetic surgery improve psychosocial wellbeing? Med J Aust 176:601–604, 2002

Center for Mental Health Services Program Guidance: Crisis Counseling and Mental Health Treatment Similarities and Differences. Rockville, MD, Center for Mental Health Services, 1994

Ching S, Thoma A, McCabe RE, et al: Measuring outcomes in aesthetic surgery: a comprehensive review of the literature. Plast Reconstr Surg 111:469–480, 2003

Clarke A, Cooper C: Psychological rehabilitation after disfiguring injury or disease: investigating the training needs of specialist nurses. J Adv Nurs 34:18–26, 2001

Craven J: Psychiatric aspects of lung transplant. The Toronto Lung Transplant Group. Can J Psychiatry 35:759–764, 1990

Curtiss CP: JCAHO: meeting the standards for pain management. Orthop Nurs 20:27–30, 41, 2001

Daniels SM, Fenley JD, Powers PS, et al: Self-inflicted burns: a ten-year retrospective study. J Burn Care Rehabil 12:144–147, 1991

Diaz V, Rodriguez J, Barrientos P, et al: Use of procholinergics in the prevention of postoperative delirium in hip fracture surgery in the elderly: a randomized controlled trial. Rev Neurol 33:716–719, 2001

Duggan M, Dowd N, O'Mara D, et al: Benzodiazepine premedication may attenuate the stress response in daycase anesthesia: a pilot study. Can J Anaesth 49:932–935, 2002

Ehde DM, Patterson DR, Wiechman SA, et al: Post-traumatic stress symptoms and distress following acute burn injury. Burns 25:587–592, 1999

Ehde DM, Patterson DR, Wiechman SA, et al: Post-traumatic stress symptoms and distress 1 year after burn injury. J Burn Care Rehabil 21:105–111, 2000

Erlandsson AL, Backman B, Stenstrom A, et al: Conscious sedation by oral administration of midazolam in paediatric dental treatment. Swed Dent J 25:97–104, 2001

Figley CR: Stress Disorder Among Vietnam Veterans: Theory, Research and Treatment. New York, Brunner/Mazel, 1978

Fisher BL, Schauer P: Medical and surgical options in the treatment of severe obesity. Am J Surg 184:9S–16S, 2002

Flacker JM, Marcantonio ER: Delirium in the elderly: optimal management. Drugs Aging 13:119–130, 1998

Flynn BW, Nelson ME: Understanding the needs of children following large-scale disasters and the role of government. Child Adolesc Psychiatr Clin North Am 7:211–227, 1998

Foertsch CE, O'Hara MW, Stoddard FJ, et al: Treatment-resistant pain and distress during pediatric burn-dressing changes. J Burn Care Rehabil 19:219–224, 1998

Fox SR, Fox KM, Srikanth MS, et al: The lap-band system in a North American population. Obes Surg 13:275–280, 2003

Fukunishi I: Relationship of cosmetic disfigurement to the severity of posttraumatic stress disorder in burn injury or digital amputation. Psychother Psychosom 68:82–86, 1999

Fulop G, Strain JJ: Medical and surgical inpatients who referred themselves for psychiatric consultation. Gen Hosp Psychiatry 7:267–271, 1985

Galanakis P, Bickel H, Gradinger R, et al: Acute confusional state in the elderly following hip surgery: incidence, risk factors and complications. Int J Geriatr Psychiatry 16:349–355, 2001

Gentilello LM, Donovan DM, Dunn CW, et al: Alcohol interventions in trauma centers: current practice and future directions. JAMA 274:1043–1048, 1995

Greenway SE, Greenway FL, III, Klein S: Effects of obesity surgery on non-insulin-dependent diabetes mellitus. Arch Surg 137:1109–1117, 2002

Greer SM, Dalton JA, Carlson J, et al: Surgical patients' fear of addiction to pain medication: the effect of an educational program for clinicians. Clin J Pain 17:157–164, 2001

Grossbart TA, Sarwer DB: Cosmetic surgery: surgical tools—psychosocial goals. Semin Cutan Med Surg 18:101–111, 1999

Guisado JA, Vaz FJ, Alarcon J, et al: Psychopathological status and interpersonal functioning following weight loss in morbidly obese patients undergoing bariatric surgery. Obes Surg 12:835–840, 2002

Gutl P, Greimel ER, Roth R, et al: Women's sexual behavior, body image and satisfaction with surgical outcomes after hysterectomy: a comparison of vaginal and abdominal surgery. J Psychosom Obstet Gynaecol 23:51–59, 2002

Hagg O, Fritzell P, Ekselius L, et al: Predictors of outcome in fusion surgery for chronic low back pain: a report from the Swedish Lumbar Spine Study. Eur Spine J 12:22–33, 2003

Hamilton JG: Needle phobia: a neglected diagnosis. J Fam Pract 41:169–175, 1995

Imbus SH, Zawacki BE: Autonomy for burned patients when survival is unprecedented. N Engl J Med 297:308–311, 1977

Inouye SK: Delirium in hospitalized older patients: recognition and risk factors. J Geriatr Psychiatry Neurol 11:118–125, 1998

Jones JD, Barber B, Engrav L, et al: Alcohol use and burn injury. J Burn Care Rehabil 12:148–152, 1991

Kain ZN, Caldwell-Andrews A, Wang SM: Psychological preparation of the parent and pediatric surgical patient. Anesthesiol Clin North Am 20:29–44, 2002

Kamolz T, Granderath FA, Pointner R: Does major depression in patients with gastro-esophageal reflux disease affect the outcome of laparoscopic antireflux surgery? Surg Endosc 17:55–60, 2003

Kaneko T, Takahashi S, Naka T, et al: Postoperative delirium following gastrointestinal surgery in elderly patients. Surg Today 27:107–111, 1997

Kelley KM, Tkachenko TA, Pliskin NH, et al: Life after electrical injury: risk factors for psychiatric sequelae. Ann N Y Acad Sci 888:356–363, 1999

Kent L, King H, Cochrane R: Maternal and child psychological sequelae in paediatric burn injuries. Burns 26:317–322, 2000

Klafta JM, Roizen MF: Current understanding of patients' attitudes toward and preparation for anesthesia: a review. Anesth Analg 83:1314–1321, 1996

Klein E, Koren D, Arnon I, et al: Sleep complaints are not corroborated by objective sleep measures in post-traumatic stress disorder: a 1-year prospective study in survivors of motor vehicle crashes. J Sleep Res 12:35–41, 2003

Koivula M, Tarkka MT, Tarkka M, et al: Fear and in-hospital social support for coronary artery bypass grafting patients on the day before surgery. Int J Nurs Stud 39:415–427, 2002

Kornfeld DS, Zimberg S, Malm JR: Psychiatric complications of open-heart surgery. N Engl J Med 273:287–292, 1965

Kudoh A, Katagai H, Takazawa T: Antidepressant treatment for chronic depressed patients should not be discontinued prior to anesthesia. Can J Anaesth 49:132–136, 2002

Kuldau JM, Rand CSW: The night eating syndrome and bulimia in the morbidly obese. Int J Eat Disord 5:143–148, 1986

Kumar V: Burnt wives: a study of suicides. Burns 29:31–35, 2003

Lieber CS: Medical disorders of alcoholism. N Engl J Med 333: 1058–1065, 1995

Lindemann E: Symptomatology and management of acute grief (1944). Am J Psychiatry 151 (suppl 6):155–160, 1994

Marcantonio ER, Flacker JM, Wright RJ, et al: Reducing delirium after hip fracture: a randomized trial. J Am Geriatr Soc 49:516–522, 2001

Marshall WR, Weaver BD, McCutcheon P: A study of the effectiveness of oral midazolam as a dental pre-operative sedative and hypnotic. Spec Care Dentist 19:259–266, 1999

Martin-Herz SP, Patterson DR, Honari S, et al: Pediatric pain control practices of North American Burn Centers. J Burn Care Rehabil 24:26–36, 2003

McGrath MH, Mukerji S: Plastic surgery and the teenage patient. J Pediatr Adolesc Gynecol 13:105–118, 2000

Milisen K, Foreman MD, Abraham IL, et al: A nurse-led interdisciplinary intervention program for delirium in elderly hip-fracture patients. J Am Geriatr Soc 49:523–532, 2001

Milstein A, Pollack A, Kleinman G, et al: Confusion/delirium following cataract surgery: an incidence study of 1-year duration. Int Psychogeriatr 14:301–306, 2002

Moesgaard F, Lykkegaard-Nielsen M: Preoperative cell-mediated immunity and duration of antibiotic prophylaxis in relation to postoperative infectious complications: a controlled trial in biliary, gastroduodenal and colorectal surgery. Acta Chir Scand 155:281–286, 1989

Moon JS, Cho KS: The effects of handholding on anxiety in cataract surgery patients under local anaesthesia. J Adv Nurs 35:407–415, 2001

Myers D: Disaster Response and Recovery: A Handbook for Mental Health Professionals (DHHS Publ No SMA 94-3010). Menlo Park, CA, Center for Mental Health Services, 1994

Mzezewa S, Jonsson K, Aberg M, et al: A prospective study of suicidal burns admitted to the Harare burns unit. Burns 26: 460–464, 2000

National Heart, Lung, and Blood Institute: Clinical Guidelines on the Identification, Evaluation, and Treatment of Overweight and Obesity in Adults. Bethesda, MD, National Institutes of Health, National Heart, Lung, and Blood Institute, June 1998

Neale MC, Walters EE, Eaves LJ, et al: Genetics of blood-injury fears and phobias: a population-based twin study. Am J Med Genet 54:326–334, 1994

Nelson S: Pre-admission education for patients undergoing cardiac surgery. Br J Nurs 5:335–340, 1996

Nir Y, Paz A, Sabo E, et al: Fear of injections in young adults: prevalence and associations. Am J Trop Med Hyg 68:341–344, 2003

North CS, Nixon SJ, Shariat S, et al: Psychiatric disorders among survivors of the Oklahoma City bombing. JAMA 282:755–762, 1999

Page AC: The role of disgust in faintness elicited by blood and injection stimuli. J Anxiety Disord 17:45–58, 2003

Paré A: The Works of That Famous Chirurgion, Ambrose Parey, translated out of the Latin and compared with the French by T. Johnson. London, England, Cotes, 1649

Powell J, Kitchen N, Heslin J, et al: Psychosocial outcomes at three and nine months after good neurological recovery from aneurysmal subarachnoid haemorrhage: predictors and prognosis. J Neurol Neurosurg Psychiatry 72:772–781, 2002

Powers PS, Santana C: Surgery, in Textbook of Psychosomatic Medicine. Edited by Levenson JL. Washington, DC, American Psychiatric Publishing, 2005, p 662

Powers PS, Cruse CW, Daniels S, et al: Safety and efficacy of debridement under anesthesia in patients with burns. J Burn Care Rehabil 14(2 Pt 1):176–180, 1993

Powers PS, Cruse CW, Daniels S, et al: Post-traumatic stress disorder in patients with burns. J Burn Care Rehabil 15:147–153, 1994a

Powers PS, Stevens B, Arias F, et al: Alcohol disorders among patients with burns: crisis and opportunity. J Burn Care Rehabil 15:386–391, 1994b

Powers PS, Rosemurgy A, Boyd F, et al: Outcome of gastric restriction procedures: weight, psychiatric diagnoses, and satisfaction. Obes Surg 7:471–477, 1997

Powers PS, Perez A, Boyd F, et al: Eating pathology before and after bariatric surgery: a prospective study. Int J Eat Disord 25:293–300, 1999

Powers PS, Cruse CW, Boyd F: Psychiatric status, prevention, and outcome in patients with burns: a prospective study. J Burn Care Rehabil 21(1 Pt 1):85–88, 2000

Prasad N, Kumar CM, Patil BB, et al: Subjective visual experience during phacoemulsification cataract surgery under sub-Tenon's block. Eye 17:407–409, 2003

Putnam FW, Hulsmann JE: Pharmacotherapy for survivors of childhood trauma. Semin Clin Neuropsychiatry 7:129–136, 2002

Regal H, Rose W, Hahnel S, et al: Evaluation of psychological stress before general anesthesia. Psychiatr Neurol Med Psychol (Leipz) 37:151–155, 1985

Rusch MD, Gould LJ, Dzwierzynski WW, et al: Psychological impact of traumatic injuries: what the surgeon can do. Plast Reconstr Surg 109:18–24, 2002

Sarwer DB, Nordmann JE, Herbert JD: Cosmetic breast augmentation surgery: a critical overview. J Womens Health Gend Based Med 9:843–856, 2000

Saunders R: Binge eating in gastric bypass patients before surgery. Obes Surg 9:72–76, 1999

Saxe G, Stoddard F, Courtney D, et al: Relationship between acute morphine and the course of PTSD in children with burns. J Am Acad Child Adolesc Psychiatry 40:915–921, 2001

Scher CS, Anwar M: The self-reporting of psychiatric medications in patients scheduled for elective surgery. J Clin Anesth 11:619–621, 1999

Scully JH, Hutcherson R: Suicide by burning. Am J Psychiatry 140:905–906, 1983

Segatore M, Dutkiewicz M, Adams D: The delirious cardiac surgical patient: theoretical aspects and principles of management. J Cardiovasc Nurs 12:32–48, 1998

Seitz HK, Simanowski UA: Ethanol and carcinogenesis of the alimentary tract. Alcohol Clin Exp Res 10 (suppl):33S–40S, 1986

Sillanaukee P: Laboratory markers of alcohol abuse. Alcohol Alcohol 31:613–616, 1996

Sjostrom B, Haljamae H, Dahlgren LO, et al: Assessment of postoperative pain: impact of clinical experience and professional role. Acta Anaesthesiol Scand 41:339–344, 1997

Smith AF, Pittaway AJ: Premedication for anxiety in adult day surgery. Cochrane Database Syst Rev 1:CD002192, 2003

Spies CD, Neuner B, Neumann T, et al: Intercurrent complications in chronic alcoholic men admitted to the intensive care unit following trauma. Intensive Care Med 22:286–293, 1996

Spies CD, Spies KP, Zinke S, et al: Alcoholism and carcinoma change the intracellular pH and activate platelet Na+/H+-exchange in men. Alcohol Clin Exp Res 21:1653–1660, 1997

Steenkamp WC, Botha NJ, Van der Merwe AE: The prevalence of alcohol dependence in burned adult patients. Burns 20:522–525, 1994

Stoddard FJ, Stroud L, Murphy JM: Depression in children after recovery from severe burns. J Burn Care Rehabil 13:340–347, 1992

Stoddard FJ, Sheridan RL, Saxe GN, et al: Treatment of pain in acutely burned children. J Burn Care Rehabil 23:135–156, 2002

Stoll C, Schelling G, Goetz AE, et al: Health-related quality of life and post-traumatic stress disorder in patients after cardiac surgery and intensive care treatment. J Thorac Cardiovasc Surg 120:505–512, 2000

Stomberg MW, Wickstrom K, Joelsson H, et al: Postoperative pain management on surgical wards—do quality assurance strategies result in long-term effects on staff member attitudes and clinical outcomes? Pain Manag Nurs 4:11–22, 2003

Strain JJ: Needs for psychiatry in the general hospital. Hosp Community Psychiatry 33:996–1001, 1982

Summers S: Evidence-based practice, part 3: acute pain management of the perianesthesia patient. J Perianesth Nurs 16:112–120, 2001

Tabares R, Peck MD: Chemical dependency in patients with burn injuries: a fortress of denial. J Burn Care Rehabil 18:283–286, 1997

Tedstone JE, Tarrier N: Posttraumatic stress disorder following medical illness and treatment. Clin Psychol Rev 23:409–448, 2003

Thomas CR, Brazeal BA, Rosenberg L, et al: Phantom limb pain in pediatric burn survivors. Burns 29:139–142, 2003

Tokita K, Tanaka H, Kawamoto M, et al: Patient-controlled epidural analgesia with bupivacaine and fentanyl suppresses postoperative delirium following hepatectomy. Masui 50: 742–746, 2001

Tønnesen H, Petersen KR, Hojgaard L, et al: Postoperative morbidity among symptom-free alcohol misusers. Lancet 340:334–337, 1992

Tønnesen H, Carstensen M, Maina P: Is carbohydrate deficient transferrin a useful marker of harmful alcohol intake among surgical patients? Eur J Surg 165:522–527, 1999

van der Schans CP, Geertzen JH, Schoppen T, et al: Phantom pain and health-related quality of life in lower limb amputees. J Pain Symptom Manage 24:429–436, 2002

Van Loey N, Van Son M: Psychopathology and psychological problems in patients with burn scars: epidemiology and management. Am J Clin Dermatol 4:245–272, 2003

van Wijk MG, Smalhout B: A postoperative analysis of the patient's view of anaesthesia in a Netherlands' teaching hospital. Anaesthesia 45:679–682, 1990

Vegter F, Hage JJ: Lack of correlation between objective and subjective evaluation of residual stigmata in cleft patients. Ann Plast Surg 46:625–629, 2001

Watkins PN, Cook EL, May SR, et al: The role of the psychiatrist in the team treatment of the adult patient with burns. J Burn Care Rehabil 13:19–27, 1992

Weisman AD, Hackett TP: Psychosis after eye surgery: establishment of a specific doctor–patient relation in the prevention and treatment of "black-patch delirium." N Engl J Med 258:1284–1289, 1958

Wilkinson CB: Aftermath of a disaster: the collapse of the Hyatt Regency Hotel sky-walks. Am J Psychiatry 140:1134–1139, 1983

Williams-Russo P, Urquhart BL, Sharrock NE, et al: Post-operative delirium: predictors and prognosis in elderly orthopedic patients. J Am Geriatr Soc 40:759–767, 1992

Yu BH, Dimsdale JE: Posttraumatic stress disorder in patients with burn injuries. J Burn Care Rehabil 20:426–433, 1999

Zatzick DF, Jurkovich GJ, Gentilello L, et al: Posttraumatic stress, problem drinking, and functional outcomes after injury. Arch Surg 137:200–205, 2002

Self-Assessment Questions

Select the single best response for each question.

1. Which of the following are the elements of informed consent that a surgeon should include in his or her discussion with a patient about a proposed surgery?

    A. Diagnosis.
    B. Why the surgery is the treatment of choice.
    C. Expected risks and benefits.
    D. Alternatives and their consequences.
    E. All of the above.

2. What percentage of patients experience significant preoperative anxiety?

    A. Less than 10%.
    B. 10%–20%.
    C. 40%–60%.
    D. 80%–90%.
    E. None of the above.

3. Risk factors for developing postoperative delirium include all of the following *except*

    A. Older age.
    B. Alcohol use.
    C. Cognitive impairment.
    D. Male gender.
    E. Type of surgery.

4. Delirium is common in burn patients. All of the following are common causes of delirium in burn patients *except*

    A. Hypernatremia.
    B. Hypophosphatemia.
    C. Fluid shifts.
    D. Opioids.
    E. Sepsis.

5. Bariatric surgery is usually performed for patients with extreme or morbid obesity. According to the National Heart, Lung, and Blood Institute guidelines, *extreme obesity* is a body mass index (BMI) of

    A. >15 kg/m^2.
    B. >20 kg/m^2.
    C. >25 kg/m^2.
    D. >30 kg/m^2.
    E. >40 kg/m^2.

14 Organ Transplantation

Andrea F. DiMartini, M.D.

Mary Amanda Dew, Ph.D.

Paula T. Trzepacz, M.D.

THE BENEFIT OF solid organ transplantation was realized in 1954 when Dr. Joseph E. Murray performed the first successful kidney transplant, with the patient's identical twin as donor. With the development of immunosuppressive medications in 1967, the first successful liver transplant was performed, followed a year later by the first successful heart transplant. Nevertheless, it was not until the early 1980s, with the advent of improved immunosuppression, that organ transplantation changed from an experimental procedure to a standard of care for many types of end-stage organ disease.

In that decade, the National Organ Transplant Act established the framework for a national system of organ transplantation, and the United Network of Organ Sharing (UNOS) was contracted by the U.S. Congress to administer the nation's only Organ Procurement and Transplantation Network (OPTN) (United Network of Organ Sharing [UNOS] 2004). In addition to facilitating organ matching and placement, UNOS collects data about every transplant performed in the United States and maintains information on every organ type (e.g., wait-list counts, survival rates) in an extensive database available on the OPTN Web site (http://www.OPTN .org) (UNOS 2004).

Although immunological barriers still exist for transplant recipients, the greatest obstacle to receiving a transplant is the shortage of donated organs. The number of wait-listed individuals is increasing far beyond the availability of donated organs (see Table 14–1) (UNOS 2004). In addition, each year, 10%–15% of liver, heart, and lung transplant candidates will die while on the waiting list (UNOS 2004). Additionally, posttransplantation graft survival rates can be significantly lower (e.g., 36.4% kidney and 45% liver graft survival after 10 years) than patient sur-

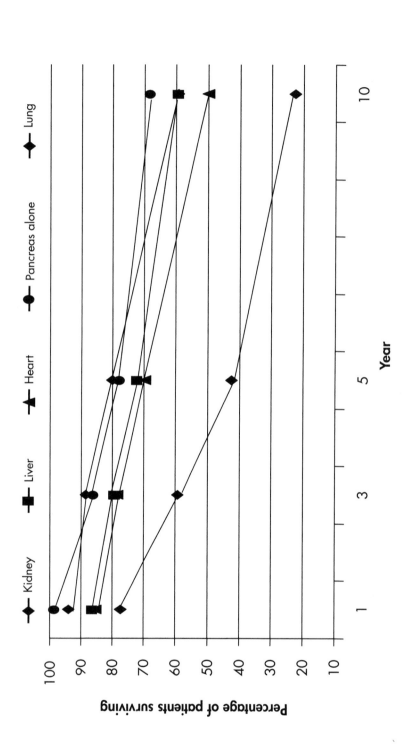

FIGURE 14–1. Survival rates of transplant recipients, by organ type.

Source. United Network of Organ Sharing (UNOS; http://www.optn.org).

TABLE 14–1. Transplant statistics for the United States for 2004

Organ	Number of patients			
	Added to list	On list	Died on list	Transplanted
Kidney	22,421	60,506	2,876	13,310
Liver	8,504	17,267	1,462	5,136
Heart	2,383	3,244	370	1,708
Pancreas	940	1,662	43	512
Kidney/pancreas	1,443	2,414	156	734
Intestine	197	195	41	126
Heart/lung	63	171	23	31
Lung	1,690	3,879	400	998
Totals	37,641	89,338	5,371	22,555

Source. United Network of Organ Sharing (UNOS; http://www.OPTN.org).

vival rates, which means that many transplant recipients will have to face a second transplant 5–10 years after their first (Figure 14–1) (UNOS 2004).

These stark facts highlight the enormous stresses facing transplant candidates, transplant recipients, and their caregivers. These issues have also created a particular environment in which hospitals must evaluate, treat, and select patients for organ transplantation. The scarcity of donated organs has driven efforts to select candidates believed to have the best chance for optimal posttransplant outcomes. Additionally, the organ shortage has increasingly led to the consideration of living kidney donors and, more recently, living liver donors (and, more rarely, living lung donors) as transplantation options.

In this chapter, we outline the essential areas of the field for psychosomatic medicine specialists and other mental health clinicians involved in the care of transplant patients—pretransplant assessment and candidate selection, emotional and psychological aspects of the transplant process, therapeutic issues, patients with complex or controversial features, psychopharmacolog-ical treatment, and neuropsychiatric side effects of immunosuppressive medications.

Pretransplantation Issues

Psychosocial/Psychiatric Assessment

Pretransplant psychosocial evaluations have been a traditional role of the psychiatric consultation team in the transplantation process. These evaluations are frequently used to assist in the determination of a candidate's eligibility for transplantation, to identify psychiatric/psychosocial problems that may need to be addressed to prepare the candidate and family for transplantation, and to identify pre- and posttransplant psychiatric and/or psychosocial needs of the candidate. These evaluations are also critical for the identification of psychiatric, behavioral, and psychosocial risk factors that may portend poor transplant outcomes (Crone and Wise 1999; Dew et al. 2000).

Although a truly comprehensive assessment of a potential transplant candidate would require a full psychiatric con-

---

TABLE 14–2.   Goals of psychosocial screening

---

1. Assess coping skills; disqualify or intervene with patients who appear to be unable to cope effectively.

2. Diagnose comorbid psychiatric conditions; provide for pre- and posttransplant monitoring and treatment.

3. Determine the candidate's capacity to understand the transplant process and to provide informed consent.

4. Evaluate the candidate's ability to collaborate with the transplant team and to adhere to treatment.

5. Assess substance use/abuse history, recovery, and ability to maintain long-term abstinence.

6. Identify health behaviors that may influence posttransplant morbidity and mortality (i.e., tobacco use, poor eating or exercise habits) and evaluate the candidate's ability to modify these behaviors over the long term.

7. Help the transplant team to understand the patient better as a person.

8. Evaluate the level of social support available to the candidate for pre- and posttransplant phases (including stable family/others committed to assisting the candidate, adequate insurance and financial resources, and logistical support).

9. Determine the psychosocial needs of the patient and family and plan for services during the waiting, recovery, and rehabilitation phases of the transplant process.

10. Establish baseline measures of mental functioning in order to be able to monitor postoperative changes.

Source.   Adapted from Levenson J, Olbrisch ME: "Psychosocial Screening and Selection of Candidates for Organ Transplantation," in *The Transplant Patient.* Cambridge, UK, Cambridge University Press, 2000, p. 23. Used with permission.

---

sultation, the current high numbers of candidates preclude this. To handle the increasing volume of evaluations, some centers employ screening batteries of patient-rated measures to identify candidates with elevated levels of psychological distress, who then undergo a full psychiatric evaluation. Screening instruments can provide baseline cognitive, affective, and psychosocial ratings for candidates; use of these instruments maximizes staff resources and minimizes costs.

A psychosocial assessment of transplant candidates provides an opportunity to identify potential problems and intervene prior to transplantation, with the goal of improving posttransplant outcomes. Transplant programs vary considerably in their psychosocial assessment criteria and procedures (see Olbrisch and Levenson 1995 for a review of methodological and philosophical issues); in gen-

eral, however, psychosocial evaluations have 10 objectives (although a given assessment may not include all 10), as enumerated in Table 14–2 (see Levenson and Olbrisch 2000).

A follow-up reassessment may be necessary to clarify relevant issues, solidify a working relationship with the patient and family, and resolve problems. A multidisciplinary approach is often used with input from psychiatrists, psychologists, psychiatric nurse clinical specialists, addiction specialists, social workers, transplant surgeons, and transplant coordinators to construct a comprehensive picture of the patient and develop a coordinated treatment plan. As with any psychiatric evaluation, verbal feedback provided to the patient and family will serve to solidify the expectations of the transplant team and the requirements of the patient for listing if indicated. Some centers also use written "contracts" to formalize these recommendations (Cupples and Steslowe 2001; Stowe and Kotz 2001). In difficult cases, these contracts serve to document expectations, thereby minimizing misinterpretation. Written contracts outline a treatment plan that can be referred to with each follow-up appointment. These contracts are particularly useful with transplant candidates who have alcohol or substance abuse/dependence problems, specifying the transplant program's requirements for addiction treatment, monitoring of compliance (e.g., documented random negative blood alcohol levels), and length of abstinence (see subsection "Alcohol and Other Substance Use Disorders" later in this chapter).

Psychosocial Instruments and Measures

Instruments that are transplant-specific (e.g., Psychosocial Assessment of Candidates for Transplant [PACT; Olbrisch et al. 1989], Transplant Evaluation Rating Scale [TERS; Twillman et al. 1993]), disease-specific (e.g., Miller Health Attitude Scale for cardiac disease [Miller et al. 1981], Quality of Life Questionnaire—Chronic Lung Disease [Guyatt et al. 1987]), and disorder-specific (e.g., High Risk Alcohol Relapse Scale for alcoholism [Yates et al. 1993]) have been used to evaluate transplant candidates and monitor their posttransplant recovery. These instruments have been used in conjunction with general instruments for rating behavior, coping, cognitive and affective states, and quality of life. Psychosocial instruments can be used to identify individuals who require further assessment (as described earlier) or to pursue evaluation of patients already identified as requiring additional screening. The evaluator's purpose for using such instruments will determine the type and specificity of the instruments chosen.

Because psychosocial selection criteria differ significantly by program and organ type, development and use of structured evaluation instruments may help to direct and standardize the transplant selection protocols used nationally. The two instruments most commonly used to assess candidates for transplantation are the PACT and the TERS. These instruments are useful in organizing patient information and can be helpful both as tools for increasing the evaluator's understanding of the candidate and for research purposes.

The PACT was the first published psychosocial structured instrument specifically designed for screening transplant candidates (Olbrisch et al. 1989). It provides an overall score and subscale scores for psychological health (psychopathology, risk for psychopathology, stable personality factors), lifestyle factors (healthy lifestyle, ability to sustain change in lifestyle, compliance, drug and alcohol use), social support (support system stability and availability), and patient educability and understanding of the transplant process. The PACT can be completed in only a few minutes by the consultant following the evaluation but requires scoring by a skilled clinician, without which the instrument's predictive power could be diminished (Presberg et al. 1995). The final rating for candidate acceptability is made by the clinician, with the freedom to weigh individual item ratings variably (Presberg et al. 1995). Thus, a single area, such as alcohol abuse, could be assigned greater weight and thus could disproportionately influence the final rating.

The TERS is used to rate patients' level of adjustment in 10 areas of psychosocial functioning: prior psychiatric history, DSM-III-R Axis I and Axis II diagnoses, substance use/abuse, compliance, health behaviors, quality of family support, prior history of coping, coping with disease and treatment, quality of affect, and mental status (Twillman et al. 1993). In one study, the TERS was significantly correlated with several clinician-reported outcome variables (compliance, health behaviors, substance use), with particularly high correlations between pretransplant TERS scores and posttransplant substance use ($r=0.64$) (Twillman et al. 1993). The instrument requires administration by a skilled clinician to maintain accuracy (Presberg et al. 1995). The TERS summary score is derived from a mathematical formula in which individual item scores are multiplied by theoretical, predetermined weightings.

The Unique Role of the Psychiatric Consultant

Unlike in most psychiatric interviews, the psychiatrist performing the pretransplant assessment primarily serves the needs of the transplant team rather than those of the patient (a possible exception is the evaluation of living organ donors; see subsection "Living Donor Transplantation" later in this chapter). The psychiatric consultant must be candid with the patient about this role. Careful delineation of specific transplant-related expectations, explanation of the importance of these requirements to the success of transplantation, and exploration of the implications of these criteria for the individual candidate serve to establish a meaningful dialogue with the patient from which the therapeutic alliance necessary for future intervention can develop.

For the clinician, the seemingly reverse nature of this role can be uncomfortable or even anxiety provoking. This is especially true if the clinician is not recommending the candidate for transplantation. Fortunately, many programs do not reject patients outright for psychosocial reasons; rather, they offer such patients the opportunity to work to bring their problematic areas into compliance with the recommendations

(i.e., through addiction counseling, behavioral changes, psychiatric treatment, identification of appropriate social supports) and then undergo reevaluation for candidacy. In these cases, the psychiatric consultant can often function as an advocate for the patient and assist in referral for appropriate treatment if indicated. Nevertheless, some patients will be unable to comply with the specified transplant requirements or will not survive to complete their efforts to meet candidacy requirements.

Philosophical, moral, ethical, legal, and therapeutic dilemmas are inherent in the role of transplant psychiatrist, as conflicting team opinions present themselves in the course of work with potential transplant candidates. Team discussions and consultation with other colleagues are the rule in complicated cases. In these instances, team discussions not only aid in resolving candidacy quandaries but also can help alleviate team members' anxiety and discomfort over declining a patient for transplantation. Group or team debriefing may also be desirable, and occasionally consultation with risk management and the legal department of the hospital is needed (e.g., when a candidate is challenging candidacy requirements or the candidacy decision of the transplant team). Thorough documentation is essential in order to delineate the issues involved, the expectations of the team for transplantation candidacy, and the efforts to work with the patient.

Psychological and Psychiatric Issues in Organ Transplantation

Psychiatric Symptoms and Disorders in Transplant Patients

Similar to other medically ill populations, transplant candidates and recipients experience a significant amount of psychological distress and are at heightened risk of developing psychiatric disorders. The prevalence rates of major depression range from 4% to 28% in liver transplant patients, 0% to 58% in heart transplant patients, and 0.4% to 20% in kidney transplant patients (Dew 2003; Dew et al. 2000). The range of rates for anxiety disorders appears to be 3% to 33% (Dew 2003; Dew et al. 2000), but there are not enough studies to identify specific types of anxiety disorders. One study found that 10% of a cohort of heart or lung transplant recipients experienced posttraumatic stress disorder (PTSD) related to their transplant experience (Köllner et al. 2002). In a prospective study of 191 heart transplant recipients, the cumulative prevalence rates for psychiatric disorders during the 3 years posttransplantation were 38% for any disorder, including 25% with major depression, 21% with adjustment disorders, and 17% with PTSD (Dew et al. 2001). Factors that increased the cumulative risk for psychiatric disorders included a pretransplant psychiatric history, a longer period of hospitalization, female gender, greater impairments in physical functioning, and fewer social supports (Dew et al. 2001).

Adaptation to Transplantation

Transplant candidates typically experience a series of adaptive challenges as they proceed through evaluation, waiting, perioperative management, postoperative recuperation, and long-term adaptation to life with a transplant (Olbrisch et al. 2002). With chronic illness, there can be progressive debility and gradual loss of vitality and of physical and social functioning. Adapting to these changes can elicit anxiety, depression, avoidance, and denial and requires working through grief (Olbrisch et al. 2002). Patients who are wait-listed may develop contraindications to transplantation (i.e., infection, serious stroke, pro-

gressive organ dysfunction), and both patients and families should be made aware that a candidate's eligibility can change over time for many reasons (Stevenson 2004). During this phase, psychiatrists may provide counseling to patients and families to help them prepare for either transplantation or death.

Much of illness behavior depends on the coping strategies and personality style of the individual. In our experience, the adaptive styles of adult transplant recipients often depend on whether the patient's pretransplant illness experience was chronic or acute, as delineated in the following broadly generalized profiles.

Patients who have dealt with chronic illness for years may adapt psychologically to the sick role and can develop coping strategies that perpetuate a dependency on being ill (Olbrisch et al. 2002). For these patients, transplantation may psychologically represent a transition from one state of illness to another, and such patients can have difficulty adjusting to or transitioning into a "state of health." They often complain that the transplant team is expecting too fast a recovery from them, and they may describe feeling pressured to get better. Some patients may develop unexplained chronic pain or other somatic complaints or may begin to evidence noncompliance with transplant team directives.

For patients with good premorbid functioning who become acutely ill, with only a short period of pretransplant infirmity, the transplant can be an unwelcome event. These patients can experience a heightened sense of vulnerability, and they may deny the seriousness of their medical situation (Olbrisch et al. 2002). These patients often wish to return to normal functioning as quickly as possible posttransplantation, and they may in fact recover more rapidly than the transplant team expects; however, they may suffer later as the result of pushing themselves too much (e.g., returning to work before they are physically ready). They may resent being a transplant recipient, with all of the restrictions and regimens inherent in that role, and may act out their anger or denial in episodes of noncompliance (Olbrisch et al. 2002).

Patients With Complex or Controversial Psychosocial and Psychiatric Issues

The stringency of selection criteria for transplantation appears to depend on the type of organ transplant being considered, and transplant programs often have strongly formed beliefs about the suitability of candidates with certain types of mental illness. Cardiac transplant programs are more likely than liver transplant programs to consider psychosocial issues as contraindications, and liver transplant programs in turn are more stringent than kidney transplant programs (Corley et al. 1998; Levenson and Olbrisch 1993). These differences may be attributable to the relative availability of specific types of organs (Yates et al. 1993); alternatively, the extent of experience with specific organ transplants may allow programs to feel more comfortable with less stringent criteria (e.g., kidney transplantation, with more than three decades of experience and nearly 300,000 kidney transplants performed in the United States) (UNOS 2004). In addition, for kidney transplantation, cost-effectiveness research has clearly demonstrated the long-term cost savings of kidney transplantation relative to dialysis (Eggers 1992). With such unequivocal evidence, insurance payers have a strong financial incentive to refer patients early for preemptive transplantation, before the high costs of dialysis begin to accumulate (Eggers 1992). In such a setting, psychosocial factors may have

less impact on transplantation candidacy. Other issues influencing the selection process include moral and ethical beliefs, societal views, personal beliefs, and even financial constraints.

Posttransplant Compliance

Lifelong immunosuppression is a prerequisite for good graft function, and noncompliance with immunosuppressive medication is often associated with late acute rejection episodes, chronic rejection, graft loss, and death. It might be assumed that transplant patients, in general, constitute a highly motivated group and that their compliance would be high. Unfortunately, overall posttransplant medical noncompliance rates of all organ types range from 20% to 50% (see Laederach-Hofmann and Bunzel 2000 for a complete review). With organ transplantation, noncompliance impairs both life quality and life span, as it is a major risk factor for graft rejection episodes and may be responsible for up to 25% of deaths after the initial recovery period (Bunzel and Laederach-Hofmann 2000). Noncompliance leads to waste, reducing the potential benefits of therapy and adding to the costs of treating avoidable consequent morbidity. Graft loss from noncompliance is also tragic, given the large numbers of patients on the waiting lists. The occurrence of clinically measurable events such as rejection episodes, organ loss, or death underrepresents the true amount of noncompliance, because some patients who are only partially compliant have not yet experienced a clinically adverse event (see Bunzel and Laederach-Hofmann 2000; De Geest et al. 1995). Although such "subclinical" noncompliance is undetectable as a medical event, it is important as an indicator of those patients having difficulty following their medical regimens (Feinstein 1990).

De Geest et al. (1995) reported a medication noncompliance rate of 22.3% in kidney transplant patients, whereas Paris et al. (1994) found a rate of 47% among heart transplant recipients. Shapiro et al. (1995) observed that of 93 heart transplant recipients, about one-third (34.4%) were noncompliant in at least some areas over the course of long-term follow-up. Dew and colleagues (1996) examined compliance in eight domains of posttransplant care in a cohort of 101 heart recipients. During the first postoperative year, the degree of noncompliance varied across time. However, they found persistent noncompliance in the domains of exercise (37%), blood pressure monitoring (34%), immunosuppressive medication (20%), smoking (19%), diet (18%), blood work completion (15%), clinic attendance (9%), and heavy drinking (6%). Dew also found that as psychosocial risk factors accumulate, compliance problems are likely to rise dramatically. These studies also identified associations between noncompliance and increased risk of morbidity and mortality in transplant recipients (De Geest et al. 1995; Dew and Kormos 1999; Dew et al. 1996; Paris et al. 1994).

Other studies have determined that psychiatric problems that persist after transplantation are highly associated with noncompliance (Paris et al. 1994; Phipps 1997). In an extensive literature review of posttransplant compliance for all organ types, Bunzel and Laederach-Hofmann (2000) found that anxiety disorders—and, in particular, untreated major depression—were significantly associated with noncompliance. In a study of 125 heart transplant recipients (Shapiro et al. 1995), compliance problems were associated with a history of substance abuse ($P=0.0007$).

Alcohol and Other Substance Use Disorders

Compared with other solid organ transplant candidates, liver transplant (LTX) candidates more often require psychiatric consultation for substance addiction assessment, due to the prevalence of alcoholic liver disease (ALD) and viral hepatitis transmitted through contaminated needles. An estimated 50% of LTX recipients have a pre-LTX history of alcohol and/or drug abuse/dependence (DiMartini et al. 2002). A survey of 69 U.S. liver transplant programs found that 83% of programs have a psychiatrist or addiction medicine specialist routinely see each patient with ALD during the evaluation phase (Everhart and Beresford 1997). In the optimal situation, the psychiatric clinician is an integral member of the transplant clinical care team and can integrate the addiction treatment plan into the patient's pre- and posttransplant care. The Cleveland Clinic Foundation has formed a chemical-dependence transplant team to assess, treat, and monitor transplant patients with addictive disorders (Stowe and Kotz 2001). This program is a model for the integration of such services.

Psychiatric consultation provides a thorough evaluation of candidates' addiction history; their understanding of their addiction (especially in the context of their health and need for transplantation, their stability in recovery, and their need for further or ongoing addiction treatment), and the presence of other psychiatric disorders. Family and social support for the candidate's continued abstinence both pre- and posttransplantation must also be evaluated. Documentation of treatment participation is desirable, as is random toxicological screening for alcohol and other substances. These measures are especially important for patients early in recovery and for those with a short period of abstinence, denial of their problem, resistance to seeking treatment, or poor social support for continuing abstinence. Periodic reassessment of sobriety is important; two studies have identified relapses in up to

25% of wait-listed ALD candidates (Iasi et al. 2003; Weinrieb et al. 2005).

One-year post-LTX drinking rates (i.e., the percentage who used any alcohol by 1 year post-LTX) range from 8% to 37% (DiMartini 2000b; Everson et al. 1997), with cumulative rates estimated at 30%–40% by 5 years post-LTX (Lucey 1999). Rates of pathological drinking, defined as drinking that results in physical injury or alcohol dependence, are 10%–15% (Everson et al. 1997; Fireman 2000). Although the rate of alcohol use appears to attenuate with the passage of time, post-LTX (Berlakovich et al. 1994; Campbell et al. 1993), dependent drinking can occur years post-LTX (DiMartini 2000a). In one study, 15% of LTX recipients had their first drink within the first 6 months post-LTX—a finding that highlights the importance of early and intensive clinical follow-up to identify alcohol use at its onset (DiMartini et al. 2001).

Consistent predictors of posttransplant alcohol use have been difficult to identify. This may be due to the heterogeneity of the ALD transplant population and the potential selection bias whereby the most stable candidates are chosen, making this population different from the general alcohol-abusing/dependent populations (DiMartini et al. 2002). For example, a pretransplant history of illicit drug use has not been consistently associated with increased risk for posttransplant alcohol relapse in ALD recipients (Coffman et al. 1997; DiMartini et al. 2002; Fireman 2000; Foster et al. 1997; Newton 1999), possibly because many ALD recipients had discontinued their drug use many years prior to transplantation (Coffman et al. 1997). In one of the few prospective studies to examine posttransplant alcohol use, a pretransplant history of alcohol dependence, a family history of alcoholism, and prior rehabilitation experience (thought to be a marker for those with more severe addiction) were all found to be associated with posttransplant alcohol use ($P<0.05$). A prior history of other substance use was associated with a higher (but not statistically significant) risk of posttransplant drinking (DiMartini 2000b).

Compared with LTX candidates with alcohol dependence, LTX candidates with polysubstance dependence are more likely to have multiple prior addiction treatments; more likely to be diagnosed with personality disorders, especially cluster B type (antisocial, narcissistic, histrionic, borderline); and less likely to have stable housing, a consistent work history, or stable social support (Fireman 2000). One of the few studies to investigate all patients with a pre-LTX addiction history found not only that patients with a pre-LTX history of polysubstance use disorders had a higher relapse rate than those with alcohol dependence alone (38% vs. 20%) but also that the majority of polysubstance users demonstrated ongoing post-LTX substance use (Fireman 2000).

After transplantation, maintaining an open, nonjudgmental dialogue with transplant recipients appears to be the most effective way to identify alcohol and/or other substance use in the posttransplant period, and most recipients are open to discussing their substance use habits with the transplant team (DiMartini et al. 2001; Weinrieb et al. 2000). In the case of alcohol use, we have found that few patients with alcoholism can drink "socially" posttransplantation (Tringali et al. 1996) and that those who take their first drink often consume moderate to heavy amounts of alcohol (DiMartini et al. 2002). Therefore, total alcohol abstinence is recommended for these patients.

Medications that may reduce cravings and potentially diminish relapse risk for alcohol (e.g., acamprosate, ondansetron, naltrexone) or opioids (naltrexone) have not been studied in transplant patients. One study that attempted to use naltrexone in actively alcohol-relapsing LTX recipients found that patients were reluctant to use naltrexone as a result of its potential, albeit small, risk of hepatotoxicity (Weinrieb et al. 2001). Naltrexone can be a direct hepatotoxin at dosages higher than recommended (>300 mg/day) and is not recommended for patients with active hepatitis or liver failure. Disulfiram has been used in nontransplant populations to provide a negative reinforcement to drinking alcohol. This agent blocks the oxidation of alcohol at the acetaldehyde stage and can create severe nausea, vomiting, and hemodynamic instability. A metabolite of disulfiram is an inhibitor of cytochrome P450 3A4 (Madan et al. 1998), and posttransplantation may cause immunosuppressive medication toxicity. Use of disulfiram in transplant recipients could place these individuals at risk for serious harm and is not recommended (Cornelius et al. 2003).

Tobacco Use

Tobacco use by transplant candidates and recipients has received surprisingly little attention. Even in lung and heart transplantation, tobacco use is not routinely reported. Tobacco use coupled with immunosuppressive therapy, which also increases cancer risk (Nabel 1999), may result in higher rates of cancer posttransplantation. For ALD liver transplant recipients in one study, the rates of oropharyngeal cancer and lung cancer were 25 and 3.7 times higher, respectively, than rates in the general nontransplant population matched for age and gender (Jain et al. 2000), presumably as a result of tobacco use.

One study of heart transplant recipients found that 26%–50% of smokers resumed smoking posttransplantation (Bell and Van Triget 1991; Nagele et al. 1997). Compared with nonsmokers, smokers had higher rates of vasculopathy and of malig-

nancies (Nagele et al. 1997); they also had significantly worse survival, with none of the smokers surviving 11.5 years posttransplantation (vs. 80% of the nonsmokers surviving). When patients were grouped by carboxy-hemoglobin level, investigators found that no patients with a level higher than 2.5% were surviving 4 years after transplantation (Nagele et al. 1997). In this cohort, smoking appeared to be much more important than other classical risk factors (Nagele et al. 1997). Similarly, a study of liver transplant recipients found a higher rate of vascular complications in patients with a history of smoking (17.8% vs. 8% in patients without such a history; $P=0.02$); furthermore, having quit smoking 2 years prior to transplantation reduced the incidence of vascular complications by 58% (Pungpapong et al. 2002). In a prospective study of ALD liver transplant recipients, 53% were found to be using tobacco posttransplantation (DiMartini et al. 2002). A study of 60 heart transplant recipients reported that 3 patients had resumed smoking within 6 months following transplantation and that all 3 had also relapsed to drug or alcohol abuse (Paris et al. 1994). Another study of heart transplant recipients found that elevated posttransplant anxiety was associated with a higher risk of resuming smoking (Dew et al. 1996). The cessation of tobacco use (both smoked and smokeless) prior to transplantation is strongly recommended, given that many pretransplant users resume use posttransplantation.

Methadone-Maintained Candidates

Transplant program acceptance of opioid-dependent patients receiving methadone maintenance treatment (MMT) is a controversial issue.

In a recent survey of U.S. liver transplant programs (Koch and Banys 2001), of the 56% of programs that reported accepting patients for evaluation who were taking methadone, a surprising 32% required patients to discontinue their methadone use prior to transplantation. Of even more concern was the overall lack of experience with such patients (i.e., only 10% of the programs had treated more than five MMT patients). Although there are no studies of pretransplant methadone cessation in liver transplant patients, there exists an abundance of evidence showing that tapering methadone in stable methadone-maintained patients results in relapse to illicit opiate use in up to 82% of these individuals (Ball and Ross 1991). Requiring methadone tapering in stable opiate-dependent patients as a prerequisite for transplant candidacy potentially heightens the risk for relapse, and those who relapse would be denied transplantation.

In regard to posttransplant outcomes of MMT patients, Koch and Banys (2001) found that of the approximately 180 transplant patients on methadone maintenance at the time of the survey, relapse to illicit opiate use was reported for less than 10% of patients. Similar to other reports of noncompliance in transplant patients (see subsection "Posttransplant Compliance" earlier in this chapter), approximately 26% of MMT patients (not necessarily those who used illicit drugs) had compliance difficulties with immunosuppressive medications (Koch and Banys 2001). In general, the transplant programs did not consider that the noncompliance necessarily affected outcomes, and the transplant coordinator's impressions were that only 7 of 180 patients had poor outcomes (Koch and Banys 2001). In two small series of MMT LTX recipients (5 in each), overall long-term patient and graft survival were found to be comparable to those of other LTX recipients at the transplant centers, with none of the MMT patients evidencing posttransplant noncompliance

or illicit drug use (Hails and Kanchana 2000; Kanchana et al. 2002). Liu et al. (2003), in a study of the largest single cohort (N=36) of MMT LTX recipients to date, concluded that patient and graft survival were comparable to national averages (they did not use a control group, however). Although 4 patients (11%) reported isolated episodes of heroin use posttransplantation, relapses were not considered to have resulted in poorer outcomes. In summary, the data to date justify neither automatic exclusion of MMT patients from transplantation nor any requirement that such patients be tapered off methadone prior to transplant.

Personality Disorders

Personality disorders are characterized by persisting and inflexible maladaptive patterns of subjective experience and behavior that may create emotional distress and interfere with the individual's interpersonal relationships and social functioning. The requirements of successful transplantation can be too difficult for such an individual, as the process requires a series of adaptations to changes in physical and social functioning and significant ability to work constructively with both caregivers and the transplant team. By identifying personality traits and disorders, the psychiatrist can potentially predict patterns of behavior, recommend treatment, develop a behavioral plan with the team to work constructively with the patient, and render an opinion as to the candidate's ability to proceed with transplantation. Patients with personality disorders can require excessive amounts of time from the transplant team, which raises the issue of resource allocation as a potential selection criterion (Carlson et al. 2000). Not surprisingly, a majority of programs (50%–60% across organ types) consider personality disorders to be a relative contraindication to transplantation (Levenson and Olbrisch

1993). Yet all personality disorders should not be viewed similarly, because the behavioral and coping styles of different personality disorders can present varying degrees of concordance with the needs of transplantation. For example, the need for structure and orderliness of a candidate with obsessive-compulsive personality disorder would be more adaptive to the demands of transplantation than the coping style of a patient with borderline personality disorder.

The incidence of personality disorders in transplant populations is similar to that in the general population, ranging from 10% to 26% (Chacko et al. 1996; Dobbels et al. 2000), although in some cohorts estimates have been as high as 57% (Stilley et al. 1997). Case reports of patients with severe character pathology demonstrate the extent of compliance problems that can arise from these disorders, resulting in significant morbidity and recipient death (Surman and Purtilo 1992; Weitzner et al. 1999). The disturbances in interpersonal relationships that can occur with personality disorders also can decrease the likelihood that patients will have stable and reliable social supports during the pre- and posttransplant phases (Yates et al. 1998). Of the personality disorders, borderline personality disorder is considered to represent the highest risk for posttransplant noncompliance (Bunzel and Laederach-Hofmann 2000).

Whereas sociopathy has not consistently been associated with substance relapse in the addiction literature (Vaillant 1997), a survey of transplant programs in the United States revealed that 4 of 14 programs (29%) would reject a candidate with comorbid antisocial personality disorder and alcohol dependence (Snyder et al. 1996). In a study of 73 ALD transplant candidates, patients with severe personality disorders had higher rates of divorce and of comorbid drug abuse/dependence, lower IQs, and higher scores

on indicators of emotional impairment, and they were more likely, although not significantly so, to return to drug use during the pretransplant follow-up period (Yates et al. 1998). However, of this cohort, 3 patients with serious personality disorders underwent liver transplantation and did not relapse or become noncompliant in the early postoperative phase (Yates et al. 1998). In contrast, another study of 91 patients transplanted for ALD and followed for up to 3 years identified 18 patients exhibiting antisocial behavior (Coffman et al. 1997). Of those with antisocial behavior, 50% returned to either alcohol ($n=6$) or prescription narcotic addiction ($n=3$) posttransplantation, which was significantly higher than the 19.8% alcohol use by the total group (Coffman et al. 1997). In a prospective study of 125 heart transplant recipients, personality disorders were associated with posttransplant compliance problems ($P=0.007$) (Shapiro et al. 1995). Although personality disorders were not associated with survival, those individuals with personality disorders tended to have more graft rejection ($P=0.06$) (Shapiro et al. 1995).

Patients with personality disorders do best with ongoing pre- and posttransplant psychotherapy, specifically cognitive and behavioral interventions to promote compliance with the care regimen and to establish a working alliance with transplant team members (Dobbels et al. 2000). These patients should be given clear and consistent instructions on rules and requirements of transplantation, reinforced by regular outpatient appointments. A limited number of transplant center staff should maintain contact with the patient, and staff should communicate regularly among themselves and the outpatient psychiatric team (Carlson et al. 2000) to coordinate care and to reduce opportunities for cognitive distortions and splitting by the patient. A formal written contract can document the expectations of the transplant team and serve as a therapeutic treatment plan whereby the patient and team agree to work together toward common goals for the transplant recipient's health (Dobbels et al. 2000).

Psychotic Disorders

Although chronic and active psychosis is thought by many to be incompatible with successful transplantation, case reports of carefully selected patients with psychosis demonstrate that such patients can successfully undergo transplantation and survive after the procedure (DiMartini and Twillman 1994; Krahn et al. 1998). A recent survey of transplant psychiatrists at national and international transplantation programs identified only 35 cases of pretransplant psychotic disorders in transplant recipients from 12 transplant centers (Coffman and Crone 2002), suggesting that such patients are highly underrepresented among transplant recipients. Results of this survey confirmed previously expressed stipulations that patients with psychotic disorders be carefully screened before acceptance. Candidates should have demonstrated good compliance with both medical and psychiatric follow-up; possess adequate social supports, especially in-residence support; and be capable of establishing a working relationship with the transplant team. In this survey (Coffman and Crone 2002), risk factors for problems with compliance after transplantation included antisocial or borderline personality disorder features, a history of assault, positive psychotic symptoms, living alone, and a family history of schizophrenia. Posttransplant noncompliance with nonpsychiatric medications was found in 20% of patients (7 of 35) and noncompliance with laboratory tests in 17% (6 of 35 patients) (Coffman and Crone 2002); however, these numbers are similar to percentages of medication and laboratory testing noncompliance in general transplant populations. Overall, noncompliance resulted in rejection episodes in 5 patients (14%) and in reduced graft function or loss in 4 patients (12%) (Coffman and Crone 2002). Thirty-seven percent of patients experienced psychotic or manic episodes posttransplantation (not necessarily associated with immunosuppression), 20% attempted suicide (with two completed suicides), 20% experienced severe depression or catatonia, 5.7% committed assaults, 5.7% were arrested for disorderly conduct, and 8.6% required psychiatric commitment (Coffman and Crone 2002).

Although concerns have been raised in regard to the potential of immunosuppressive medications to produce or exacerbate psychotic symptoms, patients with a prior psychiatric history are not necessarily more susceptible to "steroid psychosis" than are patients without such a history (Hall et al. 1979), and appropriate use of antipsychotic medication is usually adequate to manage these symptoms if they emerge. Because transplant teams often overlook the early postoperative reinstitution of antipsychotic medications, it is essential that the psychiatrist devote careful attention to this issue during the immediate postoperative phase. If quick reintegration of the patient into his or her pretransplant outpatient psychiatric treatment regimen is not possible because of infirmity, interim in-home psychiatric follow-up care should be instituted.

Special Issues During the Pretransplant Phase

Living Donor Transplantation

Despite the physical risks, discomfort and pain, expense and inconvenience, and potential psychological consequences of donating an organ, increasing numbers of people are becoming donors, and transplant programs are considering living donation as one solution to the organ shortage. In fact, in 2001 the number of living donors exceeded the number of cadaveric donors (6,526 vs. 6,081) for the first time, with the majority from kidney donors, although an increasing number are coming from living liver donors in the form of a partial hepatectomy (UNOS 2004). Currently, more than 50% of kidney transplants come from living donors (UNOS 2004). Kidneys and portions of the liver, lung, pancreas, intestine, and even the heart (through a domino procedure in which a heart–lung recipient donates his or her heart) are donated for transplantation (Oaks et al. 1994; Rodrigue et al. 2001; Taguchi and Suita 2002).

Donation of an organ—putting one's life at risk to help another—is an incredibly generous and altruistic gift. Yet the evaluation of such donors is a complex process requiring assessment of the circumstances and motives of the donor, the dynamics of the relationship between donor and recipient, the severity of the recipient's illness, and family and societal forces. Current practice guidelines require a psychosocial evaluation for each potential donor to thoroughly examine these and other issues (Table 14–3) (Olbrisch et al. 2001; Surman 2002). Donors must be fully willing, independently motivated, and completely informed about the surgery. Yet for liver donors in particular, long-term sequelae that may affect the donor's future health, functioning, and even ability to obtain health insurance (due to the presence of a preexisting condition) are not known.

Living liver donation is a much more surgically complex, more invasive, and potentially more dangerous procedure than kidney donation. Although mortality rates have been less than 1% for both kidney and liver donors (Brown et al. 2003; Najar-

---

TABLE 14–3. Areas of assessment for living donor evaluation

Reasons for donation
Relationship between donor and recipient
Donor's knowledge about the surgery
Motivation
Ambivalence
Evidence of coercion/inducement
Attitudes of significant others toward the donation
Availability of support
Financial resources
Work- and/or school-related issues (if applicable)
Donor's psychological health, including the following:

  Psychiatric disorders
  Personality disorders
  Coping resources/style
  Pain syndromes
  Prior psychological trauma/abuse
  Substance use

---

ian et al. 1992), about one-third of liver donors have complications, with serious complications occurring in 14% of donors (Brown et al. 2003; Grewal et al. 1998). There have been consensus recommendations that all potential live liver donors be evaluated by an independent physician advocate (i.e., not a member of the transplant team responsible for the recipient's care) as part of the informed consent process (Abecassis et al. 2000; Conti et al. 2002) to avoid conflicts of interest. However, in only 50% of programs does a physician who is not part of the transplant team evaluate the potential donor (Brown et al. 2003). Kidney donors should expect to miss 4–6 weeks of work and liver donors 8–12 weeks of work, especially if the job involves heavy lifting. Since the late 1990s, laparoscopic donor nephrectomy has been increasingly used, a procedure that results in less postoperative pain, shorter hospital stays, overall quicker recovery times, and more favorable cosmetic results. Future research may also show this approach has psychosocial benefits as well.

Adult-to-adult living donor liver transplantation (LDLT) is a relatively new procedure in the United States, preceded by adult-to-child transplants. Whereas only 9 such procedures had been performed in the United States prior to 1998, in 2001 more than 400 adult-to-adult LDLTs were performed. Unfortunately, too few procedures are performed at any one center—and approaches to recipients and donors are too diverse across centers—to provide reliable and generalizable information about donor and recipient outcomes. In one study that examined outcomes of parent-to-child liver donation, psychological testing was found to be useful in identifying families that were more likely to experience problems postdonation (Goldman 1993). Although donor outcomes were reported as good, with donors experiencing increased self-esteem and satisfaction, marital dissolution occurred in 2 of the 20 families following donation (Goldman 1993). In another study, one donor committed suicide 2 years after donation, and although this event was deemed by the transplantation center to be unrelated to the donation, the details were not known (Brown et al. 2003).

In contrast with the United States, Japan has extensive experience with living liver donation as a result of cultural beliefs (lack of acceptance of brain death criteria) that hamper cadaveric donation. This created an environment in which living liver donation was necessary for LTX. Fukunishi et al. (2001) first reported on psychiatric outcomes in LDLT donors and recipients, identifying post-LTX psychiatric disorders (excluding delirium) in 37% of LDLT recipients and "paradoxical reactions" (including guilt over receiving donation, avoidant coping behaviors, and psychological distress) in 34% of recipients, despite favorable medical outcomes for both

recipient and donor. Ten percent of liver donors experienced major depression within the first month after donation. Fukunishi and colleagues (2003) speculated that, predonation, the stronger sense of duty of adult children donating to their parents masked their true concerns and fears. Following donation, these concerns manifested as anxiety, fear, and pain (Fukunishi et al. 2003). The prevalence of psychiatric disorders was higher in LDLT recipients than in a comparison group of living donor kidney recipients, suggesting a potentially greater need for psychiatric evaluation and care of LDLT patients.

Altruistic donors—those donating to an unknown recipient—pose one of the most complex challenges to transplant evaluation. In these cases, the psychosocial evaluation has particular importance in determining the suitability of the donor, and some believe that the medical standards for such donors should be higher (Friedman 2002). Altruistic donors are commonly viewed with some skepticism and are evaluated with greater caution than related donors. A detailed evaluation is critical, both to understand the motives and psychological meaning of the donation to the donor and to identify any financial or other types of compensation expected for the donation. A recent study of nondirected donors reported that 21% were excluded for psychological reasons (Matas et al. 2000). Psychological outcomes of altruistic liver donors are unknown.

Psychopharmacology in End-Stage Organ Disease

Although the treatment of transplant candidates and recipients can be complicated, a thorough knowledge of psychotropic pharmacokinetics in specific types of end-stage organ failure, coupled with careful attention to medication dosing, side effects, and drug interactions, can provide the necessary foundation for pharmacological management.

Liver Disease

Liver failure affects many key steps of medication pharmacokinetics, from absorption to metabolism, distribution, and elimination, causing changes in drug levels, duration of action, and efficacy. As the liver becomes cirrhotic, collateral blood vessels develop that circumvent the liver. Intrahepatic and extrahepatic physiological or surgical shunts create portal–systemic diversion that reduces liver perfusion and particularly affects first-pass metabolism as less drug is delivered to hepatic enzymes. Loss of functional parenchyma and hepatic enzymes decreases phase I metabolism (such as the cytochrome P450 enzyme system) or phase II metabolism (conjugation enzymes). Most psychotropic medications require hepatic metabolism and are highly bound to plasma proteins. The liver's production of plasma proteins is reduced, with a resulting increase of the free and pharmacologically active fraction of highly protein-bound drugs. All of these processes will raise effective drug levels, increasing the risk of drug side effects or toxicity (Leipzig 1990; Levy 1990; Pond and Tozer 1984). Increased volume of distribution resulting from fluid retention (ascites, peripheral edema) can lower effective levels of both water-soluble and highly protein-bound drugs (because more will be in the unbound state due to hypoproteinemia) (Klotz 1976).

One semiquantitative measure of liver functioning, the Child-Pugh Score (CPS), provides a readily reproducible and standardized method for assessing the degree of liver failure and is generalizable to patients with liver disease regardless of its etiology (Albers et al. 1989) (see Table 14–4). Although the categories of the CPS may overgeneralize the complexities of drug pharmacokinetics, the indices used identify impairment in pharmacokinetic functions (i.e., protein production, portal–systemic shunting, ascites), making the CPS total rating a useful guideline for psychotropic medication dosing. Nevertheless, for the newer medications, the pharmaceutical companies typically publish detailed information on drug absorption, metabolism, and elimination, with suggested guidelines for patients with hepatic disease (often using the CPS), and these documents should be referred to for specific medication dosing. In our clinical experience, we have found that patients rated as having CPS class A liver failure are early in the disease process and can usually tolerate 75% to 100% of a standard dosage. Those with CPS class B should be dosed more cautiously, starting with a 50%–75% reduction in the normal starting dose. As a result of the prolongation of the elimination half-life and the subsequent delay in reaching steady state, more gradual increments in dosing are required. Patients with CPS class B liver failure can often obtain relief or remission of symptoms with 50% of a typical psychotropic medication dosage. Those with CPS class C commonly have some degree of hepatic encephalopathy, and medication usage must be cautiously monitored to avoid worsening of the hepatic encephalopathy symptoms.

Renal Disease

Reduced renal clearance of drugs can occur in renal insufficiency, due to primary renal disease or from hypoperfusion occurring in hepatorenal syndrome (McLean and Morgan 1991) or severe heart failure (Shammas and Dickstein 1988). Reduced renal clearance is especially important for psychotropic medications that are predominantly excreted by the kidneys (e.g., lithium, gabapentin, topiramate, meth-

TABLE 14-4. Grading of liver disease severity using the Child-Pugh Score (CPS)

	1 point	2 points	3 points
Bilirubin (mg/dL)	<2.0	2–3	>3.0
Albumin (g/dL)	>3.5	2.8–3.4	<2.7
Protime (INR)	<1.5	1.6–2.4	>2.5
Ascites	None	Mild	Moderate
Encephalopathy	None	Stage 1–2	Stage 3–4

Note. Grading: A=5–6 points; B=7–9 points; C=10–15 points. INR=international normalized ratio.
Source. Adapted from Albers et al. 1989.

ylphenidate) and also for psychotropic drugs for which renal excretion of active metabolites is the primary route of elimination (e.g., venlafaxine and its active metabolite *O*-desmethylvenlafaxine). In uremia, drug oxidation is normal or accelerated, reduction and hydrolysis are slowed, glucuronide and glycine conjugations are normal, and acetylation may be slowed (Reidenberg 1977). Excess urea may cause gastric alkalinizing effects, decreasing intestinal absorption of some medications (Levy 1990). In renal failure, hypoalbuminemia, coupled with the inhibition of drug–protein binding from uremia and the accumulation of endogenous protein-binding inhibitors (Wilkinson 1983), can increase free drug concentrations, especially for drugs with protein binding greater than 80% (i.e., most psychotropics). For patients in renal failure, dosing can be complicated, and because of decreased protein binding, it is suggested that the drug dose be decreased by two-thirds from the normal administration (Levy 1990) However, for patients with severe renal failure, renally excreted psychotropic medications should be used very cautiously.

Heart Disease

In cardiac insufficiency and congestive heart failure, organ hypoperfusion (especially the liver and kidneys) and increased volume of distribution of drugs due to "third spacing" into interstitial tissues result in decreased drug metabolism and clearance (Shammas and Dickstein 1988). In one study of patients with congestive heart failure, the half-life of midazolam was prolonged by 50% and the plasma clearance was reduced by 32% (Patel et al. 1990). Right-sided heart failure can lead to intestinal and hepatic venous congestion, which can impair drug absorption and metabolism, respectively (Shammas and Dickstein 1988). Acute hypoxia can change blood flow dynamics. Splanchnic blood flow is reduced in the liver, decreasing metabolism, and renal blood flow is also reduced (du Souich and Erill 1978). Patients with severe right-sided heart failure with passive congestion of the liver should be treated as patients with hepatic insufficiency and dosages initially reduced by 50%.

Neuropsychiatric Side Effects of Immunosuppressive Agents

Recent advances in our understanding of immunology and the development of newer strategies for immunosuppression may significantly reduce the need for—if not obviate completely—long-term maintenance immunosuppression. In the future, transplant recipients of all organ types may require immunosuppressive medication dosages only one or two times a week, or not at all (Starzl 2002). This achievement would remove the final obstacle to long-term successful outcomes for transplant recipients, given that the majority of long-term morbidity and mortality is due to chronic immunosuppression (e.g., infections, renal failure, cancer). Additionally, reduced requirements for immunosuppressive medication would aid in medication compliance and relieve some of the financial burden of long-term immunosuppression. However, for now, transplant recipients will continue to require immunosuppressive therapy and to be subject to their potential neurotoxic and neuropsychiatric side effects.

Cyclosporine

Cyclosporine (Gengraf, Neoral, Sandimmune), a lipophilic polypeptide derived from the fungus *Tolypocladium inflatum Goma*, is used as a primary immunosuppressive agent. Side effects are usually mild and include tremor, restlessness, and headache (Wijdicks et al. 1999). A smaller proportion of patients (12%) experience more serious neurotoxicity characterized by acute confusional states, psychosis, seizures, speech apraxia, cortical blindness, and coma (deGroen et al. 1987; Wijdicks et al. 1995, 1996; Wilson et al. 1988). A higher incidence (33%) of serious neurotoxic side effects was reported in one study of 52 liver transplant recipients. Seizures were experienced by 25%; less commonly reported effects included central pontine myelinolysis, delirium, cerebral abscess, and psychosis (Adams et al. 1987).

More recent evidence suggests that earlier reports of serious neurological side effects may have been attributable to intravenous administration and higher dosages (Wijdicks et al. 1999). Cyclosporine

trough levels correlate poorly with cyclosporine neurotoxicity (Wijdicks et al. 1999), although in most studies symptoms resolved when the cyclosporine was discontinued and subsequently reinstated at a lower dosage (Wijdicks et al. 1999). Anticonvulsants can successfully treat cyclosporine-induced seizures but are not required long term (Wijdicks et al. 1996), and seizures may cease with reduction or discontinuation of cyclosporine. A few patients with serious clinical neurotoxic side effects have been found to have diffuse white matter abnormalities, predominantly in the occipitoparietal region, on computed tomography (CT) scanning (deGroen et al. 1987; Gijtenbeek et al. 1999; Wijdicks et al. 1995). In one case, symptoms of cyclosporine-induced cortical blindness resolved with drug discontinuation, although pathological evidence of CNS demyelination persisted for months afterward (Wilson et al. 1988).

Several mechanisms may contribute to the CNS neurotoxicity of cyclosporine. Hypocholesterolemia has been found in a high percentage of patients with serious neurotoxicity (deGroen et al. 1987; Wijdicks et al. 1995). Access may be particularly high in the white matter, with a relatively high density of low-density lipoprotein receptors (Wijdicks et al. 1995). In addition to hypocholesterolemia, hypertension, hypomagnesemia, and the vasoactive agent endothelin may play a role in the pathogenesis of cyclosporine neurotoxicity (Gijtenbeek et al. 1999).

Tacrolimus

Tacrolimus (FK506, Prograf), a macrolide produced by *Streptomyces tsukubaensis*, is used as primary immunosuppressive therapy, as rescue therapy for patients who fail to respond to cyclosporine, and as treatment for graft-versus-host disease. It is more potent and possibly less toxic than cyclosporine, although the neuropsychiatric side effects appear to be similar (Di-Martini et al. 1991; Freise et al. 1991). As with cyclosporine, neuropsychiatric side effects are more common with intravenous administration and diminish with oral administration and dosage reduction. Common symptoms include tremulousness, headache, restlessness, insomnia, vivid dreams, hyperesthesias, anxiety, and agitation (Fung et al. 1991). Cognitive impairment, coma, seizures, dysarthria, and delirium occur less often (8.4%) and are associated with higher plasma levels (Di-Martini et al. 1997; Fung et al. 1991). FK506 can produce symptoms of akathisia (Bernstein and Daviss 1992). However, a prospective study of 25 renal transplant recipients found no correlation between FK506 plasma levels and scores on an akathisia rating scale, although higher plasma levels were associated with higher levels of subjective restlessness, tension, and autonomic and cognitive symptoms of anxiety (DiMartini et al. 1996).

FK506 has low aqueous solubility and cannot be detected in the cerebrospinal fluid of patients with suspected neurotoxicity (Venkataramanan et al. 1991). However, because FK506 has been identified in the brain tissue of animals, it is believed to cross the blood-brain barrier in humans. In addition, more serious neurotoxic side effects (focal neurological abnormalities, speech disturbances, hemiplegia, and cortical blindness) may occur from higher CNS levels in patients who have a disrupted blood-brain barrier (Eidelman et al. 1991). In a study of 294 consecutive transplant recipients on FK506, those with preexisting CNS damage (e.g., from stroke, multiple sclerosis) were at higher risk for neurotoxic side effects (Eidelman et al. 1991). A rare syndrome of immunosuppression-induced leukoencephalopathy, involving demyelination (particularly in the parieto-occipital region and centrum semiovale), has been described in transplant recipients receiving FK506 (Small et al. 1996). The clinical presentation includes generalized seizures without a clear metabolic etiology and radiographic abnormalities in the cerebral white matter of the parietal/occipital lobes. Like other serious neurotoxic side effects, this syndrome is not associated with the absolute serum level of FK506 but does resolve on discontinuation of FK506 (Small et al. 1996). The mechanism of FK506 neurotoxicity is unclear but may include direct activity at the CNS neuronal level (Dawson and Dawson 1994) or an immune-mediated cause (Wilson et al. 1994).

Corticosteroids

Although chronic corticosteroid use has become less essential in immunosuppression for most patients posttransplantation, high dosages of corticosteroids are still employed in the early postoperative phase and also as "pulsed" dosages to treat acute rejection. Behavioral and psychiatric side effects are common, but conclusions regarding the incidence or characteristics of these effects—or the specific dosages required to cause such effects—are not well established. Serious psychiatric side effects have a reported incidence of 5%–6% (Kershner and Wang-Cheng 1989; Lewis and Smith 1983) and include a wide range of cognitive, affective, psychotic, and behavioral symptoms (Hall et al. 1979; Kershner and Wang-Cheng 1989; Lewis and Smith 1983; Varney et al. 1984). These side effects are reviewed elsewhere in this book, particularly in Chapter 6, "Endocrine Disorders," and Chapter 8, "Rheumatology."

Sirolimus

Sirolimus (SRL, rapamycin, Rapamune), a macrocyclic lactone isolated from *Streptomyces hygroscopicus*, is a recent addition to the posttransplant immunosuppressive armamentarium. The side-effect profile of sirolimus so far does not include neurotoxicity (Watson et al. 1999), perhaps because sirolimus does not block calcineurin (Sindhi et al. 2001). However, a systematic evaluation of sirolimus neurotoxicity has yet to be conducted.

Drug Interactions Between Psychotropic and Immunosuppressive Medications

Several immunosuppressive medications (specifically, tacrolimus and cyclosporine) are metabolized by cytochrome P450 3A4; thus, concurrent use of psychotropic medications that strongly inhibit 3A4 should be avoided. Specific cytochrome P450 3A4 inhibitors capable of interacting adversely with immunosuppressive medications, in decreasing order of inhibition, are as follows: fluvoxamine, nefazodone > fluoxetine > sertraline, tricyclic antidepressants, paroxetine > venlafaxine. There are case reports in which nefazodone has caused toxic tacrolimus levels (Campo et al. 1998) and a 70% increase in the trough plasma level of cyclosporine (Helms-Smith et al. 1996). In a study in which fluoxetine and tricyclic antidepressants were used to treat depressed transplant recipients, no difference in cyclosporine blood level–to–dosage ratios and dose–response relationships was found between those treated and those not treated with antidepressants (Strouse et al. 1996). This finding suggests that antidepressants with less cytochrome P450 3A4 inhibition may not have clinically meaningful drug interactions with these immunosuppressive medications.

References

Abecassis M, Adams M, Adams P, et al: The Live Organ Donor Consensus Group: consensus statement on the live organ donor. JAMA 284:2919–2926, 2000

Adams DH, Ponsford S, Gunson B, et al: Neurological complications following liver transplantation. Lancet 1(8539): 949–951, 1987

Albers I, Hartmann H, Bircher J, et al: Superiority of the Child-Pugh classification to quantitative liver function tests for assessing prognosis of liver cirrhosis. Scand J Gastroenterol 24:269–276, 1989

Ball J, Ross A: The Effectiveness of Methadone Maintenance Treatment. New York, Springer-Verlag, 1991

Bell M, Van Triget P: Addictive behavior patterns in cardiac transplant patients (abstract). J Heart Lung Transplant 10: 158, 1991

Berlakovich G, Steininger R, Herbst F: Efficacy of liver transplantation for alcoholic cirrhosis with respect to recidivism and compliance. Transplantation 58:560–565, 1994

Bernstein L, Daviss S: Organic anxiety disorder with symptoms of akathisia in a patient treated with the immunosuppressant FK506. Gen Hosp Psychiatry 14:210–211, 1992

Brown RS Jr, Russo MW, Lai M: A survey of liver transplantation from living adult donors in the United States. N Engl J Med 348:818–825, 2003

Bunzel B, Laederach-Hofmann K: Solid organ transplantation: are there predictors for posttransplant noncompliance? A literature overview. Transplantation 70:711–716, 2000

Campbell D, Beresford T, Merion R, et al: Alcohol relapse following liver transplantation for alcoholic cirrhosis: long term follow-up. Proceedings of the American Society of Transplant Surgeons (May): A131, 1993

Campo JV, Smith C, Perel JM: Tacrolimus toxic reaction associated with the use of nefazodone: paroxetine as an alternative agent. Arch Gen Psychiatry 55:1050–1052, 1998

Carlson J, Potter L, Pennington S, et al: Liver transplantation in a patient at psychosocial risk. Prog Transplant 10:209–214, 2000

Chacko RC, Harper RG, Gotto J, et al: Psychiatric interview and psychometric predictors of cardiac transplant survival. Am J Psychiatry 153:1607–1612, 1996

Coffman K, Crone C: Rational guidelines for transplantation in patients with psychotic disorders. Current Opinion in Organ Transplantation 7:385–388, 2002

Coffman KL, Hoffman A, Sher L, et al: Treatment of the postoperative alcoholic liver transplant recipient with other addictions. Liver Transpl Surg 3:322–327, 1997

Conti DJ, Delmonico FL, Dubler N, et al: New York State Committee on Quality Improvement in Living Liver Donation: A Report to New York State Transplant Council and New York State Department of Health, December 2002. Available at: www.health.state.ny.us. Accessed January 14, 2004

Cornelius JR, Bukstein O, Salloum I, et al: Alcohol and psychiatric comorbidity. Recent Dev Alcohol 16:361–374, 2003

Corley MC, Westerberg N, Elswick RK Jr, et al: Rationing organs using psychosocial and lifestyle criteria. Res Nurs Health 21:327–337, 1998

Crone CC, Wise TN: Psychiatric aspects of transplantation: evaluation and selection of candidates. Crit Care Nurse 19:79–87, 1999

Cupples SA, Steslowe B: Use of behavioral contingency contracting with heart transplant candidates. Prog Transplant 11:137–144, 2001

Dawson TM, Dawson VL: Nitric oxide: actions and pathologic roles. Neuroscience (preview issue):9–20, 1994

De Geest S, Borgermans L, Gemoets H: Incidence, determinants, and consequences of subclinical noncompliance with immunosuppressive therapy in renal transplant recipients. Transplantation 59:340–347, 1995

deGroen PC, Aksamit AJ, Rakela J, et al: Central nervous system toxicity after liver transplantation: the role of cyclosporine and cholesterol. N Engl J Med 317:861–866, 1987

Dew MA: Anxiety and depression following transplantation. Presented at the Contemporary Forums Conference on Advances in Transplantation, Chicago, IL, September 2003

Dew M, Kormos R: Early posttransplant medical compliance and mental health predict physical morbidity and mortality one to three years after heart transplantation. J Heart Lung Transplant 18:549–562, 1999

Dew MA, Roth LH, Thompson ME, et al: Medical compliance and its predictors in the first year after heart transplantation. J Heart Lung Transplant 15:631–645, 1996

Dew MA, Switzer GE, DiMartini AF, et al: Psychosocial assessments and outcomes in organ transplantation. Prog Transplant 10:239–259, 2000

Dew MA, Kormos RL, DiMartini AF, et al: Prevalence and risk of depression and anxiety-related disorders during the first three years after heart transplantation. Psychosomatics 42: 300–313, 2001

DiMartini A: Monitoring alcohol use following liver transplantation. Presented at the Research Society on Alcoholism, Symposium on Liver Transplantation for the Alcohol Dependent Patient. Denver, CO, June 2000a

DiMartini A: Psychosocial variables for predicting outcomes after liver transplantation for alcoholic liver disease. Presented at the Alcohol Induced Liver Disease: The Role of Transplantation conference, University of Massachusetts Medical Center, October 20, 2000b

DiMartini A, Twillman R: Organ transplantation in paranoid schizophrenia: two case studies. Psychosomatics 35:159–161, 1994

DiMartini A, Pajer K, Trzepacz P, et al: Psychiatric morbidity in liver transplant patients. Transplant Proc 23:3179–3180, 1991

DiMartini AF, Trzepacz PT, Daviss SR: Prospective study of FK506 side effects: anxiety or akathisia? Biol Psychiatry 40:407–411, 1996

DiMartini AF, Trzepacz PT, Pager K, et al: Neuropsychiatric side effects of FK506 vs. cyclosporine A: first-week postoperative findings. Psychosomatics 38:565–569, 1997

DiMartini A, Day N, Dew M, et al: Alcohol use following liver transplantation: a comparison of follow-up methods. Psychosomatics 42:55–62, 2001

DiMartini A, Weinrieb R, Fireman M: Liver transplantation in patients with alcohol and other substance use disorders. Psychiatr Clin North Am 25:195–209, 2002

Dobbels F, Put C, Vanhaecke J: Personality disorders: a challenge for transplantation. Prog Transplant 10:226–232, 2000

du Souich P, Erill S: Metabolism of procainamide in patients with chronic heart failure, chronic respiratory failure and chronic renal failure. Eur J Clin Pharmacol 14:21–27, 1978

Eggers P: Comparison of treatment costs between dialysis and transplantation. Semin Nephrol 12:284–289, 1992

Eidelman BH, Abu-Elmagd K, Wilson J, et al: Neurologic complications of FK 506. Transplant Proc 23:3175–3178, 1991

Everhart JE, Beresford TP: Liver transplantation for alcoholic liver disease: a survey of transplantation programs in the United States. Liver Transpl Surg 3:220–226, 1997

Everson G, Bharadhwaj G, House R, et al: Long-term follow-up of patients with alcoholic liver disease who underwent hepatic transplantation. Liver Transpl Surg 3:263–274, 1997

Feinstein AR: On white-coat effects and the electronic monitoring of compliance. Arch Intern Med 150:1377–1378, 1990

Fireman M: Outcome of liver transplantation in patients with alcohol and polysubstance dependence. Presented at Research Society on Alcoholism: Symposium on Liver Transplantation for the Alcohol Dependent Patient. Denver, CO, June 2000

Foster P, Fabrega F, Karademir S, et al: Prediction of abstinence from ethanol in alcoholic recipients following liver transplantation. Hepatology 25:1469–1477, 1997

Freise CE, Rowley H, Lake J, et al: Similar clinical presentation of neurotoxicity following FK506 and cyclosporine in a liver transplant recipient. Transplant Proc 23:3173–3174, 1991

Friedman L: All donations should not be treated equally. Journal of Law, Medicine, and Ethics 30:448–451, 2002

Fukunishi I, Sugawara Y, Takayama T, et al: Psychiatric disorders before and after living-related transplantation. Psychosomatics 42:337–343, 2001

Fukunishi I, Sugawara Y, Makuuchi M, et al: Pain in liver donors. Psychosomatics 44:172–173, 2003

Fung JJ, Alessiani M, Abu-Elmagd K, et al. Adverse effects associated with the use of FK506. Transplant Proc 23:3105–3108, 1991

Gijtenbeek HJ, van den Bent MJ, Vecht CJ: Cyclosporine neurotoxicity: a review. J Neurol 246:339–346, 1999

Goldman LS: Liver transplantation using living donors: preliminary donor psychiatric outcomes. Psychosomatics 34:235–240, 1993

Grewal HP, Thistlewaite JR Jr, Loss GE, et al: Complications in 100 living-liver donors. Ann Surg 228:214–219, 1998

Guyatt GH, Berman LB, Townsend M, et al: A measure of quality of life for clinical trials in chronic lung disease. Thorax 42:773–778, 1987

Hails KC, Kanchana T: Outcome of liver transplants for patients on methadone. Poster presentation, American Psychiatric Association Annual Meeting, Chicago, IL, May 2000

Hall RC, Popkin MK, Stickney SK, et al: Presentation of the steroid psychoses. J Nerv Ment Dis 167:229–236, 1979

Helms-Smith KM, Curtis SL, Hatton RC: Apparent interaction between nefazodone and cyclosporine (letter). Ann Intern Med 125:424, 1996

Iasi MS, Vieira A, Anez CI, et al: Recurrence of alcohol ingestion in liver transplantation candidates. Transplant Proc 35:1123–1124, 2003

Jain A, DiMartini A, Kashyap R, et al: Long-term follow-up after liver transplantation for alcoholic liver disease under tacrolimus. Transplantation 70:1335–1342, 2000

Kanchana T, Kaul V, Manzarbeitia C, et al: Transplantation for patients on methadone maintenance. Liver Transplant 8:778–782, 2002

Kershner P, Wang-Cheng R: Psychiatric side effects of steroid therapy. Psychosomatics 30:135–139, 1989

Klotz U: Pathophysiological and disease-induced changes in drug distribution volume: pharmacokinetic implications. Clin Pharmacokinet 1:204–218, 1976

Koch M, Banys P: Liver transplantation and opioid dependence. JAMA 285:1056–1058, 2001

Köllner V, Schade I, Maulhardt T, et al: Posttraumatic stress disorder and quality of life after heart or lung transplantation. Transplant Proc 34:2192–2193, 2002

Krahn LE, Santoscoy G, Van Loon JA: A schizophrenic patient's attempt to resume dialysis following renal transplantation. Psychosomatics 39:470–473, 1998

Laederach-Hofmann K, Bunzel B: Noncompliance in organ transplant recipients: a literature review. Gen Hosp Psychiatry 22:412–424, 2000

Leipzig RM: Psychopharmacology in patients with hepatic and gastrointestinal disease. Int J Psychiatry Medicine 20:109–139, 1990

Levenson JL, Olbrisch ME: Psychosocial evaluation of organ transplant candidates: a comparative survey of process, criteria, and outcomes in heart, liver and kidney transplantation. Psychosomatics 34:314–323, 1993

Levenson J, Olbrisch ME: Psychosocial screening and selection of candidates for organ transplantation, in The Transplant Patient. Edited by Trzepacz PT, DiMartini AF. Cambridge, England, Cambridge University Press, 2000, pp 21–41

Levy NB: Psychopharmacology in patients with renal failure. Int J Psychiatry Med 20:325–334, 1990

Lewis DA, Smith RE: Steroid-induced psychiatric syndromes: a report of 14 cases and a review of the literature. J Affect Disord 5:319–332, 1983

Liu L, Schiano T, Lau N, et al: Survival and risk of recidivism in methadone-dependent patients undergoing liver transplantation. Am J Transplant 3:1273–1277, 2003

Lucey M: Liver transplantation for alcoholic liver disease: a progress report. Graft 2:S73–S79, 1999

Madan A, Parkinson A, Faiman MD: Identification of the human P-450 enzymes responsible for the sulfoxidation and thionooxidation of diethyldithiocarbamate methyl ester: role of P-450 enzymes in disulfiram bioactivation. Alcohol Clin Exp Res 22:1212–1219, 1998

Matas AJ, Garvey CA, Jacobs CL, et al: Nondirected donation of kidneys from living donors. N Engl J Med 343:433–436, 2000

McLean AJ, Morgan DJ: Clinical pharmacokinetics in patients with liver disease. Clin Pharmacokinet 21:42–69, 1991

Miller P, Wikoff R, McMahon M, et al: Development of a health attitude scale. Nurs Res 31:132–136, 1981

Nabel GJ: A transformed view of cyclosporine. Nature 397:471–472, 1999

Nagele H, Kalmar P, Rodiger W: Smoking after heart transplantation: an underestimated hazard? Eur J Cardiothorac Surg 12:70–74, 1997

Najarian JS, Chavers BM, McHugh LE: 20 years or more of follow-up of living kidney donors. Lancet 340:807–810, 1992

Newton SE: Recidivism and return to work posttransplant. J Subst Abuse Treat 17:103–108, 1999

Oaks TE, Aravot D, Dennis C, et al: Domino heart transplantation: the Papworth experience. J Heart Lung Transplant 13:433–437, 1994

Olbrisch ME, Levenson J: Psychosocial assessment of organ transplant candidates: current status of methodological and philosophical issues. Psychosomatics 36:236–243, 1995

Olbrisch ME, Levenson JL, Hamer R: The PACT: a rating scale for the study of clinical decision making in psychosocial screening of organ transplant candidates. Clin Transplant 3:164–169, 1989

Olbrisch ME, Benedict SM, Haller DL, et al: Psychosocial assessment of living organ donors: clinical and ethical considerations. Prog Transplant 11:40–49, 2001

Olbrisch ME, Benedict SM, Ashe K, et al: Psychological assessment and care of organ transplant patients. J Consult Clin Psychol 70:771–783, 2002

Paris W, Muchmore J, Pribil A, et al: Study of the relative incidences of psychosocial factors before and after heart transplantation and the influence of posttransplantation psychosocial factors on heart transplantation outcome. J Heart Lung Transplant 13:424–432, 1994

Patel IH, Soni PP, Fukuda EK, et al: The pharmacokinetics of midazolam in patients with congestive heart failure. Br J Clin Pharmacol 29:565–569, 1990

Phipps L: Psychiatric evaluation and outcomes in candidates for heart transplantation. Clin Invest Med 20:388–395, 1997

Pond SM, Tozer TN: First-pass elimination: basic concepts and clinical consequences. Clin Pharmacokinet 9:1–25, 1984

Presberg BA, Levenson JL, Olbrisch ME, et al: Rating scales for the psychosocial evaluation of organ transplant candidates: comparison of the PACT and TERS with bone marrow transplant patients. Psychosomatics 36:458–461, 1995

Pungpapong S, Manzarbeitia C, Ortiz J, et al: Cigarette smoking is associated with an increased incidence of vascular complications after liver transplantation. Liver Transplant 8:582–587, 2002

Reidenberg MM: The biotransformation of drugs in renal failure. Am J Med 62:482–485, 1977

Rodrigue JR, Bonk V, Jackson S: Psychological considerations of living organ donation, in Biopsychosocial Perspectives on Transplantation. Edited by Rodrigue JR. New York, Kluwer Academic/Plenum Publishers, 2001, pp 59–70

Shammas FV, Dickstein K: Clinical pharmacokinetics in heart failure: an updated review. Clin Pharmacokinet 15:94–113, 1988

Shapiro PA, Williams DL, Foray AT, et al: Psychosocial evaluation and prediction of compliance problems and morbidity after heart transplantation. Transplantation 60:1462–1466, 1995

Sindhi R, Webber S, Venkataramanan R, et al: Sirolimus for rescue and primary immunosuppression in transplanted children receiving tacrolimus. Transplantation 72:851–855, 2001

Small S, Fukui M, Bramblett G, et al: Immunosuppression-induced leukoencephalopathy from tacrolimus. Ann Neurol 40:575–580, 1996

Snyder SL, Drooker M, Strain JJ: A survey estimate of academic liver transplant teams' selection practices for alcohol-dependent applicants. Psychosomatics 37:432–437, 1996

Starzl TE: The saga of liver replacement, with particular reference to the reciprocal influence of liver and kidney transplantation (1955–1967). J Am Coll Surg 195:587–610, 2002

Stevenson LW: Indications for listing and delisting patients for cardiac transplantation (Chapter 233 [Cardiac Transplantation], reviews and editorials), in Harrison's Online. Available at: http://harrisons.accessmedicine.com. Accessed August 3, 2004

Stilley CS, Miller DJ, Tarter RE: Measuring psychological distress in candidates of liver transplantation: a pilot study. J Clin Psychol 53:459–464, 1997

Stowe J, Kotz M: Addiction medicine in organ transplantation. Prog Transplant 11:50–57, 2001

Strouse TB, Fairbanks LA, Skotzko CE, et al: Fluoxetine and cyclosporine in organ transplantation: failure to detect significant drug interactions or adverse clinical events in depressed organ recipients. Psychosomatics 37:23–30, 1996

Surman OS: The ethics of partial-liver donation (comment). N Engl J Med 346:1038, 2002

Surman OS, Purtilo R: Reevaluation of organ transplantation criteria: allocation of scarce resources to borderline candidates. Psychosomatics 33:202–212, 1992

Taguchi T, Suita S: Segmental small-intestinal transplantation: a comparison of jejunal and ileal grafts. Surgery 131:S294–S300, 2002

Tringali RA, Trzepacz PT, DiMartini A, et al: Assessment and follow-up of alcohol-dependent liver transplantation patients: a clinical cohort. Gen Hosp Psychiatry 18 (suppl): 70S–77S, 1996

Twillman RK, Manetto C, Wellisch DK, et al: The Transplant Evaluation Rating Scale: a revision of the psychosocial levels system for evaluating organ transplant candidates. Psychosomatics 34:144–153, 1993

United Network of Organ Sharing (UNOS): 2003 Annual Report of the U.S. Organ Procurement and Transplantation Network and the Scientific Registry of Transplant Recipients: Transplant Data 1994–2002. Available at: http://www.OPTJ.org. Accessed January 14, 2004.

Vaillant GE: The natural history of alcoholism and its relationship to liver transplantation. Liver Transpl Surg 3:304–310, 1997

Varney NR, Alexander B, MacIndoe JH: Reversible steroid dementia in patients without steroid psychosis. Am J Psychiatry 141:369–372, 1984

Venkataramanan R, Jain A, Warty VS, et al: Pharmacokinetics of FK 506 in transplant patients. Transplant Proc 23:2736–2740, 1991

Watson CJ, Friend PJ, Jamieson NV, et al: Sirolimus: a potent new immunosuppressant for liver transplantation. Transplantation 67:505–509, 1999

Weinrieb RM, Van Horn DH, McLellan AT, et al: Interpreting the significance of drinking by alcohol-dependent liver transplant patients: fostering candor is the key to recovery. Liver Transplant 6:769–776, 2000

Weinrieb RM, Van Horn DH, McLellan AT, et al: Alcoholism treatment after liver transplantation: lessons learned from a clinical trial that failed. Psychosomatics 42:111–115, 2001

Weinrieb R, Van Horn D, Lin Y-T, et al: A controlled study of motivation enhancement therapy vs. community alcoholism treatment for alcoholic liver transplant candidates (abstract). Alcohol Clin Exp Res 29:76A, 2005

Weitzner MA, Lehninger F, Sullivan D, et al: Borderline personality disorder and bone marrow transplantation: ethical considerations and review. Psycho-Oncology 8:46–54, 1999

Wijdicks EF, Wiesner RH, Krom RA: Neurotoxicity in liver transplant recipients with cyclosporine immunosuppression. Neurology 45:1962–1964, 1995

Wijdicks EF, Eelco FM, Plevak DJ, et al: Causes and outcome of seizures in liver transplant recipients. Neurology 47:1523–1525, 1996

Wijdicks EF, Dahlke LJ, Wiesner RH: Oral cyclosporine decreases severity of neurotoxicity in liver transplant recipients. Neurology 52:1708–1710, 1999

Wilkinson GR: Plasma and tissue binding considerations in drug disposition. Drug Metab Rev 14:427–465, 1983

Wilson JR, Conwit RA, Eidelman BH, et al: Sensorimotor neuropathy resembling CIDP in patients receiving FK506. Muscle Nerve 17:528–532, 1994

Wilson SE, deGroen PC, Aksamit AJ, et al: Cyclosporin A–induced reversible cortical blindness. J Clin Neuro-Ophthalmol 8:215–220, 1988

Yates WR, Booth BM, Reed DA, et al: Descriptive and predictive validity of a high-risk alcoholism relapse model. J Stud Alcohol 54:645–651, 1993

Yates WR, LaBrecque DR, Pfab D: Personality disorder as a contraindication for liver transplantation in alcoholic cirrhosis. Psychosomatics 39:501–511, 1998

Self-Assessment Questions

Select the single best response for each question.

1. Which of the following organ transplantations has the highest percentage of patient survival at 10 years posttransplant?

    A. Lung.
    B. Kidney.
    C. Pancreas.
    D. Heart.
    E. Liver.

2. Psychosocial rating instruments may be of value in assessing patients' psychological preparation for and adaptation to transplant surgery. All of the following are true *except*

    A. The Psychosocial Assessment of Candidates for Transplantation (PACT) provides both an overall score and a series of subscale scores.
    B. The PACT can be quickly completed but requires scoring by a skilled and experienced clinician.
    C. The Transplant Evaluation Rating Scale (TERS) rates 10 discrete areas of psychological functioning.
    D. The TERS summary score is derived from a mathematical formula.
    E. The TERS is a self-administered instrument and does not require a skilled clinician to administer it.

3. Factors that increase the risk of posttransplantation psychiatric illness include all of the following *except*

    A. Pretransplant history of psychiatric illness.
    B. Longer hospitalization.
    C. Male gender.
    D. Greater physical impairment.
    E. Fewer social supports.

4. Because of the complexity of posttransplant immunosuppressive and other ongoing medical therapy, treatment compliance is crucial to the ongoing well-being of these patients. Which of the following statements is *not* true?

    A. Medical noncompliance in posttransplant patients is estimated at 20%–50%.
    B. Noncompliance is a major risk factor for graft rejection and may account for 25% of deaths after the initial recovery period.
    C. In the Dew study of compliance in heart transplant recipients (Dew et al. 1996), nonadherence to immunosuppressive medication regimens was the most frequent area of noncompliance.
    D. Persisting psychiatric illness after transplantation is associated with medical noncompliance.
    E. In an extensive literature review of posttransplant compliance for all organ types, one research team found that anxiety disorders were significantly associated with noncompliance.

5. As is true in other areas of medical practice in which a high degree of personal investment in care is required for a successful sense of physician–patient collaboration, patients with personality disorders present special challenges for the multidisciplinary transplant team. Which of the following personality disorders is associated with the highest rate of posttransplant noncompliance?

   A. Obsessive-compulsive.
   B. Borderline.
   C. Antisocial.
   D. Narcissistic.
   E. Avoidant.

15 Neurology and Neurosurgery

Alan J. Carson, M.Phil., M.D., M.R.C.Psych.

Adam Zeman, M.A., D.M., M.R.C.P.

Lynn Myles, B.Sc., M.D., F.R.C.S.Ed.

Michael C. Sharpe, M.A., M.D., F.R.C.P., F.R.C.Psych.

PSYCHIATRISTS WORKING in a clinical neurosciences center are likely to be required to address four main categories of clinical problems:

1. Cognitive impairment—either as a primary presentation or as a secondary complication of a known condition such as multiple sclerosis.
2. Neurological disease accompanied by emotional disturbance in excess of the clinical norm.
3. Physical symptoms that do not correspond to any recognized pattern of neurological disease.
4. Postneurosurgery complications—usually involving behavioral, cognitive, or emotional disturbance.

Stroke

A cerebrovascular accident, or stroke, is a rapidly developed clinical sign of a focal disturbance of cerebral function of presumed vascular origin and of more than 24 hours' duration. One of two main pathological processes is responsible: cerebral infarction or hemorrhage. *Infarction* may result from thrombosis of vessels or emboli lodged within them. *Hemorrhage* can be either into brain tissue directly or into the subarachnoid space. Infarctions are four times more common than hemorrhages and, as a result of a lower immediate fatality rate, are a much greater source of enduring disability, with approximately

75% survival, compared with 33% survival at 1 year after hemorrhage. Strokes are the third most common cause of death in the Western world. The Oxfordshire Community Stroke Project reported a population incidence of 2 per 1,000 for first-ever stroke (Bamford et al. 1988). Age is the major risk factor, although one-quarter of persons affected are younger than 65 years. Stroke occurs more commonly in men.

Cognitive Impairment and Delirium

Delirium affects 30%–40% of patients during the first week after a stroke, especially after a hemorrhagic stroke (Gustafson et al. 1993; Langhorne et al. 2000; Rahkonen et al. 2000). It is important to distinguish delirium from focal cognitive deficits affecting declarative memory. The presence of delirium after stroke is associated with poorer prognosis, longer duration of hospitalization, and increased risk of dementia (see Gustafson et al. 1991; Henon et al. 1999).

Dementia following stroke is common, occurring in approximately one-quarter of patients at 3 months after stroke (Desmond et al. 2000; Tatimichi et al. 1994a, 1994b). This figure rises significantly if focal impairments also are considered. *Vascular dementia* is an imprecise term referring to a heterogeneous group of dementing disorders caused by impairment of the brain's blood supply. These disorders fall into three principal categories: subcortical ischemic dementia, multiinfarct dementia, and dementia due to focal "strategic" infarction. The term *strategic infarction* describes the occurrence of unexpectedly severe cognitive impairment following limited infarction, often in the absence of classic signs such as hemiplegia. Sites at which infarctions can have such an effect include the thalamus, especially the medial thalamus; the inferior genu of the internal capsule; the basal ganglia; the left angular gyrus (causing Gerstmann's syn-

drome of agraphia, acalculia, left–right disorientation, and finger agnosia); the basal forebrain; and the territory of the posterior cerebral arteries (Clark et al. 1994; Kumral et al. 1999; Rockwood et al. 1999; Tatimichi et al. 1992, 1995).

Behavioral Changes

The diverse behavioral changes following stroke are not unique to this condition and can therefore serve as a helpful model for understanding the clinical consequences of focal cerebral lesions of other causes (Bogousslavsky and Cummings 2000).

Aphasia

Global aphasia leads to the abolition of all linguistic faculties. Consequently, the physician must draw inferences about mental state from the patient's behavior and nonverbal communication (Lazar et al. 2000).

Anosognosia

Anosognosia refers to partial or complete unawareness of a deficit. It may coexist with depression (Starkstein et al. 1990), a finding that both implicates separate neural systems for different aspects of emotions (Damasio 1994) and suggests that depression after stroke cannot be explained solely as a psychological reaction to disability (Ramasubbu 1994). In extreme cases, ownership of the limb is denied or, exceptionally, phantom limb sensations can occur. Anosognosia occurs more frequently with right-sided lesions, particularly those in the region of the middle cerebral artery (Breier et al. 1995; Jehkonen et al. 2000; Meador et al. 2000).

Affective Dysprosodia

Affective dysprosodia is impairment of the production and comprehension of those language components that communicate inner emotional states in speech. These components include stresses, pauses, cadence, accent, melody, and intonation. Affective dysprosodia is not associated with an actual deficit in the ability to *experience* emotions; rather, it is associated with a deficit in the ability to *communicate* or *recognize emotions in the speech of others.*

Apathy

Patients with apathy show little spontaneous action or speech; their responses may be delayed, short, slow, or absent (Fisher 1995). Apathy is frequently associated with hypophonia, perseveration, grasp reflex, compulsive motor manipulations, cognitive and functional impairment, and older age.

Depression

Although depression following stroke is commonly defined according to DSM-IV-TR (American Psychiatric Association 2000) or ICD-10 criteria (Starkstein and Robinson 1989), the imposition of these categorical diagnoses on patients who have suffered a stroke is problematic, because it is often unclear which symptoms are attributable to the stroke and which are attributable to depression (Gainotti et al. 1997, 1999). Most clinicians take a pragmatic approach, treating depression if the patient has symptoms suggestive of low mood or anhedonia accompanied by some somatic symptoms (e.g., insomnia, anorexia) as well as signs of lack of engagement with the environment (e.g., poor participation in physiotherapy).

Most epidemiological studies have suggested an association between depression and increased disability (Andersen et al. 1994b; Herrmann et al. 1995; Parikh et al. 1990; Pohjasvaara et al. 2001) and possibly mortality (House et al. 2001; Morris et al. 1993). Some, but not all, pharmacological treatment studies have suggested that effective treatment of the depression leads to a reduction in overall disability (Andersen et al. 1994a; Lipsey et al. 1984).

There has been much speculation over the etiological mechanisms of depression after stroke, and emphasis has been placed on the site of the stroke lesion. However, a recent meta-analysis reported that the available scientific literature does not support the left frontal hypothesis (Carson et al. 2000a).

It is generally recommended that treatment for depression should be started early, in order to maximize functional outcome. However, disappointingly few randomized, controlled trials have tested this recommendation. Most studies suggest an improved outcome in mood with early treatment, but findings on measures of function have been contradictory (Andersen et al. 1994a; Chemerinski et al. 2001; Gainotti et al. 2001; Lipsey et al. 1984; Robinson et al. 2000; Wiart et al. 2000). Although both selective serotonin reuptake inhibitors (SSRIs) and tricyclic antidepressants (TCAs) have been reported to be effective, the SSRIs are probably preferable because of fewer adverse effects, particularly if cognitive or cardiac function is compromised. Nonetheless, this greater tolerability must be balanced against the finding that nortriptyline was more effective than fluoxetine in the only trial that compared these agents (Robinson et al. 2000). Psychological treatment—in particular, cognitive-behavioral therapy (CBT)—may offer an alternative, but thus far psychological approaches have received only limited evaluation (Kneebone and Dunmore 2000; Lincoln and Flannagan 2003).

Anxiety

Anxiety disorders are common after stroke and probably share the same risk factors as depression (Astrom 1996). Estimates of prevalence have varied, with the reported prevalence of generalized anxiety disorder ranging from 4% to 28% (Astrom 1996). However, the percentage of patients experiencing anxiety symptoms appears to be 25%–30% (Burvill et al. 1995).

Poststroke anxiety states may include posttraumatic stress symptoms, with compulsive and intrusive revisiting of the event, as well as health worries, with checking and reassurance-seeking about the risk of recurrence (Lyndsay 1991). Although there is a paucity of controlled-trial evidence, it is our experience that these symptoms respond to standard drug and behavioral therapies.

Emotional Lability

Emotionalism, or emotional lability, is an increase in laughing or crying that occurs with little or no warning. It is frequent in acute stroke but can also occur with delayed onset (Berthier et al. 1996). The displayed emotions are not related to the patient's internal emotional state.

It has been suggested that the neurological basis is in serotonergic systems and that there is a specific response to SSRIs (Andersen et al. 1994a). In practice, the evidence is contradictory, with reports of response to TCAs as well (Robinson et al. 1993).

Catastrophic Reactions

Catastrophic reactions manifest as disruptive emotional behavior precipitated when a patient finds a task unsolvable (K. Goldstein 1939). The sudden, dramatic appearance of such marked self-directed and stereotypical anger or frustration can be startling for both staff and relatives. Catastrophic reactions generally occur independently of depression in acute stroke; however, many patients who show early catastrophic reactions go on to develop depression (Starkstein et al. 1993).

Psychosis

The incidence of psychosis following stroke is unknown, although a rate of 1% has been reported (Starkstein et al. 1987). Old age and preexisting degenerative disease seem to increase the risk (Starkstein 1998).

Obsessive-Compulsive Disorder

Obsessive-compulsive disorder (OCD) has been reported after cerebral infarctions, particularly those affecting the basal ganglia (Maraganore et al. 1991; Rodrigo et al. 1997).

Hyposexuality

Hyposexuality is a common complaint after stroke in both men and women. The symptoms generally are nonspecific, although health worries concerning body image and fear of recurrence may also be relevant.

Parkinson's Disease

Parkinson's disease (PD) is a degenerative condition characterized by tremor, rigidity, and bradykinesis.

Incidence

Two recent incidence studies of PD, one from Minnesota (Bower et al. 1999) and one from Finland (Kupio et al. 1999), estimated 10.8 cases per 100,000 person-years and 17.2 per 100,000 population, respectively.

Cognitive Features

Dementia with Lewy bodies, PD, and PD with dementia share common features, motor symptoms, and responses to treatment. Hallucinations and delusions occur in 29%–54% of cases of PD with dementia, and in 7%–14% of cases of PD without dementia (Aarsland et al. 2001). Delusions are often paranoid in type and mainly involve persecution and jealousy. Hallucinations usually occur in the presence of intact insight and frequently are visual and phenomenologically similar to those of Charles Bonnet syndrome (Diederich et al. 2000).

More recent studies have suggested that dopaminomimetic medication is a significant risk factor for psychosis (Aarsland et al. 1999). Other studies have shown correlations between psychotic symptoms and higher rates of cognitive dysfunction and depression, but no association with dosage or length of exposure to dopaminomimetic medication has been found (Giladi et al. 2000). The most likely etiology of psychosis in PD is a combination of cortical PD pathology and age-related loss of central cholinergic function. This is corroborated by the fact that psychotic symptoms in PD are often part of non-dopaminomimetic medication–induced toxic (i.e., delirious) states and that psychosis was commonly reported in the pre-levodopa era (Wolters and Berendse 2001). Cognitive impairment and sleep disruption are predictive of the development of psychosis (Arnulf et al. 2000).

Clinically, one should distinguish a delirium of acute onset with disorientation, impaired attention, perceptive and cognitive disturbance, and alterations in the sleep-wake cycle from true dopaminomimetic psychosis, which is a subacute, gradually progressive psychotic state unaccompanied by a primary deficit of attention. The former may be induced by drugs used in the treatment of PD, such as selegiline and anticholinergic medication. For the latter, active treatment is recommended only if symptoms begin to interfere with daily functioning. Dose reduction of dopaminomimetic drugs is seldom effective, and antipsychotic drugs are often required (Wolters and Berendse 2001). The atypical antipsychotic drugs clozapine and quetiapine are preferred (Cummings 1999; Rabinstein and Shulman 2000), and high-potency typical antipsychotics should be avoided. There is also increasing interest in the role of cholinesterase inhibitors in the treatment of dementia in PD, with early studies showing promising results (McKeith et al. 2000).

Emotional Symptoms

Depression is a common symptom in PD, with a prevalence of around 40%–50%. Timing of onset shows a bimodal distribution, with peaks during early and late stages of the disease (Cummings and Masterman 1999). Several large-scale studies have demonstrated that depression is one of the major determinants of quality of life in PD (Findlay 2002; Peto et al. 1995).

The diagnosis of depression in PD is difficult, because many depressive symptoms overlap with the core features of PD—motor retardation, attention deficit, sleep disturbance, hypophonia, impotence, weight loss, fatigue, preoccupation with health, and reduced facial expression. However, anhedonia and sustained sadness are important diagnostic features, particularly if they are out of proportion to the severity of motor symptoms (Brooks and Doder 2001).

There is currently insufficient evidence to offer definitive recommendations for treatment of depression in PD (Olanow et al. 2001). Although SSRIs are popular, there have been case reports of exacerbation of motor symptoms with fluoxetine, citalopram, and paroxetine (Ceravolo et al. 2000; Chuinard and Sultan 1992; Jansen Steur 1993; Leo 1996; Tessei et al. 2000). In recent small-scale trials, TCAs have led to better motor outcomes than have SSRIs; however, TCAs with marked anticholinergic activity (e.g., amitriptyline) should be used with caution because of their potential adverse effects on cognition and autonomic function (Olanow et al. 2001). Case report data suggest that electroconvulsive therapy (ECT) can be used to treat depression in PD (George et al. 1996; Olanow et al. 2001).

Anxiety phenomena are common in PD; they tend to occur later in the disease process than depression and are more closely associated with severity of motor symptoms (Witjas et al. 2002). In particular, marked anticipatory anxiety related to freezing of gait is common. Treatment is with antidepressant drugs (Olanow et al. 2001) and CBT.

Multiple Sclerosis

Multiple sclerosis (MS) is a demyelinating disorder of the central nervous system (CNS) that causes some degree of cognitive impairment in almost half of cases and that can present with unexplained subcortical dementia. It can also be accompanied by affective disorders. The presence of high signal abnormalities on T2-weighted magnetic resonance imaging (MRI) and of oligoclonal bands of immunoglobulin in the cerebrospinal fluid (CSF) helps to confirm the diagnosis.

Cognitive Impairment

Cognitive impairment affects at least half of all patients with MS (Beatty et al. 1989a; Heaton et al. 1985; Rao 1986; Rao et al. 1991). The impairment is generally described as a subcortical dementia characterized by problems with memory, speed of processing, and executive functions (Beatty et al. 1989b; Litvan et al. 1988; Rao et al. 1984, 1989). Cortical syndromes such as aphasia, apraxia, and agnosia are relatively rare. It is important to bear in mind that depression, anxiety, and fatigue all may affect cognitive function.

Mood Disorders

Mood disorders are common in MS, with more than half of patients reporting depressive symptoms. Mania and emotional lability are also frequently reported (Joffe et al. 1987; Sadovnick et al. 1996).

It is important to distinguish depression from the fatigue and pain that are commonly associated with MS. There are few randomized, controlled trials of anti-depressant drug therapy in MS, but those available suggest modest efficacy for these agents (Feinstein 1997), similar to their efficacy for depression associated with neurological illness in general (Schiffer and Wineman 1990).

Recent studies have found no increase in depression following interferon-beta therapy (Feinstein et al. 2002; Patten and Metz 2001; Zephir et al. 2003).

Fatigue

Fatigue is the most common single symptom in MS, affecting 80% of those with the disease (Fisk et al. 1994; Freal et al. 1984). It is generally a disabling and aversive experience and affects motivation as well as physical strength (Multiple Sclerosis Council for Practice Guidelines 1998). The mechanism of fatigue is poorly understood and almost certainly multifactorial. Amantadine 100 mg twice daily has been reported to be of some benefit, and modafinil 200 mg daily (Krupp et al. 1995) and pemoline have also been suggested as useful (Krupp et al. 1995). Some patients respond to SSRIs, and cognitive-behavioral treatments have also been used (Mohr et al. 2003).

Pain

Pain, both acute and chronic, is a common and disabling complication of MS. A recent study found that one-quarter of MS patients in a large community-based sample had severe chronic pain (Ehde et al. 2003). Mechanisms may include dysesthesia, altered cognitive function, and other MS complications such as spasticity. Of the acute pain syndromes, trigeminal neuralgia is the most common and usually responds to carbamazepine (Thompson 1998). Widespread chronic pain is more frequent and harder to manage. Dysesthetic limb pain is particularly troublesome; treatment is usually with amitriptyline or gabapentin (Samkoff et al. 1997).

Amnestic Syndromes

The amnestic or amnesic syndrome is an abnormal mental state in which learning and memory are affected out of proportion to other cognitive functions in an otherwise alert and responsive patient (Victor et al. 1971). The most common cause of amnestic states is Wernicke-Korsakoff syndrome, which results from nutritional depletion, particularly thiamine deficiency. Other causes include carbon monoxide poisoning, herpes simplex encephalitis and other CNS infections, hypoxic and other acquired brain injuries, stroke, deep midline cerebral tumors, and surgical resections, particularly for epilepsy. In the majority of cases, the pathology lies in midline or medial temporal structures, but there are also case reports of amnestic disorder following frontal lobe lesions.

Wernicke-Korsakoff Syndrome

Wernicke-Korsakoff syndrome results from thiamine depletion, and any cause of such depletion can lead to the syndrome. However, the overwhelming majority of cases are associated with chronic alcohol abuse, which results in both decreased intake and decreased absorption of thiamine.

The syndrome presents acutely with Wernicke's encephalopathy, which is characterized by confusion, ataxia, nystagmus, and ophthalmoplegia. Peripheral neuropathy can also be present. Parenteral administration of high-dose B vitamins is required as *emergency* treatment if the chronic state of Korsakoff's syndrome is to be avoided. The majority of cases of Korsakoff's syndrome occur following Wernicke's encephalopathy.

On clinical examination, patients with Korsakoff's syndrome may perform well on standard tasks of attention and working memory (serial sevens and reverse digit span) (Kopelman 1985) but have a dense anterograde amnesia, affecting declarative functions, and inconsistent, poorly organized retrieval of retrograde memories with a temporal gradient (more impairment for relatively recent than for more remote memories). Confabulation commonly occurs, particularly early in the disorder. Procedural memory remains relatively intact (Schacter 1987).

Other cognitive impairments and behavioral changes may accompany the amnesia but are much less marked.

The pathological process is neuronal loss, microhemorrhages, and gliosis in the paraventricular and periaqueductal gray matter (Victor et al. 1971). The mammillary bodies, mammillothalamic tract, and the anterior thalamus are the main structures affected (Mair et al. 1979; Mayes et al. 1988).

With vitamin replacement and abstinence from alcohol, the prognosis is fair: one-quarter of patients will recover, half will improve but with some persistent impairment, and one-quarter will show no change (Victor et al. 1971). High-dose B vitamins should be given to all patients acutely and probably continued, but it is unclear how long this therapy should be maintained.

Transient Amnestic Syndromes

Transient amnesia can occur in several contexts. Transient global amnesia (TGA) is a distinctive benign disorder affecting middle-aged or elderly persons, who become amnestic for recent events and unable to lay down new memories for a period of around 4 hours (Hodges and Ward 1989). Repetitive questioning by patients of their companions is a characteristic feature. Episodes can be provoked by physical or emotional stress and are usually isolated; the medium-term recurrence rate is 3% per year (Hodges 1991). There is good evidence that TGA results from reversible medial temporal lobe dysfunction, but the etiological mechanism is uncertain (Stillhard et al. 1990). Other causes of transient amnesia include transient cerebral ischemia (usually accompanied by other neurological symptoms and signs), migraine, drug ingestion, transient epileptic amnesia, and head injury.

Dementias Accompanied by Neurological Signs

Huntington's Disease

Huntington's disease (HD) is a dominantly inherited disorder, which causes a combination of progressive motor, cognitive, psychiatric, and behavioral dysfunction. It results from an abnormality in the *IT15* gene on chromosome 4 encoding the protein huntingtin.

Epidemiology

HD occurs at a prevalence of 5–7 per 100,000 population in the United States, with wide regional variations (Chua and Chiu 1994). The sexes are affected equally. Onset can be at any age but most commonly is in young or middle adulthood (Adams et al. 1988; Farrer and Conneally 1985).

Clinical Features

Chorea is the characteristic motor disorder. As the disease progresses, other extrapyramidal features can develop, including rigidity, dystonia, and bradykinesia, as well as dysphagia, dysarthria, and pyramidal signs (Harper 1991). Epilepsy can occur. Cognitive dysfunction goes hand in hand with the motor disorder. The dementia of HD is predominantly "subcortical," with impairment of attention, executive function, speed of processing, and memory (Zakzanis 1998). Psychiatric symptoms and behavioral changes are the norm (Mendez 1994; Zappacosta et al. 1996), with depression, apathy, and aggressiveness present in most cases (Burns et al. 1990; Levy et al. 1998) and psychosis,

obsessional behavior, and suicide in a significant minority (Almqvist et al. 1999; Cummings and Cunningham 1992; Folstein et al. 1979). Progression to a state of immobility and dementia typically occurs over a period of 15–20 years (Feigin et al. 1995). Cognitive and behavioral changes may predate the clear-cut emergence of symptomatic HD (Kirkwood et al. 1999).

Pathology and Etiology

The key pathological processes of HD occur in the striatum, caudate, and putamen. The underlying genetic abnormality is expansion of a "base triplet repeat" within the huntingtin gene. Repeat lengths beyond 39 give rise to symptomatic HD over the course of a normal life span (Duyao et al. 1993). Repeat lengths between 36 and 39 can cause disease. Repeats in the 27–35 range appear to be unstable and liable to increase into the pathological range in the next generation.

Investigation and Differential Diagnosis

The diagnosis of HD can now be made with confidence by DNA analysis. Counseling by a clinical geneticist is mandatory before presymptomatic testing and should be considered in other circumstances as well (Codori et al. 1997).

Management

Chorea may require treatment. However, given the cognitive and extrapyramidal side effects of the agents used (neuroleptics, dopamine depletors such as tetrabenazine or benzodiazepines), this is often best avoided (Rosenblatt et al. 1999). Other psychiatric symptoms should be treated along standard lines (Leroi and Michalon 1998).

Wilson's Disease (Hepatolenticular Degeneration)

Wilson's disease is a very rare, autosomal recessive, progressive degenerative brain disease caused by a disorder of copper metabolism, producing personality change, cognitive decline, extrapyramidal signs, and cirrhosis of the liver.

Clinical Features

Onset most commonly occurs in childhood or adolescence but can occur as late as the fifth decade (Bearn 1957). Patients may present to psychiatrists with personality change, behavioral disturbance (including psychosis), or dementia (Akil and Brewer 1995; Dening and Berrios 1989) or to neurologists with a variety of extrapyramidal signs, including tremor, dysarthria and drooling, rigidity, bradykinesia, and dystonia (Walshe 1986; Walshe and Yealland 1992). Careful examination reveals these features and also, in virtually all symptomatic cases, the presence of *Kayser-Fleischer rings*—rings of greenish-brown copper pigment at the edge of the cornea (Wiebers et al. 1997).

Pathology and Etiology

The causative genetic mutation is in the copper-transporting P-type ATPase coded on chromosome 13 (Bull et al. 1993). The result is excessive copper deposition in the brain, cornea, liver, and kidneys and increased copper excretion in urine. The caudate and putamen are the brain regions most severely affected, but other parts of the basal ganglia and the cerebral cortex are also involved (Mochizuki et al. 1997; Starosta-Rubinstein et al. 1987).

Investigation and Differential Diagnosis

Ninety-five percent of patients with Wilson's disease have low serum levels of the copper-binding protein ceruloplasmin. Normal ceruloplasmin levels and an absence of Kayser-Fleischer rings render the diagnosis very unlikely in cases with neuropsychiatric features (Ferenci 1998). Uncertain cases may require measurement of urinary copper excretion and liver biopsy for measurement of copper content (Pfeil

and Lynn 1999). DNA analysis is becoming increasingly available.

Management

Several copper-chelating agents (penicillamine, tetraethylene tetramine, zinc acetate) are available to treat patients with Wilson's disease (Pfeil and Lynn 1999).

Leukodystrophies

Leukodystrophies—recessively inherited or X-linked disorders of myelination—can be accompanied by neuropsychiatric syndromes, usually with associated neurological features. Metachromatic leukodystrophy, caused by a deficiency of the enzyme arylsulfatase A (Hyde et al. 1992), and adrenoleukodystrophy (see also Chapter 6, "Endocrine Disorders"), an X-linked disorder associated with abnormalities of very-long-chain fatty acids (James et al. 1984), are the most commonly encountered types.

Progressive Supranuclear Palsy

Progressive supranuclear palsy is characterized by supranuclear gaze palsy (an inability to direct eye movements voluntarily, especially vertical eye movements, in the presence of normal reflex eye movements); truncal rigidity, akinesia, postural instability, and early falls; bulbar features, with dysarthria and dysphagia; subcortical dementia; and alteration of mood (including pathological crying and laughing), personality, and behavior (De Bruin and Lees 1992). Neurofibrillary tangles, consisting of tau protein, are found in neurons of the basal ganglia and brain stem. Midbrain atrophy may be apparent on MRI.

Corticobasal Degeneration

Corticobasal degeneration typically manifests as a combination of limb apraxia (usually asymmetric at onset), alien limb phenomena, limb myoclonus, parkinsonism, and cognitive decline (Rinne et al. 1994). The pathology involves neuronal loss in both the basal ganglia and the frontal and parietal cortex, with intraneuronal accumulations of tau protein resembling that seen in progressive supranuclear palsy. MRI usually reveals frontoparietal atrophy.

Transmissible Spongiform Encephalopathies (Prion Dementias)

The transmissible spongiform encephalopathies are a group of rare dementias caused by an accumulation of abnormal prion protein within the brain. Related illnesses occur in animals.

Epidemiology

All of the transmissible spongiform encephalopathies are rare. Sporadic Creutzfeldt-Jakob disease, the most common human transmissible spongiform encephalopathy, occurs with an annual incidence of one per million, usually affecting people between the ages of 55 and 70 years (P. Brown et al. 1987). At the time of this writing, variant Creutzfeldt-Jakob disease has been diagnosed in some 150 individuals, almost all of them in the United Kingdom. Variant Creutzfeldt-Jakob disease more often develops in younger subjects than does sporadic Creutzfeldt-Jakob disease: most cases have occurred during the second through fourth decade of life (Will et al. 1996).

Clinical Features

Sporadic Creutzfeldt-Jakob disease typically causes a rapidly progressive dementia, with early changes in behavior, visual symptoms, and cerebellar signs. Within weeks to months, marked cognitive impairment develops, often progressing to mutism, with pyramidal, extrapyramidal, and cerebellar signs and myoclonus (P. Brown et al. 1994). The median duration of symptom onset to death is only 4 months,

although in rare cases the disorder evolves over several years. Iatrogenic cases of Creutzfeldt-Jakob disease have occurred when CNS tissue from patients with sporadic Creutzfeldt-Jakob disease has unwittingly been transferred from patient to patient by surgical instruments or used in medical procedures as a source of growth hormone, gonadotropins, dura mater, or corneal grafts (P. Brown et al. 2000).

Variant Creutzfeldt-Jakob disease differs markedly from sporadic Creutzfeldt-Jakob disease (Spencer et al. 2002). The initial symptoms are usually psychiatric, most commonly anxiety or depression, and often of sufficient severity to lead to psychiatric referral. Limb pain or tingling is common early in the course of the illness. After some months, cognitive symptoms typically develop, causing difficulty at school or work, together with varied neurological features including pyramidal, extrapyramidal, and cerebellar signs and myoclonus. The disorder evolves more slowly than does sporadic Creutzfeldt-Jakob disease, with an average duration of 14 months from symptom onset to death.

Pathology and Etiology

The light microscope reveals "spongiform change" in the brains of patients with transmissible spongiform encephalopathies; this change is associated with neuronal loss, gliosis, and deposition of "amyloid," which is composed of a protease-resistant form of prion protein (PrP) (Prusiner 2001).

Investigation and Differential Diagnosis

In sporadic Creutzfeldt-Jakob disease, the electroencephalogram (EEG) shows 1- to 2-per-second triphasic waves in 80% of cases at some time during the course of the illness (Steinhoff et al. 1996). Detection of 14–3–3 protein in CSF has a sensitivity and specificity of approximately 90% for sporadic Creutzfeldt-Jakob disease (Hsich et al. 1996). Brain biopsy is usually diagnostic but is rarely performed. In variant Creutzfeldt-Jakob disease, characteristic MRI abnormalities (especially high signal in the pulvinar nucleus) are found in a substantial proportion of cases, with a reported sensitivity of 78% and a specificity of 100% (Zeidler et al. 2000). Tonsillar biopsy has also been used as a confirmatory test, because prion protein scrapie (PrP^{SC}) is found in lymphoid tissue in variant Creutzfeldt-Jakob disease (Hill et al. 1999).

Management

At present, there is no proven remedy for the disease.

Whipple's Disease

Whipple's disease is rare but important, because it is treatable. Infection with *Tropheryma whippelii* typically causes a multisystem disorder with prominent steatorrhea, weight loss, and abdominal pain (Fleming et al. 1988). CNS involvement is common, and neurological and psychiatric symptoms and signs occur in the absence of systemic features (A.P. Brown et al. 1990; Louis et al. 1996). Small-bowel biopsy, lymph node biopsy, brain MRI, and CSF examination, including polymerase chain reaction studies to identify the causative organism, can all be helpful in diagnosis (Louis et al. 1996). Antibiotic treatment can be effective.

Subacute Sclerosing Panencephalitis

Subacute sclerosing panencephalitis is a rare complication of childhood measles in which intraneuronal persistence of a defective form of the virus in the CNS results in a continuing immune response, with high levels of measles antibody in the CSF. Neurological signs, including myoclonus, accompany the dementia (Lishman 1997; Risk et al. 1978). Average life expectancy from onset is 1–2 years.

Progressive Multifocal Leukodystrophy

Progressive multifocal leukodystrophy is caused by activation of JC papovavirus within the CNS in an immunocompromised patient. The resulting demyelination gives rise to pyramidal signs, visual impairment, and a subcortical dementia, usually with progression to death within months (Lishman 1997; Richardson 1961).

Paraneoplastic Syndromes

Paraneoplastic "limbic encephalitis" results from an immunological cross-reaction between tumor antigens and antigens present within the CNS. It can cause a range of psychiatric presentations, including cognitive deficits, confusional states, a pure amnestic syndrome, and affective symptoms. There are also paraneoplastic syndromes that affect the cerebellum, spinal cord, and peripheral nerves (Darnell and Posner 2003). Small cell lung cancer is the most common cause of paraneoplastic syndromes, but breast, ovarian, renal, and testicular carcinoma and lymphoma can also be responsible. The tumor may be small and sometimes initially undetectable by imaging. The diagnosis is supported by detection of antineuronal antibodies in serum or CSF, most commonly "anti-Hu"; the CSF often contains oligoclonal bands of immunoglobulin.

CNS Tumors, Hydrocephalus, and Subdural Hematoma

CNS tumors, hydrocephalus, and subdural hematoma are discussed in the section "Neurosurgical Issues" later in this chapter.

Epilepsy

Epileptic seizures are transient cerebral dysfunctions resulting from an excessive and abnormal electrical discharge of neurons.

Epidemiology

Incidence rates of 40–70 per 100,000 population in developed countries and 100–190 per 100,000 in developing countries are generally accepted. Most studies show a bimodal distribution for age of incidence, with increased rates in persons younger than 10 years and older than 60 years.

A specific etiological mechanism is identified in less than one-third of cases. These mechanisms include perinatal disorders, learning disabilities, cerebral palsy, head trauma, CNS infection, cerebrovascular disease, brain tumors, Alzheimer's disease, and substance misuse. In addition, many so-called idiopathic seizures are likely to have a genetic basis.

Clinical Features

Epilepsy constitutes a heterogeneous group of disorders with multiple causes, and its clinical features reflect this diversity. The key clinical distinction is between seizures with a focal and seizures with a generalized cerebral origin. The former are more likely to be associated with a detectable and potentially remediable cerebral lesion, whereas the latter are more likely to start in childhood or adolescence and to be familial. Despite the wide variety of possible seizure manifestations, an individual patient's seizures are usually stereotyped. Their clinical features result from a recurrent pattern of cortical hyperactivity during the ictal event followed by hypoactivity in the same area postictally.

Documentation of the clinical features of the seizure is the key to diagnosis. Because firsthand observation is seldom possible unless seizures are very frequent, the history of the episode, including an eyewitness account (or a home video), is of paramount importance.

Differential Diagnosis

Differentiating epilepsy from nonepileptic attack disorder (psychogenic epilepsy, or pseudoseizures) and syncope can be difficult (Roberts 1998). Other paroxysmal disorders should also be considered; these include transient ischemic attacks, hypoglycemia, migraine, transient global amnesia, cataplexy, paroxysmal movement disorders, and paroxysmal symptoms in MS. Attacks during sleep can pose particular difficulties, as informant reports are less useful.

Nonepileptic Attack Disorder

Nonepileptic attack disorder (NEAD), also referred to as "pseudoseizures" or "psychogenic epilepsy," is the most common alternative diagnosis, accounting for about 30% of patients presenting to clinics with suspected epilepsy (Reuber and Elger 2003) and having a reported community prevalence of 33 per 100,000 population (Benbadis and Allen 2000). The terminology is confused, and it is unclear whether NEAD is a specific diagnosis or a collective term for a number of psychiatric diagnoses or symptoms that may cause seizurelike spells, including conversion, panic attacks, hyperventilation syndrome (see Chapter 3, "Lung Disease"), posttraumatic stress disorder (PTSD), and catatonia. Some patients have both epilepsy and nonepileptic attacks, but probably only around 10% of individuals with NEAD fall into this category (Benbadis et al. 2001; Reuber et al. 2002). Many of these patients are learning disabled and at increased risk of both epilepsy and psychiatric disorders.

The diagnosis of NEAD can often be made on the basis of a careful history and examination. Clinical clues include the presence of prior or current psychiatric disorders, including somatoform disorders; atypical varieties of seizure, especially the occurrence of frequent and prolonged seizures in the face of normal interictal intellectual function and EEG; a preponderance of seizures in public places, especially in clinics and hospitals; and behavior during an apparent generalized seizure that suggests preservation of awareness (e.g., resistance to attempted eye opening, persistent aversion of gaze from the examiner). Previous childhood sexual abuse is very common but not universal among those with the diagnosis (Binzer et al. 2004). When doubt remains after careful clinical assessment and standard investigations, the gold standard for diagnosis is observation of attacks during videotelemetry. A normal EEG during or immediately following an apparent generalized seizure also provides strong evidence for NEAD.

The diagnosis of NEAD is regarded as distinct from deliberate falsification of attacks (i.e., malingering or factitious disorder). The majority of patients will be cooperative with investigation and diagnosis, even when they know in advance that the purpose is to confirm NEAD and refute epilepsy (McGonigal et al. 2002).

Psychiatric Complications

Recent record-linkage studies (Bredkjaer et al. 1998; Jalava and Sillanpaa 1996) have reported an increase in psychotic symptoms, particularly schizophreniform and paranoid psychoses, in men but not women with epilepsy. Studies have also shown a fourfold increase in overall rates of psychiatric disorder in both men and women with epilepsy compared with individuals in the general population, but not compared with patients with other medical diagnoses.

Psychosis
Psychotic symptoms may be categorized as transient postictal psychosis and chronic interictal psychosis. Patients with transient postictal psychosis often present with manic grandiosity with religious and mystical features (Kanemoto et al. 1996). In general, psychotic episodes do not start immediately after a seizure, but instead occur after a lucid interval of 2–72 hours.

Antiepileptic drugs may contribute to the development of psychotic symptoms. Several of the newer drugs have significant psychiatric side effects. Vigabatrin, an irreversible inhibitor of γ-aminobutyric acid (GABA) transaminase, has been shown to precipitate psychotic and affective symptoms in 3%–10% of patients (Levinson and Devinsky 1999). This effect occurs more commonly in patients with a history of psychiatric illness.

Depressive and Anxiety Disorders
Depressive and anxiety disorders affect approximately one-third of patients with epilepsy (Jalava and Sillanpaa 1996; Kanner and Balabanov 2002; Stefansson et al. 1998). Neurobiological, psychological, social, and iatrogenic factors have all been proposed and probably all are relevant (Lambert and Robertson 1999; Weigartz et al. 1999). Depression arising from learned helplessness may occur in patients with epilepsy as a consequence of repeatedly experiencing unpredictable and unavoidable seizures (Weigartz et al. 1999). The stress of having to live with a stigmatized chronic illness may also be relevant. Finally, the antiepileptic drugs used in the treatment of epilepsy can themselves be a cause of depression. The relationship between depression and epilepsy is bidirectional (i.e., each is a risk factor for the other). Depression is an independent risk factor for unprovoked seizures (Hesdorffer et al. 2000). This effect seems to be particularly marked for partial seizures.

Similarly, anxiety in epilepsy may have a complex etiology (M.A. Goldstein and Harden 2000). Anticipatory anxiety about having a seizure without warning can lead to agoraphobic-like symptoms and behavior.

The treatment of depressive and anxiety disorders in epilepsy is the same as that of anxiety and depression in the medically ill.

Tic Disorders

Tics are habitual spasmodic muscular movements or contractions, usually of the face or extremities, that are associated with a variety of disorders.

Gilles de la Tourette's syndrome (GTS) is characterized by a combination of multiple waxing and waning motor and vocal tics. These vary from simple twitches and grunts to complex stereotypies. Premonitory sensory sensations in body parts that "need to tic" are a common feature and complicate the picture, because their temporary suppressibility lends them a voluntary component. Other features are echolalia and coprolalia, particularly in severe cases. GTS is strongly associated with OCD (Eapen et al. 1997; Miguel et al. 1997; Muller et al. 1997; Zohar et al. 1997), with symmetry, aggressive thoughts, forced touching, and fear of harming oneself as common symptoms. Depressive symptoms are common (Wodrich et al. 1997). The prevalence of GTS is about 5 per 10,000 population, with a male:female ratio of 4:1 (Staley et al. 1997). Genetic studies have suggested a strong hereditary component in the disorder. The neurobiology of GTS remains elusive, with evidence supporting dysfunctions in dopaminergic basal ganglia circuitry receiving the most attention. Structural imaging findings in GTS are usually normal; functional imaging data are contradictory at present (Robertson and Stern 1998).

A syndrome known as pediatric autoimmune neuropsychiatric disorders associated with streptococcal infection (PANDAS) has been suggested, consisting of OCD accompanied by tics with abrupt onset or exacer-

bation associated with beta-hemolytic streptococcal infection (see Chapter 10, "Infectious Diseases"). PANDAS may lie on the same clinical spectrum as Sydenham's chorea, in which OCD and vocal tics have also been reported (Mercadante et al. 1997; Swedo et al. 1998), and may cast light on the etiology of GTS.

Management of GTS is multidisciplinary, with clear need to address the educational, social, and family consequences of the disorder. Dopamine antagonists remain the mainstay of pharmacological management (Jimenez-Jimenez and Garcia Ruiz 2001; Robertson and Stern 2000). Tetrabenazine, a presynaptic monoamine depletor with postsynaptic blockade, has shown considerable efficacy in case series studies (Jankovic and Beach 1997), without a risk of dystonia or tardive dyskinesia but with a high risk of depression. In patients with comorbid restless legs syndrome, the dopamine agonist pergolide was effective in alleviating Tourette's symptoms, despite the fact that one might have predicted the opposite effect (Lipinski et al. 1997). Clonidine is used widely in the United States, but in the United Kingdom its use is generally restricted to patients with comorbid attention-deficit/hyperactivity disorder (ADHD) symptoms (Leckman et al. 1991). In establishing treatment priorities, one should bear in mind that the associated OCD and ADHD symptoms probably cause more functional and educational disability than the tics themselves (Abwender et al. 1996; De Groot et al. 1997).

Somatoform and Conversion Disorders in Neurology

Somatic symptoms unexplained by neurological disease are commonly encountered in neurological practice and may be diagnosed as somatoform disorders. Other names that are used include "medically unexplained symptoms," "psychogenic disorders," and "functional disorders." DSM-IV and its text revision, DSM-IV-TR, use the term *somatoform disorders*, although patients may prefer the term *functional disorders* (Stone et al. 2002).

Epidemiology

Neurological symptoms in the absence of neurological disease or grossly disproportionate to disease are observed in approximately one-third of patients attending neurological clinics (Carson et al. 2000b). Functional weakness and paralysis, a subgroup of neurological symptoms occurring in the absence of disease, have an incidence of at least 4 per 100,000 (Binzer and Kullgren 1998), a rate similar to that of multiple sclerosis. In less than half of patients do the symptoms remit spontaneously (Carson et al. 2003).

Clinical Features

A careful history is essential, first concentrating on the somatic symptoms and only then exploring psychological and social factors. Pain is the most common symptom (Carson et al. 2000b). Particular attention should be paid to the presence of multiple somatic symptoms (multiple symptoms make a somatoform disorder more likely), depression or anxiety (particularly panic), and a history of previous functional symptoms or of multiple surgical operations in the absence of organic pathology (Barsky and Borus 1999). Childhood abuse and neglect, personality factors, recent stressful life events, secondary gain (financial or otherwise), and illness beliefs may all be relevant to management, but their presence does not allow one to infer a diagnosis (Stone et al. 2002).

The history of the onset of the symptoms can be particularly useful. Patients with conversion weakness will often describe symptoms suggestive of depersonalization or derealization at the time of onset. These symptoms may have been associated with a panic attack, physical trauma (often minor), or unexpected physiological events (e.g., postmicturitional syncope, sleep paralysis) (Stone et al. 2002).

The neurological examination has an important role in diagnosis. Helpful signs include inconsistency, Hoover's sign (Ziv et al. 1998), collapsing ("giveaway") weakness (Gould et al. 1986), and co-contraction (Knutsson and Martensson 1985). Muscle tone and reflexes should be normal but may be mildly asymmetrical. Mild temperature and color changes in the affected limb are common in conversion disorder (Stone et al. 2002). These signs should be demonstrated to patients in a collaborative, rather than confrontational, manner.

Pathology and Etiology

The etiology of conversion disorder remains unknown, and there is value in remaining neutral about the relative contributions of biological, psychological, and social factors (Kroenke 2002). In particular, one should be aware that although Freudian theory portrays conversion disorder as a mechanism for dealing with unconscious conflict and traumatic experience, this model fits only some patients. Early functional imaging studies have yielded intriguing results (Vuilleumier et al. 2001), and numerous, although often inconsistent, biochemical abnormalities have been described (Clauw and Chrousos 1997). The psychological and social risk factors for conversion disorder are similar to those for other somatoform disorders.

Investigation and Differential Diagnosis

Diagnostic accuracy is high, with an error rate between 5% and 10%, which compares favorably with diagnostic error rates for most common neurological conditions (Carson et al. 2003). Although clinicians tend to worry about missing "organic" disease and therefore are often very conservative in making a diagnosis of conversion disorder, available evidence suggests that the reverse is more of a problem, leading to iatrogenic complications of unneeded treatment and invalidism (Fink 1992; Nimnuan et al. 2000).

Management

Patients are best managed by a psychologically sophisticated medical approach (Sharpe and Carson 2000). Key steps are, first, an explicit acceptance of the reality of the symptoms; second, a nonstigmatizing, positive explanation of the diagnosis; and third, appropriate reassurance (Thomas 1987). Such reassurance communicates to the patient that a full, but gradual, recovery may be possible and that dreaded diseases, such as stroke and MS, have been ruled out. Dismissing the symptoms as "nothing wrong" risks antagonizing or humiliating the patient and is rarely a good basis for collaborative management.

There is evidence for moderate effectiveness of antidepressant drugs, particularly TCAs, with an odds ratio for improvement of 3.4 compared with placebo (O'Malley et al. 1999). Interestingly, this effectiveness does not depend on the presence of depressive symptoms. CBT may be effective in up to 70% of cases (Kroenke and Swindle 2000).

Neurosurgical Issues

Central Nervous System Tumors

Psychiatrists generally become involved in neuro-oncology cases after tumor diagnosis, when the clinical issues are adjustment, mood disorder, or cognitive impairment.

Patients with primary and metastatic CNS tumors typically present with headache, focal neurological signs, or seizures, but these tumors can also cause cognitive impairment, and occasionally their presentation mimics a dementing illness (Lishman 1997). Some brain tumors present with predominantly psychiatric symptoms. CT scanning should reveal their presence, although diffusely infiltrating tumors are sometimes missed in the early stages.

Hydrocephalus

Hydrocephalus is caused by dilatation of the ventricles within the brain resulting from elevation of CSF pressure. Hydrocephalus is termed *communicating* when the blockage to CSF flow is outside the ventricular system, *noncommunicating* when the blockage is within the ventricles. In normal-pressure hydrocephalus (NPH), the ventricles enlarge despite apparently normal CSF pressure.

Clinical Features

Hydrocephalus can cause a wide range of psychiatric symptoms and signs. These include enlargement of the head (if hydrocephalus is present in infancy), depression, headache, sudden death due to "hydrocephalic attacks" with acute elevation of intracranial pressure, progressive visual failure, gait disturbance (often "gait apraxia"), incontinence, and subcortical cognitive impairment progressing to dementia (Hebb and Cusimano 2001). NPH in older individuals is classically associated with the triad of gait apraxia, incontinence, and cognitive decline (Hebb and Cusimano 2001).

Diagnosis

In younger persons, the radiological signs of hydrocephalus are usually clear-cut on CT scanning. This may also be the case in some elderly patients, but in other older patients apparent hydrocephalus is sometimes due to atrophy of the brain. When enlargement of the ventricles raises a suspicion of communicating hydrocephalus in an older person, determination of whether the scan appearance is relevant to the clinical problem requires specialized studies—usually either serial lumbar punctures with observation of the clinical effects or neurosurgical studies of CSF pressure (Hebb and Cusimano 2001).

Management

Shunting of hydrocephalus—diversion of CSF from a CSF space to the venous system or peritoneum—can be beneficial or even lifesaving. However, the procedure is prone to complications, including subdural hematoma and shunt infection, and should not be undertaken lightly (Hebb and Cusimano 2001).

Subdural Hematoma

Subdural hematoma is caused by accumulations of blood and blood products in the space between the fibrous dura mater and the more delicate arachnoid membrane that encloses the brain. Acute subdural hematomas accumulate rapidly following head injury; chronic hematomas can often (although not always) be traced back to a head injury.

Clinical Features

Acute subdural hematomas are diagnosed close to the time of trauma, with headache, depressed level of consciousness, focal neurological signs, or appearance on CT scan. Chronic subdural hematomas give rise to more gradually evolving symptoms and signs, including confusion and dementia (Black 1984; Lishman 1997). Marked variability is often a clue to the diagnosis. Seizures can occur. Subdural hematomas are especially common in alcoholics (Selecki 1965).

Pathology

The variability of the clinical features is explained by the tendency of the size of a chronic subdural hematoma to wax and wane as a result of alternating phases of bleeding and of breakdown of the contents of the hematoma (McIntosh et al. 1996). Subdural hematomas exert their effects both by local compression and irritation of adjacent cortical tissue and by global "brain shift."

Investigation and Differential Diagnosis

Subdural hematomas can generally be diagnosed on computed tomography (CT) scanning. They are occasionally "isodense" with brain and therefore easily missed, especially if bilateral (Davenport et al. 1994).

Management

Management requires liaison with a neurosurgical team (Bullock and Teasdale 1990).

Subarachnoid Hemorrhage

Severe, prolonged headache of abrupt onset can be due to a subarachnoid hemorrhage, usually arising from a ruptured Berry aneurysm. A diagnosis of subarachnoid hemorrhage is suggested by the rapidity of onset ("thunderclap" headache, at its worst within a minute or so) and associated loss of consciousness, photophobia, vomiting, and neck stiffness. Psychiatrists are rarely involved in the diagnosis of subarachnoid hemorrhage but are frequently asked to evaluate patients in the postacute phase, as for stroke; symptoms of irritability and anxiety may be more common after subarachnoid hemorrhage than after stroke (Lishman 1997).

Fitness for Surgery

Psychiatrists may be requested to assess patients for fitness for neurosurgery. Such requests occur most commonly for patients with epilepsy and with Parkinson's disease. A general assessment of capacity and consideration of specific issues relevant to the operation in question are required.

Epilepsy Surgery

A psychiatric opinion should be sought prior to surgery if there are significant associated behavioral or social problems. Such problems include anticipated noncompliance with medication, severe personality disturbance, psychosis, mood disorder, unrealistic expectations of surgery, and an absence of social support. The presence of mental retardation is not an absolute contraindication to surgery but can complicate postsurgical care (Sperling 1994). It is noteworthy that poor psychological outcomes occasionally accompany good postoperative seizure control, and some patients need considerable psychological help in adjusting to life without seizures (Vickrey et al. 1993).

Parkinson's Disease Surgery

Neurosurgery for Parkinson's disease is an evolving field in which a number of different surgical interventions have been suggested (Olanow 2002). Psychiatric complications can follow surgery (e.g., corticobulbar syndromes and psychic akinesia after bilateral pallidotomy) (de Bie et al. 2002; Merello et al. 2001). However, there is little in the way of guidance available for the psychiatrist asked to assess a patient's fitness for neurosurgery. It is generally agreed that patients with dementia tend to have poor outcomes; otherwise, the same principles would apply as for epilepsy surgery.

References

Aarsland D, Larsen JP, Cummins JL, et al: Prevalence and clinical correlates of psychotic symptoms in Parkinson disease: a community-based study. Arch Neurol 56:595–601, 1999

Aarsland D, Ballard C, Larsen JP, et al: A comparative study of psychiatric symptoms in dementia with Lewy bodies and Parkinson's disease with and without dementia. Int J Geriatr Psychiatry 16:528–536, 2001

Abwender DA, Como PG, Kurlan R, et al: School problems in Tourette's syndrome. Arch Neurol 53:509–511, 1996

Adams P, Falek A, Arnold J: Huntington's disease in Georgia: age at onset. Am J Hum Genet 43:695–704, 1988

Akil M, Brewer GJ: Psychiatric and behavioural abnormalities in Wilson's disease. Adv Neurol 65:171–178, 1995

Almqvist EW, Bloch M, Brinkman R, et al: A worldwide assessment of the frequency of suicide, suicide attempts and psychiatric hospitalizations following predictive testing of Huntington disease. Am J Hum Genet 64:1293–1304, 1999

American Psychiatric Association: Diagnostic and Statistical Manual of Mental Disorders, 4th Edition, Text Revision. Washington, DC, American Psychiatric Association, 2000

Andersen G, Vestergaard K, Lauritzen L: Effective treatment of post-stroke depression with the selective reuptake inhibitor citalopram. Stroke 25:1099–1104, 1994a

Andersen G, Vestergaard K, Riis J, et al: Incidence of post-stroke depression during the first year in a large unselected stroke population determined using a valid standardized rating scale. Acta Psychiatr Scand 90:190–195, 1994b

Arnulf I, Bonnet AM, Damier P, et al: Hallucinations, REM sleep and Parkinson's disease: a medical hypothesis. Neurology 55:281–288, 2000

Astrom M: Generalised anxiety disorder in stroke patients: a 3-year longitudinal study. Stroke 27:270–275, 1996

Bamford J, Sandercock P, Dennis M, et al: A prospective study of acute cerebrovascular disease in the community: the Oxfordshire Community Stroke Project 1981–86, I: methodology, demography and incident cases of first-ever stroke. J Neurol Neurosurg Psychiatry 51:1373–1380, 1988

Barsky AJ, Borus JF: Functional somatic syndromes. Ann Intern Med 130:910–921, 1999

Bearn AG: Wilson's disease: an unborn error of metabolism with multiple manifestations. Am J Med 22:747–757, 1957

Beatty WW, Goodkin DE, Monson N, et al: Cognitive disturbances in patients with relapsing-remitting multiple sclerosis. Arch Neurol 46:1113–1119, 1989a

Beatty WW, Goodkin DE, Beatty PA, et al: Frontal lobe dysfunction and memory in patients with chronic progressive multiple sclerosis. Brain Cogn 11:73–86, 1989b

Benbadis SR, Allen HW: An estimate of the prevalence of psychogenic non-epileptic seizures. Seizure 9:280–281, 2000

Benbadis SR, Agrawal V, Tatum WO: How many patients with psychogenic non-epileptic seizures also have epilepsy? Neurology 57:915–917, 2001

Berthier ML, Kulisevsky J, Gironell A, et al: Poststroke bipolar affective disorder: clinical subtypes, concurrent movement disorders, and anatomical correlates. J Neuropsychiatry Clin Neurosci 8:160–170, 1996

Binzer M, Kullgren G: Motor conversion disorder: a prospective 2–5 year follow-up study. Psychosomatics 39:519–527, 1998

Binzer M, Stone J, Sharpe M: Recent onset pseudoseizures: clues to aetiology. Seizure 13:146–155, 2004

Black DW: Mental changes resulting from subdural haematoma. Br J Psychiatry 145:200–203, 1984

Bogousslavsky J, Cummings JL: Behavior and Mood Disorders in Focal Brain Lesions. New York, Cambridge University Press, 2000

Bower JH, Maraganore DM, McDonnell SK, et al: Incidence and distribution of parkinsonism in Olmsted County, Minnesota 1976–1990. Neurology 52:1214–1220, 1999

Bredkjaer SR, Mortensen PB, Parnas J: Epilepsy and non-organic non-affective psychosis: National Epidemiological Study. Br J Psychiatry 172:235–238, 1998

Breier JI, Adair JC, Gold M, et al: Dissociation of anosognosia for hemiplegia and aphasia during left-hemisphere anaesthesia. Neurology 45:65–67, 1995

Brooks DJ, Doder M: Depression in Parkinson's disease. Curr Opin Neurol 14:465–470, 2001

Brown AP, Lane JC, Murayama S, et al: Whipple's disease presenting with isolated neurological symptoms: case report. J Neurosurg 73:623–627, 1990

Brown P, Cathala F, Raubertas RF, et al: The epidemiology of Creutzfeldt-Jakob disease: conclusion of a 15-year investigation in France and review of the world literature. Neurology 37:895–904, 1987

Brown P, Gibbs CJ Jr, Rodgers-Johnson P, et al: Human spongiform encephalopathy: the National Institutes of Health series of 300 cases of experimentally transmitted disease. Ann Neurol 35:513–529, 1994

Brown P, Preece M, Brandel J-P, et al: Iatrogenic Creutzfeldt-Jakob disease at the millennium. Neurology 55:1075–1081, 2000

Bull PC, Thomas GR, Rommens JM, et al: Wilson's disease gene is a putative copper transporting P-type ATPase similar to the Menkes gene. Nat Genet 5:327–337, 1993

Bullock R, Teasdale G: Surgical management of traumatic intracranial haematomas, in Handbook of Clinical Neurology, Vol 15. Edited by Braakman R. Amsterdam, The Netherlands, Elsevier, 1990, pp 249–298

Burns A, Folstein S, Brandt J, et al: Clinical assessment of irritability, aggression and apathy in Huntington and Alzheimer disease. J Nerv Ment Dis 178:20–26, 1990

Burvill PW, Johnson GA, Jamrozik KD, et al: Anxiety disorders after stroke: results from the Perth Community Stroke Study. Br J Psychiatry 166:328–332, 1995

Carson AJ, Machale S, Allen K, et al: Depression after stroke and lesion location: a systematic review. Lancet 356:122–126, 2000a

Carson AJ, Ringbauer B, Stone J, et al: Do medically unexplained symptoms matter? A study of 300 consecutive new referrals to neurology outpatient clinics. J Neurol Neurosurg Psychiatry 68:207–210, 2000b

Carson AJ, Postmas K, Stone J, et al: The outcome of neurology patients with medically unexplained symptoms: a prospective cohort study. J Neurol Neurosurg Psychiatry 74:897–900, 2003

Ceravolo R, Nuti A, Piccini A, et al: Paroxetine in Parkinson's disease: effects on motor and depressive symptoms. Neurology 55:1216–1218, 2000

Chemerinski E, Robinson RG, Kosier JT: Improved recovery in activities of daily living associated with remission of PSD. Stroke 32:113–117, 2001

Chua P, Chiu E: Huntington's disease, in Dementia. Edited by Burns A, Levy R. London, Chapman & Hall, 1994, pp 827–844

Chuinard G, Sultan S: A case of Parkinson's disease exacerbated by fluoxetine. Hum Psychopharmacol 7:63–66, 1992

Clark S, Assal G, Bogousslavsky J, et al: Pure amnesia after unilateral left polar thalamic infarct: tomographic and sequential neuropsychological and metabolic (PET) correlations. J Neurol Neurosurg Psychiatry 57:27–34, 1994

Clauw DJ, Chrousos GP: Chronic pain and fatigue syndromes: overlapping clinical and neuroendocrine features and potential pathogenic mechanisms. Neuroimmunomodulation 4:134–153, 1997

Codori A-M, Slavney PR, Young C, et al: Predictors of psychological adjustment to genetic testing for Huntington's disease. Health Psychol 16:36–50, 1997

Cummings JL: Managing psychosis in patients with Parkinson's disease. N Engl J Med 340:801–803, 1999

Cummings JL, Cunningham K: Obsessive-compulsive disorder in Huntington's disease. Biol Psychiatry 31:263–270, 1992

Cummings JL, Masterman DL: Depression in patients with Parkinson's disease. Int J Geriatr Psychiatry 14:711–718, 1999

Damasio AR: Emotion, Reason and the Human Brain. New York, GP Putman & Sons, 1994

Darnell RB, Posner JB: Paraneoplastic syndromes involving the nervous system. N Engl J Med 349:1543–1554, 2003

Davenport RJ, Statham PFX, Warlow CP: Detection of bilateral isodense subdural haematomas. BMJ 309:792–794, 1994

de Bie R, de Haan RJ, Schuurman PR, et al: Morbidity and mortality following pallidotomy in Parkinson's disease: a systematic review. Neurology 58:1008–1012, 2002

De Bruin VMS, Lees AJ: The clinical features of 67 patients with clinically definite Steele-Richardson-Olszeweski syndrome. Behav Neurol 5:229–232, 1992

De Groot CM, Yeates KP, Baker GB, et al: Impaired neuropsychological functioning in Tourette's syndrome subjects with co-occurring obsessive and attention deficit symptoms. J Neuropsychiatry Clin Neurosci 9:267–272, 1997

Dening TR, Berrios GE: Wilson's disease: psychiatric symptoms in 195 cases. Arch Gen Psychiatry 46:1126–1134, 1989

Desmond DW, Moroney JT, Paik MC, et al: Frequency and clinical determinants of dementia after ischemic stroke. Neurology 54:1124–1131, 2000

Diederich NJ, Pieri V, Goetz CG: Visual hallucinations in Parkinson and Charles Bonnet syndrome patients: a phenomenological and pathogenetic comparison. Fortschr Neurol Psychiatr 68:129–136, 2000

Duyao M, Ambrose C, Myers R, et al: Trinucleotide repeat length: instability and age of onset of Huntington's disease. Nat Genet 4:387–392, 1993

Eapen V, Robertson MM, Alsobrook JP, et al: Obsessive-compulsive symptoms in Gilles de la Tourette syndrome and obsessive-compulsive disorder: differences by diagnosis and family history. Am J Med Genet 74:432–438, 1997

Ehde DM, Gibbons LE, Chwastiak L, et al: Chronic pain in a large community sample of persons with multiple sclerosis. Mult Scler 9:605–611, 2003

Farrer LA, Conneally PM: A genetic model for age at onset in Huntington's disease. Am J Hum Genet 37:350–357, 1985

Feigin A, Kieburtz K, Bordwell K, et al: Functional decline in Huntington's disease. Mov Disord 10:211–214, 1995

Feinstein A: Multiple sclerosis, depression and suicide: clinicians should pay more attention to psychology. BMJ 315:691–692, 1997

Feinstein A, O'Connor P, Feinstein K: Multiple sclerosis, interferon beta-1b and depression: a prospective investigation. J Neurol 249:815–820, 2002

Ferenci P: Wilson's disease. Clin Liver Dis 2:31–49, 1998

Findlay LJ (for Global Parkinson's Disease Steering Committee): Factors impacting on quality of life in Parkinson's disease: results from an international survey. Mov Disord 17: 60–67, 2002

Fink P: Surgery and medical treatment in persistent somatizing patients. J Psychosom Res 36:439–447, 1992

Fisher CM: Abulia, in Stroke Syndromes. Edited by Bogousslavsky J, Caplan L. Cambridge, England, Cambridge University Press, 1995, pp 182–187

Fisk JD, Pontefract A, Ritvo PG, et al: The impact of fatigue on patients with multiple sclerosis. Can J Neurol Sci 21:9–14, 1994

Fleming JL, Wiesner RH, Shorter RG: Whipple's disease: clinical, biochemical and histopathological features and assessment of treatment in 29 patients. Mayo Clin Proc 63:539–551, 1988

Folstein SE, Folstein MF, McHugh PR: Psychiatric syndromes in Huntington's disease. Adv Neurol 23:281–290, 1979

Freal JE, Kraft GH, Coryell JK: Symptomatic fatigue in multiple sclerosis. Arch Phys Med Rehabil 65:135–138, 1984

Gainotti G, Azzoni A, Razzano C, et al: The Post-Stoke Depression Scale: a test specifically devised to investigate affective disorders of stroke patients. J Clin Exp Neuropsychol 19:340–356, 1997

Gainotti G, Azzoni A, Marra C: Frequency, phenomenology and anatomical-clinical correlates of major post-stroke depression. Br J Psychiatry 175:163–167, 1999

Gainotti G, Antonucci G, Marra C, et al: The relation between poststroke depression, antidepressant, therapy and rehabilitation outcome. J Neurol Neurosurg Psychiatry 71:258–261, 2001

George MS, Wassermann EM, Post RM: Transcranial magnetic stimulation: a neuropsychiatric tool for the 21st century. J Neuropsychiatry Clin Neurosci 8:373–382, 1996

Giladi N, Treves TA, Paleacu D, et al: Risk factors for dementia, depression and psychosis in long standing Parkinson's disease. J Neurol Transm 107:59–71, 2000

Goldstein K: The Organism: A Holistic Approach to Biology Derived From Pathological Data in Man. New York, American Books, 1939

Goldstein MA, Harden CL: Epilepsy and anxiety. Epilepsy Behav 1:228–234, 2000

Gould R, Miller BL, Goldberg MA, et al: The validity of hysterical signs and symptoms. J Nerv Ment Dis 174:593–597, 1986

Gustafson Y, Olsson T, Erikkson S, et al: Acute confusional states (delirium) in stroke patients. Cerebrovasc Dis 1:257–264, 1991

Gustafson Y, Olsson T, Asplund K, et al: Acute confusional state (delirium) soon after stroke is associated with hypercortisolism. Cerebrovasc Dis 3:33–38, 1993

Harper PS: Huntington's Disease. London, England, WB Saunders, 1991

Heaton RK, Nelson LM, Thompson DS, et al: Neuropsychological findings in relapsing-remitting and chronic progressive multiple sclerosis. J Consult Clin Psychol 53:103–110, 1985

Hebb AO, Cusimano MD: Idiopathic normal pressure hydrocephalus: a systematic review of diagnosis and outcome. Neurosurgery 49:1166–1186, 2001

Henon H, Lebert F, Durieu I, et al: Confusional state in stroke: relation to pre-existing dementia, patient characteristics and outcome. Stroke 30:773–779, 1999

Herrmann M, Bartels C, Schumacher M, et al: Poststroke depression: is there a pathoanatomic correlate for depression in the postacute stage of stroke? Stroke 26:850–856, 1995

Hesdorffer DC, Hauser WA, Annegers JF, et al: Major depression is a risk factor for seizures in older adults. Ann Neurol 47:246–249, 2000

Hill AF, Butterworth RJ, Joiner S, et al: Investigation of variant Creutzfeldt-Jakob disease and other human prion diseases with tonsil biopsy samples. Lancet 353:183–189, 1999

Hodges JR: Transient Amnesia: Clinical and Neuropsychological Aspects. London, WB Saunders, 1991

Hodges JR, Ward CD: Observations during transient global amnesia: a behavioural and neuropsychological study of five cases. Brain 112:595–620, 1989

House A, Knapp P, Bamford J, et al: Mortality at 12 and 24 months after stroke may be associated with depressive symptoms at 1 month. Stroke 32:696–701, 2001

Hsich G, Kenney K, Gibbs CJ Jr, et al: The 14–3-3 brain protein in cerebrospinal fluid as a marker for spongiform encephalopathies. N Engl J Med 335:924–930, 1996

Hyde TM, Ziegler JC, Weinberger DR: Psychiatric disturbances in metachromatic leukodystrophy: insights into the neurobiology of psychosis. Arch Neurol 49:401–406, 1992

Jalava M, Sillanpaa M: Concurrent illnesses in adults with childhood-onset epilepsy: a population based 35-year follow up study. Epilepsia 37:1155–1163, 1996

James AC, Kaplan P, Lees A, et al: Schizophreniform psychosis and adrenomyeloneuropathy. J R Soc Med 77:882–884, 1984

Jankovic J, Beach J: Long-term effects of tetrabenazine in hyperkinetic movement disorders. Neurology 48:358–362, 1997

Jansen Steur ENH: Increase in Parkinson disability after fluoxetine medication. Neurology 43:211–213, 1993

Jehkonen M, Ahonen JP, Dastidar P, et al: Unawareness of deficits after right hemisphere stroke: double-dissociations of anosognosias. Acta Neurol Scand 102:378–384, 2000

Jimenez-Jimenez FJ, Garcia Ruiz PJ: Pharmacological options for the treatment of Tourette's disorder. Drugs 61:2207–2220, 2001

Joffe RT, Lippert GP, Gray TA, et al: Mood disorders and multiple sclerosis. Arch Neurol 44:376–378, 1987

Kanemoto K, Takeuchi J, Kawasaki J, et al: Characteristics of temporal lobe epilepsy with mesial temporal sclerosis, with special reference to psychotic episodes. Neurology 47:1199–1203, 1996

Kanner AM, Balabanov A: Depression and epilepsy: how closely related are they? Neurology 58:S27–S39, 2002

Kirkwood SC, Siemers E, Stout JC, et al: Longitudinal cognitive and motor changes among presymptomatic Huntington disease gene carriers. Arch Neurol 56:563–568, 1999

Kneebone II, Dunmore E: Psychological management of post-stroke depression. Br J Clin Psychol 39:53–65, 2000

Knutsson E, Martensson A: Isokinetic measurements of muscle strength in hysterical paresis. Electroencephalogr Clin Neurophysiol 61:370–374, 1985

Kopelman MD: Rates of forgetting in Alzheimer-type dementia and Korsakoff's syndrome. Neuropsychologia 23:623–638, 1985

Kroenke K: Integrating psychological care into general medical practice. BMJ 324:1536–1537, 2002

Kroenke K, Swindle R: Cognitive behavioural therapy for somatization and symptom syndromes: a critical review of controlled clinical trials. Psychother Psychosom 69:205–215, 2000

Krupp LB, Coyle PK, Doscher C, et al: Fatigue therapy in multiple sclerosis: results of a double-blind, randomized, parallel trial of amantadine, permoline and placebo. Neurology 45:1956–1961, 1995

Kumral E, Evyapan D, Balkir K: Acute caudate vascular lesions. Stroke 30:100–108, 1999

Kupio AM, Marttila RJ, Helenius H, et al: Changing epidemiology of Parkinson's disease in southwestern Finland. Neurology 52:302–308, 1999

Lambert M, Robertson MM: Depression in epilepsy: etiology, phenomenology, and treatment. Epilepsia 40:S21–S47, 1999

Langhorne P, Stott DJ, Robertson L, et al: Medical complications after stroke: a multicenter study. Stroke 31:1223–1229, 2000

Lazar RM, Marshall RS, Prell GD, et al: The experience of Wernicke's aphasia. Neurology 55:1222–1224, 2000

Leckman JF, Hardin MT, Riddle MA, et al: Clonidine treatment of Gilles de la Tourette's syndrome. Arch Gen Psychiatry 48:324–328, 1991

Leo RJ: Movement disorders associated with the serotonin selective reuptake inhibitors. J Clin Psychol 57:449–454, 1996

Leroi I, Michalon M: Treatment of the psychiatric manifestations of Huntington's disease: a review of the literature. Can J Psychiatry 43:933–940, 1998

Levinson DF, Devinsky O: Psychiatric adverse events during vigabatrin therapy. Neurology 53:1503–1511, 1999

Levy ML, Cummings JL, Fairbanks LA, et al: Apathy is not depression. J Neuropsychiatry Clin Neurosci 10:314–319, 1998

Lincoln NB, Flannagan T: Cognitive behavioural psychotherapy for depression after stroke: a randomised controlled trial. Stroke 34:111–115, 2003

Lipinski JF, Sallee FR, Jackson C, et al: Dopamine agonist treatment of Tourette disorder in children: results of an open-label trial of pergolide. Mov Disord 12:402–407, 1997

Lipsey JR, Robinson RG, Pearlson GD, et al: Nortriptyline treatment of post-stroke depression: a double blind treatment trial. Lancet S2:297–300, 1984

Lishman WA: Organic Psychiatry: The Psychological Consequences of Cerebral Disorder, 3rd Edition. Oxford, UK, Blackwell Science, 1997

Litvan I, Grafman J, Vendrell P, et al: Slowed information processing in multiple sclerosis. Arch Neurol 45:281–285, 1988

Louis ED, Lynch T, Kaufmann P, et al: Diagnostic guidelines in central nervous system Whipple's disease. Ann Neurol 40: 561–568, 1996

Lyndsay J: Phobic disorders in the elderly. Br J Psychiatry 159: 531–541, 1991

Mair WGP, Warrington EK, Weiskrantz L: Memory disorder in Korsakoff's psychosis: a neuropathological and neuropsychological investigation of two cases. Brain 102:749–783, 1979

Maraganore DM, Lees AJ, Marsden CD: Complex stereotypies after right putaminal infarction: a case report. Mov Disord 6:358–361, 1991

Mayes AR, Meudell PR, Mann D, et al: Location of lesions in Korsakoff's syndrome: neuropsychological and neuropathological data on two patients. Cortex 24:367–388, 1988

McGonigal A, Oto M, Russell AJ, et al: Outpatient video EEG recording in the diagnosis of non-epileptic seizures: a randomised controlled trial of simple suggestion techniques. J Neurol Neurosurg Psychiatry 72:549–551, 2002

McIntosh TK, Smith DH, Meaney DF, et al: Neuropathological sequelae of traumatic brain injury: relationship to neurochemical and biomechanical mechanisms. Lab Invest 74: 315–342, 1996

McKeith IG, Grace JB, Walker Z, et al: Rivastigmine in the treatment of dementia with Lewy bodies: preliminary findings from an open trial. Int J Geriatr Psychiatry 15:387–392, 2000

Meador KJ, Loring DW, Feinburgh TE, et al: Anosognosia and asomatognosia during intracarotid amobarbital inactivation. Neurology 55:816–820, 2000

Mendez MF: Huntington's disease: update and review of neuropsychiatric aspects. Int J Psychiatry Med 24:189–208, 1994

Mercadante MT, Do Roasario Campos MC, Marques-Dias MJ, et al: Vocal tics in Sydenham's chorea (letter). J Am Acad Child Adolesc Psychiatry 36:305, 1997

Merello M, Starkstein S, Nouzeilles M, et al: Bilateral pallidotomy for treatment of Parkinson's disease induced corticobulbar syndrome and psychic akinesia avoidable by globus pallidus lesion combined with contralateral stimulation. J Neurol Neurosurg Psychiatry 71:611–614, 2001

Miguel EC, Bauer L, Coffey BJ, et al: Phenomenological differences appearing with repetitive behaviours in obsessive-compulsive disorder and Gilles de la Tourette disorder. Br J Psychiatry 170:140–145, 1997

Mochizuki H, Kamakura K, Mazaki T, et al: Atypical MRI features of Wilson's disease: high signal in globus pallidus on T1 weighted images. Neuroradiology 39:171–174, 1997

Mohr DC, Hart SL, Goldberg A: Effects of treatment for depression on fatigue in multiple sclerosis. Psychosom Med 65:542–547, 2003

Morris PL, Robinson RG, Andrzejewski P, et al: Association of depression with 10-year poststroke mortality. Am J Psychiatry 150:124–129, 1993

Muller N, Putz A, Kathman N, et al: Characteristics of obsessive-compulsive disorder and Parkinson's disease. Psychiatry Res 70:105–114, 1997

Multiple Sclerosis Council for Practice Guidelines: Fatigue and multiple sclerosis: evidence-based management strategies for fatigue in multiple sclerosis. Washington, DC, Paralyzed Veterans of America, 1998

Nimnuan C, Hotopf M, Wessely S: Medically unexplained symptoms: how often and why are they missed? Q J Med 93:21–28, 2000

Olanow CW: Surgical therapy for Parkinson's disease. Eur J Neurol 9:31–39, 2002

Olanow CW, Watts RL, Koller WC: An algorithm (decision tree) for the management of Parkinson's disease: treatment guidelines. Neurology 56:S1–S88, 2001

O'Malley PG, Jackson JL, Santoro J, et al: Antidepressant therapy for unexplained symptoms and symptom syndromes. J Fam Pract 48:980–990, 1999

Parikh RM, Robinson RG, Lipsey JR, et al: The impact of poststroke depression on recovery in activities of daily living over a 2-year follow-up. Arch Neurol 47:785–789, 1990

Patten SB, Metz LM: Interferon beta-1 and depression in relapsing-remitting multiple sclerosis: an analysis of depression data from the PRISMS clinical trial. Mult Scler 7:243–248, 2001

Peto V, Jenkinson C, Fitzpatrick R, et al: The development and validation of a short measure of functioning and well being for individuals with Parkinson's disease. Qual Life Res 4:241–248, 1995

Pfeil SA, Lynn JD: Wilson's disease: copper unfettered. J Clin Gastroenterol 29:22–31, 1999

Pohjasvaara T, Vataja R, Leppavuori A, et al: Depression is an independent predictor of poor long-term functional outcome poststroke. Eur J Neurol 8:315–319, 2001

Prusiner SB: Neurodegenerative disorders and prions. N Engl J Med 344:1516–1526, 2001

Rabinstein AA, Shulman LM: Management of behavioural and psychiatric problems in Parkinson's disease. Parkinsonism Relat Disord 7:41–50, 2000

Rahkonen T, Makela H, Paanila S, et al: Delirium in elderly people without severe predisposing disorders: aetiology and 1-year prognosis after discharge. Int Psychogeriatr 12:473–481, 2000

Ramasubbu R: Denial of illness and depression in stroke (letter). Stroke 25:226–227, 1994

Rao SM: Neuropsychology of multiple sclerosis. J Clin Exp Neuropsychol 8:503–542, 1986

Rao SM, Hammeke TA, McQuillen MP, et al: Memory disturbance in chronic progressive multiple sclerosis. Arch Neurol 41:625–631, 1984

Rao SM, St Aubin-Faubert P, Leo GJ: Information processing speed in patients with multiple sclerosis. J Clin Exp Neuropsychol 11:471–477, 1989

Rao SM, Leo GJ, Bernardin L, et al: Cognitive dysfunction in multiple sclerosis, I: frequency, patterns and prediction. Neurology 41:685–691, 1991

Reuber M, Elger C: Psychogenic nonepileptic seizures: review and update. Epilepsy Behav 4:205–216, 2003

Reuber M, Fernandez G, Bauer J, et al: Diagnostic delay in psychogenic non-epileptic seizures. Neurology 58:493–495, 2002

Richardson EP: Progressive multifocal leukoencephalopathy. N Engl J Med 265:815–823, 1961

Rinne JO, Lee MS, Thompson PD, et al: Corticobasal degeneration. A clinical study of 36 cases. Brain 117(pt 5):1183–1196, 1994

Risk WS, Haddad FS, Chemali P: Substantial spontaneous long-term improvement in subacute sclerosing panencephalitis: six cases from the Middle East and a review of the literature. Arch Neurol 35:494–502, 1978

Roberts R: Differential diagnosis of sleep disorders, non-epileptic attacks and epileptic seizures. Curr Opin Neurol 11: 135–139, 1998

Robertson MM, Stern JS: Tic disorders: new developments in Tourette syndrome and related disorders. Curr Opin Neurol 11: 373–380, 1998

Robertson MM, Stern JS: Gilles de la Tourette syndrome: symptomatic treatment based on evidence. Eur Child Adolesc Psychiatry 9:60–75, 2000

Robinson RG, Parikh RM, Lipsey JR, et al: Pathological laughing and crying following stroke: validation of a measurement scale and a double-blind treatment study. Am J Psychiatry 150:286–293, 1993

Robinson RG, Schultz SK, Castillo C, et al: Nortriptyline versus fluoxetine in the treatment of depression and in short-term recovery after stroke: a placebo-controlled, double-blind investigation. Am J Psychiatry 157:351–359, 2000

Rockwood K, Bowler J, Erkinjuntti T, et al: Subtypes of vascular dementia. Alzheimer Dis Assoc Disord 13 (suppl 3):S59–S65, 1999

Rodrigo EP, Adair JC, Roberts BB, et al: Obsessive-compulsive disorder following bilateral globus pallidus infarction. Biol Psychiatry 42:410–412, 1997

Rosenblatt A, Ranen NG, Nance MA, et al: A Physician's Guide to the Management of Huntington's Disease, 2nd Edition. New York, Huntington's Disease Society of America, 1999

Sadovnick AD, Remick RA, Allen J, et al: Depression and multiple sclerosis. Neurology 46:628–632, 1996

Samkoff LM, Daras M, Tuchman AJ, et al: Amelioration of refractory dysesthetic limb pain in multiple sclerosis by gabapentin. Neurology 49:304–305, 1997

Schacter DL: Implicit memory: history and current status. J Exp Psychol Learn Mem Cogn 13:501–518, 1987

Schiffer RB, Wineman NM: Antidepressant pharmacotherapy of depression associated with multiple sclerosis. Am J Psychiatry 147:1493–1497, 1990

Selecki BR: Intracranial space-occupying lesions among patients admitted to mental hospitals. Med J Aust 1:383–390, 1965

Sharpe M, Carson A: Unexplained somatic symptoms, functional syndromes and somatization: do we need a paradigm shift? Ann Intern Med 134:926–930, 2000

Spencer MD, Knight RSG, Will RG: First hundred cases of variant Creutzfeldt-Jakob disease: retrospective case note review of early psychiatric and neurological features. BMJ 324:1479–1482, 2002

Sperling MR: Who should consider epilepsy surgery? Medical failure in the treatment of epilepsy, in The Surgical Management of Epilepsy. Edited by Wyler AR, Herman BR. Boston, MA, Butterworth-Heinemann, 1994, pp 26–31

Staley D, Wand R, Shady G: Tourette's disorder: a cross-cultural review. Compr Psychiatry 38:6–16, 1997

Starkstein SE: Mood disorders after stroke, in Cerebrovascular Disease. Edited by Grinsberg M, Bogousslavsky J. Oxford, England, Blackwell Science, 1998, pp 131–138

Starkstein SE, Robinson RG: Affective disorders and cerebral vascular disease. Br J Psychiatry 154:170–182, 1989

Starkstein SE, Pearlson GD, Boston J, et al: Mania after brain injury: a controlled study of causative factors. Arch Neurol 44:1069–1073, 1987

Starkstein SE, Berthier MI, Fedoroff P, et al: Anosognosia and major depression in 2 patients with cerebrovascular lesions. Neurology 40:1380–1382, 1990

Starkstein SE, Fedoroff JP, Price TR, et al: Catastrophic reaction after cerebrovascular lesions: frequency, correlates, and validation of a scale. J Neuropsychiatry Clin Neurosci 5:189–194, 1993

Starosta-Rubinstein S, Young AB, Kluin K, et al: Clinical assessment of 31 patients with Wilson's disease: correlations with structural changes on magnetic reasoning imaging. Arch Neurol 44:365–370, 1987

Stefansson SB, Olafsson E, Hauser WA: Psychiatric morbidity in epilepsy: a case controlled study of adults receiving disability benefits. J Neurol Neurosurg Psychiatry 64:238–241, 1998

Steinhoff BJ, Racker S, Herrendorf G, et al: Accuracy and reliability of periodic sharp wave complexes in Creutzfeldt-Jakob disease. Arch Neurol 53:162–166, 1996

Stillhard G, Landis T, Schiess R, et al: Bitemporal hypoperfusion in transient global amnesia: 99m-Tc-HM-PAO SPECT and neuropsychological findings during and after an attack. J Neurol Neurosurg Psychiatry 53:339–342, 1990

Stone J, Zeman A, Sharpe M: Physical signs: functional weakness and sensory disturbance. J Neurol Neurosurg Psychiatry 73:241–245, 2002

Swedo SE, Leonard HL, Garvey M, et al: Pediatric autoimmune neuropsychiatric disorders associated with streptococcal infections: clinical description of the first 50 cases. Am J Psychiatry 155:264–271, 1998

Tatimichi TK, Desmond DW, Prohovnik I, et al: Confusion and memory loss from capsular genu infarction: a thalamocortical disconnection syndrome? Neurology 42:1966–1979, 1992

Tatimichi TK, Desmon DW, Stern Y, et al: Cognitive impairment after stroke: frequency, patterns and relationship to functional abilities. J Neurol Neurosurg Psychiatry 57:202–207, 1994a

Tatimichi TK, Paik M, Begiella E, et al: Risk of dementia after stroke in a hospitalised cohort: results of a longitudinal study. Neurology 44:1885–1891, 1994b

Tatimichi TK, Desmond DW, Prohovnik I: Strategic infarcts in vascular dementia: a clinical and brain imaging experience. Arzneimittelforschung 54:371–385, 1995

Tessei S, Antonin A, Canesi M, et al: Tolerability of paroxetine in Parkinson's disease: a prospective study. Mov Disord 15:986–989, 2000

Thomas KB: General practice consultations: is there any point in being positive? BMJ 294:1200–1202, 1987

Thompson AJ: Symptomatic treatment in multiple sclerosis. Curr Opin Neurol 11:305–309, 1998

Vickrey BG, Hays RD, Hermann BP, et al: Outcomes with respect to quality of life, in Surgical Treatment of Epilepsies, 2nd Edition. New York, Raven, 1993, pp 623–635

Victor M, Adams RD, Collins GH: The Wernicke-Korsakoff syndrome. Philadelphia, PA, FA Davis, 1971

Vuilleumier P, Chicherio C, Assal F, et al: Functional neuroanatomical correlates of hysterical sensorimotor loss. Brain 124:1077–1090, 2001

Walshe JM: Wilson's disease, in Handbook of Clinical Neurology. Edited by Vinken PJ, Bruyn GW, Klawans HL. New York, Elsevier, 1986, pp 223–238

Walshe JM, Yealland M: Wilson's disease: the problem of delayed diagnosis. J Neurol Neurosurg Psychiatry 55:692–696, 1992

Weigartz P, Seidenberg M, Woodard A, et al: Comorbid psychiatric disorder in chronic epilepsy: recognition and etiology of depression. Neurology 53:S3–S8, 1999

Wiart L, Petit H, Joseph PA, et al: Fluoxetine in early post-stroke depression: a double-blind placebo-controlled study. Stroke 31:1829–1832, 2000

Wiebers DO, Hollenhorst RW, Goldstein NP: The ophthalmologic manifestations of Wilson's disease. Mayo Clin Proc 52:409–416, 1997

Will RG, Ironside JW, Zeidler M, et al: A new variant of Creutzfeldt-Jakob disease in the UK. Lancet 347:921–925, 1996

Witjas T, Kaphan E, Azulay JP, et al: Nonmotor fluctuations in Parkinson's disease: frequent and disabling. Neurology 59:408–413, 2002

Wodrich DL, Benjamin E, Lachar D: Tourette's syndrome and psychopathology in a child psychiatry setting. J Am Acad Child Adolesc Psychiatry 26:1618–1624, 1997

Wolters ECH, Berendse HW: Management of psychosis in Parkinson's disease. Curr Opin Neurol 14:499–504, 2001

Zakzanis KK: The subcortical dementia of Huntington's disease. J Clin Exp Neuropsychol 20:565–578, 1998

Zappacosta B, Monza D, Meoni C, et al: Psychiatric symptoms do not correlate with cognitive decline, motor symptoms or CAG repeat length in Huntington's disease. Arch Neurol 53:493–497, 1996

Zeidler M, Sellar RJ, Collie DA, et al: The pulvinar sign on magnetic resonance imaging in variant CJD. Lancet 355: 1412–1418, 2000

Zephir H, De Seze J, Stojkovic T, et al: Multiple sclerosis and depression: influence of interferon beta therapy. Mult Scler 9:284–288, 2003

Ziv I, Djaldetti R, Zoldan Y, et al: Diagnosis of "nonorganic" limb paresis by a novel objective motor assessment: the quantitative Hoover's test. J Neurol 245:797–802, 1998

Zohar AH, Pauls DL, Ratzoni G, et al: Obsessive-compulsive disorder with and without tics in an epidemiological sample of adolescents. Am J Psychiatry 154:274–276, 1997

Self-Assessment Questions

Select the single best response for each question.

1. Which of the following statements concerning a cerebrovascular accident or stroke is *false?*
   A. The survival rate 1 year after cerebral hemorrhage is 33%.
   B. Cerebral hemorrhage is four times more common than cerebral infarction.
   C. The survival rate 1 year after cerebral infarction is 75%.
   D. Strokes are the third most common cause of death in the Western world.
   E. Stroke occurs more commonly in men than in women.

2. Which of the following is a category or type of vascular dementia?
   A. Subcortical ischemic dementia.
   B. Multi-infarct dementia.
   C. Dementia due to focal "strategic" infarction.
   D. A and B.
   E. A, B, and C.

3. Which of the following statements concerning psychiatric symptoms in Parkinson's disease (PD) is *true?*
   A. Hallucinations and delusions occur in 29%–54% of cases of PD without dementia.
   B. Hallucinations in PD are usually auditory and occur without insight.
   C. Depression has a prevalence rate of 40%–50% in PD.
   D. High-potency typical antipsychotics are preferred in PD because of fewer anticholinergic side effects.
   E. Anxiety is uncommon in PD and usually occurs earlier in the disease process.

4. Which of the following statements about psychiatric symptoms in multiple sclerosis (MS) is *false?*
   A. More than half of MS patients report depressive symptoms.
   B. Cortical syndromes such as aphasia, apraxia, and agnosia are relatively rare.
   C. Cognitive impairment is rare, affecting less than 10% of MS patients.
   D. Fatigue is the most common single symptom in MS.
   E. Acute and chronic pain are common and disabling complications of MS.

5. Which of the following statements concerning Huntington's disease is *true?*
   A. Has a prevalence rate of 5–7 per 100,000 population.
   B. Affects men more than women.
   C. The most common age at onset is in young or middle adulthood.
   D. A and C.
   E. A, B, and C.

16 Obstetrics and Gynecology

Nada L. Stotland, M.D., M.P.H.

Donna E. Stewart, M.D., F.R.C.P.C.

Sarah E. Munce, M.Sc.

Iram Ashraf, B.Sc.

REPRODUCTIVE EXPERIENCES and behavior are fraught with intense feelings: joy, pride, and passion, as well as shame, guilt, and fear. Therefore, interactions between obstetrics and gynecology and psychiatry are particularly important. Tradition or regulations sometimes separate a patient's obstetrics and gynecology care from her mental health care and may divide her mental health care among two or more practitioners (Fugh-Berman and Kronenberg 2003).

Since Hippocrates and the notion of the unmoored uterus causing "hysteria," physicians have linked women's reproductive functions to mental illness (Hirshbein 2003). The care of female patients requires an understanding of the anatomical and physiological substrates of reproduction, its social contexts, and the nature of obstetric and gynecological diseases and treatments.

In this chapter, we cover gender identity, infertility, contraception, sterilization, hysterectomy, abortion (both spontaneous and induced), chronic pelvic pain, psychiatric disorders during pregnancy and postpartum and their treatment, menopause, and urinary incontinence.

Note that some of the phenomena described in this chapter vary by culture and sexual orientation and that most findings are generally derived from research on presumably heterosexual women in North America and Europe. An often overlooked minority group is lesbian women. Many lesbians experience or fear disapprobation and misunderstanding in most health care settings, are reluctant to seek care, and therefore experience adverse health outcomes. Psychiatrists can help gynecologists and other primary care physicians to phrase questions about sexual orientation and activity in nonjudgmental terms and become familiar with the range of lesbian sexual practices.

Gender Identity

Reproductive organs are the first defining feature of each human being, and gender remains a core aspect of identity throughout life. Sex hormones influence not only physical development and a host of physiological functions but also brain structure and activity. Environmental factors influence developing anatomy and ongoing physiology. A lifelong, active interplay occurs among anatomy, physiology, social influences, and individual psychology.

The term *sex* refers to narrowly defined biological characteristics. The term *gender* includes social roles and an individual's sense of femininity or masculinity. Some evidence indicates that girls are aware of their sexual organs and identity as early as toddlerhood. As puberty approaches in females, the sense of gender identity is powerfully reinforced and reshaped by physical changes. With menarche come fertility and the possibility that sexual activity will lead to pregnancy. The possibility of pregnancy can be at once a worry and a wish. Although girls can be sexually abused at any age, the possibility of rape is more overt after puberty, and vulnerability to attack becomes part of gender identity. Girls who feel sexual attraction for other girls face a crisis in gender identity because society increasingly expects them to date, form relationships, and engage in sexual activity with males. Medical problems that interfere with any of these functions threaten core gender identity.

Infertility

Infertility is commonly defined as 12 months of appropriately timed unprotected inter-

course that does not result in conception. Approximately 40% of infertility problems are attributable to the female, and 60% are attributable to the male or are of unknown etiology (Klock 1998). The World Health Organization has reported that between 8% and 12% of couples experience some type of fertility problem during their reproductive lives (World Health Organization Programme of Maternal and Child Health and Family Planning Unit 1991). The rate of infertility has remained relatively stable since 1965, while the use and availability of medical services, as well as willingness to disclose and public awareness of infertility treatment options, have increased (Burns and Covington 1999). Both organic and psychological factors may be involved in infertility (Kainz 2001).

Psychological Factors Associated With Infertility

Early publications suggested that infertility without a detectable organic cause was "psychogenic." More recent studies have examined the stresses of investigation and treatment, as well as psychiatric morbidity, influencing fertility and the outcomes of infertility treatments (Verhaak et al. 2005; Smeenk et al. 2005). For example, in a study that used a nationally representative sample of 11,000 American women, generalized anxiety disorder was associated with lower fecundity, independent of treatment status (King 2003). Similarly, depressive symptoms were associated with lower pregnancy rates after in vitro fertilization (Demyttenaere et al. 1998). Eating disorders are also associated with infertility. Restrictive or purging eating behaviors are often undisclosed and result in both subfecundity and poor pregnancy outcomes (Stewart and Robinson 2001a).

Studies on gender differences in psychological reactions to infertility have shown that women report a higher degree of anxiety, depression, and loss of self-esteem compared with their partners. What is unclear is whether this plays an etiological role or is reactive to infertility labeling, investigation, or treatment (Kainz 2001). Infertile women report poorer sexual and marital adjustment; more sexual dysfunction; and more feelings of guilt, inferiority, and isolation compared with infertile men (Weaver et al. 1997; Kainz 2001).

Psychosocial Assessment in Infertility Patients

Some have suggested that current levels of distress and coping strategies should be assessed in couples before initiating infertility treatment (Lukse and Vacc 1999). The process of infertility diagnosis and treatment is grueling. Normally intimate and private behaviors are brought into the clinical situation. The psychological effects, particularly mood alterations, of fertility-enhancing drugs are underappreciated. Careful attention should be paid to recent changes in drug regimens and their potential contribution to recent-onset psychiatric symptoms such as depression, anxiety, mania, or psychosis (Lukse and Vacc 1999). Group interventions are often helpful in providing mutual support, information, and coping techniques (Kainz 2001).

Contraception

Half of the pregnancies in North America each year are unintended. Contraceptive choices and use are affected by knowledge and misinformation, by women's comfort with their own genitalia, by the preferences of sexual partners, by social custom, and by access to physicians for hormonal methods. Many women are ill-informed about the advantages of hormonal contraception (Picardo et al. 2003).

Gender and relationship power differentials play major roles in the use of contraception (Harvey et al. 2002). A psychological study of 132 heterosexual college men reported that those who had not used condoms at last intercourse stated that they had not planned on sex and had no condoms available (Franzini and Sideman 1994). In another study of students, the attitudes of men and women toward male and female contraceptive pills were compared. Of the women, 71% expressed willingness to take an oral contraceptive; for men, the figure was 20%. The authors concluded that despite their level of education, these men were not willing to assume responsibility for contraception (Laird 1994). Women who do not discuss sexual decisions with their male partners are at increased risk for contraceptive failure (Zlokovich and Snell 1997). Ethnicity plays a role as well; Hispanic women may be less likely, and African American women more likely, to use condoms than are white women (Castaneda and Collins 1998; Upchurch et al. 2003).

Psychodynamics and psychiatric conditions can interfere with a woman's use of a contraceptive technique. Unmarried women who do not approve of extramarital sexual intercourse may be able to engage in it only when "swept away" by a romantic situation and thus be unprepared to prevent pregnancy. Some women feel uncomfortable touching their own genitalia, as some contraceptive methods require. Many women have limited knowledge about their own anatomy or are too anxious to absorb the information (Sanders et al. 2003).

Unplanned pregnancy is by no means always the result of unconscious conflict. Contraceptives do fail. Some women are forced into unprotected sexual intercourse (Rickert et al. 2002). However, the myth of female control over sexuality and female seduction, as reflected in the biblical story of Adam and Eve, persists. Women are blamed for becoming pregnant at the wrong time or with the wrong partner.

New developments in contraception have important psychosocial implications (Fraser and Kovacs 2003). Emergency contraception consists of doses of oral contraceptives taken after unprotected intercourse. Although it was believed at first that the hormones had to be ingested within 24 hours, it now appears that they can be effective within at least 3, and possibly 5, days. In England and Canada, and in some parts of the United States and other countries, emergency contraceptives can be obtained without a prescription. In other areas, they can be obtained at family planning clinics, hospital emergency departments, or pharmacies by prescription. However, several barriers exist to the use of this highly effective contraceptive technique (DelBanco et al. 1997). Women who are young, especially those who are poor, may be uninformed, embarrassed, unaware of their level of risk for pregnancy, worried about side effects, and concerned about negative responses from others (Free et al. 2002). Pharmacies may decline to stock the medication, because of either moral objections, lack of demand, or disagreement over patient access without a physician prescription (N. Cooper et al. 2000).

Another new development is the use of hormonal contraceptives on a continuous, rather than intermittent, basis. Women can receive long-lasting hormone implants, use a contraceptive patch, or take contraceptive pills every day with breaks for withdrawal bleeding, which is easier to remember than the usual regimen. Depressive symptoms have been reported in some women taking depot medroxyprogesterone (Civic et al. 2000). Continuous hormonal contraception causes months of amenorrhea. Women who experience menstrual periods as painful and inconvenient welcome amenorrhea,

whereas others hold personal or cultural beliefs that bleeding is necessary to clean the uterus or confirm femininity (Glasier et al. 2003).

Patients may be so accustomed to their birth control pills or injections that they fail to report them when asked what medications they are taking. Hormonal contraceptives interact with some psychotropic medications. Implanted levonorgestrel metabolism is enhanced by phenobarbital, possibly resulting in a pregnancy (Shane-McWhorter et al. 1998). Modafinil, carbamazepine, and oxcarbazepine enhance the metabolism of oral contraceptives, decreasing their effectiveness; the oxidation of benzodiazepines and tricyclic antidepressants (TCAs) in the liver is inhibited, and their blood levels increased, by oral contraceptives (Schatzberg et al. 2003).

Inquiries about sexual behavior and protection from unwanted consequences should be part of every psychiatric treatment. Some physicians ensure that all their female patients of reproductive age who are not intending to become pregnant are supplied with either emergency contraceptive prescriptions or the pills themselves.

Sterilization

Sterilization is a permanent solution to unwanted fertility. A psychiatrist may be asked to consult when a young, nulliparous woman, or a patient with a mental illness, desires to be sterilized. The situation is paradoxical. Women may have psychotic symptoms, or a history of them, that interfere with capacity, but they also may make well-informed decisions not to have children, or more children, precisely because they recognize that their illness would interfere with their parenting. One way to approach this situation is to ask the patient to return in 3–6 months. If she is not acutely psychotic, and is persistent in her desire for sterilization, she may be as appropriate a candidate for the procedure as a woman without diagnosed psychiatric illness.

Recent studies of psychological aspects of sterilization in North America have focused almost entirely on the incidence of postsurgical regret, which ranges from 5% to 20% (Hillis et al. 1999). Risk factors include youth, marital conflict over the procedure, and subsequent changes in marital partnerships (Jamieson et al. 2002). Sexual satisfaction does not appear to be affected (Pati and Cullins 2000). The provision of clear information about the procedure is a crucial factor in patient satisfaction.

Hysterectomy

Epidemiology and Indications

Hysterectomy (the surgical removal of the uterus) is one of the most common surgical procedures performed on North American women, with rates more than double those in many European countries (Stewart et al. 2002). Variations are widespread in most countries and appear to depend on the woman's socioeconomic class, race/ethnicity, education level, religion, physician practice, reimbursement schedules, and availability of new technology (Stewart et al. 2002). The vast majority are elective procedures performed primarily to improve quality of life in women with abnormal uterine bleeding, fibroids, uterine prolapse, chronic pelvic pain, or endometriosis. The mean age of most women undergoing hysterectomy is the mid-40s, or an average of 6–7 years before the mean age of natural menopause, when some of these problems (abnormal uterine bleeding, fibroids) spontaneously resolve. The predicted advantage must be carefully weighed against the risks of surgery and other treatment alternatives such as hor-

monal therapy, endometrial ablation, and fibroid embolization (Lefebvre et al. 2002).

Psychosocial Issues

Information Needs and Decision-Making Preferences

Well-informed women who have been involved in decision making about hysterectomy have the best outcomes (Vigod and Stewart 2002). Women's decision making regarding, and response to, hysterectomy is influenced by their age, socioeconomic status, education, desire for fertility, sexual orientation, and ethnicity and by the role of their family, friends, and partners (Groff et al. 2000; Richter et al. 2000) and the severity of their symptoms. Women who require hysterectomy for the treatment of malignancies are understandably focused more on the cancer.

Variations With Ethnic, Socioeconomic, and Sexual Diversity

Qualitative analyses with Hispanic, African American, and lesbian women (Groff et al. 2000) have explored limitations on alternatives due to ethnicity, economics, education, and access. African American women undergo hysterectomy at a younger age for most diagnostic categories, and are more likely to have an abdominal hysterectomy, extended hospital stays, and higher in-hospital mortality (Lewis et al. 2000).

Psychological and Sexual Outcomes of Hysterectomy

Women with substantiated diagnoses and clear indication for hysterectomy have better physical and psychological outcomes than do women with less-defined symptoms and indicators such as chronic pelvic pain. A prospective study (Kjerulff et al. 2000) of more than 1,000 women followed for 2 years after hysterectomy for benign conditions revealed that although symptom severity, depression, and anxiety decreased significantly after hysterectomy and quality of life improved for most women, 8% reported symptoms at least as severe 1–2 years after hysterectomy as before. Over 100 studies have shown a subgroup of women (10%–20%) who report negative psychosocial outcomes (Flory et al. 2005). Presurgical characteristics that predicted lack of symptom relief included previous therapy for psychological problems, history of depression, and household income less than $35,000. Bilateral oophorectomy also predicted lack of symptom relief at 2 years after hysterectomy (Kjerulff et al. 2000).

A systematic review of English- and German-language literature on sexual outcomes after hysterectomy found no change in or an enhancement of sexuality in the women after hysterectomy (Farrell and Kieser 2000). Prehysterectomy depression was notably associated with postsurgical psychopathology (Rannestad 2005).

Women undergoing hysterectomy with oophorectomy have to confront the onset of sudden surgical menopause if estrogen therapy is not begun shortly after surgery. This sudden hormonal change may result in vasomotor symptoms, sleep loss, and depression, especially in vulnerable women with a history of depression associated with reproductive events (Stewart and Boydell 1993).

Psychiatrists should ascertain the hormonal status of women with sudden mood changes following hysterectomy and consider short-term hormonal treatment as well as antidepressants.

Abortion

Spontaneous Abortion

Abortion can be spontaneous (miscarriage) or induced (usually just termed *abortion*). Spontaneous abortion generally evokes feelings of failure and loss. A woman's body has failed to perform one of its basic functions; she has failed to produce a child for her partner and parents; she has expelled her own potential child; and she may have conceived an embryo with genetic anomalies. Decades ago, miscarriage was sometimes attributed to the woman's unconscious rejection of motherhood, but this theory has never been validated by empirical research. Spontaneous abortion, like a stillbirth or neonatal death, may precipitate pathological grief, postpartum depression, or posttraumatic stress (Engelhard et al. 2003). Women report that the failure of friends and family to acknowledge the loss complicates the grieving process. Health care providers also may fail to recognize the emotional effect of spontaneous abortion. It is often helpful for them to meet with the patient some weeks after the event to go over the medical findings, if any; the prognosis; and the state of the woman's recovery.

The loss of pregnancy through miscarriage or stillbirth is associated with an increase in anxiety during a subsequent pregnancy and with overprotectiveness toward children subsequently born (Bourne and Lewis 1984). Although patients are frequently counseled to wait 6 months or a year after such a loss, older women often conceive as soon as possible.

Induced Abortion

Psychiatric Sequelae

Approximately 1 million abortions are performed every year in the United States; approximately one in three women will have an abortion in her lifetime (Ventura et al. 2000). There is no evidence that formal mental health consultation is routinely necessary. The psychiatric ramifications of abortion are a matter of some debate, but the findings are clear once methodological confounds are taken into account. Unbiased reviews of the literature indicate that self-limited feelings of guilt and sadness are common after abortion, although the predominant reaction is one of relief, and new episodes of psychiatric illness are rare (Dagg 1991; Koop 1989). Studies corroborated findings that women's quality of life improves in the period from before to after an early abortion (Garg et al. 2001; Westhoff et al. 2003). The best outcomes prevail when women are able to make autonomous, supported choices about their pregnancies. When women seek, but are denied, abortion, the resulting children have significantly poorer mental health than their siblings or matched control subjects (Kubicka et al. 2002).

Antiabortion groups and writers claim that abortion is associated with a higher risk of serious psychiatric disorders and suicide than is childbirth (Pro-Life Action Ministries, undated; Reardon et al. 2003; Thorp et al. 2003). These publications fail to address the circumstances of, and reasons for, abortion. Sometimes they confound common, self-limited feelings of loss and guilt with diagnosable depression (Dagg 1991).

Women have abortions because they have been abandoned by the men who impregnated them, because those men threaten to leave if they continue the pregnancy, because the pregnancy is the result of rape or incest, because they are poor and overburdened with other responsibilities, or because they do not have the resources—educational, financial, emotional, or social—to provide adequate parenting. They may simply not want to be a parent. Preexisting serious psychiatric illness makes some women more vulnerable to unwanted pregnancy and less able to parent.

Risk Factors

Not surprisingly, coercion, lack of social support, poverty, rape, incest, and preexisting psychiatric illness are associated with increased risk for psychological difficulties following, but not causally related to, abortion. Women who belong to religious faiths opposed to abortion choose abortion as often as or more often than those who do not. Efforts have been made to reach out to this population, both to enlist them in antiabortion advocacy and to offer them spiritual support (Jeal and West 2003; Ventura et al. 2000). Demonstrators or fear of terrorism at an abortion facility may exacerbate stress, and the attitudes and behaviors of medical personnel during the abortion procedure have a significant influence on patients' experience (Slade et al. 2001).

The delay of abortion into the second trimester, or later, is most often secondary to denial of pregnancy, difficulties with access, or diagnosis of a serious fetal defect, each of which increases the risk for postabortion reactions. Consultation may be sought when a woman or family cannot decide, or manifests overwhelming anxiety, when making an abortion decision under these circumstances (Zlotogora 2002). Continuing a pregnancy and relinquishing the child for adoption pose a psychological burden as well (Cushman et al. 1993).

Minors and Abortion

The effect of abortion on minors, and their ability to make decisions about abortion, is another area of controversy. Term pregnancy and delivery pose greater medical and psychological risks for adolescents than does abortion. Arguments that minors are too immature to elect abortion overlook the fact that these same minors, if their pregnancies are not terminated, will soon be mothers with responsibility for infants. In Zabin's classic study of inner-city girls who obtained pregnancy tests at a school clinic, those who had abortions had better outcomes than did those who carried to term and even than did those whose pregnancy test results were negative. This may imply that the inability to tell whether one is pregnant is associated with other psychosocial problems. Marriage of the pregnant teenager to the father of the baby does not improve outcome and may worsen it (Zabin et al. 1989).

Chronic Pelvic Pain

Chronic pelvic pain is nonmenstrual pelvic pain of 6 or more months' duration that is severe enough to cause functional disability or require medical or surgical treatment (Howard 2003). It has an estimated prevalence of 3.8% in adult women, similar to that of asthma or back pain (Zondervan et al. 1999). Chronic pelvic pain may lead to disability and suffering, with loss of employment, marital discord and divorce, and an overall decline in quality of life (Howard 2003).

Etiology of Chronic Pelvic Pain

The etiology is often difficult to discern. Disorders of the reproductive, gastrointestinal, urological, musculoskeletal, and neurological systems may be associated. In many cases, however, the pain is related to a combination of physical and psychological factors, such as endometriosis, adhesions, urological problems, irritable bowel syndrome, myofascial pain, depression, anxiety, somatization, and past abusive experiences (Howard 2003; Moore and Kennedy 2001). A significant number of patients have no obvious etiology for their pain at the time of laparoscopy (Gelbaya and El-Halwagy 2001; Savidge and Slade 1997). As with other chronic syndromes, especially those with ambiguous etiology, the biopsychosocial model offers the best way of integrating physical causes of pain with psychological and social factors. Attempts to separate chronic pain into a simple cause-and-effect relation are usually unrewarding.

Psychological Factors Associated With Chronic Pelvic Pain

The relation of chronic pelvic pain to psychological state or personality style has received great attention. A comprehensive review showed that most studies have reported more depression, somatic symptoms, substance abuse, sexual dysfunction, and physical and sexual abuse in patients with chronic pelvic pain than in comparison groups (Fry et al. 1997). Both physical and sexual abuse are associated with psychological distress in women with chronic pelvic pain (Poleshuck et al. 2005). Cognitive-behavioral and psychophysiological theories have moved increasingly toward supporting complex, multicausal views. A subsequent review reported that psychological diagnoses were apparent in 60% of the women referred for chronic pelvic pain, with major depressive disorder the most common (Reiter 1998) .

Management of Chronic Pelvic Pain

A comprehensive evidence-based management review of chronic pelvic pain (Reiter 1998) recommended a multidisciplinary, individualized, multifocal approach to chronic pelvic pain, including medical therapies and cognitive-behavioral or other psychotherapeutic approaches. Focused psychotherapy may be useful. Special techniques, such as relaxation and correcting maladaptive thoughts, may increase the patient's coping ability and sense of control. Activity programs can decrease disability behaviors. Multidisciplinary management of chronic pelvic pain has significantly better outcomes than does traditional medical management (Price and Blake 1999; Reiter 1998; Savidge and Slade 1997).

Endometriosis

Endometriosis is a common gynecological condition caused by the presence of hormonally responsive endometrial tissue outside the uterine cavity. It has been proposed that retrograde menstruation occurs to some degree in all women, but that only those who are unable to clear the menstrual debris because of immune dysfunction will go on to develop endometriosis (Cramer and Missmer 2002). The mean age of women at diagnosis of endometriosis ranges from 25 to 30 years. Endometriosis is often asymptomatic but is also found in association with dysmenorrhea, dyspareunia, infertility, chronic pelvic or back pain, and rectal discomfort. The pain from the disorder is often cyclic, although it can be constant. The gold standard for diagnosis is laparoscopy; however, the intensity of pain and discomfort does not correlate well with the severity of the disease at laparoscopy (Lu and Ory 1995).

Management

Endometriosis can be treated by watchful waiting or medical or surgical management. Although surgical conservative treatment is widely used to enhance fertility, its efficacy for endometriosis-associated infertility has not yet been shown.

Role of the Psychiatrist

Some women report that their worst experience is the way in which their symptoms are trivialized and dismissed by medical professionals (Cox et al. 2003). Gonadotropin-releasing hormone agonists are often used to treat endometriosis, and depressive symptoms may be associated. Selective serotonin reuptake inhibitor (SSRI) antidepressants appear to be helpful in the treatment of mood symptoms during the course of gonadotropin-releasing hormone agonists (Warnock et al. 1998). Psychotherapy and serotonin-norepinephrine reuptake inhibitors (SNRIs) may be helpful in women with endometriosis.

Vulvodynia

Vulvodynia is chronic burning, stinging, or pain in the vulva in the absence of objective findings. Vulvodynia is divided into two classes: 1) vulvar vestibulitis, which is restricted burning and pain in the vestibular region that is solicited by touch, and 2) dysesthetic vulvodynia, which is burning or pain not limited to the vestibule, which may occur without touch or pressure. A population-based National Institutes of Health study found that approximately 16% of women reported lower genital tract discomfort persisting for 3 months or longer (Edwards 2003).

The etiology of vulvodynia is unknown, and previously suspect agents have largely been discounted. Neuropathic pain has been invoked because TCAs, SNRIs, and gabapentin have shown some promise in treating this disorder; however, to date, no randomized controlled trials have been published. Many women with vulvodynia also have comorbid disorders, such as interstitial cystitis, headaches, fibromyalgia, and irritable bowel syndrome. Depression and anxiety are common (Stewart et al. 1994), and sexual functioning is frequently impaired (Masheb et al. 2004).

Pregnancy

The entire range of psychiatric disorders occurs during pregnancy, but some conditions are unique to pregnancy.

Psychiatric Disorders Occurring During Pregnancy

Depression

The incidence of depression during pregnancy is approximately the same as that for matched nonpregnant populations (Stewart 2005). The signs and symptoms of depression must be carefully distinguished from the sleep, appetite, and energy changes often characteristic of pregnancy and from the signs and symptoms of thyroid dysfunction, anemia, or other diseases of pregnancy. Discontinuation of maintenance medication for women who have had recurrent depressions carries a high risk of relapse. Mild cases can be effectively treated with interpersonal or cognitive-behavioral psychotherapy (Grote and Frank 2003; Spinelli and Endicott 2003).

Bipolar Disorder

There is a growing literature on bipolar disorders during pregnancy (Cohen et al. 1995; Viguera et al. 2002). Some pregnant patients can forgo mood stabilizers, but a substantial proportion (up to 50%) may relapse. Episodes of mania or depression may pose a threat to the pregnancy, necessitating especially careful risk–benefit analysis with regard to psychotropic medication.

Anxiety Disorders

Panic disorder may remit or recur during pregnancy. Patients with panic disorder who wish to discontinue medication should be tapered off gradually and treated with cognitive-behavioral therapy. More than 10% of female patients with panic disorder report that their first episode occurred postpartum. Panic disorder during pregnancy may recur with subsequent pregnancies. Obsessive-compulsive disorder is likely to worsen pre- and postpartum, and withdrawal of medication is very likely to result in recurrence. Patients with moderate to severe symptoms may require maintenance medication during pregnancy; patients with milder cases can be treated with cognitive-behavioral therapy.

Psychotic Disorders

The fertility of women with psychotic disorders approximates that of the general population. Pregnancy does not ameliorate, and may exacerbate, psychotic symptoms (Davies et al. 1995). Psychotic episodes during pregnancy may be characterized by delusions that the fetus is evil or dangerous, leading the pregnant woman to stab herself in the abdomen or engage in other self-destructive behaviors. Electroconvulsive therapy (ECT) can be effective and is relatively safe for the fetus. Psychotic illness can impair a woman's ability to recognize and react appropriately to the signs and symptoms of labor (Miller and Finnerty 1996). Hospitalization toward the end of pregnancy is not completely protective against these concerns. The consulting psychiatrist can facilitate collaboration between the psychiatric and obstetrical departments in these difficult cases.

Prenatal assessment and treatment can mitigate wrenching custody disputes after the infant is born. Serious psychiatric illness, if treated, is not always incompatible with successful mothering. Psychiatrists may be called on to assist in the assessment of competency to parent an infant. When it is clear that the mother will not be able to care for the child, the psychiatrist can help her come to terms with the very real loss.

Alcohol and Substance Abuse

Standing by while a woman's behavior puts her fetus at risk is a painful situation for prenatal care professionals. The most serious and well-documented result of alcohol abuse during pregnancy is fetal alcohol syndrome. A pregnant woman who drinks the equivalent of 10 beers per day has a one-third risk of delivering a child with fetal alcohol syndrome and a similar risk of delivering a child who is retarded but does not have the full syndrome. The perinatal mortality in these circumstances is 17% (Greenfield and Sugarman 2001). Lower ingestion of alcohol in pregnancy may cause fetal alcohol effects that result in cognitive or behavioral abnormalities.

More recent studies have not substantiated early fears of an epidemic of "crack babies." It appears that most or all of the negative cognitive and behavioral findings in these children are a result of the environment in which they grow up rather than intrauterine exposure to cocaine (Chiriboga 1998). However, misinformation and rage at pregnant women who abuse substances has led to instances in which women have been imprisoned, either for the protection of the fetus or as punishment for harming the fetus.

Many or most pregnant women who abuse drugs or alcohol will accept treatment if it is practical (e.g., providing child care) and humane. Evidence indicates that the threat of coercion and punishment leads women to avoid seeking prenatal care altogether, obviating any opportunity to treat them and improve the fetus's intrauterine environment.

Situational Anxiety

New anxiety in a pregnant woman may occur because she has been frightened by the experiences of a close family member or has had a traumatic obstetrical or general medical care experience herself (Saisto and Halmesmaki 2003). Fear of labor or birth may motivate some requests for elective cesarean sections. The degree of pain a woman experiences in labor is related to many factors, including her expectations of pain (Chang et al. 2002). When the source of the anxiety is identified, it can be addressed by reviewing the past experience and plans to avoid the frightening aspects of care in the coming delivery, providing prenatal education about delivery, or using relaxation techniques or hypnosis. Domestic violence is another cause of prenatal anxiety. Literature about the effect of pregnancy on domestic violence is contradictory; in some reports, violence is increased, and in others, it is not (Johnson et al. 2003; Saltzman et al. 2003).

Issues Unique to Pregnancy

Denial of Pregnancy

Some women go into full-term labor without themselves or their families having recognized that they are pregnant. Many such patients are not psychotic, but some are women with schizophrenia who are delusional in denying pregnancy (Miller 1990). Older patients may report that they thought pregnancy was impossible at their age and attributed their amenorrhea to menopause and the sensations of fetal movement to digestive problems. Younger patients in this situation are typically passive daughters isolated in very strict families without much knowledge about reproduction. Their preconscious or unconscious fears of the consequences of pregnancy are so terrifying that they keep its signs and symptoms out of awareness (Spielvogel and Hohener 1995). They wear loose-fitting clothing and go about their usual activities. These cases generally come to psychiatric attention only if the new mother kills or abandons the infant after birth. Therefore, these young women end up in the penal rather than the mental health care system. A German study reported an incidence of up to 1 case of pregnancy denial per 475 births (Wessel et al. 2002).

Pseudocyesis

At the other end of the spectrum from the patient who does not realize she is pregnant is the patient who is convinced she is pregnant when she is not. This condition, referred to as *pseudocyesis*, is a fascinating example of psychobiological interplay. The patient ceases to have menstrual periods. Her abdomen grows, and her cervix may show signs of pregnancy. Some patients with the delusion that they are pregnant are psychotic, but that is not the case in classical pseudocyesis. Patients with pseudocyesis are a heterogeneous group, and they have no other signs or symptoms of frank psychiatric disorder (Rosch et al. 2002). They declare an expected date of delivery and move the date forward when delivery does not ensue. Their conviction may or may not be swayed by ultrasonographic evidence or physical examination. For unknown reasons, the incidence of this condition is decreasing. Frequent antecedents are pregnancy loss, infertility, isolation, naiveté, and a belief that childbearing is a woman's crucial role. These individuals have no interest in psychiatric care, and little is known about their eventual outcome (Whelan and Stewart 1990).

Hyperemesis

Pernicious vomiting in pregnancy was once thought to be the result of unconscious rejection of the pregnancy. Hyperemesis, which can result in dehydration and electrolyte imbalance and may require hospitalization and intravenous treatment, certainly could induce ambivalence about a pregnancy in a woman who had been very pleased at the prospect of becoming a mother, but no scientific evidence indicates that ambivalence induces the vomiting. Hyperemesis is no longer considered a psychiatric disorder. Mental health intervention can, however, help the patient and family cope until the condition resolves (Deuchar 1995).

Routine Psychiatric Screening

Psychiatrists may advise obstetricians that including psychiatric screening in routine antenatal care will decrease the frequency and intensity of noncompliance with antenatal care and of psychiatric emergencies during pregnancy and labor (Stewart 2005). Psychiatric illnesses can be identified and treated. Patients who might not otherwise recognize that they are in labor, and their families, can receive special education so that infants are not delivered into the toilet or in some other less-than-ideal environment. Prenatal education can prepare them for labor and delivery, so that they can best cooperate and communicate with medical staff when the time comes.

Postpartum Psychiatric Issues

Perinatal Death

Stillbirth and neonatal death provoke much the same reactions as do losses earlier in pregnancy, which are discussed earlier in this chapter, with the added stresses of full-term labor and delivery and the probability that many practical provisions for the expected infant have been made. Practice in dealing with the bereaved parents has varied over time. It is probably best to offer parents the opportunity to see the stillborn infant and to allow them to decide if they want to do so. Grief is exacerbated by the failure of friends and relatives to acknowledge the loss. For some, naming the baby and having a funeral service is a helpful ritual. A religious leader of the parents' choice may also help them.

When the cause of fetal or neonatal death is not clear, an autopsy or other tests may be performed. The obstetrician, pathologist, geneticist, and psychiatrist may want to meet with the parents some weeks later to convey the results, answer questions, observe the grieving process, and determine whether additional supports are necessary. Stillbirth increases the risk of posttraumatic stress, anxiety, and depression in a subsequent pregnancy (Bourne and Lewis 1984; Hughes et al. 1999). These sequelae generally resolve within 1 year after the birth of a subsequent healthy child (Turton et al. 2001). Premature birth or the stress of complicated, or even normal, labor can precipitate posttraumatic stress symptoms, especially in women with preexisting psychiatric symptoms and poor social supports (Czarnocka and Slade 2000; Holditch-Davis et al. 2003).

Postpartum Psychiatric Disorders

"Baby Blues"

Within days after birth, 25%–75% of newly delivered women experience significantly heightened emotional lability. After a few days, the symptoms abate (Ross et al. 2005). The phenomenon has been reported in a wide variety of cultures and is not related to demographic variables (Sakumoto et al. 2002). Although the patient may be moved to tears from time to time, none of the other signs or symptoms of depression are present. The mother also experiences periods of joy. This self-limited state may be caused by prolactin, oxytocin, or other hormones. Clinicians should offer reassurance that the condition usually lasts less than 2 weeks.

Postpartum Depression

Postpartum depression occurs in approximately 13% of mothers in North America. Some cases of postpartum depression are simply continuations of prepartum depression or baby blues. As noted earlier, depression during pregnancy is common and is the strongest predictor of postpartum depression. Symptoms generally begin later than baby blues and range from 4 weeks to 12 months postpartum. The diagnostic process can be complicated because new mothers are often tired, sleepless, distracted, and preoccupied with infant care. It is useful to ask whether the mother can sleep when the baby sleeps.

Risk factors include previous depression, especially previous antenatal or postpartum depression, and poor social supports (Robertson et al. 2004). Some evidence shows that postpartum calls and visits from health care professionals decrease the incidence of postpartum depression (Chabrol et al. 2002). Endocrine factors also play a major role; some women are particularly vulnerable to rapid changes in hormone levels.

Anxiety accompanies pre- and postpartum depression in up to 50% of cases (Ross et al. 2003). Antecedent anxiety disorders are a more important risk factor for postpartum depression than is antecedent depression (Matthey et al. 2003a).

The thought content of a woman with postpartum depression centers on mothering (e.g., ruminating that she is not a good mother or that her infant is suffering). Sometimes the woman becomes obsessed with thoughts of harm coming to the infant and vividly imagines his or her injury or death. These thoughts are profoundly upsetting to the mother; they are thoughts, not intentions, and should be distinguished from the delusionally driven infanticidal impulses of postpartum psychosis.

Reassurance of eventual recovery is crucial to patient care. One of the fears of women with postpartum depression, and their families, is that the depression is the first sign of a condition that will result in self-harm or infanticide. Relatives may be tempted to take over care of the infant of a depressed mother to allow her to rest and recuperate. This can be counterproductive, exacerbating her sense of failure and deprivation. It is preferable for them to help the mother with household tasks, allow her to care for the infant, and reinforce her sense of maternal adequacy.

Obstetric clinicians should be encouraged to increase their contacts with and availability to new mothers, both for screening and for prevention. Several validated scales are available for screening; the Edinburgh Postnatal Depression Scale (Matthey et al. 2003b) is the best known. However, a simple query about depressed mood is often successful in identifying cases (Wisner et al. 2002b). There have been attempts to convince pediatricians to screen mothers for postpartum depression.

Postpartum Psychosis

Many experts believe that most episodes of postpartum psychosis are bipolar (Attia et al. 1999; Chaudron and Pies 2003). The risk of postpartum relapse of bipolar disorder is 30%–50%.

If pregnant women with bipolar disorder discontinue medication, there should be a plan for immediate medication resumption at delivery. Third trimester or immediate postpartum treatment significantly lowers the risk of recurrence (Cohen et al. 1995).

Postpartum psychosis is characterized by extreme agitation, delirium, confusion, sleeplessness, and hallucinations and/or delusions. Onset can be sudden and usually occurs between days 3 and 14 postpartum. The overall incidence of postpartum psychosis is estimated at 0.1%–0.2%. The risk and the stakes are high enough to consider postpartum psychosis as a medical emergency and hospitalize the patient.

Media coverage of cases of infanticide disclose major misunderstandings about the state and motivation of the perpetrators. Most often, the mother in these cases has command hallucinations or delusions and/or is suicidal and does not wish to leave the child behind. Appleby et al. (1998) reported that the risk of suicide in the first postnatal year is "increased 70-fold."

Custody

Psychiatric illness in and of itself does not rule out the possibility of adequate mothering. When the question of custody arises, it is useful to perform a regular mental status examination. What are most important, however, are the parenting knowledge, attitudes, and behaviors of the newly delivered patient. Has she been able to arrange adequate accommodations for herself and the infant? How does she plan to feed the infant? Does she know approximately how often a newborn must be fed and changed? Does she have delusions about the infant?

Observation of mother–infant interaction is key. The postpartum staff should allow the mother as much observed time with the infant as possible and note how the mother responds to the infant's cries and other needs, whether she can feed the infant and change diapers, and how she relates to the infant overall.

Custody decisions can be life-or-death decisions. Removing a child from its mother, unless a well-disposed and capable relative can take over care, exposes the child to the possibility of a lifetime in transient foster care situations. Allowing a severely ill mother to retain custody exposes the child to possible abuse and neglect. Often the most appropriate approach, when available, is the provision of home help and/or visiting nurse services, which provide both support and further opportunities for observation of the parenting and the condition of the infant.

Psychotropic Drugs, Psychotherapy, and Electroconvulsive Therapy in Pregnancy and Lactation

No perfect solution exists for treating mental illness during pregnancy and lactation, and a risk–benefit decision must be made in the face of imprecise data. For example, untreated clinical depression can result in problems with maternal nutrition, sleeping, exercise, and adherence to prenatal care. Infants born to mothers with depression are more likely to have low birth weight for gestational age and to be born prematurely (Stewart and Robinson 2001b). Although mental illness of mild to moderate severity may be treated with psychotherapy, support, or environmental changes, more severe illness usually requires psychotropic medications, which carry variable and sometimes unknown risks (Hendrick et al. 2003).

Three types of adverse fetal effects may occur when psychotropics are taken during pregnancy. *Teratogenic effects* may be incurred from first trimester exposure, *neonatal toxicity and withdrawal syndromes* are related to third trimester exposure, and *behavioral or developmental effects* may manifest later in childhood (Marcus et al. 2001; Wisner et al. 2002a). Note that changes in drug metabolism and extracellular fluid volume during pregnancy may require dose adjustment for several drugs. For example, approximately twice the usual dose of lithium carbonate is often required in the second and third trimesters to achieve therapeutic serum levels (Stewart and Robinson 2001b).

Classification of Drugs

Current U.S. Food and Drug Administration (FDA) (2001) risk assignments of drugs in pregnancy range from A (no risk) through B, C, D, and X (contraindicated). This classification is primarily based on concerns about teratogenicity and neonatal toxicity, because few or no data exist for later child behavior or development. The FDA classification lags behind current data and experience. At present, bupropion, clozapine, and buspirone have a B designation (absence of human risk) with a caveat of limited data. Most SSRI antidepressants, some TCAs (including desipramine), newer antidepressants (such as mirtazapine, nefazodone, and venlafaxine), clonazepam, and most conventional and atypical antipsychotics have received a C designation (human risk should not be eliminated because of inadequate human clinical trials and no or some risk in animals). Lithium, carbamazepine, sodium valproate, most TCAs, paroxetine, and some benzodiazepines (other than clonazepam) have received a D designation, indicating evidence of fetal risk without an absolute contraindication during pregnancy. A long-standing debate has existed, with contradictory data from several studies, on whether diazepam in pregnancy is associated with cleft lip or

cleft palate. Some benzodiazepines, such as triazolam, temazepam, and flurazepam, have received an X designation, indicating complete contraindication in pregnancy (Marcus et al. 2001). Although the strength of evidence for safety of all psychotropics in pregnancy is fair to poor, expert consensus guidelines were developed (Altshuler et al. 2001). Insufficient data are available to ensure safety for most novel antipsychotics; however, high-potency antipsychotics, such as haloperidol, appear to be relatively safe in pregnancy (Patton et al. 2002).

Early reports warned of congenital heart disease in infants exposed in utero to lithium carbonate, but subsequent analyses have shown these risks to be only slightly greater than those of the general population (Altshuler et al. 1996). Other mood stabilizers such as carbamazepine and valproic acid are associated with greater teratogenicity than lithium (Stewart and Robinson 2001b). For women with unstable bipolar disorder, it is reasonable to continue lithium throughout pregnancy, while carefully monitoring serum levels. Divided doses may be safer than once-daily dosing. An ultrasound during the first trimester may be used to identify possible congenital cardiac malformations. Dosage should be reduced after delivery to avoid lithium toxicity in the early postpartum period. Lithium is contraindicated while breast-feeding (Stewart and Robinson 2001b).

Because the FDA is currently revising its method of classifying drug risk in pregnancy, physicians should consult the most recent classification, as well as other new literature. A report in 2005 described a relative risk of cardiovascular anomalies in infants exposed to paroxetine in the first trimester (Diav-Citrin et al. 2005). Other data reported in 2005 show that infants exposed in utero to SSRI antidepressants have a shorter mean gestational age, are more active and tremulous, have more startles and sudden arousals, show lower heart rate variability, and have lower peak behavioral status (Sanz 2005). In 2006, Chambers and colleagues found an odds ratio of 6.1 for persistent pulmonary hypertension of the newborn in infants exposed to SSRIs after 20 weeks' gestation. Infants exposed to tricyclic antidepressants in pregnancy or to SSRIs before 20 weeks' gestation did not have an increased risk (Chambers et al. 2006).

Disruptions in a wide range of neurobehavioral outcomes, as well as seizures and respiratory and feeding problems, prompted regulatory authorities in Canada and the United States to issue advisories suggesting increased awareness of potential complications of all SSRIs in infants who were exposed during the third trimester of pregnancy.

Adverse Effects

Only a few long-term studies of behavioral teratogenicity following exposure to psychotropic drugs have been done. More studies of fluoxetine have been published than of other SSRIs, following its use in pregnancy (Goldstein et al. 1997) and its effects on child development and behavior. Nulman et al. (2002) found no difference in social, cognitive, or motor development in children up to 86 months whose mothers had taken a variety of TCAs or fluoxetine in pregnancy. In several studies, sertraline, paroxetine, fluvoxamine, citalopram, and venlafaxine were shown as relatively safe in pregnancy when infants were assessed in the early postnatal period (Altshuler et al. 2001; Einarson et al. 2003; Heikkinen et al. 2002; Wisner et al. 2002a), but none of these studies provided longer-term follow-up. Acute withdrawal effects have been described in infants whose mothers took paroxetine during the third trimester (Stiskal et al. 2001). Only limited data are available on

the new antipsychotics (Hallberg and Sjoblom 2005; Howard et al. 2004).

Breast-Feeding and Psychotropic Drugs

The amount of drug present in breast milk is small but extremely variable over time. No controlled studies exist of the effects of psychotropic medication during breastfeeding, but several reviews provide further guidance (Altshuler et al. 1995, 2001; American Academy of Pediatrics Committee on Drugs 2001; Hendrick et al. 2001; Ilett et al. 2002; Stewart 2001; Wisner et al. 2001). In general, it appears relatively safe for depressed women to take antidepressants and typical antipsychotics while breast-feeding full-term and healthy babies. Fewer data are available for premature infants or newer antidepressants and atypical antipsychotics. Chaudron and Jefferson (2000) reviewed the literature on the use of mood stabilizers during lactation. They concluded that lithium is generally not recommended during lactation and that although carbamazepine and valproate may be considered acceptable, decisions about the care of women with a history of bipolar illness must be made on a case-by-case basis. The risk of recurrence is considerable, with significant implications for mother and child (Chaudron and Jefferson 2000).

Because new information on the use of drugs during pregnancy and lactation is frequently published, the reader is advised to consult the most recent reference in making risk–benefit decisions. The expert consensus guidelines (Altshuler et al. 2001) need updating. The clinician must be cognizant that untreated mental illness in pregnancy and postpartum also has risks to the woman and the developing fetus and newborn child. Decisions should be made in consultation with the woman (and partner, if appropriate) and other health care providers (such as obstetricians and pediatricians), and discussions should be carefully documented in the patient's chart.

Psychotherapy in Pregnancy and Postpartum

Spinelli (1997) found interpersonal psychotherapy to be effective in the treatment of depressed pregnant women. Appleby et al. (1997) compared the effects of antidepressant treatment and six sessions of cognitive-behavioral counseling for postnatal depression and found both treatments to be effective. More recent work by P. Cooper and colleagues (2003) has shown that psychotherapy has short-term benefits for maternal mood but is not superior to spontaneous remission in the long term. Murray and colleagues (2003) showed that early psychotherapy intervention was beneficial for short-term mother–infant relationships but had no effect on infant behavior problems, secure attachment, cognitive development, or any child outcome at 5 years. O'Hara and colleagues (2000) established the efficacy of interpersonal psychotherapy for postpartum depression. In general, interpersonal and cognitive-behavioral psychotherapy appear to be efficacious for mild to moderate depression. Because many women refuse to take medication while pregnant or breast-feeding, psychotherapy is often a viable alternative. However, its efficacy for severe depression in unproven.

Electroconvulsive Therapy

ECT is generally regarded as a safe and effective treatment for severe depression, affective psychosis, and catatonia in pregnancy and the puerperium. ECT is underused and should be considered in emergency situations in which the safety of the mother, fetus, or child is jeopardized; to avoid first-trimester exposure to terato-genic drugs; and in patients who are refractory to psychotropics or who have previously had successful treatment with ECT (Stewart and Robinson 2001b).

Premenstrual Psychiatric Symptoms

Background

Most women in North America, if asked, report premenstrual mood, behavior, and somatic changes. Both women and men attribute unpleasant or problematic feelings and behaviors to the menstrual cycle. However, more than half of the women presenting for care of premenstrual symptoms, when assessed with prospective ratings and careful diagnostic interviews, have symptoms unrelated to their menstrual cycles. Strong feelings and methodological difficulties have made the diagnosis of premenstrual psychiatric syndromes controversial (Sveinsdottir et al. 2002).

Etiology

Many attempts have been made, over decades, to identify circulating levels of reproductive hormones to account for mood symptoms occurring in concert with reproductive events and cycles and to treat those symptoms with hormones. Recent research links allopregnanolone to premenstrual dysphoric disorder (PMDD) in women with previous depression (Klatzkin et al. 2006). Women who report premenstrual symptoms are more likely to experience postpartum depression and may be predisposed to mood symptoms around perimenopause as well (Stewart and Boydell 1993). Premenstrual symptoms persist into the perimenopause, when they become difficult to distinguish from symptoms of perimenopause (Grady-Weliky 2003).

Diagnosis

For many years, the study of premenstrual psychiatric symptoms was complicated by the lack of a specific and uniform definition. More than 100 physical, emotional, and cognitive signs and symptoms have been attributed to premenstrual syndrome (PMS) (Janowsky et al. 2002). Currently, premenstrual psychiatric symptoms are conceptualized and treated as part of the mood disorder spectrum, and research diagnostic criteria have been developed in an attempt to describe a clinically significant condition. PMDD is listed in DSM-IV-TR as an example of a depressive disorder not otherwise specified (NOS) and is described as follows:

> In most menstrual cycles during the past year, five (or more) of the following symptoms (e.g., markedly depressed mood, marked anxiety, marked affective lability, decreased interest in activities) were present for most of the time during the last week of the luteal phase, began to remit within a few days after the onset of the follicular phase, and were absent in the week post-menses....The disturbance markedly interferes with work or school or with usual social activities and relationships with others. (American Psychiatric Association 2000, p. 774)

PMDD, as distinguished from PMS, is said to affect up to 8% of cycling women. Given the tendency to retrospectively overattribute symptoms to the menstrual cycle, prospective daily ratings and careful evaluation for other psychiatric disorders are essential (Landen and Eriksson 2003; Lane and Francis 2003).

Management

No specific, empirically supported treatments for PMS are available, but several approaches have proved helpful: reducing or eliminating caffeine and nicotine, exercising, and using stress reduction techniques. Exogenous hormones are not effective.

Like other disorders in the mood spectrum, PMDD is best treated with SSRIs (Freeman 2002; Wyatt et al. 2002). As of this writing, fluoxetine, sertraline, and paroxetine have received FDA indications for PMDD. SSRIs are apparently effective for PMDD when used only in the premenstrual phase (Halbreich et al. 2002). Symptoms recur rapidly when luteal-phase treatment is discontinued (Pearlstein et al. 2003).

In one study, cognitive-behavioral therapy was found to be equally as effective as fluoxetine in treating PMDD; fluoxetine produced more rapid results, and cognitive-behavioral therapy produced more lasting results (Hunter et al. 2002). Calcium carbonate has also produced promising results (Thys-Jacobs et al. 1998).

The possibility of cyclical changes in symptoms and/or treatment response in all diagnostic categories should be considered in all menstruating women (Lande and Karamchandani 2002).

Perimenopause and Menopause

The average age at menopause in North American and European women is 51 years, although the entire period of transition may extend over several years. By definition, menopause is said to have occurred after 12 months of amenorrhea, and perimenopause is that period of time leading up to menopause. During the perimenopause, the ovarian follicles gradually decline with age, estradiol and inhibin production by the ovary decreases, and levels of follicle-stimulating hormone and luteinizing hormone rise (through loss of feedback inhibition). These changes are orchestrated through the hypothalamic-pituitary-ovarian axis, and cyclic variability often occurs throughout the transitional period (Baram 1997).

The perimenopause may be asymptomatic, but 70%–90% of women will experience some vasomotor symptoms consisting of hot flashes and night sweats. In addition, some women will experience palpitations, dizziness, fatigue, headaches, insomnia, joint pains, and paresthesias. Women also may complain of lack of concentration and loss of memory during the transitional period, but because men also complain of these symptoms, distinguishing them from normal aging is difficult (Baram 2005).

Large community surveys show no increase in psychopathology with menopause; however, increases in depression and anxiety prevalence have been reported over the perimenopausal years (Freeman et al. 2004). These symptoms may be caused by hormonal changes, sociocultural factors, or psychological factors (Avis 2003). Sociocultural theories focus on the importance of role changes in parenting, marriage, sex, and work. In addition, attitudes toward aging and female roles vary by culture. Psychological theories focus on stress during the perimenopausal years as a result of diminished personal and family health, socioeconomic status, family and work changes, other losses, retirement, illness, and deaths (Avis 2003). A lifetime history of major depression may be associated with an early decline in ovarian function and earlier menopause (Harlow et al. 2003). Moreover, the changing hormonal milieu in transition to menopause is strongly associated with both new onset of high depressive symptoms and new onset of depressive disorder in women with no history of depression (Freeman et al. 2006).

Women seeking treatment for physical symptoms in menopause clinics report a high prevalence of depression, irritability, mood lability, anxiety, lack of concentration, short-term memory loss, and decreased libido. Subgroups of women appear to be more vulnerable to physiological hormonal changes associated with the premenstruum, postpartum, and perimenopause (Stewart and Boydell 1993). Other investigators have shown that prior depression is a risk factor for depression at perimenopause and that poor physical health, social circumstances, divorce, widowhood, and interpersonal stress are closely correlated with depression in menopausal women (Hunter 1990).

The incidence of depression in women mirrors estrogen shifts across the life cycle, at puberty, premenopause, postpartum, and perimenopause (Stahl 2001). Estrogen receptors are present throughout the body and are particularly dense in the limbic system, which mediates emotion. Estrogen is known to influence serotonin through inhibiting monoamine oxidase at high doses and displacing tryptophan from plasma albumin–binding sites, influencing serotonin receptor–binding downregulation and increasing endogenous catecholamine release. It is not surprising that the actions of estrogen in the central nervous system may affect mood and cognition (Stahl 2001).

A study by Schmidt et al. (2000) randomly assigned 34 women to estradiol-17-beta patches or placebo for 3 weeks, then crossed over the women in the placebo group to the estrogen condition. The women with both major depression and minor depression taking estrogen reported significantly improved mood, but those receiving placebo did not. In another study, 50 perimenopausal women with major depression, dysthymia, and minor depression were randomly assigned to receive transdermal patches of estradiol-17-beta 100 mg for 12 weeks. Of the women receiving estradiol, 68% showed improvement on the

Montgomery-Åsberg Rating Scale for Depression and the Blatt-Kupperman Menopause Index, compared with 20% of those taking placebo (Soares et al. 2001).

Although estrogen appears to have a salutary effect on depression in some perimenopausal women, in contrast, progesterone and progestins are known to cause dizziness, drowsiness, and sedation in many women and may be associated with negative moods (Bjorn et al. 2000).

Studies also have been conducted on the role of estrogen as an augmentation agent with antidepressants. Women who were concurrently treated with estrogen had a threefold increased chance of responding to fluoxetine (Schneider et al. 1997). Further studies of estrogen and selective estrogen receptor modulators as psychotropic or augmentation agents are needed.

Seeman (2002) and others have shown a worsening in preexisting schizophrenic illness and other psychoses associated with decreases in estradiol during perimenopause and beyond. However, the Women's Health Initiative (WHI) results have indicated that estrogen–progesterone therapy is associated with an increased risk of breast cancer, cardiovascular disease (Writing Group for the Women's Health Initiative Investigators 2002), cognitive dysfunction, and dementia (Rapp et al. 2003; Shumaker et al. 2003). The estrogen-only arm of the WHI found increased rates of stroke, dementia, and mild cognitive impairment, but not of breast cancer (Women's Health Initiative Steering Committee 2004).

Estrogen is useful to control severe vasomotor symptoms and vaginal dryness, with current FDA guidelines recommending the smallest dosage for the shortest time possible. Antidepressants such as fluoxetine, venlafaxine, and paroxetine are also known to decrease hot flashes (Loprinzi et al. 2000, 2002; Stearns et al.

2000). Phytoestrogens (soy) and black cohosh have been shown to have contradictory results in diminishing hot flashes in perimenopausal women (Kronenberg and Fugh-Berman 2002).

Personal, social, and physical factors should always be considered in assessing the individual woman, and psychotherapy may be helpful in navigating the many transitions at midlife.

Urinary Incontinence

Urinary incontinence, the involuntary loss of urine, affects up to 23% of adults (Roe et al. 1999), with a prevalence in women that is twice that in men (Melville et al. 2005a). It is highly prevalent in women across their lifespan, and its severity increases with age (Melville et al. 2005b). Many people are reluctant to seek help because they are embarrassed, are ashamed, or believe that the problem is a part of normal aging (Roe et al. 1999).

The etiology of urinary incontinence is multifactorial and may be caused by impairment of the lower urinary tract or the nervous system or by various external factors.

Psychosocial Effects

Urinary incontinence may affect quality of life, sexual function, and mood (Melville et al. 2005a). A population-based, cross-sectional study of nearly 6,000 American women between ages 50 and 69 found that 16% reported mild, moderate, or severe incontinence (Nygaard et al. 2003). Double rates of depression have been found in incontinent women (Melville et al. 2005a). Comorbid major depression also has been found to have a significant effect on patients' urinary incontinence symptom reporting, incontinent-specific quality of life, and functional status (Melville et al. 2005a; Vigod and Stewart 2006).

Role of the Psychiatrist

Given the high prevalence of incontinence, psychiatrists may wish to tactfully ask about urinary problems, as well as comorbid psychiatric conditions and adjustment problems.

TCAs and duloxetine are useful treatments for stress urinary incontinence, particularly in women who have concurrent depression (Norton et al. 2002). Treatments that have been used for urinary incontinence include behavioral training with or without biofeedback, pelvic floor exercises, other drug therapies, and surgery (Hendrix 2002).

Psychosomatic Obstetrics/ Gynecology and Men

Virtually every study of the psychosocial aspects of an obstetric and gynecological event or treatment indicates that the attitude of the partner is a (or the) major determinant of outcome. Women turn to their significant others for reaffirmation of their worthiness if infertile, for reaffirmation of their femininity after hysterectomy, and for help deciding whether to take psychotropic medications while pregnant and whether to breast-feed or bottle-feed.

Fathers, brothers, sons, and male partners can be deeply affected by the obstetrical and gynecological experiences of the women they care about, but they often feel uncomfortable and excluded (Abboud and Liamputtong 2003; Buist et al. 2003). Women are more likely to show emotion and to want to talk to friends and relatives. Men are more likely to keep their emotions to themselves and to withdraw into work or other activities. Women can mistake this behavior for a failure to care. Sometimes, one of the most useful interventions a psychiatric consultant can perform is to facilitate communication within the family.

Conclusion

Obstetricians and gynecologists are busy practitioners, challenged to deal with both specialized technological developments and primary care, and burdened by the likelihood of lawsuits. Despite the intense emotional aspects of much of their clinical work, obstetricians and gynecologists have relatively little training or time for psychiatric problems. The scope of psychosomatic medicine in the area of obstetrics and gynecology includes psychopathological aspects of normal reproductive events, psychiatric aspects of obstetrical and gynecological diseases and treatments, and psychiatric conditions specific to women's reproductive health. Gender-based medicine, which intersects psychosomatic obstetrics and gynecology at many points, is one of the most exciting and promising areas of research and clinical practice. Myriad opportunities exist for providing practical psychiatric assistance to obstetricians and gynecologists and the women who are their patients, for educating fellow psychiatrists about developments in obstetrics and gynecology, and for basic and clinical research.

References

Abboud LN, Liamputtong P: Pregnancy loss: what it means to women who miscarry and their partners. Soc Work Health Care 36:37–62, 2003

Altshuler L, Burt V, McMullen M, et al: Breast-feeding and sertraline: a 24-hour analysis. J Clin Psychiatry 56:243–245, 1995

Altshuler L, Cohen L, Szuba M, et al: Pharmacologic management of psychiatric illness during pregnancy: dilemmas and guidelines. Am J Psychiatry 153:592–606, 1996

Altshuler LL, Cohen LS, Moline ML, et al: The Expert Consensus Guideline Series. Treatment of depression in women. Postgrad Med (Spec No):1–107, 2001

American Academy of Pediatrics Committee on Drugs: Transfer of drugs and other chemicals into human milk. Pediatrics 108:776–789, 2001

American Psychiatric Association: Diagnostic and Statistical Manual of Mental Disorders, 4th Edition, Text Revision. Washington, DC, American Psychiatric Association, 2000

Appleby L, Warner R, Whitton A, et al: A controlled study of fluoxetine and cognitive-behavioral counseling in the treatment of postnatal depression. BMJ 314:932–936, 1997

Appleby L, Mortensen PB, Faragher EB: Suicide and other causes of mortality after post-partum psychiatric admission. Br J Psychiatry 173:209–211, 1998

Attia A, Downey J, Oberman M: Postpartum psychoses, in Postpartum Mood Disorders. Edited by Miller L. Washington, DC, American Psychiatric Press, 1999, pp 99–117

Avis NE: Depression during the menopausal transition. Psychol Women Q 27:91–100, 2003

Baram DA: Physiology and symptoms of menopause, in Menopause: A Mental Health Practitioner's Guide. Edited by Stewart DE. Washington, DC, American Psychiatric Publishing, 2005, pp 15–32

Bjorn I, Bixo M, Nojd K, et al: Negative mood changes during hormone replacement therapy: a comparison between two progestogens. Am J Obstet Gynecol 183:1419–1426, 2000

Bourne S, Lewis E: Delayed psychological effects of perinatal deaths: the next pregnancy and the next generation. BMJ 289:209–210, 1984

Buist A, Morse CA, Durkin S: Men's adjustment to fatherhood: implications for obstetric health care. J Obstet Gynecol Neonatal Nurs 32:172–180, 2003

Burns L, Covington S: Psychology of infertility, in Infertility Counseling. Edited by Burns LH, Covington SN. Pearl River, NY, Parthenon, 1999, pp 3–25

Castaneda DM, Collins BE: The effects of gender, ethnicity, and a close relationship theme on perceptions of persons introducing a condom. Sex Roles 39:369–390, 1998

Chabrol H, Teissedre F, Saint-Jean M, et al: Prevention and treatment of post-partum depression: a controlled randomized study of women at risk. Psychol Med 32:1039–1047, 2002

Chambers CD, Hernandez-Diaz S, Van Marker LJ, et al: Selective serotonin reuptake inhibitors and risk of persistent pulmonary hypertension of the newborn. N Engl J Med 354:579–587, 2006

Chang MY, Chen SH, Chen CH: Factors related to perceived labor pain in primiparas. Kaohsiung J Med Sci 18:604–609, 2002

Chaudron LH, Jefferson JW: Mood stabilizers during breastfeeding: a review. J Clin Psychiatry 61:79–90, 2000

Chaudron LH, Pies RW: The relationship between postpartum psychosis and bipolar disorder: a review. J Clin Psychiatry 64:1284–1292, 2003

Chiriboga CA: Neurological correlates of fetal cocaine exposure. Ann N Y Acad Sci 846:109–125, 1998

Civic D, Scholes D, Ichikawa L, et al: Depressive symptoms in users and non-users of depot medroxyprogesterone acetate. Contraception 61:385–390, 2000

Cohen LS, Sichel DA, Robertson LM, et al: Postpartum prophylaxis for women with bipolar disorder. Am J Psychiatry 152:1641–1645, 1995

Cooper N, Blackwell D, Taylor G, et al: Pharmacist's perceptions of nurse prescribing of emergency contraception. Br J Community Nurs 5:126–131, 2000

Cooper P, Murray L, Wilson A, et al: Controlled trial of the short- and long-term effect of psychological treatment of postpartum depression, I: impact on maternal mood. Br J Psychiatry 182:412–419, 2003

Cox H, Henderson L, Andersen N, et al: Focus group study of endometriosis: struggle, loss and the medical merry-go-round. Int J Nurs Pract 9:2–9, 2003

Cramer DW, Missmer SA: The epidemiology of endometriosis. Ann N Y Acad Sci 955:11–22, 2002

Cushman LF, Kalmuss K, Namerow PB: Placing an infant for adoption: the experience of young birth mothers. Soc Work 38:264–272, 1993

Czarnocka J, Slade P: Prevalence and predictors of posttraumatic stress symptoms following childbirth. Br J Clin Psychol 39:35–51, 2000

Dagg PKB: The psychological sequelae of therapeutic abortion: denied and completed. Am J Psychiatry 148:578–585, 1991

Davies A, McIvor RJ, Kumar C: Impact of childbirth on a series of schizophrenic mothers: a comment on the possible influence of oestrogen on schizophrenia. Schizophr Res 16:25–31, 1995

DelBanco SF, Mauldon J, Smith MD: Little knowledge and limited practice: emergency contraceptive pills, the public, and the obstetrician-gynecologist. Obstet Gynecol 89:1006–1011, 1997

Demyttenaere K, Bonte L, Gheldof M, et al: Coping style and depression level influence outcome in vitro fertilization. Fertil Steril 69:1026–1033, 1998

Deuchar N: Nausea and vomiting in pregnancy: a review of the problem with particular regard to psychological and social aspects. Br J Obstet Gynecol 102:6–8, 1995

Diav-Citrin O, Shechtman S, Weinbaum D, et al: Paroxetine and fluoxetine in pregnancy: a multicenter, prospective, controlled study. Reprod Toxicol 20:459, 2005

Edwards L: New concepts in vulvodynia. Am J Obstet Gynecol 189:S24–S30, 2003

Einarson A, Bonari L, Voyer-Lavigne S, et al: A multicentre prospective controlled study to determine the safety of trazodone and nefazodone use during pregnancy. Can J Psychiatry 48: 106–110, 2003

Engelhard IM, van den Hout MA, Kindt M, et al: Peritraumatic dissociation and posttraumatic stress after pregnancy loss: a prospective study. Behav Res Ther 41:67–78, 2003

Farrell SA, Kieser K: Sexuality after hysterectomy. Obstet Gynecol 95:1045–1051, 2000

Flory N, Bissonnette F, Binik YM: Psychosocial effects of hysterectomy: literature review. J Psychosom Res 59:117–129, 2005

Franzini LR, Sideman LM: Personality characteristics of condom users. J Sex Educ Ther 20:110–118, 1994

Fraser IS, Kovacs GT: The efficacy of non-contraceptive uses for hormonal contraceptives. Med J Aust 178:621–623, 2003

Free C, Lee RM, Ogden J: Young women's accounts of factors influencing their use and non-use of emergency contraception: in-depth interview study. BMJ 325:1393–1396, 2002

Freeman EW: Current update of hormonal and psychotropic drug treatment of premenstrual dysphoric disorder. Curr Psychiatry Rep 4:435–440, 2002

Freeman EW, Sammel MD, Liu L, et al: Hormones and menopausal status as predictors of depression in women in transition to menopause. Arch Gen Psychiatry 61:62–70, 2004

Freeman EW, Sammel MD, Lin H, et al: Associations of hormones and menopausal status with depressed mood in women with no history of depression. Arch Gen Psychiatry 63:375–382, 2006

Fry R, Crisp A, Beard R: Sociopsychological factors in chronic pelvic pain: a review. J Psychosom Res 42:1–15, 1997

Fugh-Berman A, Kronenberg F: Complementary and alternative medicine (CAM) in reproductive-age women: a review of randomized controlled trials. Reprod Toxicol 17:137–152, 2003

Garg M, Singh M, Mansour D: Peri-abortion contraceptive care: can we reduce the incidence of repeat abortions? J Fam Plann Reprod Health Care 27:77–80, 2001

Gelbaya T, El-Halwagy E: Focus on primary care: chronic pelvic pain in women. Obstet Gynecol Surv 56:757–764, 2001

Glasier AF, Smith KB, van der Spuy ZM, et al: Amenorrhea associated with contraception--an international study on acceptability. Contraception 67:1–8, 2003

Goldstein D, Corbin L, Sundell K: Effects of first-trimester fluoxetine exposure on the newborn. Obstet Gynecol 89: 713–718, 1997

Grady-Weliky TA: Clinical practice: premenstrual dysphoric disorder. N Engl J Med 348:433–438, 2003

Greenfield SF, Sugarman DE: Treatment and consequences of alcohol abuse and dependence during pregnancy, in Management of Psychiatric Disorders During Pregnancy. Edited by Yonkers KA, Little B. London, Edward Arnold, 2001, pp 213–227

Groff JY, Mullen PD, Byrd T, et al: Decision making, beliefs, and attitudes toward hysterectomy: a focus group study with medically underserved women in Texas. J Womens Health Gend Based Med 9:S39–S50, 2000

Grote NK, Frank E: Difficult-to-treat depression: the role of contexts and comorbidities. Biol Psychiatry 53:660–670, 2003

Halbreich U, Bergeron R, Yonkers KA, et al: Efficacy of intermittent, luteal phase sertraline treatment of premenstrual dysphoric disorder. Obstet Gynecol 100:1219–1229, 2002

Hallberg P, Sjoblom V: The use of selective serotonin reuptake inhibitors during pregnancy and breast-feeding: a review and clinical aspects. J Clin Psychopharmacol 25:59–73, 2005

Harlow BL, Wise LA, Otto MW, et al: Depression and its influence on reproductive endocrine and menstrual cycle markers associated with perimenopause: the Harvard Study of Moods and Cycles. Arch Gen Psychiatry 60:29–36, 2003

Harvey SM, Bird ST, Galavotti C, et al: Relationship power, sexual decision making and condom use among women at risk for HIV/STDS. Womens Health 36:69–84, 2002

Heikkinen T, Ekblad U, Kero P, et al: Citalopram in pregnancy and lactation. Clin Pharmacol Ther 72:184–191, 2002

Hendrick V, Altshuler L, Wertheimer A, et al: Venlafaxine and breast-feeding. Am J Psychiatry 158:2089–2090, 2001

Hendrick V, Smith L, Suri R, et al: Birth outcomes after prenatal exposure to antidepressant medication. Am J Obstet Gynecol 188:812–815, 2003

Hendrix S: Urinary incontinence and menopause: an evidence-based treatment approach. Dis Mon 48:622–636, 2002

Hillis SD, Marchbanks PA, Tylor LR, et al: Poststerilization regret: findings from the United States Collaborative Review of Sterilization. Obstet Gynecol 93:889–895, 1999

Hirshbein LD: Biology and mental illness: a historical perspective. J Am Med Womens Assoc 58:89–94, 2003

Holditch-Davis D, Bartlett TR, Blickman AL, et al: Posttraumatic stress symptoms in mothers of premature infants. J Obstet Gynecol Neonatal Nurs 32:161–171, 2003

Howard F: Chronic pelvic pain. Obstet Gynecol 101:594–611, 2003

Howard L, Webb R, Abel K: Safety of antipsychotic drugs for pregnant and breastfeeding women with non-affecive psychosis. BMJ 329:933–934, 2004 [erratum: 329: 1236, 2004]

Hughes PM, Turton P, Evans CD: Stillbirth as risk factor for depression and anxiety in the subsequent pregnancy: cohort study. BMJ 318:1721–1724, 1999

Hunter MS: Somatic experience of the menopause: a prospective study. Psychosom Med 52:357–367, 1990

Hunter MS, Ussher JM, Browne SJ, et al: A randomized comparison of psychological (cognitive behavior therapy), medical (fluoxetine) and combined treatment for women with premenstrual dysphoric disorder. J Psychosom Obstet Gynaecol 23:193–199, 2002

Ilett K, Kristensen J, Hackett L, et al: Distribution of venlafaxine and its O-desmethyl metabolite in human milk and their effects in breastfed infants. Br J Clin Pharmacol 53: 17–22, 2002

Jamieson DJ, Kaufman SC, Costello C, et al: U.S. Collaborative Review of Sterilization Working Group: a comparison of women's regret after vasectomy versus tubal sterilization. Obstet Gynecol 99:1073–1079, 2002

Janowsky DS, Rausch JL, Davis JM: Historical studies of premenstrual tension up to 30 years ago: implications for future research. Curr Psychiatry Rep 4:411–418, 2002

Jeal RR, West LA: Rolling away the stone: post-abortion women in the Christian community. J Pastoral Care Counsel 57:53–64, 2003

Johnson JK, Haider F, Ellis K, et al: The prevalence of domestic violence in pregnant women. BJOG 110:272–275, 2003

Kainz K: The role of the psychologist in the evaluation and treatment of infertility. Womens Health Issues 11:481–485, 2001

Kariminia A, Saunders DM, Chamberlain M: Risk factors for strong regret and subsequent IVF request after having tubal ligation. Aust N Z J Obstet Gynaecol 42:526–529, 2002

King R: Subfecundity and anxiety in a nationally representative sample. Soc Sci Med 56:739–751, 2003

Kjerulff KH, Langenberg PW, Rhodes JC, et al: Effectiveness of hysterectomy. Obstet Gynecol 95:319–326, 2000

Klatzkin RR, Morrow AL, Light KC, et al: Histories of depression, allopregnanolone responses to stress, and premenstrual symptoms in women. Biol Psychol 71:2–11, 2006

Klock S: Obstetric and gynecological conditions, in Clinical Handbook of Health Psychology. Edited by Camic P, Knight S. Seattle, WA, Hogrefe & Huber, 1998, pp 349–388

Koop CE: Surgeon General's report: the public health effects of abortion, 101st Cong., 1st sess. Congressional Record (March 21, 1989): E906–909

Kronenberg F, Fugh-Berman A: Complementary and alternative medicine for menopausal symptoms: a review of randomized, controlled trials. Ann Intern Med 137:805–813, 2002

Kubicka L, Roth Z, Dytrych Z, et al: The mental health of adults born of unwanted pregnancies, their siblings, and matched controls: a 35-year follow-up study from Prague, Czech Republic. J Nerv Ment Dis 190:653–662, 2002

Laird J: A male pill? Gender discrepancies in contraceptive commitment. Fem Psychol 4:458–468, 1994

Lande RG, Karamchandani V: Chronic mental illness and the menstrual cycle. J Am Osteopath Assoc 102:655–659, 2002

Landen M, Eriksson E: How does premenstrual dysphoric disorder relate to depression and anxiety disorders? Depress Anxiety 17:122–129, 2003

Lane T, Francis A: Premenstrual symptomatology, locus of control, anxiety and depression in women with normal menstrual cycles. Arch Women Ment Health 6:127–138, 2003

Lewis CL, Groff JY, Herman CJ, et al: Overview of women's decision making regarding elective hysterectomy, oophorectomy, and hormone replacement therapy. J Womens Health Gend Based Med 9:S5–S14, 2000

Loprinzi CL, Kugler JW, Sloan JA, et al: Venlafaxine in management of hot flashes in survivors of breast cancer: a randomised controlled trial. Lancet 356:2059–2063, 2000

Loprinzi CL, Sloan JA, Perez EA, et al: Phase III evaluation of fluoxetine for treatment of hot flashes. J Clin Oncol 20: 1578–1583, 2002

Lu PY, Ory SJ: Endometriosis: current management. Mayo Clin Proc 70:453–463, 1995

Lukse M, Vacc N: Grief, depression, and coping in women undergoing fertility treatment. Obstet Gynecol 93:245–251, 1999

Marcus S, Barry K, Flynn H, et al: Treatment guidelines for depression in pregnancy. Int J Obstet Gynecol 71:61–70, 2001

Masheb RM, Lozano-Blanco C, Kohorn EI, et al: Assessing sexual function and dyspareunia with the Female Sexual Function Index (FSFI) in women with vulvodynia. J Sex Marital Ther 30:315–324, 2004

Matthey S, Barnett B, Howie P, et al: Diagnosing postpartum depression in mothers and fathers: whatever happened to anxiety? J Affect Disord 74:139–147, 2003a

Matthey S, Barnett B, White T: The Edinburgh Postnatal Depression Scale. Br J Psychiatry 182:368–370, 2003b

Melville JL, Delaney K, Newton K, et al: Incontinence severity and major depression in incontinent women. Obstet Gynecol 106:585–592, 2005a

Melville JL, Katon W, Delaney K, et al: Urinary incontinence in US women: a population-based study. Arch Intern Med 165:537?542, 2005b

Miller LJ: Psychotic denial of pregnancy: phenomenology and clinical management. Hosp Community Psychiatry 41:1233–1237, 1990

Miller LJ, Finnerty J: Sexuality, pregnancy and childrearing among women with schizophrenia-spectrum disorders. Psychiatr Serv 47:502–506, 1996

Moore J, Kennedy S: Causes of chronic pelvic pain. Baillieres Best Pract Res Clin Obstet Gynaecol 14:389–402, 2001

Murray L, Cooper P, Wilson A, et al: Controlled trial of the short- and long-term effect of psychological treatment of postpartum depression, 2: impact on the mother-child relationship and child outcome. Br J Psychiatry 182:420–427, 2003

Norton P, Zinner N, Yalcin, I, et al: Duloxetine versus placebo in the treatment of stress urinary incontinence. Am J Obstet Gynecol 187:40–48, 2002

Nulman I, Rovet J, Stewart D, et al: Child development following exposure to tricyclic antidepressants or fluoxetine throughout fetal life: a prospective, controlled study. Am J Psychiatry 159:1889–1895, 2002

Nygaard I, Turvey C, Burns T, et al: Urinary incontinence and depression in middle-aged United States women. Obstet Gynecol 101:149–156, 2003

O'Hara MW, Stuart S, Gorman LL, et al: Efficacy of interpersonal psychotherapy for postpartum depression. Arch Gen Psychiatry 57:1039–1045, 2000

Pati S, Cullins V: Female sterilization: evidence. Obstet Gynecol Clin North Am 27:859–899, 2000

Patton S, Misri S, Corral M, et al: Antipsychotic medication during pregnancy and lactation in women with schizophrenia: evaluating the risk. Can J Psychiatry 47:959–965, 2002

Pearlstein T, Joliat MJ, Brown EB, et al: Recurrence of symptoms of premenstrual dysphoric disorder after the cessation of luteal-phase fluoxetine treatment. Am J Obstet Gynecol 188:887–895, 2003

Picardo CM, Nichols M, Edelman A, et al: Women's knowledge and sources of information on the risks and benefits of oral contraception. J Am Med Womens Assoc 58:112–116, 2003

Poleshuck EL, Dworkin RH, Howard FM, et al: Contributions of physical and sexual abuse to women's experiences with chronic pelvic pain. J Reprod Med 50:91–100, 2005

Price J, Blake F: Chronic pelvic pain: the assessment as therapy. J Psychosom Res 46:7–14, 1999

Pro-Life Action Ministries: What They Won't Tell You at the Abortion Clinic (flyer). St. Paul, MN, Pro-Life Action Ministries, undated

Rannestad T: Hysterectomy: effects on quality of life and psychological aspects. Best Pract Res Clin Obstet Gynaecol 19:419–430, 2005

Rapp SR, Espeland MA, Shumaker SA, et al: Effect of estrogen plus progestin on global cognitive function in postmenopausal women. The Women's Health Initiative Memory Study: a randomized controlled trial. JAMA 289:2663–2672, 2003

Reardon DC, Cougle JR, Rue VM, et al: Psychiatric admissions of low-income women following abortion and childbirth. CMAJ 168:1253–1256, 2003

Reiter R: Evidence-based management of chronic pelvic pain. Clin Obstet Gynecol 41:422–435, 1998

Richter DL, McKeown RE, Corwin SJ, et al: The role of male partners in women's decision making regarding hysterectomy. J Womens Health Gend Based Med 9:S51–S61, 2000

Rickert VI, Wiemann CM, Harrykissoon SD, et al: The relationship among demographics, reproductive characteristics, and intimate partner violence. Am J Obstet Gynecol 187:1002–1007, 2002

Robertson E, Grace SL, Wellington T, et al: Antenatal risk factors for postpartum depression: a synthesis of recent literature. Gen Hosp Psychiatry 26:289–295, 2004

Roe B, Doll H, Wilson K: Help seeking behaviour and health and social services utilization by people suffering from urinary incontinence. Int J Nurs Stud 36:245–253, 1999

Rosch DS, Sajatovic M, Sivec H: Behavioral characteristics in delusional pregnancy: a matched control group study. Int J Psychiatry Med 32:295–303, 2002

Ross LE, Gilbert Evans SE, Sellers EM, et al: Measurement issues in postpartum depression part 1: anxiety as a feature of postpartum depression. Arch Womens Ment Health 6:51–57, 2003

Ross LE, Dennis CL, Blackmore ER, et al: Postpartum Depression: A Guide for Front-line Health and Social Service Providers. Toronto, ON, Canada, Centre for Addiction and Mental Health, 2005

Saisto T, Halmesmaki E: Fear of childbirth: a neglected dilemma. Acta Obstet Gynecol Scand 82:201–208, 2003

Sakumoto K, Masamoto H, Kanazawa K: Postpartum maternity "blues" as a reflection of newborn nursing care in Japan. Int J Gynaecol Obstet 78:25–30, 2002

Saltzman LE, Johnson CH, Gilbert BC, et al: Physical abuse around the time of pregnancy: an examination of prevalence and risk factors in 16 states. Matern Child Health J 7: 31–43, 2003

Sanders SA, Graham CA, Yarber WL, et al: Condom use errors and problems among young women who put condoms on their male partners. J Am Med Womens Assoc 58:95–98, 2003

Sanz EJ, De-las-Cuevas C, Kiuru A, et al: Selective serotonin reuptake inhibitors in pregnant women and neonatal withdrawal syndrome: a database analysis. Lancet 365:482–487, 2005

Savidge C, Slade P: Psychological aspects of chronic pelvic pain. J Psychosom Res 42:433–444, 1997

Schatzberg AF, Cole JO, DeBattista C: Manual of Clinical Psychology, 4th Edition. Washington, DC, American Psychiatric Publishing, 2003

Schmidt P, Nieman L, Danaceau M, et al: Estrogen replacement in perimenopause-related depression: a preliminary report. Am J Obstet Gynecol 183:414–420, 2000

Schneider LS, Small GW, Hamilton SH, et al: Estrogen replacement and response to fluoxetine in a multicenter geriatric depression trial: Fluoxetine Collaborative Study Group. Am J Geriatr Psychiatry 5:97–106, 1997

Seeman MV: Does menopause intensify symptoms in schizophrenia? in Psychiatric Illness in Women: Emerging Treatments and Research. Edited by Lewis-Hall F, Williams TS, Panetta J, et al. Washington, DC, American Psychiatric Publishing, 2002, pp 239–248

Shane-McWhorter L, Cerveny JD, MacFarlane LL, et al: Enhanced metabolism of levonorgestrel during phenobarbital treatment and resultant pregnancy. Pharmacotherapy 18:1360–1365, 1998

Shumaker SA, Legault C, Rapp SR, et al: Estrogen plus progestin and the incidence of dementia and mild cognitive impairment in postmenopausal women. The Women's Health Initiative Memory Study: a randomized controlled trial. JAMA 289:2651–2662, 2003

Slade P, Heke S, Fletcher J, et al: Termination of pregnancy: patients' perceptions of care. J Fam Plann Reprod Health Care 27:72–77, 2001

Smeenk JM, Verhaak CM, Vingerhoets AJ, et al: Stress and outcome success in IVF: the role of self-reports and endocrine variables. Hum Reprod 20:991–996, 2005

Soares CN, Almeida OP, Joffe H, et al: Efficacy of estradiol for the treatment of depressive disorders in perimenopausal women: a double-blind, randomized, placebo-controlled trial. Arch Gen Psychiatry 58:529–534, 2001

Spielvogel AM, Hohener HC: Denial of pregnancy: a review and case reports. Birth 22:220–226, 1995

Spinelli M: Interpersonal psychotherapy for depressed antepartum women: a pilot study. Am J Psychiatry 154:1028–1030, 1997

Spinelli MG, Endicott J: Controlled clinical trial of interpersonal psychotherapy versus parenting education program for depressed pregnant women. Am J Psychiatry 160:555–562, 2003

Stahl SM: Effects of estrogen on the central nervous system. J Clin Psychiatry 62:317–318, 2001

Stearns V, Isaacs C, Rowland J, et al: A pilot trial assessing the efficacy of paroxetine hydrochloride (Paxil) in controlling hot flashes in breast cancer survivors. Ann Oncol 11:17–22, 2000

Stewart DE: Antidepressant drugs during pregnancy and lactation. Int Clin Psychopharmacol 15 (suppl 3):S19–S24, 2001

Stewart DE: Depression in pregnancy. Can Fam Physician 58:1061–1063, 2005

Stewart DE, Boydell KM: Psychologic distress during menopause: associations across the reproductive life cycle. Int J Psychiatry Med 23:157–162, 1993

Stewart DE, Robinson G: Eating disorders and reproduction, in Psychological Aspects of Women's Health Care: The Interface Between Psychiatry and Obstetrics and Gynecology, 2nd Edition. Edited by Stotland N, Stewart D. Washington, DC, American Psychiatric Press, 2001a, pp 441–456

Stewart DE, Robinson G: Psychotropic drugs and electroconvulsive therapy during pregnancy and lactation, in Psychological Aspects of Women's Health Care: The Interface Between Psychiatry and Obstetrics and Gynecology, 2nd Edition. Edited by Stotland N, Stewart D. Washington, DC, American Psychiatric Press, 2001b, pp 67–93

Stewart DE, Reicher AE, Gerulath AH, et al: Vulvodynia and psychological distress. Obstet Gynecol 84:587–590, 1994

Stewart DE, Leyland NA, Shime J, et al: Achieving Best Practices in the Use of Hysterectomy: Report of Ontario's Expert Panel on Best Practices in the Use of Hysterectomy. Ontario, Canada, Ontario Women's Health Council, 2002

Stiskal J, Kulin N, Koren G, et al: Neonatal paroxetine withdrawal syndrome. Arch Dis Child Fetal Neonatal Ed 84: F134–F135, 2001

Sveinsdottir H, Lundman B, Norberg A: Whose voice? Whose experiences? Women's qualitative accounts of general and private discussion of premenstrual syndrome. Scand J Caring Sci 16:414–423, 2002

Thorp JM Jr, Hartmann KE, Shadigian E: Long-term physical and psychological health consequences of induced abortion: review of the evidence. Obstet Gynecol Surv 58:67–79, 2003

Thys-Jacobs S, Starkey P, Bernstein D, et al: Calcium carbonate and the premenstrual syndrome: effects on premenstrual and menstrual symptoms. Premenstrual Syndrome Study Group. Am J Obstet Gynecol 179:444–452, 1998

Turton P, Hughes P, Evans CD, et al: Incidence, correlates and predictors of post-traumatic stress disorder in the pregnancy after stillbirth. Br J Psychiatry 178:556–560, 2001

Upchurch DM, Kusunoki Y, Simon P, et al: Sexual behavior and condom practices among Los Angeles women. Womens Health Issues 13:8–15, 2003

U.S. Food and Drug Administration: Current categories for drug use in pregnancy. Available at: http://www.fda.gov/fdac/features/2001/301_preg.html. Accessed September 3, 2003

Ventura SJ, Mosher WD, Curtin SC, et al: Trends in pregnancies and pregnancy rates by outcome: estimates for the United States 1976–96. Vital Health Stat 21:1–47, 2000

Verhaak CM, Smeenk JM, van Minnen A, et al: A longitudinal, prospective study on emotional adjustment before, during and after consecutive fertility treatment cycles. Hum Reprod 20:2253–2260, 2005

Vigod SN, Stewart DE: The management of abnormal uterine bleeding by northern, rural and isolated primary care physicians, part II: what do we need? BMC Womens Health 2:11, 2002

Vigod SN, Stewart DE: Major depression in female urinary incontinence. Psychosomatics 47:147–151, 2006

Viguera AC, Cohen LS, Baldessarini RJ, et al: Managing bipolar disorder during pregnancy: weighing the risks and benefits. Can J Psychiatry 47:426–436, 2002

Warnock JK, Bundren JC, Morris DW: Sertraline in the treatment of depression associated with gonadotropin-releasing hormone agonist therapy. Biol Psychiatry 43:464–465, 1998

Weaver S, Clifford E, Hay D, et al: Psychosocial adjustment to unsuccessful IVF and GFT treatment. Patient Educ Couns 31:7–18, 1997

Wessel J, Endrikat J, Buscher U: Frequency of denial of pregnancy: results and epidemiological significance of a 1-year prospective study in Berlin. Acta Obstet Gynecol Scand 81:1021–1027, 2002

Westhoff C, Picardo L, Morrow E: Quality of life following early medical or surgical abortion. Contraception 67:41–47, 2003

Whelan CI, Stewart DE: Pseudocyesis: a review and report of six cases. Int J Psychiatry Med 20:97–108, 1990

Wisner K, Findling R, Perel J: Paroxetine in breast milk. Am J Psychiatry 158:144–145, 2001

Wisner K, Gelenberg A, Leonard H, et al: Pharmacologic treatment of depression during pregnancy. JAMA 282:1264–1269, 2002a

Wisner KL, Parry BL, Piontek CM: Postpartum depression. N Engl J Med 347:194–199, 2002b

Women's Health Initiative Steering Committee: Effects of conjugated equine estrogen in postmenopausal women with hysterectomy: the Women's Health Initiative randomized controlled trial. JAMA 291:1701–1712, 2004

World Health Organization Programme of Maternal and Child Health and Family Planning Unit: Infertility: a tabulation of available data on prevalence of primary and secondary infertility (WHO/MCM/91.9). 1991. Available at: http://www.who.int/reproductive-health/publications/Abstracts/infertility.html

Writing Group for the Women's Health Initiative Investigators: Risks and benefits of estrogen plus progestin in healthy postmenopausal women: principal results from the Women's Health Initiative randomized controlled trial. JAMA 288: 321–333, 2002

Wyatt KM, Dimmock PW, O'Brien PM: Selective serotonin reuptake inhibitors for premenstrual syndrome. Cochrane Database Syst Rev 4:CD001396, 2002

Zabin LS, Hirsch MB, Emerson MR: When urban adolescents choose abortion: effects on education, psychological status, and subsequent pregnancy. Fam Plann Perspect 21:248–255, 1989

Zlokovich MS, Snell WE Jr: Contraceptive behavior and efficacy: the influence of illusion of fertility control and adult attachment tendencies. J Psychol Human Sex 9:39–55, 1997

Zlotogora J: Parental decisions to abort or continue a pregnancy with an abnormal finding after an invasive prenatal test. Prenat Diagn 22:1102–1106, 2002

Zondervan K, Yudkin P, Vessey M, et al: Patterns of diagnosis and referral in women consulting for chronic pelvic pain in UK primary care. Br J Obstet Gynecol 106:1149–1155, 1999

Self-Assessment Questions

Select the single best response for each question.

1. Infertility is a common clinical problem in obstetric/gynecological practice that is often fraught with psychosocial distress. Attention to and management of comorbid psychiatric illness may be an important part of infertility treatment. All of the following statements are true *except*

   A. The prevalence of infertility has increased steadily since 1965.
   B. Generalized anxiety disorder (GAD) is associated with lower rates of fecundity.
   C. Comorbid depression is associated with lower pregnancy rates in women undergoing in vitro fertilization.
   D. Restrictive or purging eating behaviors are often undisclosed and result in poor fecundity.
   E. The majority of infertility problems are attributable to the male or are of unknown etiology.

2. The pharmacological interactions between psychotropic medications and contraceptives may result in unwelcome clinical events. All of the following statements are true *except*

   A. Implanted levonorgestrel metabolism can be enhanced by phenobarbital, decreasing contraceptive effectiveness.
   B. Oral contraceptives inhibit the metabolism of tricyclic antidepressants, thus increasing serum levels.
   C. Oral contraceptives enhance the metabolism of benzodiazepines, decreasing their effectiveness.
   D. Modafinil increases the metabolism of oral contraceptives.
   E. Carbamazepine and oxcarbazepine both enhance the metabolism of oral contraceptives.

3. Hysterectomy is a common gynecological procedure that frequently involves significant psychiatric factors. Which of the following statements is *true?*

   A. The mean age of women undergoing hysterectomy is the early to mid-50s when menopause normally occurs.
   B. Among women who undergo hysterectomy, African American women have the procedure at an older age than do other American women, on the average.
   C. Women who undergo hysterectomy for chronic pelvic pain have better psychological outcomes than do women who undergo hysterectomy for bleeding.
   D. Women undergoing surgical hysterectomy with oophorectomy are at risk for depression, especially if they have a history of depression associated with reproductive events.
   E. Most studies show a decrease in sexuality in women following hysterectomy.

4. Psychiatric disorders that occur during pregnancy can be of great concern because of the challenges of managing a pregnant psychiatric patient. Which of the following statements is *true?*

    A. Panic disorder patients who become pregnant should continue on medication throughout pregnancy.
    B. Obsessive-compulsive disorder is likely to worsen postpartum but not prepartum.
    C. Electroconvulsive therapy (ECT) for acute psychosis during pregnancy can be effective and is generally safe for the fetus.
    D. Despite the later-appearing cognitive impairments, the perinatal mortality for fetal alcohol syndrome is less than 5%.
    E. In "crack babies," the cognitive impairments are usually due to the toxic exposure to cocaine in utero rather than to social factors.

5. Postpartum depression and psychosis are among the most serious and potentially dangerous conditions in psychiatry because of their threat to infant safety. Which of the following statements is *true?*

    A. Miscarriage increases the risk of depression in subsequent pregnancies, but stillbirth does not.
    B. Postpartum depression incidence in North America is 30%–40% of pregnancies.
    C. Symptoms of depression begin about the same time as "baby blues," normally within a few days after birth.
    D. Antecedent anxiety disorder is an important risk factor for postpartum depression.
    E. Relatives of a patient with postpartum depression should typically offer to assume total care of the newborn.

17 Pediatrics

Brenda Bursch, Ph.D.
Margaret Stuber, M.D.

Children's Developmental Understanding of Illness and Their Bodies

Children's conceptions of their bodies vary widely and are obviously influenced by experiences with illness. However, in general, children appear to follow a developmental path in their understanding of their bodies that roughly corresponds to Piaget's stages of cognitive development. *Sensorimotor children* (birth to approximately 2 years) are largely preverbal and do not have the capacity to create narratives to explain their experiences. Their perception of their bodies and of illness is therefore primarily built on sensory experiences and does not involve any formal reasoning. *Preoperational children* (approximately 2–7 years) also understand through perception, but they are able to use words and some very basic concepts of cause and effect. They tend to be most aware of parts of the body that they can directly sense, such as bones and heart (which they can feel) and blood (which they have seen

come out of their bodies). However, they do not have a clear sense of cause and effect and they are therefore inclined to see events that are temporally related as causally related. They also have no real sense of organs, but conceptualize blood and food as going into or coming out of their bodies as though the body were itself the container. This leads to many humorous but confusing assumptions and misunderstandings. *Concrete operational children* (approximately 7–11 years) are able to apply logic to their perceptions in a more integrative manner. However, the logic is quite literal or concrete and allows for only one cause for an effect. They tend to be eager to learn factual information about the body and illness at this age but will have difficulty with any concepts that require abstract reasoning. *Formal operational children* (11+ years) are able to use a level of abstract reasoning that allows discussion of systems rather than simple organs and can incorporate multiple causation of illness. It should not be assumed, however, that all adolescents approach the understanding of illness and their bodies at this level of cognition. In fact, most adults function at this level of thought only in areas of their own expertise, if at all.

As with all areas of cognition, education and experience make a difference. Children who have a medical problem (or who have a friend or family member with a medical history) may know more about the body and its function than other children. However, children will also often be able to repeat what has been said to them without any real understanding of what it means. It is always important to assess children's level of understanding by asking them to explain in their own words or give their own version of why something is happening. This can alert you and the treating team to gross misunderstandings or fears that could influence adherence to the treatment plan.

Symptoms and Psychiatric Disorders

Psychological Responses to Illness

Psychological distress in response to serious pediatric illness has been a focus of many disease-specific and noncategorical studies over the years. Often symptoms of depression, anxiety, and behavioral problems are grouped together. For example, a recent review of empirical studies of pediatric heart transplant recipients found that 20%–24% of these children experienced significant problems of psychological distress (Todaro et al. 2000). A study of children with epilepsy, using the State-Trait Anxiety Inventory and the Children's Depression Inventory (Oguz et al. 2002), found that the epileptic children reported significantly more depressed and anxious symptoms than a control group. Even in children undergoing a surgical procedure as minor as a tonsillectomy, 17% of 89 children followed prospectively had temporary symptoms consistent with a depressive epi-

sode (Papakostas et al. 2003). In some cases, the effects can be longer lasting, as was found in a study of 5,736 childhood cancer survivors, studied as young adults, who reported significantly more symptoms of depression than their sibling controls (Zebrack et al. 2002). The symptoms assessed in most of these cases would not necessarily meet criteria for a DSM diagnosis. However, these symptoms do appear to be associated with decrease in function. For example, the type of depression that is seen in association with chronic pain of various etiologies has been found to be strongly associated with functional disability (Kashikar-Zuck et al. 2001).

Social support appears to be a key element in psychological adjustment to illness. Social support was found to negatively correlate with problem behavior in adolescents with HIV over a period of 3 years (Battles and Wiener 2002). In a study of 160 pediatric rheumatology patients, children with higher classmate support had lower levels of depression (von Weiss et al. 2002). Depressed parents of chronically ill children have been found to have depressed children (Williamson et al. 2002). Social support has medical implications as well. For example, families that are less caring or are in more conflict are associated with poorer metabolic control of children with juvenile-onset diabetes (Schiffrin 2001). Serious pediatric illness or treatment may also lead to chronic as well as acute symptoms of emotional distress in the parents, which may interfere with their ability to provide support for the children. This has been found with pediatric cancer patients (Kazak et al. 1997) and pediatric transplant recipients (Young et al. 2003).

In some cases, psychological distress and behavioral problems can be directly caused by physical manifestations of the illness or the treatment. For example, mood disorders and anxiety are relatively common manifestations of involvement of the central nervous system (CNS) in pediatric systemic lupus erythematosus (Sibbitt et al. 2002). Depression, anxiety, aggression, and school problems are observed as side effects of tacrolimus, given to prevent rejection of a transplanted kidney (Kemper et al. 2003). Use of steroids for inflammatory conditions, such as rheumatoid arthritis, can have a significant impact on mood (Klein-Gitelman and Pachman 1998). Treatment of behavioral distress, depression, or anxiety in juvenile-onset diabetes mellitus must always consider the agitation that is symptomatic of hypoglycemia or the confusion associated with hyperglycemia (Goodnick et al. 1995).

Effective treatment for anxiety that persists after normal adjustment and comfort issues are addressed is similar to that provided in general psychiatric practice: cognitive-behavioral therapy (Kendall 1994; Ollendick and King 1998) and the use of selective serotonin reuptake inhibitors (SSRIs) (Research Unit on Pediatric Psychopharmacology Anxiety Study Group 2001). Individual behavioral techniques, such as exposure and systematic desensitization, can be effective for patients with simple phobias such as needle phobia or food aversion. More extensive cognitive-behavioral treatment packages that address anxiety across many dimensions (including somatic, cognitive, and behavioral problems) are indicated for children with more complex anxiety disorders (Piacentini and Bergman 2001).

Pediatricians are familiar with the use of stimulants and some antidepressants in their practice (Efron et al. 2003), but there is yet a limited literature on the use of these medications in medically ill children. The strongest research effort in child psychiatry on effective medication treatments for depression and anxiety has been with SSRIs. In a five-center trial, fluvoxamine was superior to placebo in treating pa-

tients with separation anxiety disorder, social anxiety disorder, or generalized anxiety disorder (Research Unit on Pediatric Psychopharmacology Anxiety Study Group 2001). Additionally, fluoxetine has been found to be effective for childhood obsessive-compulsive disorder (Liebowitz et al. 2002). Strong evidence does not exist to support the use of tricyclic antidepressants or benzodiazepines as a first-line treatment for child anxiety disorders (Riddle et al. 1999). Despite a lack of supporting data, benzodiazepines are frequently prescribed by pediatricians for acute anxiety or agitation in the hospital because they can have a more immediate effect than SSRIs. Therefore, it is important to note that some anxious children have agitated reactions to benzodiazepines. Psychiatric consultants can offer alternatives, including neuroleptics in cases where immediate response is necessary.

Because hospitalized and chronically ill children often experience many of the symptoms seen in depression, making a decision as to whether a pediatric patient should be treated for depression can be difficult. A depressed or irritable mood, diminished interest or pleasure in activities, significant weight loss or change in appetite, insomnia or hypersomnia, psychomotor agitation or retardation, and fatigue or loss of energy may be secondary to the medical condition or to prolonged separation from friends and family. Although medication may be indicated, often supportive and behavioral interventions can lead to significant improvements for such symptoms. Less common, and thus more concerning, are feelings of worthlessness or inappropriate guilt, diminished ability to think or concentrate, or thoughts of suicide (Goldston 1994). A careful assessment is necessary, with attention to suicidal fantasies or actions, concepts of what the child thinks would happen if suicide was attempted or achieved, previous experiences with suicidal behavior, circumstances at the time of the suicidal behavior, motivations for suicide, concepts and experiences of death, family situations, and environmental situations (Pfeffer 1986). Adolescents with suicidal intent and plan, family history of suicide, a comorbid psychiatric disorder, intractable pain, persistent insomnia, lack of social support, inadequate coping skills, a recent improvement in depressive symptoms, or impulsivity are at particular risk for suicide. Antidepressant medication should be started carefully in such cases. For some adolescents, the idea of suicide is an important source of control in the face of an unknown and uncontrollable illness course. Addressing a lack of perceived control, isolation, and distressing physical symptoms should be a high priority.

Adherence

The term *adherence* is generally used to describe the extent to which a patient's health behavior is consistent with medical recommendations. Defined as such, adherence would include not only the taking of medications and attendance at clinical appointments but also diet, exercise, and other lifestyle issues such as smoking and use of sunscreen (Lemanek et al. 2001). Adherence is measured using blood levels, pill counts, and self-report, all of which are problematic (Du Pasquier-Fediaevsky and Tubiana-Rufi 1999; Shemesh et al. 2004). With such a wide definition and different assessment strategies, the estimates vary as to the number of pediatric patients who adhere to medical regimens for chronic conditions (Rapoff 1999; Steele and Grauer 2003). Despite these problems, there is general agreement that nonadherence with medication regimens is a serious problem in pediatric patients with both acute and chronic conditions, resulting in significant clinical morbidity

(Bauman et al. 2002; DiMatteo et al. 2002; Phipps and DeCuir-Whalley 1990; Serrano-Ikkos 1998).

Many variables have been cited as potential predictors of nonadherence. Increasing age of the child is correlated with increased nonadherence, as is longer time on treatment and lack of appropriate family support in most studies across a variety of illnesses (Griffin and Elkin 2001; Lurie et al. 2000; Rapoff et al. 2002; Strunk et al. 2002). The patient's health beliefs regarding barriers to care, severity of the illness, and susceptibility to problems have been found to be related to nonadherence in some studies (Soliday and Hoeksel 2000), whereas other studies have found that parental health beliefs did not predict adherence (Steele et al. 2001). Some investigations have suggested that cultural beliefs may be equally or more important (Snodgrass et al. 2001; Tucker et al. 2002). Although lack of knowledge would seem to be an important predictor, this has proven more difficult to measure than might be expected (Ho et al. 2003; McQuaid et al. 2003). One study actually found that mild anxiety was associated with better adherence (Strunk et al. 2002), whereas others suggest that psychological distress is associated with nonadherence (Simoni et al. 1997).

Interventions to increase adherence have fallen under the general categories of educational (written and verbal instructions), organizational (simplification of regimens, improved access, increased supervision), and behavioral (reminders, incentives, and self-monitoring). A recent review of published studies of interventions to improve adherence found that different strategies appear to be more effective for specific illnesses. Although cognitive-behavioral approaches appear promising, no interventions have been found to meet criteria to be considered "well established" for improving adherence in asthma, juvenile rheumatoid arthritis, or type 1 diabetes (Lemanek et al.

2001). A provocative pilot study found that treating liver transplant recipients for posttraumatic stress disorder (PTSD) improved adherence to medication (Shemesh et al. 2000).

Death, Dying, and Bereavement

Although depression, withdrawal, and anxiety may be expected, a variety of emotional responses may be seen in terminally ill children and should be anticipated in conversations with parents. Children and adolescents may manifest their confusion and loss by negative, oppositional, aggressive, or emotional acting out, as well as with apathy and withdrawal from family and friends. They may frighten the medical staff or family as they talk about death or carry on conversations with someone who has died or with God. They may seem to know when they are going to die or "take a trip." What may initially appear to be confusion or delirium may actually be an attempt to communicate through a metaphor (Callanan and Kelley 1992). The approach of the consultant should be to allow such conversations to occur, and to support the staff and parents to tolerate these attempts of the child to cope with the process of dying. Play therapy or art therapy may be particularly helpful for younger children and for older children who prefer these modalities. In some cases, children will choose to specifically address unfinished business, such as saying good-bye, making amends, being absolved of perceived transgressions, planning their memorial service, or deciding who gets particular belongings (Gyulay 1989). Environmental interventions can relieve many physical discomforts. Interventions to improve communication and understanding can relieve many emotional discomforts and fears. If such interventions are not sufficient to resolve distressing symptoms, medications should be considered. It is important to recognize that children and parents vary in their preferences for sedation versus symptoms. It is important to understand these preferences when choosing medications. For a more thorough review of emotional and physical symptom management, see the article by Stuber and Bursch (2000) and the book by Behrman et al. (2004). For a more thorough review on the topic of talking to children about death, refer to the article by Stuber and Mesrkhani (2001).

Delirium

Although pediatric delirium has received little research attention (Turkel et al. 2003) and appears to be less often diagnosed in pediatrics than on the adult units (Manos and Wu 1997), it is still a relatively common reason for psychiatric consultation. As in adults, it sometimes may present with what are interpreted to be psychotic symptoms (Webster and Holroyd 2000). The consultation request may also be put in terms of a request for an assessment of unexplained lethargy, depression, or confusion.

In adults, delirium has been found to be the strongest predictor of length of stay in the hospital, after controlling for severity of illness, age, gender, race, and medication (Ely et al. 2001). A recent evaluation of the widely used Delirium Rating Scale found that it does appear to be applicable to children, with scores comparable to those of adults. However, the scores or diagnosis of delirium in a child may not have the same implications as in adults. The scores for children, unlike those for adults, did not predict length of hospital stay or mortality (Turkel et al. 2003). Similarly, the Glasgow Coma Scale appears to be less effective in predicting prognosis for children than adults (Lieh-Lai et al. 1992).

Common causes of delirium include infections, metabolic disturbances, and toxicity of medications. These can often be determined with a careful chart review. Other potentially severe or life-threatening causes of confusion include stroke (Kothare et al. 1998), confusional migraine (Shaabat 1996), neuropsychiatric symptoms of systemic lupus erythematosus (Turkel et al. 2001), or inflammatory encephalopathy (Vasconcellos et al. 1999). Less common causes of acute confusional state in children would be multiple sclerosis (Gadoth 2003) or thiamine deficiency (Hahn et al. 1998). Conventional and quantitative electroencephalography (EEG) have been used to evaluate the etiology of delirium in adults, particularly elderly adults (S.A. Jacobson et al. 1993). In acute pediatric confusional states, EEG appears to be useful in differentiation of hepatic encephalopathy and convulsive pathology from other causes. Certain patterns had strong prognostic value (Navelet et al. 1998). Magnetic resonance imaging (MRI) and single photon emission computed tomography have been found to be useful in used in differentiation of inflammatory encephalopathy (Hahn et al. 1998) and systemic lupus erythematosus (Turkel et al. 2001), respectively.

Even after correction or treatment of the underlying etiology, the symptoms of delirium can last 1–2 weeks (Manos and Wu 1997). Therefore, symptomatic treatment is essential. Support and orienting cues can be very helpful in reducing the fear and confusion. These include the presence of familiar objects, photographs, and people who can reassure and orient the child, as well as age-appropriate clocks, calendars, or signs. Education can help the parents understand what is happening, reduce their distress, and help them to provide support for the child rather than show irritation or fear.

Pharmacological intervention is indicated only if the child is distressed by the delirium or is becoming dangerous because of his or her lack of cooperation with care.

Because the research into pharmacological approaches to pediatric delirium is almost nonexistent, the general guidelines are pragmatic, based on the adult literature and the pediatric anesthesia literature. Intravenous haloperidol or droperidol is titrated with careful monitoring, avoiding or weaning off benzodiazepines, which appear to compound the confusion with sedation (Breitbart et al. 1996).

Factitious Disorders and Malingering

Illness Falsification

The difference between factitious behavior and malingering is the primary motivation. *Factitious disorder* is defined as the intentional production or feigning (falsification) of physical or psychological signs or symptoms to assume the sick role. *Malingering* is the intentional falsification of physical or psychological signs or symptoms to achieve external gain or to avoid unwanted responsibilities or outcomes.

Libow (2000) conducted the only literature review to date for cases of child and adolescent illness falsification. She identified 42 published cases with a mean age of 13.9 (range 8–18 years). Most patients were female (71%), with the gender imbalance greater among older children. Patients engaged in false symptom reporting and induction, including active injections, bruising, and ingestions. The most commonly falsified or induced conditions were fevers, ketoacidosis, purpura, and infections. The average duration of the falsifications before detection was about 16 months. Many admitted to their deceptions when confronted, and some had positive outcomes at followup. The children were described as bland, depressed, and fascinated with health care.

Child Victims of Illness Falsification

Child victims of illness falsification (called *Munchausen syndrome by proxy* when the abuser's behavior is due to factitious disorder not otherwise specified [NOS]) experience significant psychological problems during childhood, including feelings of helplessness, self-doubt, and poor self-esteem; self-destructive ideation; eating disorders; behavioral growth problems; nightmares; and school concentration problems (Bools et al. 1993; Libow 1995; Porter et al. 1994). Adult survivors describe emotional difficulties, including suicidal feelings, anxiety, depression, low self-esteem, intense rage reactions, and PTSD symptoms (Libow 1995). Ayoub (2002) presented longitudinal data on a sample of 40 children found by courts to be victims of illness falsification. The findings revealed that child victims frequently develop serious psychiatric symptoms that vary depending on the child's developmental age, the length and intensity of his or her exposure, and the current degree of protection and support. PTSD and oppositional disorders are significant sequelae, as are patterns of reality distortion, poor self-esteem, and attachment difficulties.

Although these children can superficially appear socially skilled and well-adjusted, they often struggle with basic relationships. Lying is common, as is manipulative illness behavior and sadistic behavior toward other children. Many remain trauma-reactive and experience cyclical anger, depression, and oppositionality. Children who fared best were separated from their biological parents and remained in a single protected placement, or had an abuser who admitted to the abuse and worked over a period of years toward reunification.

Feeding Disorders

Food Refusal, Selectivity, and Phobias

Feeding problems and eating disturbances in toddlers and young school-age children occur in 25%–40% of the population (Mayes et al. 1993). Most are transient and can be easily addressed with parent training, education about nutrition or normal child development, child–caregiver interaction advice, and suggestions for food preparation and presentation. However, severe eating disturbances requiring more aggressive treatment occur in 3%–10% of young children and are most common in children with other physical or developmental problems (Ahearn et al. 2001; Kerwin 1999). These children are at risk for aspiration, malnutrition, invasive medical procedures, hospitalizations, limitations in normal functioning and development, liver failure, and death.

Some physical factors that can impair normal eating include anatomical abnormalities, sensory perceptual impairments, oral motor dysfunctions, and chronic medical problems (such as reflux, short-gut syndrome, inflammatory bowel disease, hepatic or pancreatic disease, or cancer). Other contributing factors can include the pairing of eating with an aversive experience, inadvertent caregiver reinforcement of progressively more selective food choices, or a lack of normal early feeding experiences.

Food aversion and oral motor dysfunction are often treated by a speech pathologist and/or an occupational therapist. Effective behavioral interventions include contingency management with positive reinforcement for appropriate feeding and ignoring or guiding inappropriate responses. Desensitization techniques can be effectively used to address phobias or altered sensory processing. Although no research has directly examined the use of psychotropic medication in treating food refusal, selectivity, or phobias, it may be valuable to consider for use with children with associated anxiety disorders.

Failure to Thrive

It is helpful to think of failure to thrive (FTT) as a presenting symptom with varied and potentially multiple causes (Wren and Tarbell 1998). Parents might have a poor understanding of feeding techniques or might improperly prepare formula, or the mother might have an inadequate supply of breast milk. Biological contributors to failure to thrive include defects in food assimilation, excessive loss of ingested calories, increased energy requirements, and prenatal insults; environmental contributors include economic or emotional deprivation.

Research examining the role of the child–parent attachment reveals that feeding problems and growth deficiencies can occur within the context of organized and secure attachments; however, insecure attachment relationships may intensify feeding problems and lead to more severe malnutrition (Chatoor et al. 1998). In one study of FTT children (who had no identifiable biological contributors), 80% of the mothers reported they had a history of being victims of physical abuse (Weston et al. 1993).

Classic teaching has been that etiology can be determined by the child's ability to gain weight in the hospital, with a psychosocial etiology presumed if the child gains weight under these conditions. However, it is important to note that conclusions about likely FTT contributors cannot always be made on the basis of the child's ability to gain weight in the hospital. For example, some FTT children who have an inadequate caregiver will still lose weight in the hospital simply because they are separated from the caregiver. Former FTT children have been found to be smaller, less cognitively able, and more behaviorally disturbed than those children without a history of FTT, especially if their mothers are poorly educated (Drewett et al. 1999; Dykman et al. 2001).

The goal of treatment is to provide the medical, psychiatric, social, and environmental resources needed to promote satisfactory growth. Psychosocial treatment interventions need to be targeted at the likely

contributors. Children with feeding skills deficits or maladaptive behavior related to food are likely to benefit from behavioral interventions. Primary caregivers with a history of abuse or with current psychopathology might require specific psychiatric assessment and treatment. Interventions targeting the child–parent relationship, sometimes including in-home intervention, might be effective for selected families (Black et al. 1995; Steward 2001). Interventions targeting the social–economic burdens of the family can be critical. In some cases of inadequate parenting, foster care is required while the parent receives needed parent training and psychiatric care. In such cases, the return to home should be closely monitored and based on the parents' demonstrated ability and resources to adequately care for their child.

Psychosocial Short Stature

Short stature can typically be attributed to defects in the growing tissues, abnormalities of the environment of the growing tissues (e.g., nutritional insufficiency or organ disease), or endocrine abnormalities. Psychosocial short stature is relatively rare, often confused with FTT, and not well studied (Wren and Tarbell 1998). It is distinguished from FTT in that it is considered a direct result of adverse social–environmental factors on endocrine functioning (suppression of normal pulsatile growth hormone [GH] secretion) that results in a failure to make expected gains in *height* or *length*, as opposed to weight. Examples of adverse social–environmental factors are physical abuse, extreme deprivation, or a seriously disturbed child–parent relationship. Other behavioral and emotional disturbances, also induced by adverse social–environmental issues, are common. One diagnostic feature is that psychosocial short stature is reversible, with rapid acceleration in growth and development often observed, when the child is removed from the environment.

Consequently, the primary intervention is often placement in a safe, structured, stimulating environment with ample opportunity to develop new attachments (Green et al. 1984). Distress related to separation is less likely to temporarily hinder progress in psychosocial short stature (when compared with FTT), because of the severity of the adverse social–environmental factors endured before separation. Other treatments should be geared toward the specific symptoms and experiences of the child but may include individual psychotherapy, family therapy, school assessment and intervention, and psychotropic medication. Case reports suggest that attempts at in-home intervention must be intensive and comprehensive to be effective. The involvement of child protective services is often essential.

Pica

Pica is defined as eating nonnutritious substances on a continued basis over a period of at least 1 month (Wren and Tarbell 1998). It is most frequently found in children with mental retardation or a pervasive developmental disorder. Pica also has a high prevalence in children with sickle cell disease, with preliminary studies suggesting that over 30% are affected (Bond et al. 1994; Ivascu et al. 2001). Mouthing and occasional eating of nonnutritious substances are considered normal in children under 3 years. Young children with pica are most likely to eat sand, bugs, paint, plaster, paper, or other items within reach. Adolescents are more likely to eat clay, soil, paper, or similar substances. Pica can be a conditioned behavior, an indication of distress or environmental neglect, or evidence of a vitamin or mineral deficiency. Medical assessment includes screening for ingestion of toxic substances and evaluation for possible nutritional deficits. An evaluation and treatment plan to reduce psychosocial stress are also clearly im-

portant. Behavioral interventions have been shown to be effective in targeting the pica behavior include food-versus-nonfood discrimination training; these interventions include response interruption and positive practice overcorrection, habit reversal, and brief-duration physical restraint (Fisher et al. 1994; Johnson et al. 1994; Paniagua et al. 1986; Winton and Singh 1983; Woods et al. 1996). Psychiatric medications are not generally used to treat pica unless it is comorbid with another psychiatric disorder.

Rumination

Rumination syndrome is the effortless regurgitation into the mouth of recently ingested food followed by rechewing and reswallowing or expulsion (Clouse et al. 1999; Malcolm et al. 1997). Associated behavioral signs can include aversive posturing or gaze avoidance (Berkowitz 1999). Rumination can be conditioned after an illness, a sign of general distress, or a form of self-stimulation or self-soothing that appears to be associated with pleasure. It is most commonly seen in infants and the developmentally disabled but also occurs in children and adolescents with normal intelligence (O'Brien et al. 1995; Soykan et al. 1997).

Patients with rumination syndrome can be misdiagnosed as having bulimia nervosa, gastroesophageal reflux disease, or upper gastrointestinal motility disorders (such as gastroparesis or chronic intestinal pseudo-obstruction). They might undergo extensive, costly, and invasive medical testing before diagnosis. Complications can include weight loss, fatal malnutrition, dental erosions, halitosis, dehydration, school absenteeism, hospitalizations, and iatrogenic problems from the extensive diagnostic testing (O'Brien et al. 1995). Evaluation for gastroesophageal reflux disease is warranted if the rumination is accompanied by apnea, reactive airway disease, hematemesis, or food refusal.

In cases of rumination because of environmental neglect, the primary caretaker–child relationship and possible psychiatric disturbance in the primary caretaker should be evaluated and addressed. Operant behavioral methods can be used for conditioned rumination. Postmeal chewing gum has been used successfully to treat adolescents with rumination (Weakley et al. 1997). Habit reversal using diaphragmatic breathing as the competing response can also be effective in older children and adolescents (Chial et al. 2003; Kerwin 1999; Wagaman et al. 1998). Rumination in the presence of other psychosocial problems or psychiatric disorders in the child or primary caretaker may require additional therapeutic interventions. Later experiences of stress, loss, or isolation can trigger a relapse, requiring the reinstitution of the previously effective intervention (Berkowitz 1999).

Chronic Somatic Symptoms

Children and adolescents often report persistent physical concerns that are not clearly accounted for by identifiable medical illness (Campo and Fritsch 1994; Garber et al. 1991). In fact, the most common reason for a pediatric psychiatry consultation is for evaluation of unexplained physical symptoms (Simonds 1977; Tsai et al. 1995). Somatoform disorders can be considered the severe end of a continuum that includes functional somatic symptoms in the middle and minor transient symptoms at the other end (Fritz et al. 1997). Examples of disorders on this continuum include atypical migraines, cyclic vomiting, chronic nausea, dizziness, fibromyalgia, chronic fatigue, functional abdominal pain, irritable bowel syndrome, myofascial pain, palpitations, conversion paralysis, and pseudoseizures (Caplan 1998; Heruti et al. 2002; Krilov et al. 1998; Li and Balint 2000; Schanberg et al. 1998; Volkmar et al. 1984). Disabling somatic symp-

toms can occur in the presence or absence of an identifiable etiology and in the presence or absence of other medical or psychiatric disorders.

It is helpful to remember that experiences of somatic symptoms are the result of an integration of biological processes, psychological and developmental factors, and social context (Bennett 1999; Li and Balint 2000; Mailis-Gagnon et al. 2003; Peyron et al. 2000; Terre and Ghiselli 1997; Walker and Jones 2005; Zeltzer et al. 1997). Traditionally, disability and symptoms in excess of what would be expected given the amount of tissue pathology have been considered psychogenic. Children and families are informed that the symptom has no physiological basis, with the intended or unintended suggestion that the child is fabricating the symptom. It is misleading and often confusing to families to dichotomize symptoms as organic versus nonorganic because all symptoms are associated with neurosensory changes and influenced by psychosocial factors. Maintaining the organic versus nonorganic dichotomy can lead to unnecessary tests and treatments or to an unhelpful lack of empathy.

Psychiatric assessment is geared toward identifying psychiatric symptoms, behavioral reinforcements, and psychosocial stressors that could be exacerbating the symptoms. Common comorbid findings include anxiety disorders, alexithymia, depression, unsuspected learning disorders (in high-achieving children), developmental or communication disorders, social problems, physical or emotional trauma, family illness, and family distress (Bursch and Zeltzer 2002; Campo et al. 1999, 2002; Egger et al. 1998; Fritz et al. 1997; Garber et al. 1990; Hodges et al. 1985a, 1985b; Hyman et al. 2002; Lester et al. 2003; Livingston 1993; Livingston et al. 1995; Schanberg et al. 1998; Stuart and Noyes 1999; Zuckerman et al. 1987).

The family and treatment team often worry about missing a life-threatening problem or a diagnosis that could be easily remedied. This fear is particularly strong when the patient exhibits significant distress about the symptoms. The treatment team must feel that a reasonable evaluation has been completed so that they can clearly communicate to the family that no further evaluation is indicated to understand and treat the problem. A rehabilitation approach can improve independent and normal functioning, enhance coping and self-efficacy, and serve to prevent secondary disabilities (Bursch et al. 1998; Campo and Fritz 2001; Heruti et al. 2002). Functioning, rather than symptoms, should be tracked to determine whether progress is being made. As functioning, coping skills, and self-efficacy improve, symptoms and the distress related to the symptoms often remit.

Specific treatment plans target the biological, psychological, and social factors that are exacerbating or maintaining the symptoms and disability. Treatment techniques designed to target underlying sensory signaling mechanisms and specific symptoms can include cognitive-behavioral strategies (e.g., psychotherapy, hypnosis, biofeedback, or meditation), behavioral techniques, family interventions, physical interventions (e.g., massage, yoga, acupuncture, transcutaneous electrical nerve stimulation [TENS], physical therapy, heat or cold therapies, occupational therapy), sleep hygiene, and pharmacological interventions (Fritz et al. 1997; Minuchin et al. 1978; Robins et al. 2005; Sanders et al. 1989, 1994; Zeltzer and Bursch 2002). In general, interventions that promote active coping are preferred over those that require passive dependency.

Most of the currently employed pharmacological strategies are extrapolated from adult trials without evidence of efficacy in children. Classes of medications to consider include tricyclic antidepressants or anticonvulsants for neuropathic pain or irritable bowel syndrome, SSRIs for symptoms of anxiety or depression, muscle relaxants for myofascial pain, and low-dose antipsychotics (especially those with low potency) for acute anxiety, multiple somatic symptoms with significant distress, and chronic nausea. Benzodiazepines sometimes elicit paradoxical reactions in those children who are hypervigilant to their bodies and concerned about losing control. Blocks, trigger point injections, epidurals, and other invasive assessments and treatments that further stimulate the CNS can sometimes exacerbate the problem. Evidence-based treatments should be used whenever available. For example, in adolescent migraine headache, cognitive-behavioral interventions have better evidence for efficacy than triptans, and ibuprofen appears to be more effective than acetaminophen.

Specific Medical Disorders

Oncology

Despite the numerous stressors, pediatric oncology patients report relatively few depressive symptoms during the time of active treatment. Children with cancer report fewer symptoms of depression than healthy schoolchildren or children with asthma, and self-esteem concerns and somatic symptoms do not differentiate between depressed and nondepressed children with cancer (Gizynski and Shapiro 1990; Worchel et al. 1988). In fact, pediatric cancer patients report so few symptoms that clinical researchers have hypothesized that these children use an avoidant coping style to deal with their emotional response to cancer (Phipps and Srivastava 1997, 1999) or that their emotional response is shaped by traumatic avoidance (Erickson and Steiner 2000). Interventions that address the contextual issues that are precipitating distress are generally sufficient for the depressive symptoms seen during active treatment (Kazak et al. 2002).

One area of intervention that has been extensively researched is preparation for the many invasive procedures children experience during cancer treatment. Cognitive-behavioral techniques, including imagery, relaxation, distraction, modeling, desensitization, and positive reinforcement, are well established as effective (Kazak 2005; Powers 1999). This is consistent with the literature that suggests depressive attributional style and avoidance coping are major predictors of anxiety and depression in pediatric oncology patients (Frank et al. 1997). Although all children have some distress with painful procedures, some appear to be more sensitive to pain and have differential responses to psychological interventions for procedural distress (Chen et al. 2000). In cases of children with severe distress, integration of pharmacological interventions has proven useful (Jay et al. 1991; Kazak et al. 1998). Topical anesthetic cream has been used with some success to alleviate the pain of venipuncture or the topical pain of other invasive procedures with pediatric oncology patients (Robieux et al. 1990). In comparisons of conscious sedation and general anesthesia for lumbar punctures, the outcomes were similar, and the conscious sedation was generally preferred, as well as less expensive. However, for some children, the procedure could only be performed under general anesthesia because they were too distressed to cooperate (Ljungman et al. 2001). For conscious sedation, the amnestic effect of midazolam, as well as the ability to administer it nasally, rectally, or orally, has made it popular with anesthesiologists and intensivists. In a double-blind study, midazolam was shown to significantly reduce children's procedural anxiety, discomfort, and pain

(Ljungman et al. 2000). For brief general anesthesia, a combination of midazolam and ketamine has been found effective (Parker et al. 1997).

With increasing survival of childhood cancer patients, the long-term impact of cancer has become a major focus of psychooncology research over the past 20 years. Here again, depression does not seem to be a problem (Zebrack et al. 2002). However, a rapidly growing area is investigations of PTSD. A study of 309 childhood cancer survivors (ages 8–20), an average of almost 6 years after cancer treatment, found similar rates of PTSD symptoms in the cancer and comparison groups (219 healthy children) (Kazak et al. 1997). However, in a study of 78 young adult (ages 18–37) survivors of childhood cancer, approximately 20% of the young adult survivors reported symptoms meeting diagnostic criteria for PTSD (Hobbie et al. 2000). Furthermore, PTSD in the young adults appeared predictive of adverse consequences. The young adult survivors who met the criteria for PTSD were less likely to be married (none, compared with 23% of the non-PTSD group) and reported more psychological distress and poorer quality of life across all domains. The greatest differences reported were in social functioning, emotional well-being, and role limitations caused by emotional health and pain. Survivors without PTSD did not differ from population norms (Meeske and Stuber 2001). These findings indicate a need to prevent and intervene with children during the time of acute treatment, to prevent long-term consequences in much the same way that medical treatments are being adapted in light of the late effects of radiation and chemotherapy.

Parents report significant distress both during and after their children's cancer treatment (Best et al. 2002). Specific problem-solving therapy has been found to be effective in helping mothers deal with the stresses of treatment (Sahler et al. 2002), as have brief stress reduction techniques (Streisand et al. 2001). Rates of PTSD in parents of children off treatment appear comparable to those of adult cancer survivors (Manne et al. 1998). In a large study of pediatric cancer survivors' parents, 3% of the survivors' mothers reported severe, and 18.2% reported moderate, symptoms of PTSD; whereas 7% of the survivors' fathers reported severe, and 28.3% reported moderate, PTSD symptoms (Kazak et al. 1997).

Cystic Fibrosis

Cystic fibrosis (CF) affects approximately 30,000 children and adults in the United States and is the most common hereditary disease in white children. More than 80% of patients with CF are diagnosed by age 3; however, almost 10% are diagnosed at age 18 or older. The median age of survival is 33.4 years, and nearly 40% of those with CF are adults. Many people with CF lead remarkably normal lives and maintain hope with the possibilities of gene therapy and organ transplantation in case of severe deterioration. Although early research suggested that eating disorders may be more prevalent in those with CF, recent work has suggested that this is not true. Similarly, rates of other psychiatric disorders among those with CF do not appear to be greater than the prevalence reported in the general population (Kashani et al. 1988a; Raymond et al. 2000). In one study of CF adolescents' health values, it was revealed that they are willing to trade very little of their life expectancy or take more than a small risk of death to obtain perfect health (Yi et al. 2003). Although there is little research on this topic, there are no apparent contraindications for standard assessment and treatment approaches for psychiatric disorders in those with CF. There is some data to suggest that family interventions can be successfully used to improve maternal mental health and treatment adherence among those at high risk (Goldbeck and Babka 2001; Ireys et al. 2001).

Asthma

Asthma is the most common pediatric chronic illness, and both prevalence and morbidity are rising, despite better pharmacological treatments. Comorbid psychiatric problems and increased levels of stress are cited as possible factors for the increases (Wamboldt and Gavin 1998). Comorbid psychiatric disorders may reduce asthma treatment compliance, impair daily functioning, or have a direct effect on autonomic reactions and pulmonary function (Norrish et al. 1977). While the literature contains some contradictory findings about the prevalence and type of comorbid psychiatric problems, it appears that internalizing disorders are more common and that over one-third of asthmatic children have anxiety disorders. Additionally, those with moderate to severe asthma appear to be at a higher risk for anxiety disorders compared to those with mild disease. Adolescents with asthma and their parents, especially those adolescents who have experienced a life-threatening event, have high levels of posttraumatic stress symptoms (Kean et al. 2006). Although depression has been less consistently identified as a comorbid psychiatric disorder among pediatric asthma patients, the literature suggests that depression, along with other psychosocial problems, may be a risk factor for death in children with asthma. Consequently, the presence of depression in a child with uncontrolled or severe asthma requires serious attention (Bussing et al. 1996; Butz and Alexander 1993; Graham et al. 1967; Kashani et al. 1988b; MacLean et al. 1988; McNichol et al. 1973; Mrazek et al. 1985; Steinhausen et al. 1983; Strunk et al. 1985; Vila et al. 1999).

Twin studies suggest that there may be a genetic relationship between atopic disorders and internalizing disorders (Wamboldt et al. 1998). One possible explanation is that panic anxiety acts as an asphyxia alarm system that is triggered by central chemoreceptors monitoring $PaCO_2$. Children with a genetic vulnerability for panic disorder who also have periodic increased $PaCO_2$ from asthma exacerbations may thus have panic anxiety triggered by their asthma attacks. Left undiagnosed and untreated, this anxiety can develop into panic disorder. Indeed, prospective epidemiological studies indicate the primary risk factor for development of panic disorder in young adulthood is history of asthma as a child (Goodwin et al. 2003). Other reasons for increased comorbidity include the fact that most asthma medications (e.g., steroids and beta agonists) are known to cause symptoms that appear psychiatric in nature. An inflammatory allergic response may release cytokines and other mediators that cause fatigue, trouble concentrating, and irritability that could also be interpreted as depression. The physiological response accompanying strong emotions can trigger wheezing in some patients. Recent research indicates that not only can stress lead to increased asthma exacerbations, but those children with atopic illnesses have a reduced cortisol response to stress (Wamboldt et al. 2003). Stressors may thus have a direct effect on increased inflammation, leading to asthma symptoms or an increase in upper respiratory infections, which also exacerbate asthma. Depression and anxiety may indirectly influence asthma because distressed asthmatics tend to misperceive anxiety symptoms as asthma symptoms, often leading to unnecessary medication usage.

Vocal cord dysfunction (VCD) can mimic asthma and commonly occurs comorbidly with asthma. It is a condition of involuntary paradoxical adduction of the vocal cords during the inspiratory phase of the respiratory cycle (Wamboldt and Gavin 1998). It is often associated with anxiety or chronic stress; however, sexual abuse in this population is not as prevalent as previously believed (Brugman et al. 1994; Gavin et al. 1998). Patients with VCD frequently present with stridulous breathing, experience tightness in their throats, and feel short of breath. It can be quite anxiety-provoking that their symptoms are unrelieved by asthma medications.

Clinicians should assess for 1) psychosocial disruption and psychiatric symptoms, especially symptoms of anxiety and depression (including medical trauma); 2) likelihood of nonadherence; 3) ability to perceive symptoms; and 4) presence of VCD. Asthma can increase family burden, and having depressed primary caretakers increases the risk of poorer treatment adherence. New electronic monitoring of adherence with inhaled medications helps determine how much nonadherence is undermining outcome. Having patients guess their peak flow or rate their symptoms before spirometry or after a methacholine challenge is one way to assess if the patient is an accurate perceiver or not. Patients who have difficulty with symptom perception (either under- or overperceiving symptoms) can be trained to use objective assessment methods, such as peak flow meters. Clinicians can assess for VCD by asking patients where they feel short of breath and if there is throat tightness. A flow volume loop can be helpful in showing VCD, especially on the inspiratory part of the loop. Definitive diagnosis of VCD is made by visualization of adducted cords during an acute episode using laryngoscopy. Provocation of symptoms during laryngoscopy has been achieved using methacholine, histamine, or exercise challenges.

Pharmacological and psychological treatments with efficacy to treat anxiety and depression in children are largely applicable to those with asthma. Focused family therapy to improve asthma management skills has been shown to be effective and efficient (Godding et al. 1997; Gustafsson et al 1986; Lask and Matthew 1979; Panton and Barley 2000). The primary treatment for VCD is speech therapy or hypnotherapy geared toward increasing awareness and control of breathing and throat muscles (Wamboldt and Gavin 1998). Although some concern has been raised about the concurrent use of tricyclic antidepressants with medicines used in treating asthma, they appear to be safe, and the anticholinergic effects can sometimes be helpful (Wamboldt et al. 1997). Beta-receptor agonists are often used to treat asthma, which makes beta-blockers potentially dangerous. There is no contraindication for using neuroleptics, and they may be particularly indicated for steroid-induced psychosis. Lithium increases theophylline clearance, requiring that levels of both drugs be monitored (Wamboldt and Gavin 1998). Some children with asthma have difficulty tolerating stimulants. Bupropion has shown efficacy in the treatment of attention-deficit/hyperactivity disorder in young patients in controlled trials (Barrickman et al. 1995; Conners et al. 1996) and does not interact with asthma medications.

Sickle Cell Anemia

Although children and adolescents with sickle cell disease do not appear to have a greater risk for psychiatric disorders than those in the same-race outpatient clinic control group, children attending outpatient medical clinics are at a higher risk for mental disorders than nonmedical populations (Cepeda et al. 1997; Yang et al. 1994). Most well-designed studies report a prevalence rate of 25%–30% for psychiatric disorders among pediatric sickle cell patients, with internalizing disorders being most prevalent (Cepeda et al. 1997), simi-

lar to other pediatric outpatients (Costello and Shugart 1992; Costello et al. 1988). Psychosocial factors have accounted for more variability than biomedical ones in both depressive symptoms and anxiety, with social assertion, self-esteem, use of social support, and family factors accounting for a significant amount of the variability in adaptation (Burlew et al. 2000; Telfair 1994). Two studies suggest that pica (not often assessed) has a relatively high prevalence (up to 30%) in children with sickle cell disease (Bond et al. 1994; Ivascu et al. 2001).

Psychiatric assessment should look for 1) psychosocial disruption or psychiatric symptoms, especially related to pica, anxiety, and depression; 2) school or social problems that could reflect subtle neurocognitive problems; and 3) chronic pain problems. Pharmacological and psychological treatments with efficacy to treat psychiatric disorders in children are applicable to those with sickle cell anemia. Problems with academic or social functioning might be assessed via neurocognitive testing and addressed within the school system with an Individualized Education Program (IEP). Pain in sickle cell patients is most commonly medically managed pharmacologically with nonsteroidal anti-inflammatory drugs, opioids, and adjuvant medications (American Pain Society 1999). Chronic as well as acute pediatric pain can also be reduced with behavioral, psychological, or physical interventions (American Pain Society 1999). Behavioral interventions might include relaxation, deep breathing, biofeedback, behavioral modification, or exercise. Psychological interventions might include cognitive therapies, hypnotherapy, imagery, distraction, or social support. Physical interventions might include hydration, heat, massage, hydrotherapy, ultrasound, acupuncture, TENS, or physical therapy. Successful treatment of anxiety symptoms can reduce pain and pain-related distress. Although there are no contraindications for the use of psychotropic medications with this population, it is important to remember that phenothiazines may antagonize the analgesic effects of opiate agonists and that tricyclic antidepressants, monoamine oxidase inhibitors, and other CNS depressants may potentiate adverse effects of opioids. It is important to note, however, that these agents may also serve to successfully augment pain control efforts and should be considered if needed.

Renal Disease

Pediatric patients with chronic renal failure exhibit more problems in psychiatric adjustment than do healthy children, with a trend toward more psychological difficulties in those with higher illness severity (Garralda et al. 1988). However, even less severely physically ill children appear to have increased difficulties in school adjustment and feelings of loneliness (Garralda et al. 1988). Separation anxiety disorder in particular may be a relatively common disorder (up to 65.4%) among children on continuous ambulatory peritoneal dialysis (Fukunishi and Kudo 1995). This may be due to the forced dependence on parents for daily renal care. The burden for families caring for children with end-stage renal disease (ESRD) can be significant, especially when it involves dialysis. Disruption of family life, marital strain, and a tendency for more mental health problems in the parents also appear to be related to the severity of the child's renal illness and its associated care burdens (Reynolds et al. 1988). Children with ESRD (with or without transplant) have been shown to have lower-than-expected IQs and achievement scores. Lower achievement test scores were predicted by younger age at the time of renal disease diagnosis, increased time on dialysis, and

caregiver's lower achievement (Brouhard et al. 2000; Fennell et al. 1984; Qvist et al. 2002). Overall, former pediatric ESRD adults appear to have a long-term favorable adjustment, with lower self-esteem related to early onset of the disease and to educational and social dysfunction (Morton et al. 1994).

Pediatric kidney transplantation is associated with improved physical health, emotional health, and family functioning; however, poor peer relationships, school maladjustment, and other adjustment problems (as well as adherence problems) can remain after transplant (Fukunishi and Kudo 1995; Reynolds et al. 1991). Living with a transplant is a lifelong process requiring daily medications and monitoring for rejection. Medication nonadherence rates for pediatric renal transplant patients can be as high as 64% (Ettenger et al. 1991). Adverse consequences of nonadherence include medical complications and hospitalizations, higher health care costs and family stress, and increased risks for loss of the organ (Arbus et al. 1993; Bittar et al. 1992; Fukunishi and Honda 1995; Salvatierra et al. 1997; Swanson et al. 1992).

Diabetes

The complexity of the management of type 1 diabetes mellitus leads to frequent problems with adherence to medical instructions. Additionally, the physiological changes of puberty can lead to increased insulin resistance. The importance of peer acceptance and the withdrawal of parental supervision with the normal developmental focus on identity and autonomy also lead to significant adherence problems during adolescence (Hauser et al. 1990). Poor control of diabetes has been repeatedly demonstrated using HbA1c (glycosylated hemoglobin), which allows one to get an estimate of glycemic control over the past 3 months. The medical consequences of such poor control were demonstrated in a study of 78 adolescents with type 1 diabetes, ages 11–18 years, followed for 8 years. Their mean HbA1c peaked in late adolescence. Serious diabetic complications were seen in 38% of the females and 25% of the males (Bryden et al. 2001).

Studies of the utility of intervention with pediatric diabetic patients have found that interventions to enhance adherence must be intense and early to make a significant difference in long-term outcome. A study of 1,441 patients, ages 13–39 years, followed for a mean of 6.5 years demonstrated a decrease in long-term complications with intensive treatment. However, there was a two- to fourfold increase in experiencing severe hypoglycemia, as well as a twofold increase in becoming overweight in the intensive treatment group (DCCT Research Group 1993, 1994).

Psychiatric comorbidity in diabetic individuals is also a major issue for psychiatric consultants to pediatrics. Some moodiness and feelings of isolation and of loss or grief, as well as mild anxiety about the future, are to be expected as normal responses to diabetes. However, assessment for possible intervention is indicated if patients demonstrate aggression, school absences, hopelessness, or nonadherence to the insulin regimen (A.M. Jacobson 1996). Children at higher risk of developing psychiatric comorbidity appear to be those who are in the first year after diagnosis and those who had preexisting anxiety or mothers with psychopathology (Kovacs et al. 1997). Eating disorders are also relatively common (Rydall et al. 1997).

Treatment of comorbid psychiatric disorders with medications requires careful monitoring because most antidepressant, mood stabilizer, and atypical antipsychotic medications may stimulate appetite or affect glucose tolerance, inducing hypoglycemia or hyperglycemia. Beta-blockers should be avoided, as they mask the early warning signs of hypoglycemia, eliminating the window of opportunity for patients to address the problem themselves before requiring the assistance of others (Goodnick et al. 1995).

Effective behavioral interventions for children with diabetes and their parents include identifying readiness for change and improving self-efficacy, the belief that one can maintain behavior change despite regular challenges (Anderson et al. 1996, 1999). In 110 young adults (ages 18–35) with insulin-dependent diabetes mellitus, self-efficacy was more predictive than self-esteem of self-care and metabolic control. Factoring in previous adherence, self-efficacy continues to be predictive of self-care and HbA1c (Johnston-Brooks et al. 2002). A growing area of research is the application of motivational interviewing to work with adolescents with diabetes mellitus (Berg-Smith et al. 1999; Dunn et al. 2001; Williams et al. 1998).

Cardiac Disease and Congenital Heart Defects

Overall, it appears that children with heart disease psychiatrically resemble a normal population without elevations in anxiety, depression, or behavioral problems (Connolly et al. 2002; DeMaso et al. 2000; Visconti et al. 2002). However, similar to the case in healthy or other chronically ill children, socioeconomic factors, medical severity, and family distress appear to be related to symptoms of depression, anxiety, or behavioral problems (Alden et al. 1998; Visconti et al. 2002; Yildiz et al. 2001). DeMaso et al. (2000) studied pediatric patients with recurrent cardiac arrhythmias who underwent radiofrequency catheter ablation of ectopic myocardial foci. Although these patients psychiatrically resembled a normal population before the procedure, they demonstrated reductions in their "fear of their heart problem" and increases in "the things that they enjoy" after the ablation (DeMaso et al. 2000, p. 134). Those who experienced a curative ablation had better functioning than those who did not experience improvement.

Fetal Alcohol Syndrome and Alcohol-Related Neurological Disorder

Prenatal alcohol exposure represents one of the leading preventable causes of congenital neurological impairment, affecting as many as 1 in 100 children born in the United States yearly (May and Gossage 2001), with severe lifelong consequences for affected individuals. Fetal alcohol syndrome (FAS) is defined by a characteristic pattern of facial anomalies, growth retardation, and CNS dysfunction in one or more of the following areas: decreased cranial size at birth, structural brain abnormalities, and neurological hard or soft signs (Stratton et al. 1996). However, alcohol exposure to the fetus can result in neurocognitive changes even when none of the characteristic facial anomalies are present (Streissguth and O'Malley 2000).

The facial characteristics most frequently described in individuals with FAS include short palpebral fissures and abnormalities in the premaxillary zone, including a thin upper lip and flattened philtrum (Astley and Clarren 2001; Stratton et al. 1996). Neurocognitive changes include structural changes in the brain (Roebuck et al. 1998); verbal learning and memory problems; attention deficits; problems in executive functioning characterized by difficulties in planning, organizing, and sequencing behavior; and problems in abstract and practical reasoning (Adnams et al. 2001), complex nonverbal problem solving (Goodman et al. 1999), flexible thinking (Schonfeld et al. 2001), and behavioral inhibition (Mattson et al. 1999). These changes appear to last into adult-

hood (Streissguth and O'Malley 2000). Secondary disabilities include high levels of psychiatric illness, school failure, social problems, delinquency, and trouble with the law. No safe level of prenatal alcohol consumption has been established, making abstinence the best policy for those who are hoping to conceive. Because many women are often not aware of when they conceived and may continue to drink alcohol at least until pregnancy recognition, preconception counseling is suggested for all women of childbearing age who consume alcohol.

References

Adnams CM, Kodituwakku PW, Hay A, et al: Patterns of cognitive-motor development in children with fetal alcohol syndrome from a community in South Africa. Alcohol Clin Exp Res 25:557–562, 2001

Ahearn WH, Castine T, Nault K, et al: An assessment of food acceptance in children with autism or pervasive developmental disorder–not otherwise specified. J Autism Dev Disord 31:505–511, 2001

Alden B, Gilljam T, Gillberg C: Long-term psychological outcome of children after surgery for transposition of the great arteries. Acta Paediatr 87:405–410, 1998

American Pain Society: Guideline for the management of acute and chronic pain in sickle-cell disease. Glenview, IL, American Pain Society, 1999

Anderson B, Ho J, Brackett J, et al: Parental involvement in diabetes management tasks: relationships to blood glucose monitoring adherence and metabolic control in young adolescents with insulin-dependent diabetes mellitus. J Pediatr 130:257–265, 1996

Anderson BJ, Bracett J, Ho J, et al: An office-based intervention to maintain parent-adolescent teamwork in diabetes management: impact on parent involvement, family conflict, and subsequent glycemic control. Diabetes Care 22:713–721, 1999

Arbus GS, Sullivan EK, Tejani A: Hospitalization in children during the first year after kidney transplantation. Kidney Int Suppl 43:83–86, 1993

Astley SJ, Clarren SK: Measuring the facial phenotype of individuals with prenatal alcohol exposure: correlations with brain dysfunction. Alcohol Alcohol 36:147–159, 2001

Ayoub CC: Munchausen by Proxy: Child Placement and Emotional Health. Denver, CO, The 14th International Congress for the Prevention of Child Abuse and Neglect, 2002

Barrickman LL, Perry PJ, Allen AJ, et al: Bupropion versus methylphenidate in the treatment of attention-deficit hyperactivity disorder. J Am Acad Child Adolesc Psychiatry 34:649–657, 1995

Battles HB, Wiener LS: From adolescence through young adulthood: psychosocial adjustment associated with long-term survival of HIV. J Adolesc Health 30:161–168, 2002

Bauman LJ, Wright E, Leickly FE, et al: Relationship of adherence to pediatric asthma morbidity among inner-city children. Pediatrics 110(1 pt 1):e6, 2002

Behrman RE, Kliegman RM, Jenson HB (eds): Nelson Textbook of Pediatrics, 17th Edition. Philadelphia, PA, JB Saunders, 2004

Bennett RM: Emerging concepts in the neurobiology of chronic pain: Evidence of abnormal sensory processing in fibromyalgia. Mayo Clin Proc 74:385–398, 1999

Berg-Smith SM, Stevens VJ, Brown KM, et al: A brief motivational intervention to improve dietary adherence in adolescents. Health Educ Res 14:339–410, 1999

Berkowitz C: Nonorganic failure to thrive and infant rumination syndrome, in Pediatric Functional Bowel Disorders. Edited by Hyman P. New York, Academy of Professional Information Services, 1999, pp 4.1–4.9

Berkowitz RI, Wadden TA, Tershakovec AM, et al: Behavior therapy and sibutramine for the treatment of adolescent obesity: a randomized controlled trial. JAMA 289:1805–1812, 2003

Best M, Streisand R, Catania L, et al: Parental distress during pediatric leukemia and parental posttraumatic stress symptoms after treatment ends. J Pediatr Psychol 26:299–307, 2002

Bittar AE, Keitel E, Garcia CD, et al: Patient noncompliance as a cause of late renal graft failure. Transplant Proc 24:2720–2721, 1992

Black MM, Dubowitz H, Hutcheson J, et al: A randomized clinical trial of home intervention for children with failure to thrive. Pediatrics 95:807–814, 1995

Bond S, Conner-Warren R, Sarnaik SA: Prevalence of pica in children with sickle cell disease. Paper presented at the 19th Annual Meeting of the National Sickle Cell Disease Program, New York, NY, March 25, 1994

Bools CN, Neale BA, Meadow SR: Follow up of victims of fabricated illness (Munchausen syndrome by proxy). Arch Dis Child 69:625–630, 1993

Breitbart W, Marotta R, Platt MM, et al: A double-blind trial of haloperidol, chlorpromazine, and lorazepam in the treatment of delirium in hospitalized AIDS patients. Am J Psychiatry 153:231–237, 1996

Brouhard BH, Donaldson LA, Lawry KW, et al: Cognitive functioning in children on dialysis and post-transplantation. Pediatr Transplant 4:261–267, 2000

Brugman SM, Howell JH, Mahler JL, et al: The spectrum of pediatric vocal cord dysfunction. Am Rev Respir Dis 149: A353, 1994

Bryden KS, Peveler RC, Stein A, et al: Clinical and psychological course of diabetes from adolescence to young adulthood. Diabetes Care 24:1536–1540, 2001

Burlew K, Telfair J, Colangelo L, et al: Factors that influence adolescent adaptation to sickle cell disease. J Pediatr Psychol 25:287–299, 2000

Bursch B, Walco G, Zeltzer LK: Clinical assessment and management of chronic pain and pain-associated disability syndrome (PADS). J Dev Behav Pediatr 19:44–52, 1998

Bursch B, Zeltzer LK: Autism spectrum disorders presenting as chronic pain syndromes: case presentations and discussion. Journal of Developmental and Learning Disorders 6:41–48, 2002

Bussing R, Burket RC, Kelleher ET: Prevalence of anxiety disorders in a clinic-based sample of pediatric asthma patients. Psychosomatics 37:108–115, 1996

Butz AM, Alexander C: Anxiety in children with asthma. J Asthma 30:199–209, 1993

Callanan M, Kelley P: Final Gifts: Understanding the Special Awareness, Needs, and Communications of the Dying. New York, NY, Bantam, 1992

Campo JV, Fritsch SL: Somatization in children and adolescents. J Am Acad Child Adolesc Psychiatry 33:1223–1235, 1994

Campo JV, Fritz G: A management model for pediatric somatization. Psychosomatics 42:467–476, 2001

Campo JV, Jansen-McWilliams L, Comer DM, et al: Somatization in pediatric primary care: association with psychopathology, functional impairment and use of services. J Am Acad Child Adolesc Psychiatry 38:1093–1101, 1999

Campo JV, Comer DM, Jansen-McWilliams L, et al: Recurrent pain, emotional distress, and health service use in childhood. J Pediatr 141:76–83, 2002

Caplan R: Epilepsy syndromes in childhood, in Textbook of Pediatric Neuropsychiatry. Edited by Coffey CE, Brumback RA. Washington, DC, American Psychiatric Association, 1998, pp 977–1010

Cepeda ML, Yang YM, Price CC, et al: Mental disorders in children and adolescents with sickle cell disease. South Med J 90:284–287, 1997

Chatoor I, Ganiban J, Colin V, et al: Attachment and feeding problems: a reexamination of nonorganic failure to thrive and attachment insecurity. J Am Acad Child Adolesc Psychiatry 37:1217–1224, 1998

Chen E, Craske MG, Katz ER, et al: Pain-sensitive temperament: does it predict procedural distress and response to psychological treatment among children with cancer? J Pediatr Psychol 25:269–278, 2000

Chial HJ, Camilleri M, Williams DE, et al: Rumination syndrome in children and adolescents: diagnosis, treatment, and prognosis. Pediatrics 111:158–162, 2003

Clouse RE, Richter JE, Heading RC, et al: Functional esophageal disorders. Gut 45 (suppl 2):II31–II36, 1999

Conners CK, Casat CD, Gualtieri CT, et al: Bupropion hydrochloride in attention deficit disorder with hyperactivity. J Am Acad Child Adolesc Psychiatry 35:1314–1321, 1996

Connolly D, Rutkowski M, Auslender M, et al: Measuring health-related quality of life in children with heart disease. Appl Nurs Res 15:74–80, 2002

Costello EJ, Shugart MA: Above and below the threshold: severity of psychiatric symptoms and functional impairment in a pediatric sample. Pediatrics 90:359–368, 1992

Costello EJ, Costello AJ, Edelbrock C, et al: Psychiatric disorders in pediatric primary care. Prevalence and risk factors. Arch Gen Psychiatry 45:1107–1116, 1988

DCCT Research Group: The effects of intensive treatment of diabetes on the development and progression of long-term complications in insulin-dependent diabetes mellitus. N Engl J Med 329:977–986, 1993

DCCT Research Group: Effects of intensive diabetes treatment on the development and progression of long-term complications in adolescents with insulin-dependent diabetes mellitus: Diabetes Control and Complications Trial. J Pediatr 125:177–188, 1994

DeMaso DR, Spratt EG, Vaughan BL, et al: Psychological functioning in children and adolescents undergoing radiofrequency catheter ablation. Psychosomatics 41:134–139, 2000

DiMatteo MR, Giordani PJ, Lepper HS, et al: Patient adherence and medical treatment outcomes: a meta-analysis. Med Care 40:794–811, 2002

Drewett RF, Corbett SS, Wright CM: Cognitive and educational attainments at school age of children who failed to thrive in infancy: a population-based study. J Child Psychol Psychiatry 40:551–561, 1999

Du Pasquier-Fediaevsky L, Tubiana-Rufi N: Discordance between physician and adolescent assessments of adherence to treatment: influence of HbA1c level. The PEDIAB Collaborative Group. Diabetes Care 22:1445–1449, 1999

Dunn C, Deroo L, Rivara F: The use of brief interventions adapted from motivational interviewing across behavioral domains: a systemic review. Addiction 96:1725–1742, 2001

Dykman RA, Casey PH, Ackerman PT, et al: Behavioral and cognitive status in school-aged children with a history of failure to thrive during early childhood. Clin Pediatr (Phila) 40:63–70, 2001

Efron D, Hiscock H, Sewell JR, et al: Prescribing of psychotropic medications for children by Australian pediatricians and child psychiatrists. Pediatrics 111:372–375, 2003

Egger HL, Angold A, Costello EJ: Headaches and psychopathology in children and adolescents. J Am Acad Child Adolesc Psychiatry 37:951–958, 1998

Ely EW, Gautam S, Margolin R, et al: The impact of delirium in the intensive care unit on hospital length of stay. Intensive Care Med 27:1892–1900, 2001

Erickson SJ, Steiner H: Trauma spectrum adaptation: somatic symptoms in long-term pediatric cancer survivors. Psychosomatics 41:339–346, 2000

Ettenger RB, Rosenthal JT, Marik JL, et al: Improved cadaveric renal transplant outcome in children. Pediatr Nephrol 5:137–142, 1991

Fennell RS 3rd, Rasbury WC, Fennell EB, et al: Effects of kidney transplantation on cognitive performance in a pediatric population. Pediatrics 74:273–278, 1984

Fisher WW, Piazza CC, Bowman LG, et al: A preliminary evaluation of empirically derived consequences for the treatment of pica. J Appl Behav Anal 27:447–457, 1994

Frank NC, Blount RL, Brown RT: Attributions, coping, and adjustment in children with cancer. J Pediatr Psychol 22:563–576, 1997

Fritz GK, Fritsch S, Hagino O. Somatoform disorders in children and adolescents: a review of the past 10 years. J Am Acad Child Adolesc Psychiatry 36:1329–1338, 1997

Fukunishi I, Honda M: School adjustment of children with end-stage renal disease. Pediatr Nephrol 9:553–557, 1995

Fukunishi I, Kudo H: Psychiatric problems of pediatric end-stage renal failure. Gen Hosp Psychiatry 17:32–36, 1995

Gadoth N: Multiple sclerosis in children. Brain Dev 25:229–232, 2003

Garber J, Zeman J, Walker L: Recurrent abdominal pain in children: psychiatric diagnoses and parental psychopathology. J Am Acad Child Adolesc Psychiatry 29:648–656, 1990

Garber J, Walker LS, Zeman J: Somatization symptoms in a community sample of children and adolescents: further validation of the children's somatization inventory. J Consult Clin Psychol 3:588–595, 1991

Garralda ME, Jameson RA, Reynolds JM, et al: Psychiatric adjustment in children with chronic renal failure. J Child Psychol Psychiatry 29:79–90, 1988

Gavin LA, Wamboldt M, Brugman S, et al: Psychological and family characteristics of adolescents with vocal cord dysfunction. J Asthma 35:409–417, 1998

Gizynski M, Shapiro V: Depression and childhood illness. Child Adolesc Social Work J 7:179–197, 1990

Godding V, Kruth M, Jamart J: Joint consultation for high-risk asthmatic children and their families, with pediatrician and child psychiatrist as co-therapists: model and evaluation. Fam Process 36:265–280, 1997

Goldbeck L, Babka C: Development and evaluation of a multi-family psychoeducational program for cystic fibrosis. Patient Educ Couns 44:187–192, 2001

Goldston DB, Kovacs M, Ho VY, et al: Suicidal ideation and suicide attempts among youth with insulin-dependent diabetes mellitus. J Am Acad Child Adolesc Psychiatry 33:240, 1994

Goodman AM, Mattson SN, Lang AR, et al: Concept formation and problem solving in children with heavy prenatal alcohol exposure. Alcohol Clin Exp Res 23 (suppl 5):32A, 1999

Goodnick PJ, Henry JH, Buki VM: Treatment of depression in patients with diabetes mellitus. J Clin Psychiatry 56:128–136, 1995

Goodwin RD, Pine DS, Hoven CW: Asthma and panic attacks among youth in the community. J Asthma 40:139–145, 2003

Graham PJ, Rutter ML, Pless IB: Childhood asthma: a psychosomatic disorder? Some epidemiological considerations. Br J Prev Soc Med 2:78–85, 1967

Green WH, Campbell M, David R: Psychosocial dwarfism: a critical review of the evidence. J Am Acad Child Psychiatry 23:39–48, 1984

Griffin KJ, Elkin TD: Non-adherence in pediatric transplantation: a review of the existing literature. Pediatr Transplant 5:246–249, 2001

Gustafsson PA, Kjellman NI, Cederblad M: Family therapy in the treatment of severe childhood asthma. J Psychosom Res 30:369–374, 1986

Gyulay JE: Home care for the dying child. Issues Compr Pediatr Nurs 12:33–69, 1989

Hahn JS, Berquist W, Alcorn DM, et al: Wernicke encephalopathy and beriberi during total parenteral nutrition attributable to multivitamin infusion shortage. Pediatrics 101:E10, 1998

Hauser ST, Jacobson AM, Lavori P, et al: Adherence among children and adolescents with insulin-dependent diabetes mellitus over a four-year longitudinal follow-up, II: immediate and long-term linkages with the family milieu. J Pediatr Psychol 15:527–542, 1990

Heruti RJ, Levy A, Adunski A, et al: Conversion motor paralysis disorder: overview and rehabilitation model. Spinal Cord 40:327–334, 2002

Ho J, Bender BG, Gavin LA, et al: Relations among asthma knowledge, treatment adherence, and outcome. J Allergy Clin Immunol 111:498–502, 2003

Hobbie W, Stuber M, Meeske K, et al: Symptoms of posttraumatic stress in young adult survivors of childhood cancer. J Clin Onc 18:4060–4066, 2000

Hodges K, Kline JJ, Barbero G, et al: Depressive symptoms in children with recurrent abdominal pain and in their families. J Pediatr 107:622–626, 1985a

Hodges K, Kline JJ, Barbero G, et al: Anxiety in children with recurrent abdominal pain and their parents. Psychosomatics 26:859, 862–866, 1985b

Hyman PE, Bursch B, Lopez E, et al: Visceral pain-associated disability syndrome: A descriptive analysis. J Pediatr Gastroenterol Nutr 35(5):663–668, 2002

Ireys HT, Chernoff R, DeVet KA, et al: Maternal outcomes of a randomized controlled trial of a community-based support program for families of children with chronic illnesses. Arch Pediatr Adolesc Med 155: 771–777, 2001

Ivascu NS, Sarnaik S, McCrae J, et al: Characterization of pica prevalence among patients with sickle cell disease. Arch Pediatr Adolesc Med 155:1243–1247, 2001

Jacobson AM: The psychological care of patients with insulin-dependent diabetes mellitus. N Engl J Med 334:1249–1253, 1996

Jacobson SA, Leuchter AF, Walter DO: Conventional and quantitative EEG in the diagnosis of delirium among the elderly. J Neurol Neurosurg Psychiatry 56:153–158, 1993

Jay SM, Elliott CH, Woody PD, et al: An investigation of cognitive–behavioral therapy combined with oral Valium for children undergoing painful medical procedures. Health Psychol 10:317–322, 1991

Johnson CR, Hunt FM, Siebert MJ: Discrimination training in the treatment of pica and food scavenging. Behav Modif 18: 214–229, 1994

Johnston-Brooks CH, Lewis MA, Garg S: Self-efficacy impacts self-care and HbA1c in young adults with type 1 diabetes. Psychosom Med 64:43–51, 2002

Kashani JH, Barbero GJ, Wilfley DE, et al: Psychological concomitants of cystic fibrosis in children and adolescents. Adolescence 23:873–880, 1988a

Kashani JH, König P, Shepperd JA, et al: Psychopathology and self-concept in asthmatic children. J Pediatr Psychol 13: 509–520, 1988b

Kashikar-Zuck S, Goldschneider KR, Powers SW, et al: Depression and functional disability in chronic pediatric pain. Clin J Pain 17:341–349, 2001

Kazak A, Penati B, Brophy P, et al: Pharmacological and psychological interventions for procedural pain. Pediatrics 102: 59–66, 1998

Kazak A, Simms S, Rourke M: Family systems practice in pediatric psychology. J Pediatr Psychol 27:133–143, 2002

Kazak AE, Barakat LP, Meeske K, et al: Posttraumatic stress symptoms, family functioning, and social support in survivors of childhood leukemia and their mothers and fathers. J Consult Clin Psychol 65:120–129, 1997

Kazak AE: Evidence-based interventions for survivors of childhood cancer and their families. J Pediatr Psychol 30:29–39, 2005

Kean EM, Kelsay K, Wamboldt F, et al: Posttraumatic stress in adolescents with asthma and their parents. J Am Acad Child Adolesc Psychiatry 45:78–86, 2006

Kemper MJ, Sparta G, Laube GF, et al: Neuropsychologic side-effects of tacrolimus in pediatric renal transplantation. Clin Transplant 17:130–134, 2003

Kendall P: Treating anxiety disorders in children: results of a randomized clinical trial. J Consult Clin Psychol 62:100–110, 1994

Kerwin ME: Empirically supported treatments in pediatric psychology: severe feeding problems. J Pediatr Psychol 24: 193–214, 1999

Klein-Gitelman MS, Pachman LM: Intravenous corticosteroids: adverse reactions are more variable than expected in children. J Rheumatol 25:1995–2002, 1998

Kothare SV, Ebb DH, Rosenberger PB, et al: Acute confusion and mutism as a presentation of thalamic strokes secondary to deep cerebral venous thrombosis. J Child Neurol 13:300–303, 1998

Kovacs M, Goldston D, Obrosky DS, et al: Psychiatric disorders in youth with IDDM: rates and risk factors. Diabetes Care 20:36–44, 1997

Krilov LR, Fisher M, Friedman SB, et al: Course and outcome of chronic fatigue in children and adolescents. Pediatrics 102(2 Pt 1):360–366, 1998

Lask B, Matthew D: Childhood asthma. A controlled trial of family psychotherapy. Arch Dis Child 54:116–119, 1979

Lemanek KL, Kamps J, Chung MB: Empirical supported treatments in pediatric psychology: regimen adherence. J Pediatr Psychol 26:253–275, 2001

Lester P, Stein JA, Bursch B: Developmental predictors of somatic symptoms in adolescents of parents with HIV: a 12-month follow-up. J Dev Behav Pediatr 24:242–250, 2003

Li B, Balint JP: Cyclic vomiting syndrome: the evolution of understanding of a brain-gut disorder. Adv Pediatr 47:117–160, 2000

Libow JA: Munchausen by proxy victims in adulthood: a first look. Child Abuse Negl 19:1131–1142, 1995

Libow JA: Child and adolescent illness falsification. Pediatrics 105:336–342, 2000

Liebowitz MR, Turner SM, Piacentini J, et al: Fluoxetine in children and adolescents with OCD: a placebo-controlled trial. J Am Acad Child Adolesc Psychiatry 41: 1431–1438, 2002

Lieh-Lai MW, Theodorou AA, Sarnaik AP, et al: Limitations of the Glasgow Coma Scale in predicting outcome in children with traumatic brain injury. J Pediatr 120(2 pt 1):195–199, 1992

Livingston R: Children of people with somatization disorder. J Am Acad Child Adolesc Psychiatry 3:36–544, 1993

Livingston R, Witt A, Smith GR: Families who somatize. J Dev Behav Pediatr 16:42–46, 1995

Ljungman G, Gordh T, Sorensen S, et al: Lumbar puncture in pediatric oncology: conscious sedation vs. general anesthesia. Med Pediatr Oncol 36:372–379, 2001

Ljungman G, Kreuger A, Andreasson S, et al: Midazolam nasal spray reduces procedural anxiety in children. Pediatrics 105(1 pt 1):73–78, 2000

Ljungman G, Gordh T, Sorensen S, et al: Lumbar puncture in pediatric oncology: conscious sedation vs. general anesthesia. Med Pediatr Oncol 36:372–379, 2001

Lurie S, Shemesh E, Sheiner PA, et al: Nonadherence in pediatric liver transplant recipients—an assessment of risk factors and natural history. Pediatr Transplant 4:200–206, 2000

MacLean W Jr, Perrin J, Gortmarkers S, et al: Psychological adjustment of children with asthma: effects of illness severity and recent stressful life events. J Pediatr Psychol 17:159–171, 1988

Mailis-Gagnon A, Giannoylis I, Downar J, et al: Altered central somatosensory processing in chronic pain patients with "hysterical" anesthesia. Neurology 60: 1501–1507, 2003

Malcolm A, Thumshirn MB, Camilleri M, et al: Rumination syndrome. Mayo Clin Proc 72:646–652, 1997

Manne SL, Du Hamel K, Gallelli K, et al: Posttraumatic stress disorder among mothers of pediatric cancer survivors: diagnosis, comorbidity, and utility of the PTSD checklist as a screening instrument. J Pediatr Psychol 23:357–366, 1998

Manos PJ, Wu R: The duration of delirium in medical and postoperative patients referred for psychiatric consultation. Ann Clin Psychiatry 9:219–226, 1997

Mattson SN, Goodman AM, Caine C, et al: Executive functioning in children with heavy prenatal alcohol exposure. Alcohol Clin Exp Res 23:1808–1815, 1999

May PA, Gossage JP: Estimating the prevalence of fetal alcohol syndrome. Alcohol Health Res World 25:159–167, 2001

Mayes L, Volkmar F, Hooks M, et al: Differentiating pervasive developmental disorder not otherwise specified from autism and language disorders. J Autism Dev Disord 23:79–90, 1993

McNichol K, Williams H, Allan J, et al: Spectrum of asthma in children, III: psychological and social components. BMJ 4:16–20, 1973

McQuaid EL, Kopel SJ, Klein RB, et al: Medication adherence in pediatric asthma: reasoning, responsibility, and behavior. J Pediatr Psychol 28:323–333, 2003

Meeske K, Stuber ML: PTSD, Quality of life and psychological outcome in young adult survivors of pediatric cancer. Oncol Nurs Forum 28:481–489, 2001

Minuchin S, Rosman B, Baker L: Psychosomatic Families. Boston, MA, Harvard University Press, 1978

Morton MJ, Reynolds JM, Garralda ME, et al: Psychiatric adjustment in end-stage renal disease: a follow up study of former paediatric patients. J Psychosom Res 38:293–303, 1994

Mrazek DA, Anderson IS, Strunk RC: Disturbed emotional development of severely asthmatic preschool children. J Child Psychol Psychiatry 4:81–94, 1985

Navelet Y, Nedelcoux H, Teszner D, et al: Emergency pediatric EEG in mental confusion, behavioral disorders and vigilance disorders: a retrospective study. Neurophysiol Clin 28:435–443, 1998

Norrish M, Tooley M, Godfry S: Clinical, physiological, and psychological study of asthmatic children attending a hospital clinic. Arch Dis Child 52:912–917, 1977

O'Brien MD, Bruce BK, Camilleri M: The rumination syndrome: clinical features rather than manometric diagnosis. Gastroenterology 108:1024–1029, 1995

Oguz A, Kurul S, Dirik E: Relationship of epilepsy-related factors to anxiety and depression scores in epileptic children. J Child Neurol 17:37–40, 2002

Ollendick TH, King NJ: Empirically supported treatments for children with phobic and anxiety disorders: current status. J Clin Child Psychol 27:156–167, 1998

Paniagua FA, Braverman C, Capriotti RM: Use of a treatment package in the management of a profoundly mentally retarded girl's pica and self-stimulation. Am J Ment Defic 90:550–557, 1986

Panton J, Barley EA: Family therapy for asthma in children. Cochrane Database Syst Rev (2):CD000089, 2000

Papakostas K, Moraitis D, Lancaster J, et al: Depressive symptoms in children after tonsillectomy. Int J Pediatr Otorhinolaryngol 67:127–132, 2003

Parker RI, Mahan RA, Giugliano D, et al: Efficacy and safety of intravenous midazolam and ketamine as sedation for therapeutic and diagnostic procedures in children. Pediatrics 99: 427–431, 1997

Peyron R, Laurent B, Garcia-Larrea L: Functional imaging of brain responses to pain. A review and meta-analysis 2000. Neurophysiol Clin 30:263–288, 2000

Pfeffer CR: Suicide prevention. Current efficacy and future promise. Ann N Y Acad Sci 487:341–350, 1986

Phipps S, DeCuir-Whalley S: Adherence issues in pediatric bone marrow transplantation. J Pediatr Psychol 15:459–475, 1990

Phipps S, Srivastava DK: Repressive adaptation in children with cancer. Health Psychol 16:521–528, 1997

Phipps S, Srivastava DK: Approaches to the measurement of depressive symptomatology in children with cancer: attempting to circumvent the effects of defensiveness. Development and Behavioral Pediatrics 20:150–156, 1999

Piacentini J, Bergman RL: Developmental issues in cognitive therapy for childhood anxiety disorders. Journal of Cognitive Psychotherapy 15:165–182, 2001

Porter GE, Heitsch GM, Miller MD: Munchausen syndrome by proxy: unusual manifestations and disturbing sequelae. Child Abuse Negl 18:789–794, 1994

Powers SW: Empirically supported treatments in pediatric psychology: Procedure-related pain. J Pediatr Psychol 24:131–145, 1999

Qvist E, Pihko H, Fagerudd P, Valanne L, et al: Neurodevelopmental outcome in high-risk patients after renal transplantation in early childhood. Pediatr Transplant 6:53–62, 2002

Rapoff MA: Adherence to Pediatric Medical Regimens. New York, Kluwer/Plenum, 1999

Rapoff MA, Belmont J, Lindsley C, et al: Prevention of nonadherence to nonsteroidal anti-inflammatory medications for newly diagnosed patients with juvenile rheumatoid arthritis. Health Psychol 21:620–623, 2002

Raymond NC, Chang PN, Crow SJ, et al: Eating disorders in patients with cystic fibrosis. J Adolesc 23:359–363, 2000

Research Unit on Pediatric Psychopharmacology Anxiety Study Group: Fluvoxamine for the treatment of anxiety disorders in children and adolescents. N Engl J Med 344: 1279–1285, 2001

Reynolds JM, Garralda ME, Jameson RA, et al: How parents and families cope with chronic renal failure. Arch Dis Child 63:821–826, 1988

Reynolds JM, Garralda ME, Postlethwaite RJ, et al: Changes in psychosocial adjustment after renal transplantation. Arch Dis Child 66:508–513, 1991

Riddle MA, Bernstein GA, Cook EH, et al: Anxiolytics, adrenergic agents, and naltrexone. J Am Acad Child Adolesc Psychiatry 38:546–556, 1999

Robieux IC, Kumar R, Rhadakrishnan S, et al: The feasibility of using EMLA (eutectic mixture of local anaesthetics) cream in pediatric outpatient clinics. Can J Hosp Pharm 43:235–236, xxxii, 1990

Robins PM, Smith SM, Glutting JJ, et al: A randomized controlled trial of a cognitive-behavioral family intervention for pediatric recurrent abdominal pain. J Pediatr Psychol 30:397–408, 2005

Roebuck RM, Mattson SN, Riley EP: Behavioral and psychosocial profiles of alcohol-exposed children. Alcohol Clin Exp Res 22:339–344, 1998

Rydall AC, Rodin GM, Olmsted MP, et al: Disordered eating behavior and microvascular complications in young women with insulin-dependent diabetes mellitus. N Engl J Med 336:1849–1854, 1997

Sahler OJ, Varni JW, Fairclough DL, et al: Problem-solving skills training for mothers of children with newly diagnosed cancer: a randomized trial. J Dev Behav Pediatr 23:77–86, 2002

Salvatierra O, Alfrey E, Tanne, DC, et al: Superior outcomes in pediatric renal transplantation. Arch Surg 132:842–847, 1997

Sanders MR, Rebyetz M, Morrison M, et al: Cognitive-behavioral treatment of recurrent nonspecific abdominal pain in children: an analysis of generalization, maintenance and side effects. J Consult Clin Psychol 57:294–300, 1989

Sanders MR, Shepherd RW, Cleghorn G, et al: The treatment of recurrent abdominal pain in children: a controlled comparison of cognitive-behavioral family intervention and standard pediatric care. J Consult Clin Psychol 62:306–314, 1994

Schanberg LE, Keefe FJ, Lefebvre JC, et al: Social context of pain in children with Juvenile Primary Fibromyalgia Syndrome: parental pain history and family environment. Clin J Pain 14:107–115, 1998

Schiffrin A: Psychosocial issues in pediatric diabetes. Curr Diab Rep 1:33–40, 2001

Schonfeld A, Mattson SN, Lang A, Delis DC, Riley EP: Verbal and nonverbal fluency in children with heavy prenatal alcohol exposure. J Stud Alcohol 62:239–246, 2001

Serrano-Ikkos E, Lask B, Whitehead B, et al: Incomplete adherence after pediatric heart and heart-lung transplantation. J Heart Lung Transplant 17:1177–1183, 1998

Shaabat A: Confusional migraine in childhood. Pediatr Neurol 15:23–25, 1996

Shemesh E, Lurie S, Stuber ML, et al: A pilot study of posttraumatic stress and nonadherence in pediatric liver transplant recipients. Pediatrics 105:E29, 2000

Shemesh E, Shneider BL, Savitzky JK, et al: Medication adherence in pediatric and adolescent liver transplant recipients. Pediatrics 113:825–832, 2004

Sibbitt WL Jr, Brandt JR, Johnson CR, et al: The incidence and prevalence of neuropsychiatric syndromes in pediatric onset systemic lupus erythematosus. J Rheumatol 29:1536–1542, 2002

Simonds JF: Psychiatric consultations for 112 pediatric inpatients. South Med J 70:980–984, 1977

Simoni JM, Asarnow JR, Munford PR, et al: Psychological distress and treatment adherence among children on dialysis. Pediatr Nephrol 11:604–606, 1997

Snodgrass SR, Vedanarayanan VV, Parker CC, et al: Pediatric patients with undetectable anticonvulsant blood levels: comparison with compliant patients. J Child Neurol 16: 164–168, 2001

Soliday E, Hoeksel R: Health beliefs and pediatric emergency department after-care adherence. Ann Behav Med 22:299–306, 2000

Soykan I, Chen J, Kendall BJ, et al: The rumination syndrome: clinical and manometric profile, therapy, and long-term outcome. Dig Dis Sci 42:1866–1872, 1997

Steele RG, Grauer D: Adherence to antiretroviral therapy for pediatric HIV infection: review of the literature and recommendations for research. Clin Child Fam Psychol Rev 6:17–30, 2003

Steele RG, Anderson B, Rindel B, et al: Adherence to antiretroviral therapy among HIV-positive children: examination of the role of caregiver health beliefs. AIDS Care 13:617–630, 2001

Steinhausen HC, Schindler HP, Stephan H: Comparative psychiatric studies on children and adolescents suffering from cystic fibrosis and bronchial asthma. Child Psychiatry Hum Dev 14:117–130, 1983

Steward DK: Behavioral characteristics of infants with nonorganic failure to thrive during a play interaction. MCN Am J Matern Child Nurs 26:79–85, 2001

Stratton K, Howe C, Battaglia F (eds): Fetal Alcohol Syndrome: Diagnosis, Prevention, and Treatment. Washington, DC, National Academy Press, 1996

Streisand R, Braniecki S, Tercyak KP, et al: Childhood illness-related parenting stress: the pediatric inventory for parents. J Pediatr Psychol 26:155–162, 2001

Streissguth AP, O'Malley K: Neuropsychiatric implications and long-term consequences of fetal alcohol spectrum disorders. Semin Clin Neuropsychiatry 5:177–190, 2000

Strunk RC, Mrazek DA, Wolfson Fuhrmann GS, et al: Psychologic and psychological characteristics associated with death due to asthma in childhood. A case-controlled study. JAMA 254:1193–1198, 1985

Strunk RC, Bender B, Young DA, et al: Predictors of protocol adherence in a pediatric asthma clinical trial. J Allergy Clin Immunol 110:596–602, 2002

Stuart S, Noyes R: Attachment and interpersonal communication in somatization. Psychosomatics 40:34–43, 1999

Stuber ML, Bursch B: Psychiatric care of the terminally ill child, in Psychiatric Dimensions of Palliative Medicine. Edited by Chochinov HM, Breitbart W. New York, NY, Oxford University Press, 2000, pp 225–264

Stuber ML, Mesrkhani VH: "What do we tell the children?": understanding childhood grief. West J Med 174:187–191, 2001

Swanson M, Hall D, Bartas S, et al: Economic impact of noncompliance in kidney transplant recipients. Transplant Proc 24:2723–2724, 1992

Telfair J: Factors in the long term adjustment of children and adolescents with sickle cell disease: conceptualizations and review of the literature. J Health Soc Policy 5:69–96, 1994

Terre L, Ghiselli W: A developmental perspective on family risk factors in somatization. J Psychosom Res 42:197–208, 1997

Todaro JF, Fennell EB, Sears SF, et al: Review: cognitive and psychological outcomes in pediatric heart transplantation. J Pediatr Psychol 25:567–576, 2000

Tsai SJ, Lee YC, Chang K, et al: Psychiatric consultations in pediatric inpatients. Zhonghua Min Guo Xiao Er Ke Yi Xue Hui Za Zhi 36:411–414, 1995

Tucker CM, Fennell RS, Pedersen T, et al: Associations with medication adherence among ethnically different pediatric patients with renal transplants. Pediatr Nephrol 17:251–256, 2002

Turkel SB, Miller JH, Reiff A: Case series: neuropsychiatric symptoms with pediatric systemic lupus erythematosus. J Am Acad Child Adolesc Psychiatry 40:482–485, 2001

Turkel SB, Braslow K, Tavare CJ, et al: The delirium rating scale in children and adolescents. Psychosomatics 44:126–129, 2003

Vasconcellos E, Pina-Garza JE, Fakhoury T, et al: Pediatric manifestations of Hashimoto's encephalopathy. Pediatr Neurol 20:394–398, 1999

Vila G, Nollet-Clemencon C, Vera M, Robert JJ, et al: Prevalence of DSM-IV disorders in children and adolescents with asthma versus diabetes. Can J Psychiatry 44:562–569, 1999

Visconti KJ, Saudino KJ, Rappaport LA, et al: Influence of parental stress and social support on the behavioral adjustment of children with transposition of the great arteries. J Dev Behav Pediatr 23:314–321, 2002

Volkmar FR, Poll J, Lewis M: Conversion reactions in childhood and adolescence. J Am Acad Child Adolesc Psychiatry 23:424–430, 1984

von Weiss RT, Rapoff MA, Varni JW, et al: Daily hassles and social support as predictors of adjustment in children with pediatric rheumatic disease. J Pediatr Psychol 27:155–165, 2002

Wagaman JR, Williams DE, Camilleri M: Behavioral intervention for the treatment of rumination. J Pediatr Gastroenterol Nutr 27:596–598, 1998

Walker LS, Jones DS: Psychosocial factors: impact on symptom severity and outcomes of pediatric functional gastrointestinal disorders. J Pediatr Gastroenterol Nutr 41 (suppl 1):S51–S52, 2005

Wamboldt MZ, Gavin L: Pulmonary disorders, in Handbook of Pediatric Psychology and Psychiatry, Vol I: Disease, Injury and Illness. Edited by Ammerman R, Campo J. Needham Heights, MA, Allyn & Bacon, 1998, pp 266–297

Wamboldt MZ, Yancey AG Jr, Roesler TA: Cardiovascular effects of tricyclic antidepressants in childhood asthma: a case series and review. J Child Adolesc Psychopharmacol 7:45–64, 1997

Wamboldt MZ, Schmitz S, Mrazek D: Genetic association between atopy and behavioral symptoms in middle childhood. J Child Psychol Psychiatry 39:1007–1016, 1998

Wamboldt MZ, Laudenslager M, Wamboldt FS, et al: Adolescents with atopic disorders have an attenuated cortisol response to laboratory stress. J Allergy Clin Immunol 111:509–514, 2003

Weakley MM, Petti TA, Karwisch G: Case study: chewing gum treatment of rumination in an adolescent with an eating disorder. J Am Acad Child Adolesc Psychiatry 36:1124–1127, 1997

Webster R, Holroyd S: Prevalence of psychotic symptoms in delirium. Psychosomatics 41:519–522, 2000

Weston JA, Colloton M, Halsey S, et al: A legacy of violence in nonorganic failure to thrive. Child Abuse Negl 17:709–714, 1993

Williams GC, Freedman ZR, Deci EL: Supporting autonomy to motivate patients with diabetes for glucose control. Diabetes Care 21:1644–1651, 1998

Williamson GM, Walters AS, Shaffer DR: Caregiver models of self and others, coping, and depression: predictors of depression in children with chronic pain. Health Psychol 21: 405–410, 2002

Winton AS, Singh NN: Suppression of pica using brief-duration physical restraint. J Ment Defic Res 27(pt 2):93–103, 1983

Woods DW, Miltenberger RG, Lumley VA: A simplified habit reversal treatment for pica-related chewing. J Behav Ther Exp Psychiatry 27:257–262, 1996

Worchel FF, Nolan BF, Wilson VL, et al: Assessment of depression in children with cancer. J Pediatr Psychol 13:101–112, 1988

Wren F, Tarbell S: Feeding and growth disorders, in Handbook of Pediatric Psychology and Psychiatry, Vol I: Disease, Injury and Illness. Edited by Ammerman R, Campo J. Needham Heights, MA, Allyn & Bacon, 1998, pp 133–165

Yang YM, Cepeda M, Price C, et al: Depression in children and adolescents with sickle-cell disease. Arch Pediatr Adolesc Med 148:457–460, 1994

Yi MS, Britto MT, Wilmott RW, et al: Health values of adolescents with cystic fibrosis. J Pediatr 142:133–140, 2003

Yildiz S, Savaser S, Tatlioglu GS: Evaluation of internal behaviors of children with congenital heart disease. J Pediatr Nurs 16:449–452, 2001

Young GS, Mintzer LL, Seacord D, et al: Symptoms of posttraumatic stress disorder in parents of transplant recipients: incidence, severity, and related factors. Pediatrics 111(6 pt 1): e725–e731, 2003

Zebrack B, Zeltzer L, Whitton J, et al: Psychological outcomes in long-term survivors of childhood leukemia, Hodgkin's disease, and non-Hodgkin's lymphoma: a report from the childhood cancer survivors study. Pediatrics 110:42–52, 2002

Zeltzer LK, Bursch B: Psychological management strategies for functional disorders. J Pediatr Gastroenterol Nutr 32:S40–S41, 2002

Zeltzer LK, Bursch B, Walco GA: Pain responsiveness and chronic pain: a psychobiological perspective. J Dev Behav Pediatr 18:413–422, 1997

Zuckerman B, Stevenson J, Bailey V: Stomachaches and headaches in a community sample of preschool children. Pediatrics 79:677–682, 1987

Self-Assessment Questions

Select the single best response for each question.

1. Which of the following is *not* one of Piaget's stages of cognitive development?

   A. Concrete operations.
   B. Informal operations.
   C. Sensorimotor operations.
   D. Preoperational thought.
   E. Formal operations.

2. Which of the following statements concerning failure to thrive (FTT) children is *incorrect?*

   A. Feeding problems and growth deficiencies can occur.
   B. Mothers of FTT children are reported to have experienced high rates of physical abuse.
   C. If a FTT child gains weight in the hospital, a psychosocial cause of the FTT should be presumed.
   D. Former FTT children have more behavioral problems than do children without a history of FTT.
   E. None of the above.

3. Which of the following statements about cystic fibrosis is *correct?*

   A. Rates of psychiatric disorders among patients with cystic fibrosis are twice that of the general population.
   B. Approximately 250,000 children and adults in the United States have cystic fibrosis.
   C. Less than 10% of patients with cystic fibrosis are adults.
   D. More than 80% of patients with cystic fibrosis are diagnosed by age 3 years.
   E. The median age of survival is 15 years.

4. Vocal cord dysfunction

   A. Commonly occurs comorbidly with asthma.
   B. Is often associated with anxiety.
   C. Can mimic asthma.
   D. Is associated with chronic stress.
   E. All of the above.

5. Which of the following statements concerning juvenile-onset diabetes is *incorrect?*

   A. Puberty can lead to increased insulin resistance.
   B. Poor control commonly occurs during adolescence.
   C. Children at higher risk for developing psychiatric comorbidity are those 5–10 years after diagnosis.
   D. Beta-blockers should not be used to treat anxiety because they mask the early warning signs of hypoglycemia.
   E. Self-efficacy types of behavioral interventions have been shown to be particularly effective in fostering adherence to treatment.

18 Physical Medicine and Rehabilitation

Jesse R. Fann, M.D., M.P.H.

Richard Kennedy, M.D.

Charles H. Bombardier, Ph.D.

PHYSICAL MEDICINE AND rehabilitation, or *rehabilitation medicine*, is concerned with helping people reach the fullest physical, psychological, social, vocational, and educational potential consistent with their physiological or anatomic impairment, environmental limitations, and desires and life plans (DeLisa et al. 1998). The patients encountered in the rehabilitation setting are highly diverse, and their problems include those listed in Table 18–1. Striving for maximum independence is central to the goal of maximizing quality of life.

Rehabilitation is generally a multi- or interdisciplinary effort. Rehabilitation medicine physicians (physiatrists) usually lead the team of other specialized professionals, including physical therapists, occupational therapists, speech pathologists, clinical and neuropsychologists, vocational rehabilitation counselors, recreation therapists, social workers, and

nurses. Rehabilitation programs often have a dedicated psychologist on staff whose job is to conduct psychological and neuropsychological assessments; provide counseling to patients and families; oversee behavioral programs; and generally assist staff in the management of cognitive, behavioral, affective, and social aspects of rehabilitation.

Psychiatrists have an increasing role in the care of patients in the rehabilitation setting. As advances in medical care have increased survival in many medical and traumatic conditions that previously were fatal—the so-called epidemic of survival—opportunities and challenges have emerged that did not previously exist in the rehabilitation of thousands of individuals each year. Data from the 2000 National Health Interview Survey suggest that 12% of the U.S. population has a physical limitation in one or more activities (Schoenborn et al. 2003).

TABLE 18–1.   Problems treated in rehabilitation medicine

Stroke
Traumatic brain injury
Multiple sclerosis
Spinal cord injury
Degenerative movement disorders
Cancer
HIV/AIDS
Cardiac disease
Respiratory dysfunction
Chronic pain
Spinal and muscle pain
Osteoporosis
Rheumatological disorders
Peripheral vascular disease
Peripheral neuropathy and myopathy
Motor neuron diseases
Burn injury
Organ transplantation
Sports injuries
Occupational disorders
Cumulative trauma disorders
Total hip and knee replacements
Hand trauma and disorders
Visual impairment
Hearing impairment
Vestibular disorders

The World Health Organization has shifted its framework for classifying functioning, health, and health-related states from an emphasis on "consequences of disease" found in the previous *International Classification of Impairments, Disabilities and Handicaps* (ICIDH) (World Health Organization 1980) to an emphasis on "components of health" in the current *International Classification of Functioning, Disability and Health* (ICF) (World Health Organization 2001). The ICF conceptually differentiates health and health-related components of the disabling process at the levels of 1) *body structures* (anatomic parts of the body, such as organs, limbs, and their components) and *functions* (physiological functions of body systems,

including psychological functions), and 2) *activities* (execution of a task or an action by an individual) and *participation* (involvement in a life situation). The ICF defines *impairments* as problems in body function or structure, such as a significant deviation or loss, and focuses on *activity limitations* rather than disabilities and *participation limitations* rather than handicaps. A further change has been the inclusion of a section on *environmental factors* as part of the classification, with the recognition of the important role of environment in either facilitating functioning or creating barriers for people with disabilities. Environmental factors interact with a health condition to restore functioning or create a disability, depending on whether the environmental factor is a facilitator or barrier.

In this chapter, we focus on the psychiatric issues encountered in the treatment of traumatic brain injury (TBI) and spinal cord injury (SCI), two common and highly complex rehabilitation problems with aspects that may require psychiatric intervention. Although many of the other disorders encountered in the rehabilitation setting are covered in other chapters of this text, many of the principles discussed in this chapter also apply to them.

Traumatic Brain Injury

Epidemiology

TBI is a significant problem from both an individual and a public health perspective. An estimated 1.4 million Americans sustain TBI each year; of these, approximately 235,000 are hospitalized and survive, 50,000 die, and 80,000–90,000 experience the onset of long-term disability (Langlois et al. 2006). Although about 80% of TBIs are mild in severity, many of these individuals experience long-term somatic and psychiatric problems that may lead to disability (Brown et al. 1994; Guerrero et al. 2000). TBI is often referred to as the "silent epidemic" because TBI-related disabilities are not readily visible to the general public.

With improved medical care, TBI mortality and hospitalizations have declined 20% and 50%, respectively, since 1980 (Thurman et al. 1999), leading to more long-term morbidity and disability. The peak incidence of TBI is in 15- to 24-year-olds (mostly from motor vehicle accidents), with a secondary peak among those 60 years and older (mostly from falls) (Langlois et al. 2006). Because TBI affects a predominantly younger population, the effects of disability are much greater than for illnesses occurring later in life. Figures reported in 1999 showed total costs for acute care and rehabilitation of TBI were $9–$10 billion per year (National Institutes of Health Consensus Development Panel on Rehabilitation of Persons With Traumatic Brain Injury 1999), and about $13.5 billion was necessary for continuing care of those who experienced TBI in previous years (J.F. Kraus and McArthur 1999). Long-term disability has primarily been attributed to neurobehavioral factors (Sander et al. 1997; Witol et al. 1996). Thus, many psychiatrists will be involved at some level in the care of individuals with TBI.

Severity and Classification

Original severity classifications for TBI focused on the Glasgow Coma Scale (GCS) (Jennett and Bond 1975) because of its widespread use. A TBI with a lowest postresuscitation GCS score of 3–8 is considered severe, 9–12 is moderate, and 13–15 is mild. However, although the GCS is useful for predicting mortality after TBI, it has less utility in predicting level of disability and neurobehavioral outcome, particularly at the upper end of the scale. It is recognized

that the group of individuals with GCS scores of 13–15 are quite heterogeneous in levels of impairment and outcome (Dikmen et al. 2001; Williams et al. 1990). Durations of coma and of posttraumatic amnesia are also used to describe TBI severity.

The American Congress of Rehabilitation Medicine has put forth a definition of mild TBI that is widely used, requiring loss of consciousness (LOC) of 30 minutes or less, posttraumatic amnesia of 24 hours or less, and any alteration of mental state at the time of the injury (including feeling dazed, disoriented, or confused) or a focal neurological deficit, in addition to a GCS score of 13–15 (Kay et al. 1993). Patients with a GCS score of 13–15 who have imaging evidence of intracranial pathology have outcomes more similar to those of moderate TBI and are often classified as "complicated mild" injuries (see Williams et al. 1990).

Functional Pathophysiology

There has been considerable progress in understanding the pathophysiological mechanisms of TBI in recent years. The physical forces in TBI initiate mechanical and chemical changes that lead to neurological dysfunction. These are divided into *primary damage*, which occurs at the moment of injury, and *secondary damage*, which is initiated at injury but evolves over time. The latter is subdivided into direct injury, occurring within the neuron itself, and indirect injury, occurring outside the neuron but affecting its function.

Primary damage consists of injuries such as skull fractures, brain contusions and lacerations, and intracranial hemorrhage (McIntosh et al. 1996). Because these occur at the time of injury, the key treatment is prevention. Diffuse axonal injury is the predominant mechanism of injury in most cases of TBI (Meythaler et al. 2001).

Direct secondary injury occurs via neurochemical changes evolving over time after the mechanical disruption of neuronal pathways (McIntosh et al. 1996). The acute phase of this process has been well described, with a global increase in cerebral metabolism after injury (Bergsneider et al. 2001; Yoshino et al. 1991). This is accompanied by a period of excessive activity of neurotransmitters, including acetylcholine, glutamate, dopamine, norepinephrine, and various growth factors (Hayes et al. 1992; McIntosh et al. 1996). A key event in the early phase of injury is excessive influx of calcium (Gennarelli and Graham 1998), which may lead to gene activation, triggering preprogrammed cell death and enzyme activation, leading to damage to the cellular cytoskeleton and free radical generation.

The neurochemical changes in the subacute phase of TBI have been less intensively investigated, but current evidence indicates that this phase is associated with a dramatic reversal of acute processes (Hamm et al. 2000; Hayes and Dixon 1994). Research in animal models of TBI has successfully identified pharmacotherapies to reduce behavioral and histological complications (McIntosh et al. 1998). However, clinical investigations of such agents have been disappointing (Povlishock 2000).

Psychiatric Disorders in Traumatic Brain Injury

Although useful data have been collected in recent years regarding the epidemiology of psychiatric disorders after TBI, the numbers of studies and subjects for each disorder remain small. Other limitations of many studies include selection bias (examining only hospitalized subjects or those referred for psychiatric evaluation), varying assessment periods, use of unstructured psychiatric interviews, and limited assessment of premorbid psychiatric history (Van Reekum et al. 2000). Such factors lead to wide variation in the estimates of incidence and prevalence of psychiatric disorders after TBI. Other complex disturbances seen after TBI are not adequately captured by current diagnostic systems such as DSM-IV-TR (American Psychiatric Association 2000). Some symptoms, such as fatigue or impulsivity, may cause significant impairment but may not fit into a specific diagnosis. Also, individuals with TBI may lack insight into, and not report, their deficits. In addition to these general concerns, there may be differences in the presentation and phenomenology of specific disorders in the context of TBI.

The development of psychiatric disorders involves a complex interplay between premorbid biological and psychological factors, postinjury biological changes, and psychosocial and environmental factors. A review by Rao and Lyketsos (2002) compiled risk factors for the development of psychiatric sequelae in general (shown in Table 18–2). These are divided into highly significant risk factors (sufficient evidence exists for their role in psychiatric disorders) and less significant risk factors (evidence is still controversial). In a large unselected primary care population, Fann et al. (2004) found psychiatric history to be a highly significant risk factor for psychiatric illness in the 3 years following TBI. Their data suggested that moderate to severe TBI may be associated with higher initial risk for psychiatric problems, whereas mild TBI and prior psychiatric illness may increase the risk for more persistent psychiatric problems. The authors hypothesized that psychiatric symptoms that arise immediately after TBI may be etiologically related to the neurophysiological effects of the injury, consistent with the early relation between TBI severity and psychiatric risk, whereas other factors, such as psychological vulnerability, self-awareness of

TABLE 18–2.   **Risk factors for psychiatric illness after traumatic brain injury**

Highly significant risk factors

  Preinjury psychiatric history
  Preinjury social impairments
  Increased age
  Alcohol abuse
  Arteriosclerosis

Less significant risk factors

  More severe injury
  Poor neuropsychological functioning
  Marital discord
  Financial instability
  Poor interpersonal relationships
  Low preinjury level of education
  Compensation claims
  Female gender
  Short time since injury
  Lesion location (especially left prefrontal)

Source. Adapted from Rao V, Lyketsos CG: "Psychiatric Aspects of Traumatic Brain Injury." *Psychiatric Clinics of North America* 25:43–69, 2002. Copyright © 2002. Used with permission of Elsevier.

deficits, social influences, and secondary gain, may play roles over time, particularly in individuals with prior psychiatric illness and prior injury.

Although several psychiatric disorders are common after TBI, establishing a causal link between these remains difficult. Van Reekum and colleagues (2000, 2001) noted that there is some evidence for causality, in that studies (particularly in experimental animals) have shown that TBI disrupts neuronal systems involved in mood and behavior. However, other lines of evidence are inconclusive. The following suggestive findings point to other possible associations: 1) the psychiatric disorder increases the risk for TBI (Fann et al. 2002); 2) the risk for both TBI and the psychiatric disorder is due to a common third factor, such as substance abuse; and 3) a postinjury condition, such as pain or change in family status, contributes to the

psychiatric disorder. Evidence for a biological gradient, in which more severe injuries are associated with higher risk for psychiatric disorders, is mixed.

Depression

Several studies have used structured interviews to examine rates of depression. Fann and colleagues (1995) used the National Institute of Mental Health Diagnostic Interview Schedule to assess 50 consecutive outpatients presenting to a rehabilitation clinic for evaluation of TBI. Of these, 26% were diagnosed with major depression, and another 28% had had major depression with onset after injury that had since resolved. Hibbard and colleagues (1998) administered the Structured Clinical Interview for DSM-IV (SCID) to 100 patients with TBI who were randomly selected from a larger quality-of-life study. Depression was found in 61%, with the onset of depression after injury in 48%. Deb et al. (1999) examined 164 outpatients previously admitted to the emergency department with a diagnosis of TBI. Assessment based on the Schedules for Clinical Assessment in Neuropsychiatry (SCAN) indicated the rate of depression was 18%. Ashman et al. (2004) administered the SCID to 188 outpatients 3 months to 4 years after injury as part of a longitudinal follow-up of TBI. Major depression was present in 20% of patients before injury and in 24%–35% of patients during the first year of follow-up.

In a systematic examination of depression after TBI, Federoff and colleagues (1992) examined 66 consecutive trauma center admissions with the Present State Examination (PSE), a forerunner of the SCAN. Approximately 1 month after injury, 26% had symptoms that met criteria for major depression. Jorge and colleagues (1993a, 1993c) carried out follow-up examinations on this cohort. At 3 months after injury, 12 of 54 patients (22%) had major depression; at 6 months, 10 of 43 (23%) had major depression; and at 12 months, 8 of 43 (19%) had major depression. Jorge et al. (2004) subsequently replicated these results in another cohort of 91 consecutive hospital admissions for TBI, showing 33% of the patients developing major depression during the first year after injury: 17% at initial evaluation, 10% at 3 months, and 6% at 6 months.

In their cohort, Jorge and colleagues (1993c) noted those with depression were significantly more likely to have a premorbid history of psychiatric disorders. Subjects with depression had significantly poorer social functioning prior to injury, and poor social functioning was the strongest and most consistent correlate of depression on follow-up. In the original study (Federoff et al. 1992), depression at 1 month was strongly associated with lesions in the left dorsolateral frontal and/or left basal ganglia regions on computed tomographic scanning. Right parieto-occipital lesions were associated with depression to a lesser extent. Pure cortical lesions were associated with a decreased probability of depression. However, no relation was found between lesion location and depression in subsequent follow-ups (Jorge et al. 1993a). In their later study (Jorge et al. 2004), major depression was associated with reduced volume in the left prefrontal cortex at 3-month follow-up. Replication is needed to confirm these correlations.

Fann et al. (2004) found that patients with mild TBI had a higher risk for affective disorders (including depressive and anxiety disorders) than did patients with moderate to severe TBI (e.g., relative risk 2.7 vs. 1.0 in the first 6 months following TBI) among 939 health maintenance organization enrollees with TBI.

Early studies of major depression showed high rates of vegetative symptoms among individuals with TBI that exceeded

the reported rate of depression in these patients. The "inclusive," "etiological," "substitutive," and "exclusive" approaches used in the medically ill have similar advantages and disadvantages in the TBI population. Jorge et al. (1993a) found that TBI patients who reported depressed mood had higher rates of both physical and psychological symptoms of depression (as assessed with the PSE) than did those without depressed mood. The group with depressed mood also endorsed more DSM-III-R (American Psychiatric Association 1987) symptoms of major depression than did those without depressed mood. The symptoms of suicidal ideation, inappropriate guilt, anergia, psychomotor agitation, and weight loss or poor appetite occurred with significantly greater frequency in the depressed group. Thus, it appears that the diagnosis of major depression can be accurately made with DSM criteria in brain-injured patients. Although there are few studies examining the validity of self-report depression screening instruments in the TBI population, the Patient Health Questionnaire–9 (Kroenke et al. 2001) has been found to be valid when compared with the SCID (Fann et al. 2005). The Neurobehavioral Functioning Inventory (Kreutzer et al. 1999) also performs well (Kennedy et al. 2005) and has been used in large-scale studies of depression after TBI (Kreutzer et al. 2001; Seel et al. 2003).

Jorge and colleagues (1993b) estimated that the mean duration of depression was 4.7 months. Subjects with anxious depression had a significantly longer duration of symptoms than did those with depression and no anxiety (7.5 months vs. 1.5 months) (Jorge et al. 1993c). In their follow-up study, the mean duration of depression was 4.7 months for those who received antidepressants and 5.8 months for those who did not (Jorge et al. 2004). Collectively, these data show that the onset of depression is not immediately linked to the occurrence of TBI in a significant number of individuals.

Mania

A prevalence of 2% was reported by Hibbard et al. (1998), with all occurring after TBI; and Jorge et al. (1993d) reported that 9% of their subjects met the criteria for mania at some point during the year after injury. In contrast, none of the subjects developed bipolar disorder in the study by Fann et al. (1995). Thus, although TBI may increase the risk for developing bipolar disorder, it still appears to be a relatively rare consequence of injury.

Phenomenologically, all forms of bipolar disorder, including bipolar I, bipolar II, and rapid-cycling variants, have been reported (McAllister and Ferrell 2002). The largest study addressing this topic suggested that patients are more likely to present with irritable than with euphoric mood (Shukla et al. 1987). Shukla and colleagues (1987) observed that mania after TBI was associated with posttraumatic seizures but not with family history of bipolar disorder. Jorge and colleagues (1993d) noted that mania after TBI was significantly related to basopolar temporal lesions. The duration of the manic episode was only 2 months, but elevated or expansive mood persisted for a mean of 5.7 months.

Anxiety

A recent area of interest and controversy has been the development of acute stress disorder and posttraumatic stress disorder (PTSD) after TBI. Early opinion was that PTSD could not develop after TBI; investigators argued that LOC or posttraumatic amnesia would prevent patients from having reexperiencing and avoidance because memories were not encoded (Harvey et al. 2003). This was supported by the studies of Mayou et al. (1993), Sbordone and Liter (1995), and Warden et al. (1997). However, some experts have raised concerns that these studies did not adequately assess for PTSD.

Studies with more detailed, structured assessments of PTSD have yielded different results. Hibbard et al. (1998) noted that 19% of their subjects had symptoms that met criteria for PTSD. Mayou and colleagues (2000) examined consecutive admissions to an emergency department with the PTSD Symptom Scale. Ten of the 21 subjects (48%) with definite LOC met the criteria for PTSD at 3 months, compared with 9 of 39 (23%) with probable LOC, and 179 of 796 (22%) without LOC. At 1-year follow-up, the rates of PTSD were 33%, 14%, and 17%, respectively. Levin and colleagues (2001) interviewed a sample of 69 patients with mild to moderate TBI drawn from admissions to a major trauma center. Twelve percent of the patients received diagnoses of PTSD at 3 months according to the SCID, which was identical to the rate in general trauma control subjects. Ashman et al. (2004) found that 10% of their subjects met criteria for PTSD prior to injury, with 18%–30% meeting criteria during the first year of follow-up.

A series of studies by Bryant and Harvey represents the most extensive exploration of the topic. Bryant and Harvey (1995) examined 38 hospital admissions with mild TBI with the PTSD Interview, a structured interview for DSM-III-R symptoms of PTSD. Approximately 27% of the subjects met the criteria for diagnosis, although these were not consecutive admissions. In another study, Harvey and Bryant (1998) reported on 79 consecutive hospital admissions with mild TBI. According to the Acute Stress Disorder Interview, a structured clinical interview based on DSM-IV symptoms of acute stress disorder, 14% fulfilled diagnostic criteria. Seventy-one of these subjects participated in follow-up at 6 months (Bryant and Harvey 1998). Rates of PTSD were 25% at 6 months and

22% at 2 years. Bryant and colleagues (2000) also examined 96 subjects drawn from admissions to a brain injury rehabilitation unit with severe TBI. Approximately 27% of the subjects met the criteria for PTSD on the basis of the PTSD Interview; however, again, subjects were not consecutive admissions, and these data cannot be used to estimate overall prevalence of PTSD after TBI.

Bryant and Harvey (1998) noted that 82% of the mild TBI patients who met criteria for acute stress disorder went on to develop PTSD, whereas only 11% of those without acute stress disorder eventually developed PTSD. It is not entirely clear whether memory of the traumatic event is necessary for the development of PTSD (Gil et al. 2005). In some cases, those who are "amnestic" for the event will actually have "islands" of traumatic memories that are involved in PTSD. In other cases, patients who do not recall their injury may develop PTSD around traumatic experiences involved in hospitalization, which they do recall. This area clearly warrants further investigation to determine the appropriateness of a PTSD diagnosis for such individuals.

It seems rather certain that those who do have memories of traumatic events are at increased risk for developing PTSD and should be monitored accordingly (Gil et al. 2005; Hiott and Labbate 2002). This is particularly important in light of research suggesting that PTSD occurring after TBI may be less likely to spontaneously remit (Harvey and Bryant 2000).

Other anxiety disorders also may be common. Fann et al. (1995) found that 24% of subjects met the criteria for generalized anxiety disorder (GAD) and 4% had panic disorder after TBI. In the study by Jorge et al. (1993c), 7 subjects (11%) met the criteria for GAD, with all 7 also having major depression. In the follow-up study by Jorge et al. (1993c), 23 (76.7%) of the patients with major depression also met criteria for comorbid anxiety disorder, compared with 9 (20.4%) of the patients without major depression. Hibbard et al. (1998) reported rates of 14% for obsessive-compulsive disorder (OCD), 11% for panic disorder, 7% for phobias, and 8% for GAD after injury. Deb et al. (1999) noted that 9% of their subjects had panic disorder, 3% had GAD, 2% had OCD, and 1% had phobias. Finally, Ashman et al. (2004) found that 16% of their subjects met criteria for other anxiety disorders besides PTSD prior to injury, with 19%–27% having other anxiety disorders during the first year of follow-up.

Psychosis

Relatively few studies have examined psychosis after TBI. Davison and Bagley (1969) reviewed eight studies before 1960, showing between 0.7% and 9.8% of the patients with TBI having a schizophrenia-like psychosis (but diagnosis was not based on structured criteria). In a different approach, Wilcox and Nasrallah (1987) performed a retrospective review of 659 hospital admissions, finding a significantly higher rate of prior head trauma in patients with schizophrenia compared with control subjects admitted for depression, mania, or general surgery. Malaspina and colleagues (2001) found individuals with a history of TBI were significantly more likely to develop schizophrenia than other first-degree relatives of patients having schizophrenia or bipolar disorder. This suggested a synergistic relation between schizophrenia and TBI, in which familial factors among schizophrenic patients and their relatives increased the risk of TBI, and TBI further increased the risk of schizophrenia in those with genetic vulnerability.

Only a few studies have examined other forms of psychosis. Violon and DeMol (1987) performed a retrospective review of

530 patients with TBI admitted to a neurosurgical unit, noting that 3% had delusions during follow-up. Fann et al. (2004) also found a higher rate of psychotic disorders among persons with TBI, compared with matched non-TBI control subjects, especially in those with moderate to severe TBI and with prior psychiatric illness.

Risk factors and phenomenology are similarly understudied. Sachdev and colleagues (2001) noted that auditory hallucinations and paranoid delusions were more common than negative symptoms. Fujii and Ahmed (2002) reviewed descriptions of psychosis after TBI in 69 patients from 39 publications, with particular emphasis on studies that used neuroimaging or neurophysiological measures. Delusions, most commonly persecutory, were much more common than hallucinations, and hallucinations were more likely to be observed in delayed-onset psychosis.

In their review, Davison and Bagley (1969) identified several risk factors for psychosis, including left hemisphere and temporal lobe lesions, closed head injury, and increasing severity of TBI. Others have noted that more extensive brain injury, greater cognitive impairment, male gender, and having TBI in childhood are associated with psychosis (Fujii and Ahmed 2002; Sachdev et al. 2001).

Electroencephalogram abnormalities (especially in the temporal lobe) were common, and the rates for seizure disorder among individuals with psychosis after TBI were much higher than estimates for the rate of seizures after TBI in general (Fujii and Ahmed 2002). Neuroimaging lesions (predominantly in the frontal and temporal lobes) were also frequent. Finally, the severity and duration of psychosis occurring after TBI may be less than that of idiopathic psychotic disorders, with only about one-third having a chronic course similar to schizophrenia in the studies examining this issue (Hillbom

1960; Violon and DeMol 1987). The onset of psychotic symptoms is typically gradual and delayed, often occurring more than a year after injury (Fann et al. 2004; Fujii and Ahmed 2002; Sachdev et al. 2001).

Anger, Aggression, and Agitation

Many patients with TBI have difficulty modulating emotional reactions and controlling impulses (Rao and Lyketsos 2002), often described in the TBI literature as *posttraumatic agitation* (Sandel and Mysiw 1996). However, as noted by Yudofsky et al. (1997), *agitation* is a poorly defined term encompassing behaviors ranging from "constant unwarranted requests" to assaultiveness. Brooke and colleagues (1992b) used the Overt Aggression Scale (Yudofsky et al. 1986) to measure agitation in 100 patients with severe TBI. Only 11% of the patients had agitation; an additional 35% were classified as "restless" but not severely enough to be labeled "agitated." Bogner and Corrigan (1995) examined 100 consecutive patients admitted to an inpatient TBI unit. Of these, 42% had agitation (as measured by the Agitated Behavior Scale) during at least one shift.

Although aggression may be a symptom of many disorders, several features are characteristic of aggression after TBI (Yudofsky et al. 1990). Such behavior is typically *nonreflective*, occurring without any premeditation or planning, and *nonpurposeful*, achieving no particular goals for the individual. It is also *reactive*, triggered by a stimulus, but often a stimulus that would not normally provoke a strong reaction. Aggression after TBI is *periodic*, occurring at intervals with relatively calm behavior in between, and *explosive*, occurring without a prodromal buildup. Finally, it is *ego-dystonic*, creating a great deal of distress for the patient.

Agitation is more likely to occur with frontotemporal injuries (Van der Naalt et al. 1999). Disorientation, comorbid medical illness, and use of anticonvulsant medications are also associated with agitation (Galski et al. 1994). Risk of aggression is increased with a premorbid history of impulsive aggression (Greve et al. 2001), arrest (Kreutzer et al. 1995), substance abuse (Dunlop et al. 1991), or depression (Jorge et al. 2004). For these risk factors, it is often difficult to ascertain whether the aggression is a direct result of TBI, premorbid character pathology, or both (Kim 2002). It appears that agitation and aggression may be chronic problems not confined to the early stage of recovery (Silver and Yudofsky 1994a).

Substance Use Disorders

Substance abuse and dependence are of great concern in the TBI population, at the time of injury and afterward. Literature reviews have shown that in higher-quality studies, 44%–66% of the patients with TBI have a history of significant alcohol-related problems before injury and that 36%–51% are intoxicated at the time of injury (Bombardier 2000; Corrigan 1995). Those with a history of significant alcohol-related problems before injury are 11 times more likely to have alcohol problems after injury compared with those without alcohol problems before injury (Bombardier et al. 2003). A history of illicit drug use is found in 21%–37% (Bombardier et al. 2002; Kolakowsky-Hayner et al. 1999; Kreutzer et al. 1991, 1996; Ruff et al. 1990).

Substance abuse declines after TBI but remains significant. Rates of remission from alcohol problems range from 31% to 56% during the first year after injury (Bombardier et al. 2003). After TBI, about 22%–29% of patients are moderate to heavy drinkers (Bombardier et al. 2002; Horner et al. 2005; Kreutzer et al. 1996) or meet the criteria for substance abuse or dependence (Hibbard et al. 1998). However, some stud-

ies report much lower rates of substance abuse or dependence—8% by Fann and colleagues (1995), 4% by Deb and colleagues (1999), and 10%–14% by Ashman and colleagues (2004). Timing of assessment, sensitivity of screening measures, and the issue of whether patients were unselected or from referral populations may play critical roles in explaining some of these variations. Risk factors for postinjury substance abuse include history of legal problems related to substance abuse, substance abuse problems among family and/or friends, age younger than 25 years, and less severe injuries (Taylor et al. 2003).

Brain injury rehabilitation may represent a window of opportunity for intervening in substance abuse disorders (Bombardier et al. 1997). Several potentially effective interventions, including TBI-specific education, physician advice to cut down or abstain, and brief motivational interventions, should be considered within rehabilitation (Bombardier 2000). Referral to outside substance abuse treatment programs also may be considered, especially when staff at available programs are comfortable with the cognitive and physical disabilities associated with TBI.

Cognitive Impairment

Much effort has been devoted to characterizing the cognitive deficits that occur after TBI. Some have suggested that deficits can be divided into four time periods (Rao and Lyketsos 2000). The first is the period of LOC that results from the injury. After emerging from unconsciousness, many individuals enter a phase consisting of multiple cognitive and behavioral deficits, which some have described as posttraumatic delirium (Kwentus et al. 1985; Trzepacz 1994). The third period is a rapid recovery of cognitive function, which plateaus over time. This leads to the fourth period of permanent cognitive deficits. TBI is associated with deficits in multiple domains, including impaired memory, language deficits, reduced attention and concentration, slowed information processing, and executive dysfunction (Capruso and Levin 1996).

Although TBI is associated with an acute decrement in cognitive function that typically improves over time, recovery is very individualized, and there is no universally applicable description of the recovery process. Rao and Lyketsos (2000) offer the following general timeline: the first two periods of recovery will last from a few days to a month, the third period will last 6–12 months, and the fourth period will last 12–24 months. Such guidelines are more characteristic of moderate to severe injuries. By definition, individuals with mild TBI will have LOC of less than 30 minutes, with many having none at all (Kay et al. 1993). It is also estimated that about 95% of patients with mild TBI will recover to baseline status within 3–6 months and not enter the fourth phase of permanent deficits (Binder et al. 1997). Even among individuals with moderate to severe TBI, some recovery of cognitive function may occur 2 years or more after injury, although the gains are typically small (Millis et al. 2001). A few patients may experience decline late in the course of recovery, perhaps caused by depression (Millis et al. 2001). Thus, these time frames must be considered general approximations only.

Descriptions of the period of recovery from TBI vary in the rehabilitation literature. One classical term is *posttraumatic amnesia*, which occurs "from injury until recovery of full consciousness and the return of ongoing memory" (Grant and Alves 1987). This would include the first two periods described above and potentially extend into the third. However, characterization of the deficits after TBI as purely amnestic is an oversimplification because multiple cognitive deficits occur (D.I. Katz 1992). Stuss and colleagues

(1999) advocated discarding *posttraumatic amnesia* for the concept of *posttraumatic confusion*, although this has not gained widespread use in the TBI literature. Most definitions of posttraumatic amnesia would be consistent with a period of delirium followed by an amnestic phase (Trzepacz and Kennedy 2005).

The long-term diffuse cognitive deficits seen after TBI would be categorized as dementia due to head trauma or cognitive disorder not otherwise specified under DSM-IV-TR. This would include the fourth period described earlier and potentially the third period when the recovery process is slow. Rehabilitation experts have expressed concern with use of the term *dementia* in the TBI population (Leon-Carrion 2002). The impairments seen after TBI, unlike those seen in most dementias, tend to either remain static or improve over time.

Several risk factors for delirium in the medical-surgical population would likely apply to individuals with TBI (Trzepacz and Kennedy 2005), who are at increased risk for several medical illnesses (Kalisky et al. 1985; Shavelle et al. 2001). Risk factors for prolonged posttraumatic amnesia include older age, low initial GCS score, nonreactive pupils, coma duration, higher number of lesions detected by neuroimaging, and use of phenytoin (Ellenberg et al. 1996; Wilson et al. 1994). These would likely be risk factors for delirium as well.

For dementia, severity of injury is consistently associated with the degree and duration of cognitive impairments. The extent of impairment is also influenced by premorbid intellectual abilities and the time after injury at which the patient is assessed (Dikmen et al. 1995). As with other dementias, the cognitive domains affected will vary from patient to patient (Kreutzer et al. 1993). Patients with TBI also may be at increased risk for developing dementia from other causes, such as Alzheimer's disease (Amaducci et al. 1986; Graves et al. 1990).

Postconcussive Syndrome

The diagnosis of postconcussive syndrome has been a source of wide controversy. It is important to differentiate postconcussive *symptoms* from postconcussive *syndrome*. The *symptoms* of postconcussive syndrome are very nonspecific and include disturbances such as headache, dizziness, irritability, fatigue, and insomnia (Boake et al. 2005; Caveness 1966; Gouvier et al. 1988; McLean et al. 1983; Tuohimaa 1978). Most experts concur that the diagnosis of postconcussive syndrome requires the presence of multiple concurrent symptoms (Brown et al. 1994; Mittenberg and Strauman 2000), although disagreement may remain over which specific symptoms are required. DSM-IV-TR lists provisional criteria for postconcussional disorder, indicating that the diagnosis may still undergo refinement. The ICD-10 (World Health Organization 1992) also has published criteria.

Because postconcussive symptoms are not specific to TBI, it is important to consider their differential diagnosis. Alexander (1995) and Mittenberg and Strauman (2000) noted that postconcussive syndrome has significant overlap with psychiatric disorders. Thus, the presence of psychiatric disorders may lead to high rates of reporting of postconcussive symptoms, regardless of TBI history (Fox et al. 1995; Suhr and Gunstad 2002; Trahan et al. 2001). Careful history taking and diagnosis are needed to avoid mislabeling these patients as having postconcussive syndrome. The clinician also must keep in mind that individuals may have both postconcussive syndrome and a psychiatric disorder, which may blur the boundaries between the two.

Most studies of postconcussive syndrome have focused on individuals with mild TBI, although postconcussive syndrome can occur with more severe injuries as well. The symptoms of postconcussive syndrome are extremely common after mild TBI, with 80%–100% of patients experiencing one or more symptoms in the immediate postinjury period (Levin et al. 1987b). Several studies have shown that such symptoms resolve completely within 3 months in most patients (Alves et al. 1986; R.W. Evans 1996; Leininger et al. 1990). However, other prospective studies have shown that 20%–66% of patients have persistent symptoms at 3 months (Alves et al. 1986; Englander et al. 1992) and that 1%–50% have persistent symptoms at 1 year (Middleboe et al. 1992; Rutherford et al. 1979). For many studies, the lack of an appropriate control group makes it difficult to determine how many symptoms could be attributed to the TBI itself.

Currently, the acute syndrome is thought to be related to neurological factors, whereas chronic symptoms are more likely to persist because of psychological factors (Larrabee 1997; Mittenberg and Strauman 2000). It is not known how these putative neurological injuries, which should resolve quickly, transition into chronic postconcussive syndrome. Symptom expectations, in which patients fear that their symptoms will not resolve, may play a role (King 2003; Mittenberg and Strauman 2000; Mittenberg et al. 1996). However, the precise role of psychological factors in persistent postconcussive syndrome is far from clear (Dikmen et al. 1989). Thus, the risk factors for postconcussive syndrome are a mixture of biological and psychological.

The more commonly reported risk factors are female gender (Bazarian et al. 1999; Fenton et al. 1993; McCauley et al. 2001; McClelland et al. 1994), older age (Alexander 1997; McCauley et al. 2001), history of previous TBI (Alexander 1997; McCauley et al. 2001), psychosocial stress (Fenton et al. 1993; Moss et al. 1994; Radanov et al. 1991), and poor social support (Fenton et al. 1993; McCauley et al. 2001). Low socioeconomic status and ongoing litigation also increase risk (Alexander 1997; Binder and Rohling 1996; McCauley et al. 2001).

However, for the latter, it should be noted that few individuals involved in litigation have improvement in postconcussive syndrome after settlement (King 2003).

A significant association is seen between depression and postconcussive symptoms, including those postconcussive symptoms that do not overlap with depression (Fann et al. 1995; King 2003), and severity of depressive symptoms predicts risk for postconcussive syndrome (McCauley et al. 2001).

Although the vast majority of the persons with mild TBI experience good recovery (Binder et al. 1997), Ruff (1999) identified a "miserable minority" of 10%–20% of mild TBI patients with poor outcome, and Malec (1999) noted that 20%–40% of mild TBI patients have residual long-term symptoms or disability. In many cases, such individuals complain of symptoms of postconcussive syndrome, indicating that ongoing postconcussive syndrome may be an important source of disability. Studies of such patients also have found significant deficits on a variety of neuropsychological tests (Bohnen et al. 1992; Guilmette and Rasile 1995; Leininger et al. 1990). These data suggest that individuals with persistent postconcussive syndrome differ in significant respects from most individuals with TBI, although the reasons for these differences remain unexplained. Investigators also have found that high rates of postconcussive symptoms were better predictors of neuropsychological test performance than was actual history of mild TBI (Hanna-Pladdy et al. 1997; Pinkston et al. 2000). These results cast further doubt on the contention that the cognitive impairment in persistent postconcussive syndrome is due to TBI.

Psychological Aspects

In addition to the defined DSM-IV-TR psychiatric disorders, TBI is associated with psychological challenges that may not fit into specific diagnostic categories. Four areas of importance are the neurological disorder and resultant cognitive deficits, the psychological meaning of deficits and effect on the patient, psychological factors that exist independently of TBI, and the broader social context (Lewis 1991).

Deficits due to neurological impairment may have a direct effect on psychological functioning. Between 76% and 97% of TBI patients show some degree of impaired self-awareness (Sherer et al. 1998a, 2003). Many individuals with TBI also have deficits in awareness of their behavioral limitations (Prigatano and Altman 1990), which may be one of their most troubling problems (Ben-Yishay et al. 1985; Prigatano and Fordyce 1986). Awareness of cognitive and emotional changes tends to be worse than awareness of physical dysfunction (Sherer et al. 1998a). Patients are also less likely to report deficits when asked general questions rather than specific ones (Gasquione 1992; Sherer et al. 1998b).

Impaired awareness has both neurological and psychological dimensions. At one extreme is anosognosia, wherein the person has no awareness of neurological impairments (Prigatano 1999). At the other extreme is "defensive denial," which represents the person's attempt to cope with overwhelming anxiety associated with neurological impairment by minimizing the implications. Apparent impaired awareness also can be the result of moderate to severe memory impairment that prevents the person from consolidating and acting on new information about his or her condition. Interventions designed to address denial and psychological causes may be ineffective when the decreased awareness is due to neurological dysfunction that cannot be reversed.

The patient's psychological state and the perceived meaning of physical and cognitive deficits may be strongly linked.

Patients with depression or anxiety appear to perceive their injury and associated cognitive problems as more severe (Fann et al. 1995, 2000). Many patients with TBI experience grief in reaction to their disability and loss of their "former self." For many years, rehabilitation researchers have relied on bereavement concepts to explain the adjustment-to-disability process (Stewart and Shields 1985; Vargo 1978). However, advances in the understanding of grief following loss of a loved one, with few exceptions (Niemeier and Burnett 2001), have not yet been applied to the emotional experience of individuals with functional and cognitive losses due to illness or injury.

Psychological defenses and adaptations used by the patient prior to TBI are also important. However, in some instances, coping mechanisms used before the injury may no longer be available because of the degree of neurocognitive impairment; this can cause considerable distress for the patient. Many behavioral traits are exacerbated by TBI rather than developing *de novo* after injury (Prigatano 1991). Such alterations would be diagnosed as personality change due to TBI in DSM-IV-TR.

Finally, as with many other chronic illnesses, TBI has a significant effect on family and social functioning. Patients with TBI may be unable to return to their former roles as breadwinner, parent, or spouse, placing significant demands on other members of the family system (Kay and Cavallo 1994). In general, neurobehavioral disturbances are the most important source of stress for the family, but this effect can be mediated by good social support (Ergh et al. 2002; Groom et al. 1998). Family members are at significantly increased risk for psychiatric disorders, particularly anxiety, depression, and increased substance use (Hall et al. 1994; Kreutzer et al. 1994; Livingston et al. 1985). Caregivers may experience problems such as unemployment or financial loss, placing additional stresses on the patient and family (Hall et al. 1994). Sexual dysfunction after TBI stresses intimate relationships (Hibbard et al. 2000a), and partners may be uncomfortable with the dual role of caregiver (parentlike) and sexual partner (spouse) (Gosling and Oddy 1999). Rates of separation and divorce are also elevated for individuals with TBI (Webster et al. 1999).

Spinal Cord Injury

Epidemiology

SCI is an uncommon but often catastrophic injury with an annual incidence of 30–40 per million and a point prevalence of 183,000–230,000 in the United States (Go et al. 1995). Those who sustain spinal cord injuries are predominantly males (80%), young (half are ages 16–30), and Caucasian (89%). At the time that they are injured, those sustaining SCI are less likely to be married, twice as likely to be divorced, and slightly less educated than the general population. The most common causes of SCI are motor vehicle crashes (44.5%), falls (18.1%), sports activities (12.7%), and violence (16.6%).

Early survival and overall life expectancy rates for persons with SCI have improved dramatically over the last 30 years. However, life expectancy with SCI remains below that of the general population, especially among those that are ventilator dependent (DeVivo et al. 1999). Death from suicide is approximately five times more common in people with SCI than in the general population (59.2 per 100,000) and represents about 9% of deaths (DeVivo et al. 1999).

Severity and Classification

Tetraplegia (or quadriplegia) denotes SCI that affects all four limbs, whereas *paraplegia* denotes injuries affecting only the lower extremities. The level of injury re-

---

TABLE 18-3.　American Spinal Injury Association (ASIA) Impairment Scale

A　Complete—No sensory or motor function is preserved in the sacral segments S4/5.

B　Sensory Incomplete—Sensory but no motor function is preserved below the neurological level and includes the sacral segments S4/5.

C　Motor Incomplete—Motor function is preserved below the neurological level, and more than half of the key muscles below the neurological level have muscle grade less than 3 (active movement against gravity). There must be some sparing of sensory and/or motor function in the sacral segments S4/5.

D　Motor Incomplete—Motor function is preserved below the neurological level, and at least half of the key muscles below the neurological level have a muscle grade greater than or equal to 3. There must be some sparing of sensory and/or motor function in the sacral segments S4/5.

E　Normal—Sensory and motor functions are normal. Patient may have abnormalities of reflex examination.

Source. Reprinted from American Spinal Injury Association: *International Standards for Neurological and Functional Classification of Spinal Cord Injury.* Chicago, IL, American Spinal Injury Association, 1996. Used with permission.

---

fers to the most caudal segment with normal motor or sensory function. More than half of all injuries (54%) result in tetraplegia. Injury severity is described according to the American Spinal Injury Association (ASIA) Impairment Scale (Table 18–3). Approximately half of all injuries are considered ASIA-A, or "complete." Those admitted with an SCI classified as ASIA-A, B, or C have about a 2%, 35%, or 71% chance, respectively, of regaining functional motor ability below the level of their injury (Marino et al. 1999).

Secondary Complications

Pain is a common problem; 25% complain of severe pain, and 44% report that pain interferes with daily activities (Staas et al. 1998). Several different types of pain are noted, including radicular pain, central or diffuse pain, visceral pain, musculoskeletal pain, and "psychogenic" pain (Staas et al. 1998). Of the patients with recent SCI, 10%–60% may have cognitive impairment (Davidoff et al. 1992). Cognitive deficits may be attributable to a variety of factors, including preinjury learning disabilities and substance abuse as well as traumatic or hypoxic brain injury sustained at the time

of SCI. Behavior problems such as noncompliance, anger, and agitation may be attributable to premorbid traits or undetected brain injury. A severe complication for people with midthoracic or higher spinal cord injuries is autonomic dysreflexia. Autonomic dysreflexia is often triggered by a noxious stimulus below the level of lesion that leads to sympathetic discharge uninhibited by descending neural control. Immediate steps must be taken to control hypertension and to identify and reverse the triggering stimulus. The most common secondary medical complication during the first year postinjury is pressure ulcers (McKinley et al. 1999).

Adjustment to Spinal Cord Injury

Following discharge from acute rehabilitation, 91% of the people with SCI are discharged to a home environment (Eastwood et al. 1999). Estimates of employment rates after SCI have varied from 13% to 69%. Recent data show that, overall, 27% were employed, with 14% employed within 1 year and 35% employed within 10 years postinjury (Krause et al. 1999). More than 90% of the people living in the community with high tetraplegia, including those with ventilator dependence, report that they are "glad to be alive" (Gerhart et al. 1994). Nevertheless, people with SCI tend to report lower subjective quality of life compared with non-disabled persons (Gerhart et al. 1994). Quality of life is generally unrelated to level of injury or injury severity, weakly related to physical impairment, and more strongly related to one's ability to carry out day-to-day tasks and participate in school, work, or other community activities (Dijkers 1997). Quality of life is higher among those with a longer time since injury, those who are working, and those with few or no medical problems, especially pain (Westgren and Levi 1998).

Common biased expectations among rehabilitation staff and their misapplication of stage models have interfered with appropriate understanding and intervention to promote psychological adjustment to SCI (Elliott and Frank 1996; Trieschmann 1988). In numerous studies, rehabilitation staff have been found to regularly overestimate depressed mood in SCI patients (Trieschmann 1988). Rehabilitation staff also tend to view signs of depression as a normal, even necessary, stage of grief. Empirical data contradict popular conceptualizations of grief. Most people who sustain significant losses (including SCI) do not become depressed and do not go through traditional "stages of grief" (Bonanno et al. 2002; Wortman and Silver 1989). Viewing persisting depression as a normal or even healing part of the grief process may interfere with appropriate recognition and treatment of major depression. Conversely, staff may judge the absence of depression to be pathological, a sign of denial or poor adjustment and an indication that the staff should confront the patient more forcefully with the implications of his or her impairments.

In the absence of empirically supported approaches to manage grief and poor adjustment, the consultant is advised to avoid approaches that may only damage relatively healthy defenses or increase patient resistance. We recommend tolerance of adjustment patterns that are not interfering with rehabilitation. We also attempt to educate staff and family members about countertherapeutic myths of coping with loss, such as the belief that it is necessary to "work through" the loss, that patients should reach a state of "acceptance," and that the absence of grief is pathological (Wortman and Silver 1989).

Psychiatric Disorders in Spinal Cord Injury

Depression

Major depressive disorder is probably the most common psychiatric disorder after SCI (Fullerton et al. 1981). The prevalence of major depression after SCI ranges from 23% to more than 30% in 12 separate studies (see Elliott and Frank 1996 for review). Depression may be more common soon after injury but may remit after several months (Kishi et al. 1994, 1995). In unselected cases, mood tends to improve over the first year after injury (Richards 1986). However, other studies suggest that a subgroup of about 30% of patients develop significant depressive and anxiety symptoms soon after injury and remain highly depressed and anxious through at least 2 years after injury (Craig et al. 1994). Both somatic and psychological symptoms should be considered in diagnosing depression (Bombardier et al. 2004).

Depression is a significant and disabling problem for persons with SCI. Depression is associated with longer lengths of hospital stay and fewer functional improvements (Malec and Neimeyer 1983) as well as less functional independence and mobility at discharge (Umlauf and Frank 1983). Depression is associated with the occurrence of pressure sores and urinary tract infections (Herrick et al. 1994), poorer self-appraised health (Bombardier et al. 2004; Schulz and Decker 1985), less leisure activity (Elliott and Shewchuck 1995), poorer community mobility and social integration, and fewer meaningful social pursuits (Furher et al. 1993; MacDonald et al. 1987). Persons with SCI and significant depression spend more days in bed and fewer days outside the home, require greater use of paid personal care, and incur greater medical expenses (Tate et al. 1994). Moreover, symptoms consistent with depression, such as documented expressions of despondency, hopelessness, shame, and apathy, are the variables most predictive of suicide 1–9 years after SCI (Charlifue and Gerhart 1991).

Anxiety

Relatively few studies have examined PTSD or other anxiety disorders in this population. Rates of current PTSD range from 14% to 22% of the patients with SCI (Kennedy and Evans 2001; Radnitz et al. 1998). Rates of PTSD appear to vary as a function of level of injury, with lower rates found among those with tetraplegia (2%) compared with those with paraplegia (22%; Radnitz et al. 1998). This variability has been attributed to diminished experience of psychophysiological arousal, which may occur in higher-level injuries (Kennedy and Duff 2001). Current PTSD appears to be no more prevalent in persons with SCI than in other trauma survivors. Elevated levels of general anxiety also have been found in people with SCI (Craig et al. 1994; Kennedy and Rogers 2000), particularly in a subgroup of patients with chronic comorbid depression.

Substance Use Disorders

High rates of alcohol and drug abuse problems are found among trauma patients generally and SCI patients specifically (Bombardier 2000). Preinjury alcohol problems are common (35%–49%) (Bombardier and Rimmele 1998; Heine-

mann et al. 1988). Rates of alcohol intoxication at the time of injury range from 36% to 40% (Heinemann et al. 1988; Kiwerski and Krauski 1992). After SCI, substance abuse appears to decline but remains somewhat higher than in the general population and, importantly, may be more harmful because of its association with poorer health maintenance behaviors (Krause 1992).

Sexual Dysfunction

SCI affects erectile functioning, ejaculation, and emission in males, and lubrication in females, as a function of level (upper motor neuron vs. lower motor neuron) and completeness of injury (Table 18–4). Clinicians must test the integrity of the sacral reflex arc to determine whether injury at the level of sacral roots is upper motor neuron or lower motor neuron.

Recent laboratory research confirms that women with complete upper motor lesions affecting the sacral segments are likely to have vaginal lubrication from reflexive but not psychogenic mechanisms. Incomplete upper motor lesions affecting the sacral segments retain the capacity for reflex lubrication but will have psychogenic lubrication only if they have intact pinprick sensation in the T11–L2 dermatomes. Women with incomplete lower motor lesions affecting the sacral segments are expected to achieve psychogenic lubrication in 25% of cases and no reflex lubrication.

By contrast, achieving orgasm is less well studied but appears to be relatively independent of level and completeness of injury. Among males with SCI, 38%–47% report achieving orgasm, which may be experienced as similar to or different from preinjury experiences. In a laboratory study, about 50% of the women with SCI reported experiencing orgasm, with longer stimulation, greater sexual knowledge, and higher sexual drive associated with higher rates of orgasm (Sipski et al. 1995).

TABLE 18–4.   Male sexual functioning by level and type of lesion

Male sexual functioning	Psychogenic erection (%)	Reflex erection (%)	Anterograde ejaculation (%)
Upper motor neuron—complete	0	70–93	4
Upper motor neuron—incomplete	19	80	32
Lower motor neuron—complete	26–50	0	18
Lower motor neuron—incomplete		67–95	70

Source.   Adapted from Sipski and Alexander 1997.

Numerous treatments are available for sexual dysfunction related to SCI. Erectile dysfunction can be managed with sildenafil and other selective phosphodiesterase inhibitors, vacuum erection devices, pharmacological penile injections, and penile implants. Ejaculatory dysfunction and related infertility are treated with vibratory or electroejaculation procedures in conjunction with intrauterine insemination, in vitro fertilization, or intracytoplasmic sperm injection, depending on sperm quality and motility. A free online manual of resources for male infertility related to SCI is available at www.scifertility.com (Amador et al. 2000). Decreased lubrication in females can be managed by water-based lubricants. Regarding sexual enjoyment, patients can benefit from many standard counseling strategies adapted for people with SCI.

Personality and Psychological Testing

Personality assessment among persons with SCI has received justifiable criticism. Critics allege that clinicians are guilty of a negative bias, of overreliance on measures designed only to detect pathology, and of attributing behavior patterns only to intrapsychic and not to situational or environmental factors (Elliott and Umlauf 1995). Measures such as the Minnesota Multiphasic Personality Inventory and the Hopkins Symptom Checklist–90 should be interpreted cautiously and with the aid of norms correcting for disability-related factors

(Barncord and Wanlass 2000). Nonpathological measures such as the NEO Personality Inventory, the 16 Personality Factor Questionnaire, and the Myers-Briggs Type Indicator may be more appropriate tests of personality functioning in this population (Elliott and Shewchuck 1995). Yet evidence indicates that certain premorbid personality characteristics are more prominent among individuals with SCI than in the uninjured population. Nearly two-thirds of the patients with SCI have personality characteristics suggesting a strong physical orientation, difficulty expressing emotion, a preference for working with things rather than people, and a dislike of intellectual or academic interests (Rohe and Krause 1998). Neuropsychological evaluation that documents areas of cognitive impairment and strength can be critical in guiding treatment and vocational rehabilitation, especially when comorbid TBI is suspected.

Treatment of Psychiatric Disorders in Traumatic Brain Injury and Spinal Cord Injury

General Principles

A patient's specific physical (e.g., spasticity) and cognitive impairments (e.g., defects in executive functions) must be considered in designing a treatment plan for psychiatric disorders in the rehabilitation setting. A detailed understanding of the patient's physical and psychological stage in rehabilitation and functional goals will help in choosing the most appropriate psycho-pharmacological or psychotherapeutic treatment modality. Consulting with other members of the multidisciplinary rehabilitation team will provide clues as to the patient's motivation and treatment limitations. Knowledge of the patient's current functional, social, and vocational status is required to tailor the psychiatric treatment to specific practical needs and limitations.

Once rapport has been established, it is helpful to discuss the events that led up to the patient's impairment in order to explore the psychodynamic significance of these events. For example, patients will often blame themselves for their predicament, with such self-attribution leading to guilt and depression. In contrast, the patient may not associate his or her psychiatric symptoms with his or her physical impairment, which may affect readiness for psychotherapy.

Interviewing the patient's family, friends, and caregivers can provide critical information about the patient's past and present mental state. How patients handled prior losses and health problems can provide clues as to how resilient they will be during rehabilitation. Moreover, patients may report different symptoms from those observed by those close to them. For example, a patient often focuses on physical and cognitive deficits, whereas family members may consider the patient's emotional changes as more disabling (Hendryx 1989; Oddy et al. 1978; Sherer et al. 1998b). Patients often report significantly less frequent symptoms of depression, aggression, and memory and attention problems on self-rating compared with ratings by their significant others (Hart et al. 2003). Close communication with family and other caregivers and acquaintances can provide critical longitudinal information about the progress of psychiatric treatment.

Because SCI may result in marked weight loss, alterations in appetite and sleep, and reduced energy and activity, diagnosing depression can be complicated. However, vegetative symptoms should not be dismissed because altered psychomotor activity, appetite change, and sleep disturbance are predictive of major depression (Clay et al. 1995). The patient's own experience and interpretation of the vegetative symptoms can aid the diagnostic process (Elliott and Frank 1996).

Although psychopathology based on DSM-IV-TR criteria should be thoroughly explored, psychiatric symptoms that do not meet DSM diagnostic criteria but that still lead to significant functional impairment are common in the rehabilitation setting (e.g., the depressed TBI patient who has four depressive symptoms but shows apathy that affects his or her level of functioning, or the severely anxious SCI patient with few autonomic symptoms). These syndromes, or symptom clusters, still may warrant close monitoring and treatment to maximize functioning. Therefore, in addition to monitoring and documenting psychiatric signs and symptoms, functional status (e.g., activities of daily living, progress in physical and occupational therapy, role functioning) should be monitored closely as an indicator of overall progress. Consistent with the rehabilitation process's basic tenet of working toward realistic and measurable goals, psychiatric intervention should begin with defining treatment end points according to measurable outcomes. Examples of useful measures include the Patient Health Questionnaire (Spitzer et al. 1999) for depression and anxiety, the Neurobehavioral Rating Scale (Levin et al. 1987b) for behavior and cognition, and the Rivermead Postconcussion Symptoms Questionnaire (King et al. 1995) or the Overt Aggression Scale (Yudofsky et al. 1986) for severe agitation.

Collaboration with rehabilitation psychologists and counselors can provide significant depth of assessment and breadth of intervention. Attending rehabilitation team meetings is often a valuable and efficient way of communicating and coordinating needs and treatment. Because the patient probably is already feeling overwhelmed about his or her situation, framing the psychiatric consultation and intervention as another modality, similar to, for example, occupational or speech therapy, that can help him or her achieve the rehabilitation goals during a period of intense stress and adaptation can quickly put the patient at ease. Often, appropriately applied treatments may not have been given ample time to work. This problem may be exacerbated by recently imposed pressures on rehabilitation centers to work within predetermined payment structures and lengths of stay on the basis of medical diagnoses (Carter et al. 2000).

Treatment of psychiatric problems in the rehabilitation setting typically warrants a combination of pharmacological and psychosocial interventions. Because treatments for most chronic diseases are covered in other chapters, the following treatment recommendations focus on TBI and SCI.

Psychopharmacology

Several common physiological changes in SCI (Table 18–5), often more pronounced in tetraplegia than in paraplegia, can have an effect on the pharmacokinetics and tolerability of many psychotropic medications. The goals and potential side effects of pharmacotherapy should be explained thoroughly to the patient and caregivers because unanticipated symptoms caused by medications may be viewed as a sign that the underlying condition is worsening. For example, urinary retention from an anticholinergic psychotropic drug may signal to the patient with SCI that the spinal le-

TABLE 18–5. Common physiological changes associated with spinal cord injury

Increased body fat and glucose intolerance
Decreased gastrointestinal motility
Reduced cardiac output
Anemia
Orthostatic hypotension
Bradyarrhythmia
Decreased blood flow to skeletal muscle
Venous thrombosis
Osteoporosis

sion is progressing. Medications that can cause weight gain, constipation, dry mouth, orthostatic hypotension, or sexual dysfunction also may exacerbate already present pathophysiology. Medications that are sedating are of particular concern in TBI and SCI because they may impair mobility and cognition, increase risk for pressure sores, and interfere with rehabilitation. Sedation is a frequent problem because many patients with TBI and SCI are taking multiple central nervous system (CNS) depressants, such as anticonvulsants, muscle relaxants, and opioid analgesics (for discussion of interactions between neurological and psychiatric drugs, see Chapter 15, "Neurology and Neurosurgery").

Because patients with TBI or SCI are often more susceptible to sedative, extrapyramidal, anticholinergic, epileptogenic, and spasticity effects (Fann 2002), psychotropic dosages should be started at lower-than-standard levels and be titrated slowly. Despite this need for caution, some patients still may ultimately need full standard doses (Silver and Yudofsky 1994b).

Neuropsychiatric polypharmacy is common in TBI patients and should be critically examined. When multiple psychotropics are needed, they should be initiated one at a time, when possible, to accurately determine the therapeutic and adverse effects of each medication.

Because few randomized, placebo-controlled studies exist that tested pharmacotherapy for psychiatric conditions in TBI and SCI populations, many of the following recommendations are based on case series or are extrapolated from other neurological populations. Heterogeneous study populations, including those varying in time elapsed since injury, confound the interpretation of study results. When TBI or SCI occurs in the context of a preexisting psychiatric illness, it is logical to continue a previously effective medication regimen, but previously absent side effects may emerge that require changes in dosages and/or drugs. Electroconvulsive therapy for refractory depression (Crow et al. 1996), mania (Clark and Davison 1987), and prolonged posttraumatic delirium and agitation (Kant et al. 1995) may be considered. However, efforts should be made to lessen cognitive dysfunction in TBI patients (e.g., by using high-dose unilateral electrode placement or twice-weekly treatment frequency), and caution should be exercised in treating patients with SCI who may have unstable spinal columns.

Depression, Apathy, and Fatigue

Because of a favorable side-effect profile, a selective serotonin reuptake inhibitor (SSRI) usually is the first-line antidepressant for patients with TBI. A single-blind, placebo run-in study of 15 patients (Fann et al. 2000) and a case series of 9 patients (Cassidy 1989) suggested that SSRIs are efficacious and well tolerated in TBI populations. The study by Fann et al. found that 67% had remission of their major depression after 8 weeks of sertraline and that treatment also was associated with improvements in postconcussive symptoms, neuropsychological functioning, functional status, and self-ratings of injury severity and distress. The areas of cognitive functioning that improved included short-term memory, mental flexibility,

cognitive efficiency, and psychomotor speed. In a 4-week study of depressed patients, H. Lee et al. (2005) found both sertraline and methylphenidate to be superior to placebo in decreasing depression scores. Perino et al. (2001) assessed 20 depressed post-TBI patients before and after administration of citalopram and carbamazepine and found that depression, anxiety, inappropriate and labile affect, and somatic overconcern improved significantly. SSRIs should be started at about half their usual starting dose and titrated slowly. SSRI-induced akathisia sometimes can be mistaken for TBI-related agitation (Hensley and Reeve 2001). Escitalopram, citalopram, and sertraline all have low potential for significant drug–drug interactions. For patients at high risk for noncompliance (e.g., because of cognitive impairment), fluoxetine should be considered because of its lower risk for withdrawal symptoms.

No clinical trials of antidepressants in persons with SCI are available to help guide pharmacotherapy. Combining an antidepressant and psychotherapy may be effective for major depression (Kemp et al. 2004). Although SSRIs are likely efficacious in patients with SCI, the risk for spasticity is increased (Stolp-Smith and Wainberg 1999).

The data on the efficacy and tolerability of tricyclic antidepressants (TCAs) and monoamine oxidase inhibitors (MAOIs) after TBI are more inconsistent (Dinan and Mobayed 1992; Saran 1985; Wroblewski et al. 1996). Because of the potentially problematic adverse effects of TCAs and MAOIs (e.g., sedation, hypotension, and anticholinergic effects) in patients with CNS impairment and their narrow therapeutic index (which can lead to inadvertent overdose in patients with cognitive impairment), these medications should be used with extreme caution in TBI patients. Autonomic dysfunction in patients with SCI makes them more vulnerable to TCA-related anticho-linergic and orthostatic side effects. If a TCA is chosen, nortriptyline or desipra-mine may cause the fewest side effects.

Although not yet systematically stud-ied, venlafaxine is likely safe and effective in patients with TBI. Mirtazapine, nefazo-done, and trazodone may prove to be too sedating for some patients, particularly if they have cognitive impairment or gait in-stability, but if insomnia is a major prob-lem, these drugs may be helpful. Venlafax-ine and mirtazapine have low drug–drug interaction potential. Moclobemide, a re-versible inhibitor of monoamine oxidase A, showed efficacy in an open subgroup analysis of 26 depressed patients with TBI (Newburn et al. 1999).

Some data suggest that antidepressants, especially TCAs and bupropion, are associ-ated with an increased risk of seizures (Davidson 1989), a particular concern fol-lowing severe TBI (Wroblewski et al. 1990); however, if the drugs are titrated cau-tiously, most patients will not experience in-creased seizures, particularly if they are tak-ing an anticonvulsant (Ojemann et al. 1987).

The symptoms of apathy and fatigue, often associated with CNS impairment, can occur concomitantly with or inde-pendently of depression and are often mistaken for primary depression (Marin 1991). For apathy and fatigue, medica-tions that augment dopaminergic activity appear to be the most useful (Marin et al. 1995). Methylphenidate and dextroam-phetamine are generally safe at standard dosages (Alban et al. 2004) (e.g., meth-ylphenidate 10–30 mg/day in divided doses) and have been used successfully to enhance participation in rehabilitation (Gualtieri and Evans 1988). Methylpheni-date and dextroamphetamine also have been shown in case series and double-blind studies to be effective in improving some aspects of mood, mental speed, attention, and behavior, although im-

provement was not always sustained long term (Bleiberg et al. 1993; R.W. Evans et al. 1987; Gualtieri and Evans 1988; Kaelin et al. 1996; Mooney and Haas 1993; Plenger et al. 1996; Speech et al. 1993; Whyte et al. 1997). Dextroamphetamine may exacerbate dystonia and dyskinesia in some cases. Therapeutic use of these oral psychostimulants in the medically ill rarely leads to abuse in patients without a personal or family history of substance abuse (Masand and Tesar 1996), but substance abuse is overrepresented in the TBI and SCI populations.

Modafinil has been efficacious in treat-ing fatigue in patients with multiple scle-rosis (Rammahan et al. 2000; Terzoudi et al. 2000; Zifko et al. 2002) and excessive daytime sleepiness in patients with TBI (Teitelman 2001). It has also been used in two cases of SCI to improve self-esteem (Mukai and Costa 2005). Bupropion (Marin et al. 1995) and dopamine agonists, such as amantadine (Cowell and Cohen 1995; Gualtieri et al. 1989; M.F. Kraus and Maki 1997; Nickels et al. 1994), bro-mocriptine (Catsman-Berrevoets and Harskamp 1988; Eames 1989; Gupta and Mlcoch 1992), and levodopa/carbidopa (Lal et al. 1988), have been used for apathy states, fatigue, and cognitive impairment. Bupropion's stimulating properties may be of particular benefit in the fatigued or ap-athetic depressed patient. Stimulants and dopamine agonists can increase the risk for delirium and psychosis and thus should be used with caution in more vulnerable patients. Amantadine has been associated with an increased risk of seizures (Gual-tieri et al. 1989), but methylphenidate, dextroamphetamine, and bromocriptine do not appear to lower seizure threshold at typical doses. The TCA protriptyline also has been used to improve arousal and be-havior (Wroblewski et al. 1993).

There is great interest in pharmaco-logical agents that could improve not only arousal and attention following TBI but also memory; however, data are lacking. Preliminary evidence indicates that the acetylcholinesterase inhibitor donepezil may improve memory and global functioning (Taverni et al. 1998; Whelan et al. 2000; Whitlock 1999).

Another secondary benefit of some antidepressants in TBI and SCI patients is their analgesic properties (Onghena and Van Houdenhove 1992) (see also Chapter 19, "Pain"). TCAs have been shown to be effective for the treatment of chronic nonmalignant pain, including neuropathic pain (McQuay et al. 1996). SSRIs have not been shown to be effective in neuropathic pain (Jung et al. 1997). Venlafaxine and duloxetine may be effective in treating a variety of pain syndromes, including neuropathic pain (Diamond 1995; Lang et al. 1996; Schreiber et al. 1999).

Mania

For mania following TBI, the mood stabilizers lithium carbonate (Oyewumi and Lapierre 1981; Stewart and Nemsath 1988), valproic acid (Pope et al. 1988), and carbamazepine (Stewart and Nemsath 1988) all have been used successfully. Clonidine (Bakchine et al. 1989) and electroconvulsive therapy (Clark and Davison 1987) also can be used as second-line modalities. Dikmen et al. (2000) have shown that valproic acid is well tolerated following TBI, but lithium and carbamazepine have been associated with neurocognitive adverse effects (Hornstein and Seliger 1989; Schiff et al. 1982). Lithium has a narrow therapeutic window and also can lower the seizure threshold; thus, caution is required when lithium is used in TBI patients whose cognitive impairment may lead to poor adherence or inadvertent overdosage. Although serum blood levels of valproic acid and carbamazepine help in monitoring adherence and absorption, dosing should be guided primarily by thera-

peutic response and side effects. Carbamazepine, gabapentin, and clonazepam also can be effective for the treatment of neuropathic pain.

Anxiety

Benzodiazepines are the treatment of choice for acute anxiety in TBI, but they should be used initially at lower doses because of their propensity to exacerbate or cause cognitive impairment and oversedation. The high prevalence of substance abuse in patients with TBI and SCI adds to the risk of benzodiazepine use and may preclude their use in some patients. Although few studies exist in TBI patients, antidepressants also appear to be effective for anxiety, particularly in the context of depression. SSRIs also have been found to be effective in decreasing mood lability after brain injury (Nahas et al. 1998; Sloan et al. 1992), although this effect may take as long as their antidepressant effects. Valproic acid and gabapentin may be of benefit, especially in patients with concomitant mood lability or seizures (Pande et al. 1999, 2000). Buspirone is another option for generalized anxiety symptoms; however, it has been associated, albeit rarely, with seizures and movement disorders (Levitt et al. 1993).

Sleep Disorders

Sleep apnea is fairly common in TBI (Castriotta and Lai 2001; Masel et al. 2001) and SCI (Burns et al. 2000), and nocturnal periodic leg movements are frequent in SCI (Dickel et al. 1994). Fichtenberg et al. (2000) found that insomnia often appeared to be associated with depression in post–acute TBI patients. No specific data exist on treating insomnia or other sleep disorders in TBI or SCI, but trazodone is widely used in these patients for middle or late insomnia. Trazodone-associated orthostatic hypotension may be particularly problematic in the rehabilitation setting, however. Antihistamines such as diphenhydramine should be avoided because of their anticholinergic properties.

Anger, Aggression, and Agitation

Anger, aggression, and agitation are common following TBI and can occur in isolation or as part of delirium or other psychiatric disorders. The published literature regarding their treatment is often not diagnostically specific and consists of largely case reports, case series, and reviews (e.g., Burnett et al. 1999; Krieger et al. 2003; Maryniak et al. 2001; McAllister and Ferrell 2002; Stanislav and Childs 2000).

Treatment can be divided into acute treatment, in which the goal is timely management of behavior to prevent injury to self or others, and chronic treatment, in which the goal is long-term management and prevention (Silver et al. 2002). Many agents take from 2 to 8 weeks to gain full effectiveness. It is important to keep in mind that medications that worsen cognition or sedation can actually worsen confusion and may, therefore, worsen agitation during the confusional state of posttraumatic amnesia after TBI. Because the effects of medications on the patient with TBI can be unpredictable, and their side effects actually may potentiate the behavior problem (e.g., akathisia from antipsychotics), systematically eliminating certain medications, including those that were initially prescribed to treat the behavioral dyscontrol, can prove beneficial. A rationale for such an approach is the clinical observation that some patients have a natural course of recovery and that some medication efficacy may decrease over time.

The atypical antipsychotics afford the clinician many more options in the acute setting than were available a decade ago (Battaglia et al. 2003; Currier and Simpson 2001; Lesem et al. 2001). The efficacy of the atypical antipsychotics in treating aggression and agitation in TBI patients is undocumented; however, evidence is mounting to support their efficacy in treating other agitated states associated with neurological syndromes (M.A. Lee et al. 2001; Meehan et al. 2002). The typical antipsychotics given orally or intramuscularly also may be useful in the acute setting (Stanislav and Childs 2000), but the elevated risks of extrapyramidal and anticholinergic effects in TBI patients must be considered.

Antipsychotic use for chronic agitation should be reserved for situations when aggression occurs in the context of psychotic symptoms. Risperidone (Cohen et al. 1998; De Deyn et al. 1999; I.R. Katz et al. 1999; McDougle et al. 1998) and olanzapine (Street et al. 2000) show promise in neuropsychiatric patients, although efficacy data are lacking in TBI patients for these and the other atypical antipsychotics. Clozapine use in TBI patients is limited by its seizure risk, although it has been found to be effective for chronic aggression (Duffy and Kant 1996; Michals et al. 1993).

The benzodiazepines offer rapid sedation that may be useful in the acute setting; however, they also have a high potential for neurocognitive effects, such as mental slowing, amnesia, disinhibition, and impaired balance, in patients with TBI. As a result, low doses of a short-acting agent, such as lorazepam 1–2 mg orally or parenterally, should be used initially and titrated as needed. If agitation is frequent, a longer-acting agent, such as clonazepam 0.5–1.0 mg two or three times a day, may be used for short durations. The combination of haloperidol and low-dose lorazepam (e.g., 0.5–1.0 mg) may offer a synergistic calming effect for some acutely agitated patients.

Serotonergic antidepressants, such as the SSRIs, trazodone, and amitriptyline, have been used to treat agitation and aggression in TBI populations (Mysiw et al. 1988; Rowland et al. 1992). In 8-week non-randomized trials with sertraline, Fann et al. (2000) showed that improved depression was associated with improved anger and aggression scores in patients with mild TBI, whereas Kant et al. (1998) found improved aggression independent of depression scores. SSRIs are also effective in treating emotional incontinence, such as pathological crying or laughter (Muller et al. 1999; Nahas et al. 1998; Sloan et al. 1992).

Buspirone also has shown some efficacy for agitation in patients with TBI and other neurological patients (Gualtieri 1991; Silver and Yudofsky 1994a; Stanislav et al. 1994) and can be particularly useful when anxiety also is present. Although one 6-week placebo-controlled trial found that methylphenidate significantly reduced anger an average of 27 months after severe TBI (Mooney and Haas 1993), stimulants should be used with caution in the agitated TBI patient because of the risks of exacerbating agitation and psychosis and of abuse.

Among the anticonvulsants, carbamazepine (Azouvi et al. 1999; Chatham-Showalter 1996) and valproic acid (Chatham-Showalter and Kimmel 2000; Lindenmayer and Kotsaftis 2000; Wroblewski et al. 1997) have been studied the most for treatment of behavioral dyscontrol in TBI populations. Although evidence of seizures or epileptiform activity on electroencephalogram is a strong indication for anticonvulsant use in the agitated patient, these agents also have shown efficacy in those without electroencephalographic abnormalities. Oxcarbazepine, gabapentin, lamotrigine, and topiramate also may be efficacious, although data are more limited. Some TBI patients may experience paradoxical agitation with gabapentin (Childers and Holland 1997). Lamotrigine should be monitored for possible exacerbation of aggression, as is seen in some reports in mentally retarded patients with epilepsy (Beran and Gibson 1998; Et-

tinger et al. 1998). Evidence indicates that cognitive functioning may worsen with topiramate in some cases (Martin et al. 1999; Shorvon 1996; Tatum et al. 2001). Topiramate has also been found to attenuate binge eating behavior in some patients (Dolberg et al. 2004). Some patients may need to achieve serum levels of anticonvulsants that exceed therapeutic levels used for seizure prophylaxis to ensure adequate behavioral control. Lithium is also an effective mood stabilizer and has antiaggressive properties in TBI patients, according to case reports; however, its narrow therapeutic window and high potential for neurotoxicity limit its routine use, particularly in those with significant cognitive impairment or history of seizures.

When anger, aggression, or agitation occurs without signs of other psychiatric syndromes, beta-blockers such as propranolol, pindolol, and nadolol should be considered. Placebo-controlled studies have shown their efficacy in treating agitation in TBI patients (Brooke et al. 1992a; Greendyke and Kanter 1996; Greendyke et al. 1996). A Cochrane review (Fleminger et al. 2003) concluded that among the drugs used to treat agitation and aggression in TBI, beta-blockers have the best evidence for efficacy. Although dosages of propranolol in the range of 160–320 mg/day have been effective, Yudofsky et al. (1987) proposed titrating the dosage as high as 12 mg/kg or 800 mg/day. Bradycardia and hypotension are potential side effects; contraindications include asthma, chronic obstructive pulmonary disease, type 1 diabetes mellitus, congestive heart failure, persistent angina, significant peripheral vascular disease, and hyperthyroidism (Yudofsky et al. 1987). Pindolol is less likely to cause bradycardia.

Psychosis

Because of the increased susceptibility of patients with TBI to experience anticholinergic and extrapyramidal side effects and patients with SCI to experience problematic anticholinergic sequelae, the newer-generation atypical antipsychotics are the drugs of first choice for psychotic symptoms that emerge after TBI or SCI (Burnett et al. 1999). Clozapine carries a risk of seizures and should be used with extreme caution in TBI patients, particularly when compliance is in question.

Cognitive Impairment

Little evidence is available to guide pharmacological treatments to enhance cognitive recovery following TBI; most data are derived from theoretical or animal models or case reports. Medications targeting the dopaminergic, cholinergic, and noradrenergic neurotransmitter systems have been tried (McElligott et al. 2003). Dopaminergic agents include levodopa/carbidopa, bromocriptine, amantadine, pergolide, the newer dopamine agonists (ropinirole, pramipexole), catecholamine-O-methyltransferase (COMT) inhibitors (entacapone, tolcapone), and the monoamine oxidase–B (MAO-B) inhibitor selegiline (Meythaler et al. 2002; Zafonte et al. 2001). The SSRI sertraline, which has some dopaminergic activity, may have a cognition-enhancing effect in addition to its antidepressant effect (Fann et al. 2001), although larger, controlled studies are needed to confirm this finding and to determine whether this effect is independent of its influence on depression. Medications that enhance cholinergic activity include cholinergic precursors such as lecithin and acetylcholinesterase inhibitors such as physostigmine (Cardenas et al. 1994) and donepezil (Khateb et al. 2005; Taverni et al. 1998; Whelan et al. 2000; Whitlock 1999). The noradrenergic agents most commonly used to enhance cognition, perhaps by improving arousal and awareness, are the psychostimulants methylphenidate (Lee et al. 2005) and

dextroamphetamine, which also have dopaminergic effects. Modafinil, a treatment for narcolepsy whose mechanism of action is unclear, also may show some benefit. The opioid antagonist naltrexone helped improve TBI-associated memory impairment in a case series (Tennant and Wild 1987).

Psychological Treatment

Traumatic Brain Injury

A widely accepted model of psychological effects of TBI distinguishes among symptoms that are reactions to the effects of TBI (e.g., depression, anxiety, irritability, anger, hopelessness, helplessness, social withdrawal, distrust, and phobias), symptoms that are neurologically based (e.g., affective lability, impulsivity, agitation, paranoia, unawareness), and symptoms that reflect long-standing personality traits (e.g., obsessiveness, antisocial behavior, work attitude, social connectedness, dependence, entitlement) (Prigatano 1986). Although the genesis of symptoms can be multifactorial, it is useful to consider the potential contributions of all three factors to observed problem behaviors.

Empirically supported psychotherapies have been adapted for use in brain-injured individuals (e.g., modified cognitive-behavioral therapy [CBT] for anxiety [Hibbard et al. 2000b] and depression [Hibbard et al. 1992]). Psychological interventions are more likely to require involvement of family members or caregivers to help cue follow-through and generalization to real-world situations. Psychotherapy has been used with selected patients to foster insight in comprehensive post–acute neurorehabilitation programs (Prigatano and Ben-Yishay 1999). Insight-focused psychotherapy often begins with providing the patient with a simple model to explain what has happened.

When insight and self-management approaches are not feasible, applied behavioral analysis can be used to manage a wide variety of brain injury–related behavioral deficits or excesses, such as emotional lability, anger management, and impulsivity (Horton and Howe 1981). In some cases, such as anger management, self-control and environmental control strategies can be combined to achieve better outcomes (Uomoto and Brockway 1992).

Therapy for impaired awareness is in its infancy but has included several different strategies. Mildly impaired patients may benefit from information about the effects of brain injury coupled with test data and observations about the specific ways they have been affected, including limited awareness. With more severe or persistent problems, treatment may include more comprehensive, coordinated, and real-time feedback about impairments, such as via videotaping. With intractable unawareness, it may be essential to enlist relatives and friends to create a protective environment by ensuring 24-hour supervision, removing access to cars or other dangerous equipment, contacting employers, and providing a written letter signed by the physician that lists all the behavioral restrictions to support caregivers when the restrictions are challenged.

Cognitive rehabilitation. The science of cognitive rehabilitation has grown tremendously in the past 15 years to the point that evidence-based guidelines have been derived from significant efficacy and effectiveness trials (Cicerone et al. 2000, 2005). Empirically validated approaches are available for remediation of visuoperceptual deficits, language deficits, and impaired pragmatic communication and for memory compensation in patients with mild memory impairment. Some evidence suggests that attention training, including computer-based training modules, is ef-

fective (Park and Ingles 2001). Effective strategies are available to train patients to improve visual scanning, reading comprehension, language formation, and problem solving. Optional rehabilitation strategies that may be effective include the use of memory books for persons with moderate to severe impairment, verbal self-instructional training, and self-questioning and self-monitoring to address deficits in executive functioning. Isolated use of computer-based training procedures is not recommended for any form of impairment (Cicerone et al. 2000).

Spinal Cord Injury

Three types of problems may require psychological interventions in the context of SCI: 1) primary psychiatric disorders, 2) problems with adjustment to disability, and 3) problems with adherence to medical and rehabilitation therapies.

For depression and anxiety disorders, brief CBT is often indicated in conjunction with initiating pharmacotherapy. Rehabilitation activities should afford the patient numerous opportunities to practice CBT skills, such as identification of irrational thoughts and positive reframing within a supportive context. The consultant also can work within the rehabilitation team to accomplish additional therapy goals by proxy. For example, the recreation therapist can carry out graded exposure to being in a motor vehicle for a patient with acute PTSD–related anxiety and avoidance of cars.

Craig and colleagues (1997) used a group-based skills-oriented approach to teaching relaxation, cognitive restructuring, social skills, assertiveness, pleasant activity scheduling, and ways to begin sexual adjustment. Group-based interventions provide unique opportunities to capitalize on the positive coping abilities modeled by participants with better adjustment. Therefore, group-based coping skills training is recommended for people with significant anxiety or depressive symptoms after SCI as an adjunct to or in lieu of individual psychotherapy.

Poor adjustment to disability and management of grief are also common reasons for referrals. Clinicians should resist the temptation to confront patients with their prognosis when they, for example, insist that they are going to walk again. It should be recognized that statements labeled as *denial* may simply reflect the common, understandable hope or wish for neurological recovery rather than psychopathology. Overly direct confrontation may damage defenses needed by patients, increase resistance, and risk eliciting excessive distress. We recommend tolerance of verbal denial and other adjustment patterns that do not interfere with rehabilitation progress for more than a day or so. For these patients, staff education about the range of normal adjustment may be the main intervention. When verbal denial is accompanied by behavioral denial (e.g., refusing to learn adaptive strategies such as wheelchair use and self-catheterization) or persistently interferes with rehabilitation progress, more directive interventions may be needed. In such cases, the psychiatrist may recommend that patients review information about the nature and extent of their injury (including radiographic evidence), prognosis for recovery, and current SCI research with the attending physician, possibly with the consultant present.

Given the action-oriented behavioral style of many patients with SCI, we believe that much adjustment is behaviorally mediated. That is, rather than verbally processing losses associated with SCI, patients accommodate to their impairments largely through physical and occupational therapy wherein they repeatedly experience their abilities and limitations through activities. To the extent that therapists can set attainable incremental goals and maximize the patients' sense of mastery, positive adjustment can be facilitated. Therapies also can be organized to help patients resume participation in their most meaningful, rewarding, and pleasant life activities.

Nonadherence to treatment and the associated conflicts with staff often trigger psychiatric consultation. Causes of nonadherence are varied and include depression, amotivational states due to concomitant TBI, antisocial personality traits, ongoing substance abuse, and unrealistic staff expectations. Environmental factors may be particularly salient in cases of nonadherence. Once primary psychiatric disorders are ruled out, the consultant should examine how adherence to prescribed therapies may not be as rewarding for the patient as it should be, perhaps because of pain, withdrawal of social contact, or relinquishment of a sense of control. In some cases, nonadherence may inadvertently be rewarded by engaging staff in negative social interactions, asserting independence, or avoiding unwanted responsibilities. One example is patients with dependent traits not improving toward independence because staff attention and expressions of support are contingent on dependent behavior.

Conclusion

As society's attitudes toward disability continue to evolve and researchers work toward better understanding the potent effects of psychosocial factors in disability, psychiatrists will have an increasing role in the rehabilitation setting. To achieve comprehensive evaluation and treatment of persons with TBI and SCI, psychiatrists must appreciate and address the multiple complex facets of these conditions, from the acute neurological injury and attendant psychological trauma through the chronic neurological, medical, psychiatric, and social sequelae of the injury.

References

Alban JP, Hopson MM, Ly V, et al: Effect of methylphenidate on vital signs and adverse effects in adults with traumatic brain injury. Am J Phys Med Rehabil 83:131–137, 2004

Alexander MP: Mild traumatic brain injury: pathophysiology, natural history, and clinical management. Neurology 45:1253–1260, 1995

Alexander MP: Minor traumatic brain injury: a review of physiogenesis and psychogenesis. Semin Clin Neuropsychiatry 2:177–187, 1997

Alves WM, Colohan ART, O'Leary TJ, et al: Understanding posttraumatic symptoms after minor head injury. J Head Trauma Rehabil 1:1–12, 1986

Amador M, Lynne C, Brackett N: A Guide and Resource Directory to Male Fertility Following Spinal Cord Injury/Dysfunction: Miami Project to Cure Paralysis. Miami, FL, University of Miami, 2000

Amaducci LA, Fratiglioni L, Rocca WA, et al: Risk factors for clinically diagnosed Alzheimer's disease: a case-control study of an Italian population. Neurology 36:922–931, 1986

American Psychiatric Association: Diagnostic and Statistical Manual of Mental Disorders, 3rd Edition, Revised. Washington, DC, American Psychiatric Association, 1987

American Psychiatric Association: Diagnostic and Statistical Manual of Mental Disorders, 4th Edition, Text Revision. Washington, DC, American Psychiatric Association, 2000

Ashman TA, Spielman LA, Hibbard MR, et al: Psychiatric challenges in the first 6 years after traumatic brain injury: cross-sequential analyses of Axis I disorders. Arch Phys Med Rehabil 85 (4 suppl 2):S36–S42, 2004

Azouvi P, Jokic C, Attal N, et al: Carbamazepine in agitation and aggressive behaviour following severe closed-head injury: results of an open trial. Brain Inj 13:797–804, 1999

Bakchine S, Lacomblez L, Benoit N, et al: Manic-like state after bilateral orbitofrontal and right temporoparietal injury: efficacy of clonidine. Neurology 39:777–781, 1989

Barncord SW, Wanlass RL: A correction procedure for the Minnesota Multiphasic Personality Inventory–2 for persons with spinal cord injury. Arch Phys Med Rehabil 81: 1185–1190, 2000

Battaglia J, Lindborg SR, Alaka K, et al: Calming versus sedative effects of intramuscular olanzapine in agitated patients. Am J Emerg Med 21:192–198, 2003

Bazarian JJ, Wong T, Harris M, et al: Epidemiology and predictors of post-concussive syndrome after minor head injury in an emergency population. Brain Inj 13:173–189, 1999

Ben-Yishay Y, Rattok J, Piasetsky EB, et al: Neuropsychologic rehabilitation: quest for a holistic approach. Semin Neurol 5:252–259, 1985

Beran RG, Gibson RJ: Aggressive behavior in intellectually challenged patients with epilepsy treated with lamotrigine. Epilepsia 39:280–282, 1998

Bergsneider M, Hovda DA, McArthur DL, et al: Metabolic recovery following human traumatic brain injury based on FDG-PET: time course and relationship to neurological disability. J Head Trauma Rehabil 16:135–148, 2001

Binder LM, Rohling ML: Money matters: meta-analytic review of the effects of financial incentives on recovery after closed head injury. Am J Psychiatry 153:7–10, 1996

Binder LM, Rohling ML, Larrabee GJ: A review of mild head trauma, part I: meta-analytic review of neuropsychological studies. J Clin Exp Neuropsychol 19:421–431, 1997

Bleiberg J, Garmoe W, Cederquist J, et al: Effects of dexedrine on performance consistency following brain injury: a double-blind placebo crossover case study. Neuropsychiatry Neuropsychol Behav Neurol 6:245–248, 1993

Boake C, McCauley SR, Levin HS, et al: Diagnostic criteria for postconcussional syndrome after mild to moderate traumatic brain injury. J Neuropsychiatry Clin Neurosci 17:350–356, 2005

Bogner J, Corrigan JD: Epidemiology of agitation following brain injury. Neurorehabilitation 5:293–297, 1995

Bohnen N, Jolles J, Twijnstra A: Neuropsychological deficits in patients with persistent symptoms six months after mild head injury. Neurosurgery 30:692–696, 1992

Bombardier CH: Alcohol and traumatic disability, in The Handbook of Rehabilitation Psychology. Edited by Frank R, Elliott T. Washington, DC, American Psychological Association Press, 2000, pp 399–416

Bombardier CH, Rimmele C: Alcohol use and readiness to change after spinal cord injury. Arch Phys Med Rehabil 79: 1110–1115, 1998

Bombardier CH, Kilmer J, Ehde D: Screening for alcoholism among persons with recent traumatic brain injury. Rehabil Psychol 42:259–271, 1997

Bombardier CH, Rimmele C, Zintel H: The magnitude and correlates of alcohol and drug use before traumatic brain injury. Arch Phys Med Rehabil 83:1765–1773, 2002

Bombardier CH, Temkin N, Machamer J, et al: The natural history of drinking and alcohol-related problems after traumatic brain injury. Arch Phys Med Rehabil 84:185–191, 2003

Bombardier CH, Richards JS, Krause JS, et al: Symptoms of major depression in people with spinal cord injury: implications for screening. Arch Phys Med Rehabil 85:1749–1756, 2004

Bonanno GA, Wortman CB, Lehman DR, et al: Resilience to loss and chronic grief: a prospective study from preloss to 18-months postloss. J Pers Soc Psychol 83: 1150–1164, 2002

Brooke MM, Questad KA, Patterson PR, et al: Agitation and restlessness after closed head injury: a prospective study of 100 consecutive admissions. Arch Phys Med Rehabil 73:320–323, 1992a

Brooke MM, Patterson DR, Questad KA, et al: The treatment of agitation during initial hospitalization after traumatic brain injury. Arch Phys Med Rehabil 73:917–921, 1992b

Brown SJ, Fann JR, Grant I: Postconcussional disorder: time to acknowledge a common source of neurobehavioral morbidity. J Neuropsychiatry Clin Neurosci 6:15–22, 1994

Bryant RA, Harvey AG: Acute stress response: a comparison of head injured and non-head injured patients. Psychol Med 25:869–873, 1995

Bryant RA, Harvey AG: Relationship between acute stress disorder and posttraumatic stress disorder following mild traumatic brain injury. Am J Psychiatry 155:625–629, 1998

Bryant RA, Marosszeky JE, Crooks J, et al: Posttraumatic stress disorder following severe traumatic brain injury. Am J Psychiatry 157:629–631, 2000

Burnett DM, Kennedy RE, Cifu DX, et al: Using atypical neuroleptic drugs to treat agitation in patients with a brain injury: a review. Neurorehabilitation 13:165–172, 1999

Burns SP, Little JW, Hussey JD, et al: Sleep apnea syndrome in chronic spinal cord injury: associated factors and treatment. Arch Phys Med Rehabil 81:1334–1339, 2000

Capruso DX, Levin HS: Neurobehavioral outcome of head trauma, in Neurology and Trauma. Edited by Evans RW. Philadelphia, PA, WB Saunders, 1996, pp 201–221

Cardenas DD, McLean A, Farrell-Robers L, et al: Oral physostigmine and impaired memory in adults with brain injury. Brain Inj 8:579–587, 1994

Carter GM, Relles DA, Wynn BO, et al: Interim report on an inpatient rehabilitation facility prospective payment system. Rand Corp, DRU-2309-HCFA, July 2000

Cassidy JW: Fluoxetine: a new serotonergically active antidepressant. J Head Trauma Rehabil 4:67–69, 1989

Castriotta RJ, Lai JM: Sleep disorders associated with traumatic brain injury. Arch Phys Med Rehabil 82:1403–1406, 2001

Catsman-Berrevoets CE, Harskamp FV: Compulsive pre-sleep behavior and apathy due to bilateral thalamic stroke: response to bromocriptine. Neurology 38:647–649, 1988

Caveness WF: Posttraumatic sequelae, in Head Injury Conference Proceedings. Edited by Caveness WF, Walker A. Philadelphia, PA, JB Lippincott, 1966, pp 209–219

Charlifue SW, Gerhart KA: Behavioral and demographic predictors of suicide after traumatic spinal cord injury. Arch Phys Med Rehabil 72:488–492, 1991

Chatham-Showalter PE: Carbamazepine for combativeness in acute traumatic brain injury. J Neuropsychiatry Clin Neurosci 8:96–99, 1996

Chatham-Showalter PE, Kimmel DN: Agitated symptom response to divalproex following acute brain injury. J Neuropsychiatry Clin Neurosci 12:395–397, 2000

Childers MK, Holland D: Psychomotor agitation following gabapentin use in brain injury. Brain Inj 11:537–540, 1997

Cicerone K, Dahlberg C, Kalmar K, et al: Evidence-based cognitive rehabilitation: recommendations for clinical practice. Arch Phys Med Rehabil 81:1596–1615, 2000

Cicerone KD, Dahlberg C, Malec JF, et al: Evidence-based cognitive rehabilitation: updated review of the literature from 1998 through 2002. Arch Phys Med Rehabil 86:1681–1692, 2005

Clark AF, Davison K: Mania following head injury: a report of two cases and a review of the literature. Br J Psychiatry 150:841–844, 1987

Clay DL, Hagglund KJ, Frank RG, et al: Enhancing the accuracy of depression diagnosis in patients with spinal cord injury using Bayesian analysis. Rehabil Psychol 40:171–180, 1995

Cohen SA, Ihrig K, Lott RS, et al: Risperidone for aggression and self-injurious behavior in adults with mental retardation. J Autism Dev Disord 28:229–233, 1998

Corrigan JD: Substance abuse as a mediating factor in outcome from traumatic brain injury. Arch Phys Med Rehabil 76: 302–309, 1995

Cowell LC, Cohen RF: Amantadine: a potential adjuvant therapy following traumatic brain injury. J Head Trauma Rehabil 10:91–94, 1995

Craig AR, Hancock KM, Dickson HG: A longitudinal investigation into anxiety and depression in the first 2 years following a spinal cord injury. Paraplegia 32:675–679, 1994

Craig AR, Hancock K, Dickson H, et al: Long-term psychological outcomes in spinal cord injured persons: results of a controlled trial using cognitive behavior therapy. Arch Phys Med Rehabil 78:33–38, 1997

Crow S, Meller W, Christensen G, et al: Use of ECT after brain injury. Convuls Ther 12:113–116, 1996

Currier GW, Simpson GM: Risperidone liquid concentrate and oral lorazepam versus intramuscular haloperidol and intramuscular lorazepam for treatment of psychotic agitation. J Clin Psychiatry 62:153–157, 2001

Davidoff GN, Roth EJ, Richards JS: Cognitive deficits in spinal cord injury: epidemiology and outcome. Arch Phys Med Rehabil 73:275–284, 1992

Davidson J: Seizures and bupropion: a review. J Clin Psychiatry 50:256–261, 1989

Davison K, Bagley CR: Schizophrenia-like psychosis associated with organic disorders of the central nervous system. Br J Psychiatry 114:113–184, 1969

De Deyn PP, Rabheru K, Rasmussen A, et al: A randomized trial of risperidone, placebo, and haloperidol for behavioral symptoms of dementia. Neurology 53:946–955, 1999

Deb S, Lyons I, Koutzoukis C, et al: Rate of psychiatric illness 1 year after traumatic brain injury. Am J Psychiatry 156:374–378, 1999

DeLisa JA, Currie DM, Martin GM: Rehabilitation medicine: past, present, and future, in Rehabilitation Medicine: Principles and Practice, 3rd Edition. Philadelphia, PA, Lippincott Williams & Wilkins, 1998, pp 3–32

DeVivo MJ, Krause JS, Lammertse DP: Recent trends in mortality and causes of death among persons with spinal cord injury. Arch Phys Med Rehabil 80:1411–1419, 1999

Diamond S: Efficacy and safety profile of ven-lafaxine in chronic headache. Headache Quarterly 6:212–214, 1995

Dickel MJ, Renfrow SD, Moore PT, et al: Rapid eye movement sleep periodic leg movements in patients with spinal cord injury. Sleep 17:733–738, 1994

Dijkers M: Quality of life after spinal cord injury: a meta-analysis of the effects of disablement components. Spinal Cord 35:829–840, 1997

Dikmen SS, Temkin N, Armsden G: Neuro-psychological recovery: relationship to psychosocial functioning and postconcus-sional complaints, in Mild Head Injury. Edited by Levin HS, Eisenberg HM, Benton AL. New York, Oxford University Press, 1989, pp 229–241

Dikmen S, Machamer JE, Winn HR, et al: Neuropsychological outcome at 1-year post head injury. Neuropsychology 9: 80–90, 1995

Dikmen SS, Machamer JE, Winn HR, et al: Neuropsychological effects of valproate in traumatic brain injury: a randomized trial. Neurology 54:895–902, 2000

Dikmen S, Machamer J, Temkin N: Mild head injury: facts and artifacts. J Clin Exp Neuropsychol 23:729–738, 2001

Dinan TG, Mobayed M: Treatment resistance of depression after head injury: a prelimi-nary study of amitriptyline response. Acta Psychiatr Scand 85:292–294, 1992

Dolberg OT, Barkai G, Gross Y, et al: Differ-ential effects of topiramate in patients with traumatic brain injury and obesity: a case series. Psychopharmacology 179:838–845, 2004

Duffy JD, Kant R: Clinical utility of clozapine in 16 patients with neurological disease. J Neuropsychiatry Clin Neurosci 8:92–96, 1996

Dunlop TW, Udvarhelyi GB, Stedem AFA, et al: Comparison of patients with and with-out emotional/behavioral deterioration during the first year after traumatic brain injury. J Neuropsychiatry Clin Neurosci 3:150–156, 1991

Eames P: The use of Sinemet and bromocrip-tine. Brain Inj 3: 319–320, 1989

Eastwood EA, Hagglund KJ, Ragnarsson KT, et al: Medical rehabilitation length of stay and outcomes for persons with traumatic spinal cord injury: 1990–1997. Arch Phys Med Rehabil 80:1457–1463, 1999

Ellenberg JH, Levin HS, Saydjari C: Posttrau-matic amnesia as a predictor of outcome after severe closed head injury. Arch Neurol 53:782–791, 1996

Elliott TR, Frank RG: Depression following spinal cord injury. Arch Phys Med Rehabil 77:816–823, 1996

Elliott T, Shewchuck R: Social support and lei-sure activities following severe physical disability: testing the mediating effects of depression. Basic Appl Soc Psychol 16:471–587, 1995

Elliott T, Umlauf R: Measurement of personal-ity and psychopathology in acquired dis-ability, in Psychological Assessment in Medical Rehabilitation Settings. Edited by Cushman L, Scherer M. Washington, DC, American Psychological Association, 1995, pp 325–358

Englander J, Hall K, Simpson T, et al: Mild traumatic brain injury in an insured popu-lation: subjective complaints and return to employment. Brain Inj 6:161–166, 1992

Ergh TC, Rapport LJ, Coleman RD, et al: Pre-dictors of caregiver and family functioning following traumatic brain injury: social support moderates caregiver distress. J Head Trauma Rehabil 17:155–174, 2002

Ettinger AB, Weisbrot DM, Saracco J, et al: Positive and negative psychotropic effects of lamotrigine in patients with epilepsy and mental retardation. Epilepsia 39:874–877, 1998

Evans RW: The postconcussion syndrome and the sequelae of mild head injury, in Neurol-ogy and Trauma. Edited by Evans RW. Philadelphia, PA, WB Saunders, 1996, pp 91–116

Evans RW, Gualtieri CR, Patterson D: Treat-ment of chronic closed head injury with psychostimulant drugs: a controlled case study and an appropriate evaluation pro-cedure. J Nerv Ment Dis 175:106–110, 1987

Fann JR: Neurological effects of psychopharmacological agents. Semin Clin Neuropsychiatry 7:196–206, 2002

Fann JR, Katon WJ, Uomoto JM, et al: Psychiatric disorders and functional disability in outpatients with traumatic brain injuries. Am J Psychiatry 152:1493–1499, 1995

Fann JR, Uomoto JM, Katon WJ: Sertraline in the treatment of major depression following mild traumatic brain injury. J Neuropsychiatry Clin Neurosci 12:226–232, 2000

Fann JR, Uomoto JM, Katon WJ: Cognitive improvement with treatment of depression following mild traumatic brain injury. Psychosomatics 42:48–54, 2001

Fann JR, Leonetti A, Jaffe K, et al: Psychiatric illness and subsequent traumatic brain injury: a case-control study. J Neurol Neurosurg Psychiatry 72:615–620, 2002

Fann JR, Burington B, Leonetti A, et al: Psychiatric illness following traumatic brain injury in an adult health maintenance organization population. Arch Gen Psychiatry 61: 53–61, 2004

Fann JR, Bombardier CH, Dikmen S, et al: Validity of the Patient Health Questionnaire-9 in assessing depression following traumatic brain injury. J Head Trauma Rehabil 20:501–511, 2005

Federoff JP, Starkstein SE, Forrester AW, et al: Depression in patients with acute traumatic brain injury. Am J Psychiatry 149:918–923, 1992

Fenton G, McClelland R, Montgomery A, et al: The postconcussional syndrome: social antecedents and psychological sequelae. Br J Psychiatry 162:493–497, 1993

Fichtenberg NL, Millis SR, Mann NR, et al: Factors associated with insomnia among post-acute traumatic brain injury survivors. Brain Inj 14:659–667, 2000

Fleminger S, Greenwood RJ, Oliver DL: Pharmacological management for agitation and aggression in people with acquired brain injury (Cochrane Review), in The Cochrane Library, Issue 1, Oxford, Update Software, 2003

Fox DD, Lees-Haley PR, Earnest K, et al: Post-concussive symptoms: base rates and etiology in psychiatric patients. Clin Neuropsychol 9:89–92, 1995

Fuhrer M, Rintala D, Hart K, et al: Depressive symptomatology in persons with spinal cord injury who reside in the community. Arch Phys Med Rehabil 74:255–260, 1993

Fujii D, Ahmed I: Characteristics of psychotic disorder due to traumatic brain injury: an analysis of case studies in the literature. J Neuropsychiatry Clin Neurosci 14:130–140, 2002

Fullerton D, Harvey R, Klein M, et al: Psychiatric disorders in patients with spinal cord injury. Arch Gen Psychiatry 32:369–371, 1981

Galski T, Palasz J, Bruno RL, et al: Predicting physical and verbal aggression on a brain trauma unit. Arch Phys Med Rehabil 75:380–383, 1994

Gasquione PG: Affective state and awareness of sensory and cognitive effects after closed head injury. Neuropsychology 4:187–196, 1992

Gennarelli TA, Graham DI: Neuropathology of the head injuries. Semin Clin Neuropsychiatry 3:160–175, 1998

Gerhart KA, Koziol-McLain J, et al: Quality of life following spinal cord injury: knowledge and attitudes of emergency care providers. Ann Emerg Med 23:807–812, 1994

Gil S, Caspi Y, Ben-Ari IZ, et al: Does memory of a traumatic event increase the risk for posttraumatic stress disorder in patients with traumatic brain injury? A prospective study. Am J Psychiatry 162:963–969, 2005

Go BK, DeVivo MJ, Richards JS: The epidemiology of spinal cord injury, in Spinal Cord Injury: Clinical Outcomes from the Model Systems. Edited by Stover S, DeLisa JA, Whiteneck GG. Gaithersburg, MD, Aspen, 1995, pp 21–55

Gosling J, Oddy M: Rearranged marriages: marital relationships after head injury. Brain Inj 13:785–796, 1999

Gouvier WD, Uddo-Crane M, Brown LM: Base rates of postconcussional symptoms. Arch Clin Neuropsychol 3:273–278, 1988

Grant I, Alves W: Psychiatric and psychosocial disturbances in head injury, in Neurobehavioral Recovery from Head Injury. Edited by Levin HS, Grafman J, Eisenberg HM. New York, Oxford University Press, 1987, pp 234–235

Graves AB, White E, Koepsell TD, et al: The association between head trauma and Alzheimer's disease. Am J Epidemiol 131:491–501, 1990

Greendyke RM, Kanter DR: Therapeutic effects of pindolol on behavioral disturbances associated with organic brain disease: a double-blind study. J Clin Psychiatry 47:423–426, 1996

Greendyke RM, Kanter DR, Schuster DB, et al: Propranolol treatment of assaultive patients with organic brain disease: a double-blind, crossover, placebo-controlled study. J Nerv Ment Dis 174:290–294, 1996

Greve KW, Sherwin E, Stanford MW, et al: Personality and neurocognitive correlates of impulsive aggression in long-term survivors of severe traumatic brain injury. Brain Inj 15:255–262, 2001

Groom KN, Shaw TG, O'Connor ME, et al: Neurobehavioral symptoms and family functioning in traumatically brain-injured adults. Arch Clin Neuropsychol 13:695–711, 1998

Gualtieri CT: Buspirone for the behavior problems of patients with organic brain disorders. J Clin Psychopharmacol 11: 280–281, 1991

Gualtieri CT, Evans RW: Stimulant treatment for the neurobehavioural sequelae of traumatic brain injury. Brain Inj 2:273–290, 1988

Gualtieri T, Chandler M, Coons TB, et al: Amantadine: a new clinical profile for traumatic brain injury. Clin Neuropharmacol 12:258–270, 1989

Guilmette TJ, Rasile D: Sensitivity, specificity, and diagnostic accuracy of three verbal memory measures in the assessment of mild brain injury. Neuropsychology 9:338–344, 1995

Guerrero J, Thurman DJ, Sniezek JE: Emergency department visits associated with traumatic brain injury: United States, 1995–1996. Brain Inj 14:181–186, 2000

Gupta SR, Mlcoch AG: Bromocriptine treatment of nonfluent aphasia. Arch Phys Med Rehabil 73:373–376, 1992

Hall KM, Karzmark P, Stevens M, et al: Family stressors in traumatic brain injury: a two-year follow-up. Arch Phys Med Rehabil 75:876–884, 1994

Hamm RJ, Temple MD, Buck DL, et al: Cognitive recovery from traumatic brain injury: results of post-traumatic experimental interventions, in Neuroplasticity and Reorganization of Function After Brain Injury. Edited by Levin HS, Grafman J. New York, Oxford University Press, 2000, pp 49–67

Hanna-Pladdy B, Gouvier WD, Berry ZM: Postconcussional symptoms as predictors of neuropsychological deficits (abstract). Arch Clin Neuropsychol 12:329–330, 1997

Hart T, Whyte J, Polansky M, et al: Concordance of patient and family report of neurobehavioral symptoms at 1 year after traumatic brain injury. Arch Phys Med Rehabil 84:204–213, 2003

Harvey AG, Bryant RA: Acute stress disorder following mild traumatic brain injury. J Nerv Ment Dis 186:333–337, 1998

Harvey AG, Bryant RA: A two-year prospective evaluation of the relationship between acute stress disorder and posttraumatic stress disorder following mild traumatic brain injury. Am J Psychiatry 157:626–628, 2000

Harvey AG, Brewin CR, Jones C, et al: Coexistence of posttraumatic stress disorder and traumatic brain injury: towards a resolution of the paradox. J Int Neuropsychol Soc 9:663–676, 2003

Hayes RL, Dixon CE: Neurochemical changes in mild head injury. Semin Neurol 14:25–31, 1994

Hayes RL, Jenkins LW, Lyeth BG: Neurotransmitter-mediated mechanisms of traumatic brain injury: acetylcholine and excitatory amino acids. J Neurotrauma 9 (suppl 1):173–187, 1992

Heinemann A, Keen M, Donohue R, et al: Alcohol use in persons with recent spinal cord injuries. Arch Phys Med Rehabil 69:619–624, 1988

Hendryx PM: Psychosocial changes perceived by closed-head-injured adults and their families. Arch Phys Med Rehabil 70:526–530, 1989

Hensley PL, Reeve A: A case of antidepressant-induced akathisia in a patient with traumatic brain injury. J Head Trauma Rehabil 16:302–305, 2001

Herrick S, Elliott T, Crow F: Social support and the prediction of health complications among persons with SCI. Rehabil Psychol 39:231–250, 1994

Hibbard MR, Grober SE, Stein PN, et al: Poststroke depression, in Comprehensive Casebook of Cognitive Therapy. Edited by Freeman A, Dattilio F. New York, Guilford, 1992, pp 303–310

Hibbard MR, Uysal S, Kepler K, et al: Axis I psychopathology in individuals with traumatic brain injury. J Head Trauma Rehabil 13:24–39, 1998

Hibbard MR, Gordon WA, Flanagan S, et al: Sexual dysfunction after traumatic brain injury. Neurorehabilitation 15:107–120, 2000a

Hibbard MR, Gordon WA, Kothera LM: Traumatic brain injury, in Cognitive-Behavioral Strategies in Crisis Intervention, 2nd Edition. Edited by Dattilio F, Freeman A. New York, Guilford, 2000b, pp 219–242

Hillbom E: After-effects of brain-injuries: research on the symptoms causing invalidism of persons in Finland having sustained brain-injuries during the wars of 1939–1940 and 1941–1944. Acta Psychiatr Scand 35 (suppl 142):1–95, 1960

Hiott DW, Labbate L: Anxiety disorders associated with traumatic brain injuries. Neurorehabilitation 17:345–355, 2002

Horner MD, Ferguson PL, Selassie AW, et al: Patterns of alcohol use 1 year after traumatic brain injury: a population-based, epidemiological study. J Int Neuropsychol Soc 11:322–330, 2005

Hornstein A, Seliger G: Cognitive side effects of lithium in closed head injury (letter). J Neuropsychiatry Clin Neurosci 1:446–447, 1989

Horton A, Howe N: Behavioral treatment of the traumatically brain injured: a case study. Percept Motor Skills 53:349–350, 1981

Jennett B, Bond M: Assessment of outcome after severe brain damage. Lancet 1:480–484, 1975

Jorge R, Robinson RG: Mood disorders following traumatic brain injury. Neurorehabilitation 17:311–324, 2002

Jorge RE, Robinson RG, Arndt S: Are there symptoms that are specific for depressed mood in patients with traumatic brain injury? J Nerv Ment Dis 181:91–99, 1993a

Jorge RE, Robinson RG, Arndt SV, et al: Depression following traumatic brain injury: a 1 year longitudinal study. J Affect Disord 27:233–243, 1993b

Jorge RE, Robinson RG, Starkstein SE, et al: Depression and anxiety following traumatic brain injury. J Neuropsychiatry Clin Neurosci 5:369–374, 1993c

Jorge RE, Robinson RG, Starkstein SE, et al: Secondary mania following traumatic brain injury. Am J Psychiatry 150:916–921, 1993d

Jorge RE, Robinson RG, Moser D, et al: Major depression following traumatic brain injury. Arch Gen Psychiatry 61:42–50, 2004

Jung AC, Staiger T, Sullivan M: The efficacy of selective serotonin reuptake inhibitors for the management of chronic pain. J Gen Intern Med 12:384–389, 1997

Kaelin DL, Cifu DX, Matthies B: Methylphenidate effect on attention deficit in the acutely brain-injured adult. Arch Phys Med Rehabil 77:6–9, 1996

Kalisky Z, Morrison DP, Meyers CA, et al: Medical problems encountered during rehabilitation of patients with head injury. Arch Phys Med Rehabil 66:25–29, 1985

Kant R, Bogyi AM, Carosella NW, et al: ECT as a therapeutic option in severe brain injury. Convuls Ther 11:45–50, 1995

Kant R, Smith-Seemiller L, Zeiler D: Treatment of aggression and irritability after head injury. Brain Inj 12:661–666, 1998

Katz DI: Neuropathology and neurobehavioral recovery from closed head injury. J Head Trauma Rehabil 7:1–15, 1992

Katz IR, Jeste DV, Mintzer JE, et al: Comparison of risperidone and placebo for psychosis and behavioral disturbances associated with dementia: a randomized, double-blind trial. J Clin Psychiatry 60:107–115, 1999

Kay T, Cavallo MM: The family system: impact, assessment and intervention, in Neuropsychiatry of Traumatic Brain Injury. Edited by Hales RE. Washington, DC, American Psychiatric Press, 1994, pp 533–568

Kay T, Harrington DE, Adams R, et al: Definition of mild traumatic brain injury. J Head Trauma Rehabil 8:86–87, 1993

Kemp BJ, Kahan JS, Krause JS, et al: Treatment of major depression in individuals with spinal cord injury. J Spinal Cord Med 27:22–28, 2004

Kennedy P, Duff J: Post traumatic stress disorder and spinal cord injuries. Spinal Cord 39:1–10, 2001

Kennedy P, Evans MJ: Evaluation of post traumatic distress in the first 6 months following SCI. Spinal Cord 39:381–386, 2001

Kennedy P, Rogers BA: Anxiety and depression after spinal cord injury: a longitudinal analysis. Arch Phys Med Rehabil 81:932–937, 2000

Kennedy P, Duff J, Evans M, et al: Coping effectiveness training reduces depression and anxiety following traumatic spinal cord injuries. Br J Clin Psychol 42:41–52, 2003

Kennedy RE, Livingston L, Riddick A, et al: Evaluation of the Neurobehavioral Functioning Inventory as a depression screening tool after brain injury. J Head Trauma Rehabil 20:512–526, 2005

Khateb A, Ammann J, Annoni JM, et al: Cognitive-enhancing effects of donepezil in traumatic brain injury. Eur Neurol 54:39–45, 2005

Kim E: Agitation, aggression, and disinhibition syndromes after traumatic brain injury. Neurorehabilitation 17:297–310, 2002

King NS: Post-concussion syndrome: clarity amid the controversy? Br J Psychiatry 183:276–278, 2003

King NS, Crawford S, Wenden FJ, et al: The Rivermead Post Concussion Symptoms Questionnaire: a measure of symptoms commonly experienced after head injury and its reliability. J Neurol 242:587–592, 1995

Kishi Y, Robinson RG, Forrester AW: Prospective longitudinal study of depression following spinal cord injury. J Neuropsychiatry Clin Neurosci 6:237–244, 1994

Kishi Y, Robinson RG, Forrester AW: Comparison between acute and delayed onset major depression after spinal cord injury. J Nerv Ment Dis 183:286–292, 1995

Kiwerski J, Krauski M: Influence of alcohol intake on the course and consequences of spinal cord injury. Int J Rehab Res 15:240–245, 1992

Kolakowsky-Hayner SA, Gourley EV III, Kreutzer JS, et al: Pre-injury substance abuse among persons with brain injury and persons with spinal cord injury. Brain Inj 13:571–581, 1999

Kraus JF, McArthur DL: Incidence and prevalence of, and costs associated with, traumatic brain injury, in Rehabilitation of the Adult and Child with Traumatic Brain Injury, 3rd Edition. Edited by Rosenthal M, Kreutzer JS, Griffith ER, et al. Philadelphia, FA Davis, 1999, pp 3–18

Kraus MF, Maki PM: Effect of amantadine hydrochloride on symptoms of frontal lobe dysfunction in brain injury: case studies and review. J Neuropsychiatry Clin Neurosci 9:222–230, 1997

Krause J: Delivery of substance abuse services during spinal cord injury rehabilitation. Neurorehabilitation 2:45–51, 1992

Krause JS, Kewman D, DeVivo MJ, et al: Employment after spinal cord injury: an analysis of cases from the Model Spinal Cord Injury Systems. Arch Phys Med Rehabil 80:1492–1500, 1999

Kreutzer JS, Wehman PH, Harris JA, et al: Substance abuse and crime patterns among persons with traumatic brain injury referred for supported employment. Brain Inj 5:177–187, 1991

Kreutzer JS, Gordon WA, Rosenthal M, et al: Neuropsychological characteristics of patients with brain injury: preliminary findings from a multicenter investigation. J Head Trauma Rehabil 8:47–59, 1993

Kreutzer JS, Gervasio AH, Camplair PS: Primary caregivers' psychological status and family functioning after traumatic brain injury. Brain Inj 8:197–210, 1994

Kreutzer JS, Marwitz JH, Witol AD: Interrelationship between crime, substance abuse, and aggressive behaviours among persons with traumatic brain injury. Brain Inj 9:757–768, 1995

Kreutzer JS, Witol AD, Marwitz JH: Alcohol and drug use among young persons with traumatic brain injury. J Learn Disabil 29:643–651, 1996

Kreutzer J, Seel RT, Marwitz JH: The Neurobehavioral Functioning Inventory. San Antonio, TX, Psychological Corporation, 1999

Kreutzer JS, Seel RT, Gourley E: The prevalence and symptom rates of depression after traumatic brain injury: a comprehensive examination. Brain Inj 15:563–576, 2001

Krieger D, Hansen K, McDermott C, et al: Loxapine versus olanzapine in the treatment of delirium following traumatic brain injury. Neurorehabilitation 18:205–208, 2003

Kroenke K, Spitzer RL, Williams JB: The PHQ-9: validity of a brief depression severity measure. J Gen Intern Med 16:606–613, 2001

Kwentus JA, Hart RP, Peck ET, et al: Psychiatric complications of closed head trauma. Psychosomatics 26:8–17, 1985

Lal S, Merbitz CP, Grip JC: Modification of function in head-injured patients with Sinemet. Brain Inj 2:225–233, 1988

Lang E, Hord AH, Denson D: Venlafaxine hydrochloride (Effexor) relieves thermal hyperalgesia in rats with an experimental mononeuropathy. Pain 68:151–155, 1996

Langlois JA, Rutland-Brown W, Thomas KE: Traumatic Brain Injury in the United States: Emergency Department Visits, Hospitalizations, and Deaths. Atlanta, GA, Centers for Disease Control and Prevention, National Center for Injury Prevention and Control, 2006

Larrabee GJ: Neuropsychological outcome, post concussion symptoms and forensic considerations in mild closed head injury. Semin Clin Neuropsychiatry 2:196–206, 1997

Lee H, Kim SW, Kim JM, et al: Comparing effects of methylphenidate, sertraline and placebo on neuropsychiatric sequelae in patients with traumatic brain injury. Hum Psychopharmacol Clin Exp 20:97–104, 2005

Lee MA, Leng MEF, Tierman EJJ: Risperidone: a useful adjunct for behavioural disturbance in primary cerebral tumours. Palliative Med 15:255–256, 2001

Leininger BE, Gramling SE, Farrell AD, et al: Neuropsychological deficits in symptomatic minor head injury patients after concussion and mild concussion. J Neurol Neurosurg Psychiatry 53:293–296, 1990

Leon-Carrion J: Dementia due to head trauma: an obscure name for a clear neurocognitive syndrome. Neurorehabilitation 17:115–122, 2002

Lesem MD, Zajecka JM, Swift RH, et al: Intramuscular ziprasidone, 2 mg versus 10 mg, in the short-term management of agitated psychotic patients. J Clin Psychiatry 62:12–18, 2001

Levin HS, High WM, Goethe KE, et al: The Neurobehavioral Rating Scale: assessment of the behavioral sequelae of head injury by the clinician. J Neurol Neurosurg Psychiatry 50:183–193, 1987a

Levin HS, Mattis S, Ruff RM, et al: Neurobehavioral outcome following minor head injury: a three-center study. J Neurosurg 66:234–243, 1987b

Levin HS, Brown SA, Song JX, et al: Depression and posttraumatic stress disorder at three months after mild to moderate traumatic brain injury. J Clin Exp Neuropsychol 23:754–769, 2001

Levitt P, Henry W, McHale D: Persistent movement disorder induced by buspirone. Mov Disord 8:331–334, 1993

Lewis L: A framework for developing a psychotherapy treatment plan with brain-injured patients. J Head Trauma Rehabil 6:22–29, 1991

Lindenmayer JP, Kotsaftis A: Use of sodium valproate in violent and aggressive behaviors: a critical review. J Clin Psychiatry 61:123–128, 2000

Livingston MG, Brooks DN, Bond MR: Patient outcome in the year following severe head injury and relatives' psychiatric and social functioning. J Neurol Neurosurg Psychiatry 48: 876–881, 1985

MacDonald M, Nielson W, Cameron M: Depression and activity patterns of spinal cord injured persons living in the community. Arch Phys Med Rehabil 68:339–343, 1987

Malaspina D, Goetz RR, Friedman JH, et al: Traumatic brain injury and schizophrenia in members of schizophrenia and bipolar disorder pedigrees. Am J Psychiatry 158: 440–446, 2001

Malec JF: Mild traumatic brain injury: scope of the problem, in The Evaluation and Treatment of Mild Traumatic Brain Injury. Edited by Varney NR, Roberts RJ. Mahwah, NJ, Lawrence Erlbaum Associates, 1999, pp 15–38

Malec J, Neimeyer R: Psychologic prediction of duration of inpatient spinal cord injury rehabilitation performance of self care. Arch Phys Med Rehabil 64:359–363, 1983

Marin RS: Apathy: a neuropsychiatric syndrome. J Neuropsychiatry Clin Neurosci 3:243–254, 1991

Marin RS, Fogel BS, Hawkins J, et al: Apathy: a treatable syndrome. J Neuropsychiatry Clin Neurosci 7:23–30, 1995

Marino RJ, Ditunno JF Jr, Donovan WH, et al: Neurologic recovery after traumatic spinal cord injury: data from the Model Spinal Cord Injury Systems. Arch Phys Med Rehabil 80:1391–1396, 1999

Martin R, Kuzniecky R, Ho S, et al: Cognitive effects of topiramate, gabapentin, and lamotrigine in healthy young adults. Neurology 52:321–327, 1999

Maryniak O, Manchanda R, Velani A: Methotrimeprazine in the treatment of agitation in acquired brain injury patients. Brain Inj 15:167–174, 2001

Masand PS, Tesar GE: Use of stimulants in the medically ill. Psychiatr Clin North Am 19:515–547, 1996

Masel BE, Scheibel RS, Kimbark T, et al: Excessive daytime sleepiness in adults with brain injuries. Arch Phys Med Rehabil 82:1526–1532, 2001

Mayou R, Bryant B, Duthie R: Psychiatric consequences of road traffic accidents. BMJ 307:647–651, 1993

Mayou R, Black J, Bryant B: Unconsciousness, amnesia and psychiatric symptoms following road traffic accident injury. Br J Psychiatry 177:540–545, 2000

McAllister TW: Neuropsychiatric sequelae of head injuries. Psychiatr Clin North Am 15:395–413, 1992

McAllister TW, Ferrell RB: Evaluation and treatment of psychosis after traumatic brain injury. Neurorehabilitation 17:357–368, 2002

McCauley SR, Boake C, Levin HS, et al: Postconcussional disorder following mild to moderate traumatic brain injury: anxiety, depression, and social support as risk factors and comorbidities. J Clin Exp Neuropsychol 23:792–808, 2001

McClelland RJ, Fenton GW, Rutherford W: The post-concussional syndrome revisited. J R Soc Med 87:508–510, 1994

McDougle CJ, Holmes JP, Carlson DC, et al: A double-blind, placebo-controlled study of risperidone in adults with autistic disorder and other pervasive developmental disorders. Arch Gen Psychiatry 55:633–641, 1998

McElligott JM, Greenwald BD, Watanabe TK: Congenital and acquired brain injury. 4. New frontiers: neuroimaging, neuroprotective agents, cognitive-enhancing agents, new technology, and complementary medicine. Arch Phys Med Rehabil 84 (suppl 1):18–22, 2003

McIntosh TK, Smith DH, Meaney DF, et al: Neuropathological sequelae of traumatic brain injury: relationship to neurochemical and biomechanical mechanisms. Lab Invest 74: 315–342, 1996

McIntosh TK, Juhler M, Wieloch T: Novel pharmacological strategies in the treatment of experimental traumatic brain injury. J Neurotrauma 15:731–769, 1998

McKinley WO, Seel RT, Hardman JT: Nontraumatic spinal cord injury: incidence, epidemiology, and functional outcome. Arch Phys Med Rehabil 80:619–623, 1999

McLean A Jr, Temkin NR, Dikmen S, et al: The behavioral sequelae of head injury. J Clin Neuropsychol 5:361–376, 1983

McQuay HJ, Tramer M, Nye BA, et al: A systematic review of antidepressants in neuropathic pain. Pain 68:217–227, 1996

Meehan KM, Wang H, David SR, et al: Comparison of rapidly acting intramuscular olanzapine, lorazepam, and placebo: a double-blind, randomized study in acutely agitated patients with dementia. Neuropsychopharmacology 26:494–504, 2002

Meythaler JM, Peduzzi JD, Eleftheriou E, et al: Current concepts: diffuse axonal injury-associated traumatic brain injury. Arch Phys Med Rehabil 82:1461–1471, 2001

Meythaler JM, Brunner RC, Johnson A, et al: Amantadine to improve neurorecovery in traumatic brain injury-associated diffuse axonal injury: a pilot double-blind randomized trial. J Head Trauma Rehabil 17:300–313, 2002

Michals ML, Crismon ML, Robers S, et al: Clozapine response and adverse effects in nine brain-injured patients. J Clin Psychopharmacol 13:198–203, 1993

Middleboe T, Anderson HS, Birket-Smith M, et al: Minor head injury: impact on general health after one year. Acta Neurol Scand 85:5–9, 1992

Millis SR, Rosenthal M, Novack TA, et al: Long-term neuropsychological outcome after traumatic brain injury. J Head Trauma Rehabil 16:343–355, 2001

Mittenberg W, Strauman S: Diagnosis of mild head injury and the postconcussion syndrome. J Head Trauma Rehabil 15:783–791, 2000

Mittenberg W, Tremont G, Zielinski RE, et al: Cognitive-behavioral prevention of postconcussion syndrome. Arch Clin Neuropsychol 11:139–145, 1996

Mooney GF, Haas LJ: Effect of methylphenidate on brain injury-related anger. Arch Phys Med Rehabil 74:153–160, 1993

Moss NE, Crawford S, Wade DT: Postconcussion symptoms: is stress a mediating factor? Clin Rehabil 8:149–156, 1994

Mukai A, Costa JL: The effect of modafinil on self-esteem in spinal cord injury patients: a report of 2 cases and review of the literature. Arch Phys Med Rehabil 86:1887–1889, 2005

Muller U, Murai T, Bauer-Wittmund T, et al: Paroxetine versus citalopram treatment of pathological crying after brain injury. Brain Inj 13:805–811, 1999

Mysiw WJ, Jackson RD, Corrigan JD: Amitriptyline for post-traumatic agitation. Am J Phys Med Rehabil 67:29–33, 1988

Nahas Z, Arlinghaus KA, Kotrla KJ, et al: Rapid response of emotional incontinence to selective serotonin reuptake inhibitors. J Neuropsychiatry Clin Neurosci 10:453–455, 1998

National Institutes of Health Consensus Development Panel on Rehabilitation of Persons With Traumatic Brain Injury: Rehabilitation of persons with traumatic brain injury. JAMA 282:974–983, 1999

Newburn G, Edwards R, Thomas H, et al: Moclobemide in the treatment of major depressive disorder (DSM-3) following traumatic brain injury. Brain Inj 13:637–642, 1999

Nickels JL, Schneider WN, Dombovy ML, et al: Clinical use of amantadine in brain injury rehabilitation. Brain Inj 8:709–718, 1994

Niemeier JP, Burnett DM: No such thing as "uncomplicated bereavement" for patients in rehabilitation. Disabil Rehabil 23:645–653, 2001

Oddy M, Humphrey M, Uttley D: Stresses upon the relatives of head-injured patients. Br J Psychiatry 133:507–513, 1978

Ojemann LM, Baugh-Bookman C, Dudley DL: Effect of psychotropic medications on seizure control in patients with epilepsy. Neurology 37:1525–1527, 1987

Onghena P, Van Houdenhove B: Antidepressant-induced analgesia in chronic nonmalignant pain: a meta-analysis of 39 placebo-controlled studies. Pain 49:205–219, 1992

Oyewumi LK, Lapierre YD: Efficacy of lithium in treating mood disorder occurring after brain stem injury. Am J Psychiatry 138:110–112, 1981

Pande AC, Davidson JR, Jefferson JW, et al: Treatment of social phobia with gabapentin: a placebo-controlled study. J Clin Psychopharmacol 19:341–348, 1999

Pande AC, Pollack MH, Crockatt J, et al: Placebo-controlled study of gabapentin treatment of panic disorder. J Clin Psychopharmacol 20:467–471, 2000

Park NW, Ingles JL: Effectiveness of attention rehabilitation after an acquired brain injury: a meta-analysis. Neuropsychology 15:199–210, 2001

Perino C, Rago R, Cicolini A, et al: Mood and behavioural disorders following traumatic brain injury: clinical evaluation and pharmacological management. Brain Inj 15:139–148, 2001

Pinkston JB, Gouvier WD, Santa Maria MP: Mild head injury: differentiation of long-term differences on testing. Brain Cogn 44:74–78, 2000

Plenger PM, Dixon CE, Castillo RM, et al: Subacute methylphenidate treatment for moderate to moderately severe traumatic brain injury: a preliminary double-blind placebo-controlled study. Arch Phys Med Rehabil 77:536–540, 1996

Pope HG Jr, McElroy SL, Satlin A, et al: Head injury, bipolar disorder, and response to valproate. Compr Psychiatry 29:34–38, 1988

Povlishock JT: Pathophysiology of neural injury: therapeutic opportunities and challenges. Clin Neurosurg 46:113–126, 2000

Prigatano GP: Personality and psychosocial consequences of brain injury, in Neuropsychological Rehabilitation After Brain Injury. Edited by Prigatano GP, Fordyce DJ, Zeiner HK, et al. Baltimore, MD, Johns Hopkins University Press, 1986, pp 29–50

Prigatano GP: Disordered mind, wounded soul: the emerging role of psychotherapy in rehabilitation after brain injury. J Head Trauma Rehabil 6:1–10, 1991

Prigatano GP: Principles of Neuropsychological Rehabilitation. New York, Oxford University Press, 1999

Prigatano GP, Altman IM: Impaired awareness of behavioral limitations after traumatic brain injury. Arch Phys Med Rehabil 71:1058–1064, 1990

Prigatano GP, Ben-Yishay Y: Psychotherapy and psychotherapeutic interventions in brain injury rehabilitation, in Rehabilitation of the Adult and Child With Traumatic Brain Injury. Edited by Rosenthal M, Griffith ER, Kreutzer JS, et al. Philadelphia, PA, FA Davis, 1999, pp 271–283

Prigatano GP, Fordyce DJ: Cognitive dysfunction and psychosocial adjustment after brain injury, in Neuropsychological Rehabilitation after Brain Injury. Edited by Prigatano GP, Fordyce DJ, Zeiner HK, et al. Baltimore, MD, Johns Hopkins University Press, 1986, pp 1–17

Radanov BP, di Stefano G, Schnidrig A, et al: Role of psychosocial stress in recovery from common whiplash. Lancet 338:712–715, 1991

Radnitz CL, Hsu L, Tirch DD, et al: A comparison of posttraumatic stress disorder in veterans with and without spinal cord injury. J Abnorm Psychol 107:676–680, 1998

Rammahan KW, Rosenberg JH, Pollak CP, et al: Modafinil: efficacy for the treatment of fatigue in patients with multiple sclerosis (abstract). Neurology 54 (suppl 3):24, 2000

Rao V, Lyketsos C: Neuropsychiatric sequelae of traumatic brain injury. Psychosomatics 41:95–103, 2000

Rao V, Lyketsos CG: Psychiatric aspects of traumatic brain injury. Psychiatr Clin North Am 25:43–69, 2002

Richards JS: Psychologic adjustment to spinal cord injury during first postdischarge year. Arch Phys Med Rehabil 67:362–365, 1986

Rohe DE, Krause JS: Stability of interests after severe physical disability: an 11-year longitudinal study. J Vocat Behav 52:45–58, 1998

Rowland T, Mysiw WJ, Bogner J, et al: Trazodone for post traumatic agitation (abstract). Arch Phys Med Rehabil 73:963, 1992

Ruff RM, Marshall LF, Klauber MR, et al: Alcohol abuse and neurological outcome of the severely head injured. J Head Trauma Rehabil 5:21–31, 1990

Ruff RM: Discipline-specific approach versus individual care, in The Evaluation and Treatment of Mild Traumatic Brain Injury. Edited by Varney NR, Roberts RJ. Mahwah, NJ, Lawrence Erlbaum Associates, 1999, pp 99–114

Rutherford WH, Merrett JD, McDonald JR: Symptoms at one year following concussion from minor head injuries. Injury 10:225–230, 1979

Sachdev P, Smith JS, Cathcart S: Schizophrenia-like psychosis following traumatic brain injury: a chart-based descriptive and case-control study. Psychol Med 31:231–239, 2001

Sandel ME, Mysiw WJ: The agitated brain injured patient, part 1: definitions, differential diagnosis, and assessment. Arch Phys Med Rehabil 77:617–623, 1996

Sander AM, Kreutzer JS, Fernandez CC: Neurobehavioral functioning, substance abuse, and employment after brain injury: implications for vocational rehabilitation. J Head Trauma Rehabil 12:28–41, 1997

Saran AS: Depression after minor closed head injury: role of dexamethasone suppression test and antidepressants. J Clin Psychiatry 46:335–338, 1985

Sbordone RJ, Liter JC: Mild traumatic brain injury does not produce post-traumatic stress disorder. Brain Inj 9:405–412, 1995

Schiff HB, Sabin TD, Geller A, et al: Lithium in aggressive behavior. Am J Psychiatry 139:1346–1348, 1982

Schoenborn CA, Adams PF, Schiller JS: Summary health statistics for the U.S. population: National Health Interview Survey, 2000. National Center for Health Statistics. Vital Health Stat 10:214, 2003

Schreiber S, Backer MM, Pick CG: The antinociceptive effect of venlafaxine in mice is mediated through opioid and adrenergic mechanisms. Neurosci Lett 273:85–88, 1999

Schulz R, Decker S: Long-term adjustment to physical disability: the role of social support, perceived control, and self-blame. J Pers Soc Psychol 48:1162–1172, 1985

Seel RT, Kreutzer JS, Rosenthal M, et al: Depression after traumatic brain injury: a National Institute on Disability and Rehabilitation Research Model Systems multicenter investigation. Arch Phys Med Rehabil 84:177–184, 2003

Shavelle RM, Strauss D, Whyte J, et al: Long-term causes of death after traumatic brain injury. Am J Phys Med Rehabil 80:510–516, 2001

Sherer M, Bergloff P, Levin E, et al: Impaired awareness and employment outcome after traumatic brain injury. J Head Trauma Rehabil 13:52–61, 1998a

Sherer M, Boake C, Levin E, et al: Characteristics of impaired awareness after traumatic brain injury. J Int Neuropsychol Soc 4:380–387, 1998b

Sherer M, Hart T, Nick TG, et al: Early impaired self-awareness after traumatic brain injury. Arch Phys Med Rehabil 84:168–176, 2003

Shorvon SD: Safety of topiramate: adverse events and relationships to dosing. Epilepsia 37 (suppl 2):18–22, 1996

Shukla S, Cook BL, Mukherjee S, et al: Mania following head trauma. Am J Psychiatry 144:93–96, 1987

Silver JM, Yudofsky SC: Aggressive disorders, in Neuropsychiatry of Traumatic Brain Injury. Edited by Silver JM, Yudofsky SC, Hales RE. Washington, DC, American Psychiatric Press, 1994a, pp 313–353

Silver JM, Yudofsky SC: Psychopharmacology, in Neuropsychiatry of Traumatic Brain Injury. Edited by Silver JM, Yudofsky SC, Hales RE. Washington, DC, American Psychiatric Press, 1994b, pp 631–670

Silver JM, Hales RE, Yudofsky SC: Neuropsychiatric aspects of traumatic brain injury, in The American Psychiatric Publishing Textbook of Neuropsychiatry and Clinical Neurosciences, 4th Edition. Edited by Yudofsky SC, Hales RE. Washington, DC, American Psychiatric Publishing, 2002, pp 625–672

Sipski M, Alexander C: Sexual function in people with disabilities and chronic illness. Gaithersburg, MD, Aspen Publishers, 1997

Sipski ML, Alexander CJ, Rosen RC: Orgasm in women with spinal cord injuries: a laboratory-based assessment. Arch Phys Med Rehabil 76:1097–1102, 1995

Sloan RL, Brown KW, Pentland B: Fluoxetine as a treatment for emotional lability after brain injury. Brain Inj 6:315–319, 1992

Speech TJ, Rao SM, Osmon DC, et al: A double-blind controlled study of methylphenidate treatment in closed head injury. Brain Inj 7:333–338, 1993

Spitzer RL, Kroenke K, Williams JB: Validation and utility of a self-report version of PRIME-MD: the PHQ primary care study. Primary Care Evaluation of Mental Disorders. Patient Health Questionnaire. JAMA 282:1737–1744, 1999

Staas W, Formal C, Freedman M, et al: Spinal cord injury and spinal cord injury medicine, in Rehabilitation Medicine: Principles and Practice. Edited by DeLisa J, Gans BM. Philadelphia, PA, Lippincott-Raven Publishers, 1998, pp 1259–1291

Stanislav SW, Childs A: Evaluating the usage of droperidol in acutely agitated persons with brain injury. Brain Inj 14:261–265, 2000

Stanislav SW, Fabre T, Crismon ML, et al: Buspirone's efficacy in organic-induced aggression. J Clin Psychopharmacol 14:126–130, 1994

Stewart JT, Nemsath RH: Bipolar illness following traumatic brain injury: treatment with lithium and carbamazepine. J Clin Psychiatry 49:74–75, 1988

Stewart T, Shields CR: Grief in chronic illness: assessment and management. Arch Phys Med Rehabil 66:447–450, 1985

Stolp-Smith K, Wainberg K: Antidepressant exacerbation of spasticity. Arch Phys Med Rehabil 80:339–342, 1999

Street JS, Clark WS, Gannon KS, et al: Olanzapine treatment of psychotic and behavioral symptoms in patients with Alzheimer disease in nursing care facilities: a double-blind, randomized, placebo-controlled trial. The HGEU Study Group. Arch Gen Psychiatry 57:968–976, 2000

Stuss DT, Binns MA, Carruth FG, et al: The acute period of recovery from traumatic brain injury: posttraumatic amnesia or posttraumatic confusional state? J Neurosurg 90:635–643, 1999

Suhr JA, Gunstad J: Postconcussive symptom report: the relative influence of head injury and depression. J Clin Exp Neuropsychol 24:981–993, 2002

Tate DG, Stiers W, Daugherty J, et al: The effects of insurance benefits coverage on functional and psychosocial outcomes after spinal cord injury. Arch Phys Med Rehabil 75:407–414, 1994

Tatum WO, French JA, Faught E, et al: Postmarketing experience with topiramate and cognition. Epilepsia 42:1134–1140, 2001

Taverni JP, Seliger G, Lichtman SW: Donepezil mediated memory improvement in traumatic brain injury during post acute rehabilitation. Brain Inj 12:77–80, 1998

Taylor LA, Kreutzer JS, Demm SR, et al: Traumatic brain injury and substance abuse: a review and analysis of the literature. Neuropsychological Rehabilitation 13:165–188, 2003

Teitelman E: Off-label uses of modafinil (letter). Am J Psychiatry 158:8, 2001

Tennant FS, Wild J: Naltrexone treatment for postconcussional syndrome. Am J Psychiatry 144:813–814, 1987

Terzoudi M, Gavrielidou P, Heilakos G, et al: Fatigue in multiple sclerosis: evaluation of a new pharmacological approach (abstract). Neurology 54 (suppl 3):A61–A62, 2000

Thurman DJ, Alverson C, Dunn KA, et al: Traumatic brain injury in the United States: a public health perspective. J Head Trauma Rehabil 14:602–615, 1999

Trahan DE, Ross CE, Trahan SL: Relationships among postconcussional-type symptoms, depression, and anxiety in neurologically normal young adults and victims of mild brain injury. Arch Clin Neuropsychol 16: 435–445, 2001

Trieschmann RB: Spinal Cord Injuries: Psychological, Social and Vocational Rehabilitation. New York, Demos Publication, 1988

Trzepacz PT: Delirium, in Neuropsychiatry of Traumatic Brain Injury. Edited by Silver JM, Yudofsky SC, Hales RE. Washington, DC, American Psychiatric Press, 1994, pp 189–218

Trzepacz PT, Kennedy RE: Delirium and posttraumatic amnesia, in Textbook of Traumatic Brain Injury. Edited by Silver JM, McAllister TW, Yudofsky SC. Washington, DC, American Psychiatric Publishing, 2005, pp 175–200

Tuohimaa P: Vestibular disturbances after acute mild head injury. Acta Otolaryngol Suppl 359:3–67, 1978

Umlauf R, Frank RG: A cluster-analytic description of patient subgroups in the rehabilitation setting. Rehabil Psychol 28:157–167, 1983

Uomoto J, Brockway J: Anger management training for brain injured patients and their family members. Arch Phys Med Rehabil 73:674–679, 1992

Van der Naalt J, Van Zomeren AH, Sluiter WJ, et al: Acute behavioral disturbances related to imaging studies and outcome in mild-to-moderate head injury. Brain Inj 14:781–788, 1999

Van Reekum R, Cohen T, Wong J: Can traumatic brain injury cause psychiatric disorders? J Neuropsychiatry Clin Neurosci 12:316–327, 2000

Van Reekum R, Streiner DL, Conn DK: Applying Bradford Hill's criteria for causation to neuropsychiatry: challenges and opportunities. J Neuropsychiatry Clin Neurosci 13:318–325, 2001

Vargo JW: Some psychological effects of physical disability. Am J Occup Ther 32:31–34, 1978

Violon A, DeMol J: Psychological sequelae after head trauma in adults. Acta Neurochir (Wien) 85:96–102, 1987

Warden DL, Labbate LA, Salazar AM, et al: Posttraumatic stress disorder in patients with traumatic brain injury and amnesia for the event? J Neuropsychiatry Clin Neurosci 9:18–22, 1997

Webster G, Daisley A, King N: Relationship and family breakdown following acquired brain injury: the role of the rehabilitation team. Brain Inj 13:593–603, 1999

Westgren N, Levi R: Quality of life and traumatic spinal cord injury. Arch Phys Med Rehabil 79:1433–1439, 1998

Whelan FJ, Walker MS, Schultz SK: Donepezil in the treatment of cognitive dysfunction associated with traumatic brain injury. Ann Clin Psychiatry 12:131–135, 2000

Whitlock JA Jr: Brain injury, cognitive impairment and donepezil. J Head Trauma Rehabil 14:424–427, 1999

Whyte J, Hart T, Schuster K, et al: Effects of methylphenidate on attentional function after traumatic brain injury: a randomized placebo-controlled trial. Am J Phys Med Rehabil 76:440–450, 1997

Wilcox JH, Nasrallah HA: Childhood head trauma and psychosis. Psychiatry Res 21:303–306, 1987

Williams DH, Levin HS, Eisenberg HM: Mild head injury classification. Neurosurgery 27:422–428, 1990

Wilson JT, Teasdale GM, Hadley DM, et al: Posttraumatic amnesia: still a valuable yardstick. J Neurol Neurosurg Psychiatry 57:198–201, 1994

Witol AD, Sander AM, Seel RT, et al: Long-term neurobehavioral characteristics after brain injury: implications for vocational rehabilitation. J Voc Rehabil 7:159–167, 1996

World Health Organization: International Classification of Impairments, Disabilities and Handicaps: ICIDH. Geneva, Switzerland, World Health Organization, 1980

World Health Organization: International Statistical Classification of Diseases and Related Health Problems, 10th Revision. Geneva, Switzerland, World Health Organization, 1992

World Health Organization: International Classification of Functioning, Disability and Health: ICF. Geneva, Switzerland, World Health Organization, 2001

Wortman CB, Silver RC: The myths of coping with loss. J Consult Clin Psychol 57:349–357, 1989

Wroblewski BA, McColgan K, Smith K, et al: The incidence of seizures during tricyclic antidepressant drug treatment in a brain-injured population. J Clin Psychopharmacol 10:124–128, 1990

Wroblewski B, Glenn MB, Cornblatt R, et al: Protriptyline as an alternative stimulant medication in patients with brain injury: a series of case reports. Brain Inj 7:353–362, 1993

Wroblewski BA, Joseph AB, Cornblatt RR: Antidepressant pharmacotherapy and the treatment of depression in patients with severe traumatic brain injury: a controlled, prospective study. J Clin Psychiatry 57:582–587, 1996

Wroblewski BA, Joseph AB, Kupfer J, et al: Effectiveness of valproic acid on destructive and aggressive behaviors in patients with acquired brain injury. Brain Inj 11:37–47, 1997

Yoshino A, Hovda DA, Kawamata T, et al: Dynamic changes in local cerebral glucose utilization following cerebral concussion in rats: evidence of hyper- and subsequent hypometabolic state. Brain Res 561:106–119, 1991

Yudofsky SC, Silver JM, Jackson W, et al: The Overt Aggression Scale for the objective rating of verbal and physical aggression. Am J Psychiatry 143:35–39, 1986

Yudofsky SC, Silver JM, Schneider SE: Pharmacologic treatment of aggression. Psychiatr Ann 17:397–407, 1987

Yudofsky SC, Silver JM, Hales RE: Pharmacologic management of aggression in the elderly. J Clin Psychiatry 51:22–28, 1990

Yudofsky SC, Kopecky HJ, Kunik M, et al: The Overt Agitation Severity Scale for the objective rating of agitation. J Neuropsychiatry Clin Neurosci 9:541–548, 1997

Zafonte RD, Lexell J, Cullen N: Possible applications for dopaminergic agents following traumatic brain injury: part 2. J Head Trauma Rehabil 16:112–116, 2001

Zifko UA, Rupp M, Schwarz S, et al: Modafinil in treatment of fatigue in multiple sclerosis: results of an open-label study. J Neurol 249:983–987, 2002

Self-Assessment Questions

Select the single best response for each question.

1. Which of the following is considered a *less* significant risk factor for psychiatric illness following traumatic brain injury (TBI)?

   A. Poor neuropsychological functioning.
   B. Preinjury psychiatric history.
   C. Preinjury social impairment.
   D. Increased age.
   E. Alcohol abuse.

2. Regarding post-TBI psychosis, which of the following statements is *true?*

   A. In TBI-associated psychosis, hallucinations are more commonly reported than are delusions.
   B. Right hemisphere lesions are more common than left-sided lesions in TBI-associated psychosis.
   C. Seizure disorder rates in patients with post-TBI psychosis are higher than estimates for rates of post-TBI seizure disorders in general.
   D. The onset of psychotic symptoms is typically within 3 months of injury, with delayed onset after 1 year rarely reported.
   E. Negative symptoms are more common in post-TBI psychosis than are positive symptoms.

3. All of the following are considered risk factors for postconcussive syndrome *except*

   A. Older age.
   B. Previous TBI.
   C. Psychosocial stress.
   D. Male gender.
   E. Ongoing litigation.

4. Numerous psychotropic medications can be used to treat the symptoms of apathy and fatigue in central nervous system injury. Which of the following medications used for this purpose carries a risk of inducing seizures at usual doses?

   A. Modafinil.
   B. Methylphenidate.
   C. Dextroamphetamine.
   D. Bromocriptine.
   E. Amantadine.

5. Which anticonvulsant/mood stabilizer has been associated with paradoxical agitation in TBI and should thus be used with some caution and careful monitoring?

   A. Oxcarbazepine.
   B. Topiramate.
   C. Valproate.
   D. Lithium.
   E. Gabapentin.

6. The use of atypical antipsychotic agents in TBI may be helpful in controlling problematic psychotic and agitation symptoms. However, TBI patients are prone to delirium from anticholinergic drug effects and may also have an increased risk of seizures. For these reasons, which of the following antipsychotics should be used only with extreme caution in this population?

   A. Clozapine.
   B. Olanzapine.
   C. Risperidone.
   D. Quetiapine.
   E. Ziprasidone.

19 Pain

Michael R. Clark, M.D., M.P.H.

Definition and Assessment

Pain has been defined by the International Association for the Study of Pain (IASP) as "an unpleasant sensory and emotional experience associated with actual or potential tissue damage, or described in terms of such damage" (Merskey et al. 1986, p. S217). Other terms relevant to pain are defined in Table 19–1. Pain is the most common reason a patient presents to a physician for evaluation (Kroenke 2003; Kroenke and Mangelsdorff 1989). If the patient suffers from chronic pain, defined as "pain without apparent biological value that has persisted beyond the normal tissue healing time (usually 3 months)," many specialists may be required in the successful care of the patient (Bonica 1990, p. 19). Chronic pain and its consequences are now recognized complications of many illnesses, such as spinal cord injury, amputations, cerebral palsy, multiple sclerosis, HIV, Parkinson's disease, stroke, neuromuscular diseases, cancer, peripheral vascular disease, neuropathy, temporal arteritis, arthritis, and postherpetic neuralgia (Ehde et al. 2003; Foley 1994).

Pain is a complex experience that varies demographically; is influenced by affective, cognitive, and behavioral factors; and has an extensive neurobiology (Meldrum 2003). Pain is difficult to assess, especially in patients with terminal illness or cognitive impairment (Parmelee 1996). Patients' compliance with pain diaries is often poor, with only 11% actually following instructions, despite 90% of patients reporting compliance in one recent study (Stone et al. 2002). Pain rating scales attempt to measure the severity of pain. Generally, there are poor correlations among pain reporting, tissue pathology, disability, and treatment response (Turk 1999). Scores on simple numerical rating scales reflect the affective or emotional aspects of pain much more than the sensory intensity (W.C. Clark et al. 2002).

A comprehensive evaluation should be performed for any patient who reports pain (M.R. Clark 2000a; M.R. Clark and Cox 2002). This evaluation should incorporate simple standardized tools for rating pain severity; observations of pain-related behaviors, including any problems with activities of daily living that would indicate

TABLE 19–1. Definitions relating to pain sensations

Allodynia	Pain from a stimulus that does not normally provoke pain
Deafferentation pain	Pain resulting from loss of sensory input into the central nervous system
Dysesthesia	An unpleasant, abnormal sensation that can be spontaneous or evoked
Hyperalgesia	An increased response to a stimulus that is normally painful
Hyperesthesia	Increased sensitivity to stimulation that excludes the special senses
Hyperpathia	Pain characterized by an increased reaction to a stimulus, especially a repetitive stimulus, and an increased threshold
Hypoesthesia	Diminished sensitivity to stimulation that excludes the special senses
Nociception	Detection of tissue damage by transducers in skin and deeper structures and the central propagation of this information via A delta and C fibers in the peripheral nerves
Paresthesia	An abnormal sensation, spontaneous or evoked, that is not unpleasant
Sensitization	Lowered threshold and prolonged/enhanced response to stimulation

Source. Adapted from Merskey et al. 1986.

the presence of pain; and a clinical examination to elicit evidence of pain and the signs of possible etiologies.

Epidemiology

The prevalence of chronic pain reported in the general population ranges from 10% to 55%, with an estimate of severe chronic pain of approximately 11% among adults (Nickel and Raspe 2001; Ospina and Harstall 2002; Verhaak et al. 1998). In the most recent World Health Organization (WHO) review from multiple countries, the weighted mean prevalence of chronic pain was 31% in men, 40% in women, 25% in children up to age 18 years, and 50% in the elderly older than 65 years (Ospina and Harstall 2002). During a 2-week period, 13% of the U.S. workforce reported a loss in productivity due to a chronic pain condition (Stewart et al. 2003).

An 8-year follow-up survey by the U.S. Center for Health Statistics found that 32.8% of the general population experienced chronic pain symptoms (Magni

et al. 1993). In another WHO study of more than 25,000 primary care patients in 14 countries, 22% of patients suffered from pain that had been present for most of the time for at least 6 months (Gureje et al. 1998). In a study of 6,500 individuals ages 15–74 years in Finland, 14% experienced daily chronic pain that was independently associated with lower self-rated health (Mantyselka et al. 2003). A retrospective analysis of 14,000 primary care patients in Sweden reported that approximately 30% of patients seeking treatment had some kind of defined pain problem, with almost two-thirds diagnosed with musculoskeletal pain (Hasselstrom et al. 2002).

Selected Chronic Pain Conditions

Postherpetic Neuralgia

Postherpetic neuralgia is defined as pain persisting or recurring at the site of shingles at least 3 months after the onset of the acute varicella zoster viral rash (Bowsher 1997b). Postherpetic neuralgia occurs in about 10% of patients with acute herpes zoster. More than half of patients over 65 years of age with shingles develop postherpetic neuralgia, and it is more likely to occur in patients with cancer, diabetes mellitus, and immunosuppression. Other risk factors include greater acute pain and rash severity, sensory impairment, and psychological distress (Schmader 2002). Most cases gradually improve over time, with only about 25% of patients with postherpetic neuralgia experiencing pain at 1 year after diagnosis.

Although degeneration and destruction of motor and sensory fibers of the mixed dorsal root ganglion characterize acute varicella zoster, other neurological damage may include inflammation of the spinal cord, myelin disruption, axonal damage, and decreases in the number of nerve endings from the affected skin. These injuries persist in postherpetic neuralgia patients. Studies have suggested the role of both peripheral and central mechanisms resulting from the loss of large-caliber neurons and subsequent central sensitization or adrenergic receptor activation and alterations in C-fiber activity (Fields et al. 1998). Early treatment of varicella zoster with low-dose amitriptyline reduced the prevalence of pain at 6 months by 50% (Bowsher 1996, 1997a). Tricyclic antidepressants (TCAs), anticonvulsants, and opioids are the most common effective treatments for postherpetic neuralgia and may have potential for its prevention (Dworkin and Schmader 2003; Johnson and Dworkin 2003).

Peripheral Neuropathy Pain

Sensory neurons are damaged by many diseases, both directly and indirectly (Scadding 1994). Approximately 25% of patients with diabetes mellitus will experience painful diabetic neuropathy, with duration of illness and poor glycemic control as contributing risk factors. If C-fiber input is preserved but large-fiber input is lost, paresthesias and pain are the predominant sensory experiences. The pain of a peripheral neuropathy can range from a constant burning to pain that is episodic, paroxysmal, and lancinating in quality (Mendell and Sahenk 2003). These phenomena are primarily the result of axonal degeneration and segmental demyelination. Sites of ectopic impulse generation can be found at any point along the peripheral nerve.

The paroxysms of pain that result from stimulation of hyperexcitable damaged neurons and subsequent recruitment of nearby undamaged sensory afferents may be explained by several forms of nonsynaptic (ephaptic) and prolonged (afterdischarge) impulse transmission described in models of peripheral neuropathic pain. Voltage-dependent sodium channels in the dorsal root ganglion undergo both up- and downregulation depending on the subpopulation (Rizzo 1997). When a peripheral nerve is damaged, central sensitization amplifies and sustains neuronal activity. Pharmacological treatments are similar to those used for postherpetic neuralgia.

Parkinson's Disease

Pain is the most common sensory manifestation of Parkinson's disease and reported by half of patients (Starkstein et al. 1991). The pain is typically described as cramping and aching, located in the lower back and extremities, but not associated with muscle contraction or spasm. These pains often decrease when the patient is treated with levodopa, which suggests a central origin. The loss of dopaminergic input could explain how pain is produced, perhaps through a loss of descending inhibition in the spinal cord (Burkey et al. 1996).

Central Poststroke Pain

Approximately 5% of patients who have suffered a stroke experience intractable pain (Bowsher 1995). Patients typically have hemibody sensory deficits and pain associated with dysesthesias, allodynia, and hyperalgesia. Radiographic lesions are present in the thalamus, although other sites are often involved. Excitatory amino acids may be involved in the development of this syndrome. Pharmacological treatment is usually not effective, and even ketamine, an N-methyl-D-aspartate (NMDA) receptor antagonist, reduced pain in less than 50% of patients (Yamamoto et al. 1997). In contrast, patients with spinal cord injury experienced reductions in continuous and evoked pain with ketamine and mu opioid receptor agonists, suggesting different mechanisms in different central pain states (Eide et al. 1995).

Migraine and Chronic Daily Headache

The peak incidence of migraine occurs between the third and sixth decades of life and then decreases with age. Over the life span, 18% of women and 6% of men will suffer from migraine (Lipton et al. 1997). Theories of pathogenesis include the involvement of the trigeminovascular system and plasma protein extravasation, antagonism of serotonin receptors, modulation of central aminergic control mechanisms, stabilizing effects on membranes through action at voltage-sensitive calcium channels, and involvement of substance P (Goadsby 1997). Common migraine is defined as a unilateral pulsatile headache, which may be associated with other symptoms such as nausea, vomiting, photophobia, and phonophobia (Szirmai 1997). The classic form of migraine adds visual prodromal symptoms such as scintillating scotomata. Complicated migraine includes focal neurological signs.

Calcium channel blockers, beta-blockers, antidepressants, and anticonvulsants are the treatments with best-documented efficacy (Mathew 2001). A group-based multidisciplinary treatment consisting of stress management, supervised exercise, dietary education, and massage therapy significantly improved pain characteristics, functional status, quality of life, depression, and pain-related disability in patients with migraine (Lemstra et al. 2002).

Headache is the most common pain condition reported by the U.S. workforce as the reason for lost productive time (Stewart et al. 2003). Chronic daily headache affects about 5% of the population and is composed of constant (transformed) migraine, chronic tension-type headaches, new-onset daily persistent headache, and hemicrania continua (Lake and Saper 2002). Patients with chronic daily headache are more likely to overuse medication, leading to rebound headache; have psychiatric comorbidity such as depression and anxiety; report functional disability; and experience stress-related headache exacerbations (Lake 2001).

In addition to the traditional prophylactic agents, treatments include serotonin agonists, serotonin antagonists, and α_2-adrenergic agonists. Olanzapine decreased headache severity and frequency in patients with refractory headaches who did not respond to at least four preventive medications (Silberstein et al. 2002). Topiramate decreased migraine frequency, severity, number of headache days, and use of abortive medications in episodic and transformed migraine (Mathew et al. 2002). TCAs and stress management therapy significantly reduced headache activity, analgesic medication use, and disability (Holroyd et al. 2001). Combined medication and cognitive-behavioral psychotherapy are more effective than either treatment alone (Lake 2001; Lipchik and Nash 2002).

Low Back Pain

Low back pain (LBP) is one of the most common physical symptoms, and the most expensive condition when including lost productivity and health care costs (Stewart et al. 2003). Psychological factors associated with LBP include distress, depressed mood, and somatization, which predict the transition from acute to chronic LBP (Pincus et al. 2002). In one prospective cohort study of 1,246 patients with acute LBP who sought treatment, about 8% had chronic, continuous symptoms for 3 months, and less than 5% had unremitting pain for 22 months (Carey et al. 2000). Two-thirds of patients with chronic LBP at 3 months exhibited functional disability at 22 months. The most powerful predictor of chronicity was poor functional status 4 weeks after seeking treatment. Both economic and social rewards were associated with higher levels of disability and depression (Ciccone et al. 1999). Depression is a presurgical risk factor associated with poor outcome in long-term follow-up of compensated workers who underwent posterolateral lumbar fusion (DeBerard et al. 2001). Anxiety, depression, and occupational mental stress predicted lower rates of return to work in patients undergoing lumbar surgeries (Schade et al. 1999; Trief et al. 2000).

The presence of a depressive disorder has been demonstrated to increase the risk of developing chronic musculoskeletal pain 3 years later (Leino and Magni 1993; Magni et al. 1993, 1994; Von Korff et al. 1993). In a 15-year prospective study of workers in an industrial setting, initial depression symptom scores were predictive of LBP in men (Leino and Magni 1993). In a study of health care workers examined over 3 years with the Zung Depression Index, affective distress contributed to new-onset LBP (Adams et al. 1999). In a community-based sample, depression was associated with a fourfold increase in the likelihood of seeking a consultation at follow-up for the new complaint of back pain lasting longer than 3 months (Waxman et al. 1998). In a 13-year follow-up study that examined the longitudinal relationship, depressive disorder was a significant risk factor for incident LBP (Larson et al. 2004). While it is understandable that patients with LBP would experience reactive affective distress, a significant relationship between LBP and the subsequent onset of incident depressive disorder was not found. In another prospective analysis, as much as 16% of LBP in the general population may be attributable to psychological distress (Croft et al. 1996).

The treatment of chronic LBP has been pursued with multiple modalities alone and in combination (Deyo and Weinstein 2001). Although treatments often produce symptom reductions, there is conflicting evidence about their ability to improve functional status, particularly returning to work (Pfingsten et al. 1997; Staiger et al. 2003). Conservative interventions such as education, exercise, massage, and transcutaneous electrical nerve stimulation (TENS) produce inconsistent results (Pengel et al. 2002). Multidisciplinary rehabilitation programs usually offer the best outcomes (Huppe and Raspe 2003; Karjalainen et al. 2003; Lang et al. 2003). The patient's perception of disability is a critical factor that must be addressed for treatment to succeed.

Complex Regional Pain Syndrome (Causalgia and Reflex Sympathetic Dystrophy)

The term *complex regional pain syndrome* (CRPS) now replaces reflex sympathetic dystrophy (CRPS type I) and causalgia (CRPS type II) (Stanton-Hicks et al. 1995). Type I involves ongoing spontaneous burning pain that is precipitated by a specific noxious trauma or cause of immobilization and is usually associated with hyperalgesia or allodynia to cutaneous stimuli. The symptoms are not limited to a single peripheral nerve, and there is often evidence of edema, blood flow abnormalities, or sudomotor dysfunction in the region of pain, usually an extremity. Motor changes such as tremor, weakness, and limitations in movement are common. If nerve injury is present, CRPS type II is appropriately diagnosed. Three clinical stages are classically described. Stage 1 (acute, early) is characterized by an inflammatory onset with constant aching or burning pain. Stage 2 (dystrophic, intermediate) is notable for cool, pale, and cyanotic skin. Stage 3 (atrophic, late) manifests as atrophy and wasting of multiple soft tissues, fixed joint contractures, and osteoporosis. If pain is relieved by blockade of the efferent sympathetic nervous system, sympathetically maintained pain is present and patients often report hyperalgesia to cold stimuli (Wesselmann and Raja 1997).

Patients with CRPS often exhibit emotional distress and psychological dysfunction. The prevalence of psychiatric disorders in CRPS ranges from 18% to 64% (Bruehl and Carlson 1992). Examination using the Structured Clinical Interview for DSM-IV (SCID) found affective (46%), anxiety (27%), and substance abuse disorders (14%) in patients with CRPS (Rommel et al. 2001). Nonanatomical and expansive areas of hypoesthesia or hyperalgesia with normal peripheral sensory nerve conduction or somatosensory evoked potentials in patients with CRPS type I are probably psychogenic in origin. Neurophysiological investigation suggests that certain positive motor signs (dystonia, tremors, spasms, irregular jerks) identified in patients with CRPS type I represent pseudoneurological illness (Verdugo and Ochoa 2000).

Depression, anxiety, and fear of movement are common, but no unique personality profile predisposes one to develop CRPS (Bruehl and Carlson 1992; Lynch 1992). In patients with CRPS, a study of daily diaries demonstrated that the prior day's depressed mood contributed to the present day's increased pain and that yesterday's pain also contributed to today's depression, anxiety, and anger (Feldman et al. 1999). Treatment for CRPS usually combines a variety of anesthetic blocks, typically regional sympathetic blocks, with oral sympatholytics, reactivating physical therapies, adjuvant analgesic medications, electrical stimulation, and possibly even surgical sympathectomy (Lee and Benzon 1999).

Orofacial Pain

Trigeminal neuralgia (tic douloureux) is a chronic pain syndrome with severe, paroxysmal, recurrent, lancinating pain in the distribution of cranial nerve V that is unilateral and most commonly involves the mandibular division (Elias and Burchiel 2002). Sensory or motor deficits are not usually present. Pain can be spontaneous or evoked by nonpainful stimuli to trigger zones, activities such as talking or chewing, or environmental conditions. Between episodes, patients are typically pain-free. Less common syndromes involving the intermedius branch of the facial nerve or the glossopharyngeal nerve present with pain that can involve the ear, posterior pharynx, tongue, or larynx (Zakrzewska 2002).

Cluster headache occurs predominantly in men with onset before age 25; it presents with episodic excruciating pain, unilaterally surrounding the eye, that lasts minutes to hours and is associated with autonomic symptoms. Short-lasting, unilateral, neuralgiform pain with conjunctival injection and tearing (SUNCT) syndrome is a rare condition that commonly affects older males. Tolosa-Hunt syndrome manifests as pain in the ocular area accompanied by ipsilateral paresis of oculomotor nerves and improves with steroids. Atypical facial pain is more commonly associated with psychological factors that amplify the patient's pain, distress, and disability (Kapur et al. 2003).

The majority of patients with classical trigeminal neuralgia show evidence of trigeminal nerve root compression by blood vessels (85%), mass lesions, or other diseases that cause demyelination and hyperactivity of the trigeminal nucleus (multiple sclerosis, herpes zoster, postherpetic neuralgia) (Love and Coakham 2001). Afferent fibers become hyperexcitable as a result of injury, and paroxysms of pain are the manifestation of synchronized afterdischarge activity (Devor et al. 2002). Pharmacological treatment includes anticonvulsants, antidepressants, baclofen, mexiletine, lidocaine, and opioids (Cheshire 2002; Sindrup and Jensen 2002). When pharmacological treatments fail, a variety of surgical procedures, such as microvascular decompression via suboccipital craniectomy, percutaneous gangliolysis, and stereotactic radiosurgery, may be undertaken.

Temporomandibular disorder (TMD) is a general term referring to complaints that involve the temporomandibular joint, muscles of mastication, and other orofacial musculoskeletal structures. Pain most commonly arises from the muscles of mastication and is precipitated by jaw function, such as opening the mouth or chewing. Associated symptoms include feelings of muscle fatigue, weakness, and tightness as well as changes in bite (malocclusion) or the ability to open/close the jaw.

Psychological distress is common in patients with TMD (McCreary et al. 1991). Patients with pain of muscular origin are usually more distressed and depressed, with greater levels of disability, than those with TM joint pain (Auerbach et al. 2001). Patients with TMD classified as either "dysfunctional" or "interpersonally distressed" were at higher risk to develop chronic pain (Epker and Gatchel 2000). In treatment trials for patients with TMD, the dysfunctional group showed the best response to multidisciplinary treatment, with greater improvements in pain

intensity, interference, catastrophizing, and depression (Rudy et al. 1995). Patients with low levels of psychosocial dysfunction experienced significantly decreased pain, pain-related interference, and visits for TMD treatment (Dworkin et al. 2002).

Burning mouth syndrome (BMS) is characterized as pain in oral and pharyngeal cavities, especially the tongue, often associated with dryness and taste alterations. Most cases are idiopathic but may coincide with conditions such as bruxism, poorly fitting dentures, oral candidiasis, xerostomia, malnutrition, food allergies and contact dermatitis, gastroesophageal reflux disease, diabetes mellitus, hypothyroidism, neoplasia, menopause, and psychiatric conditions such as depression, anxiety, and somatoform disorders (Drage and Rogers 2003). The condition mainly affects middle-aged and postmenopausal women, and the oral mucosa is usually normal. Psychological factors such as severe life events have been associated with the condition (Bogetto et al. 1998). Potential underlying etiologies—such as depression/anxiety, nutritional deficiencies (iron, folate, B_{12}, and other B vitamins), maladaptive oral habits, and iatrogenic causes such as medications—should be identified and treated (Bogetto et al. 1998; Pinto et al. 2003). Treatment with TCAs or anticonvulsants has brought pain relief in some patients with BMS (Pinto et al. 2003; Zakrzewska et al. 2001).

Psychiatric Comorbidity

Pain Disorder and Somatization

Pain "caused" by emotional factors was first operationalized in DSM-II under psychophysiological disorders (American Psychiatric Association 1968). DSM-III introduced *psychogenic pain disorder*, in which pathophysiology was either absent or insufficient to explain the severity and duration of pain (American Psychiatric Association 1980). In DSM-III-R *somatoform pain disorder*, psychological factors were no longer required as an etiology of pain (American Psychiatric Association 1987). A preoccupation with pain, instead of the pain itself, was established as the core criterion in conjunction with the absence of adequate physical findings. DSM-IV refined this diagnosis as *pain disorder* (American Psychiatric Association 1994, 2000). The primary criteria require that pain be the chief complaint and that the pain cause significant distress or functional impairment. Psychological factors are recognized as having an important role in the pain (Aronoff et al. 2000; King 2000; Sullivan 2000).

The lifetime prevalence of somatoform pain disorder (DSM-III-R) in the general population was 34% with a 6-month prevalence of 17% (Grabe et al. 2003). However, when the DSM-IV requirement of significant distress or psychosocial impairment was added to make the diagnosis, the lifetime prevalence was only 12% and the 6-month prevalence decreased to 5%, with the female-to-male ratio remaining 2:1. Injured workers who developed somatoform pain disorder were characterized by more sites of pain, spread of pain beyond the area of the original injury, more opioid and benzodiazepine use, and greater involvement with compensation and litigation (Streltzer et al. 2000).

Although the actual diagnosis of somatization disorder is rare in patients with chronic pain, multiple pain complaints are present in somatization disorder by definition. Most patients with multiple unexplained symptoms have subsyndromal forms of somatization disorder, such as multisomatoform disorder, which has a prevalence in primary care of 4%–18% (Dickinson et al. 2003; Kroenke et al. 1997). Such patients are more likely to exhibit catastrophic thinking, believe the cause of their pain to be a mystery, have feelings of losing control, and think that physicians believe their pain is imaginary. Patients with chronic pain and medically unexplained symptoms also are at risk for iatrogenic consequences of excessive diagnostic tests, inappropriate medications, and unneeded surgery.

Substance Use

The prevalence of substance use disorders in patients with chronic pain is higher than in the general population (Dersh et al. 2002; Weaver and Schnoll 2002). In a study of primary care outpatients with chronic noncancer pain who received at least 6 months of opioid prescriptions during 1 year, behaviors consistent with opioid abuse were recorded in approximately 25% of patients (Reid et al. 2002). Almost 90% of patients attending a pain management clinic were taking medications and 70% were prescribed opioid analgesics (Kouyanou et al. 1997). In this population, 12% met DSM-III-R criteria for substance abuse or dependence. In another study of 414 chronic pain patients, 23% met criteria for active alcohol, opioid, or sedative misuse or dependence; current dependency was most common for opioids (13%) (Hoffman et al. 1995). In reviews of substance dependence or addiction in patients with chronic pain, the prevalence ranges from 3% to 19% in high-quality studies (Fishbain et al. 1992; Nicholson 2003).

Diagnostic criteria and definitions for problematic medication use behaviors and substance use disorders were recently revised (American Academy of Pain Medicine et al. 2001; Chabal et al. 1997; Savage et al. 2003). The core criteria for a substance use disorder in patients with chronic pain include the loss of control in the use of the medication, excessive preoccupation with it despite adequate analgesia, and adverse consequences associated with its use (Compton et al. 1998). The best predictors of addiction in a sample of patients with problematic medication use were 1) the patients believing they were addicted, 2) increasing analgesic dose/frequency, and 3) a preferred route of administration. The presence of maladaptive behaviors must be demonstrated to diagnose addiction, because physical dependence and tolerance alone are normal physiological phenomena.

Determining whether patients with chronic pain are abusing prescribed controlled substances is a routine but challenging issue in care (Compton et al. 1998; Savage 2002). Studies of opioid therapy have found that patients who developed problems with their medication all had a history of substance abuse (Portenoy and Foley 1986). However, inaccurate reporting and underreporting of medication use by patients complicate assessment (Fishbain et al. 1999b). Not infrequently, prior substance abuse history emerges only after current misuse has been identified, thus requiring physicians to be vigilant over the course of treatment. In patients with chronic pain who did develop new substance use disorders, the problem most commonly involved the medications prescribed by their physicians (Long et al. 1988).

The causes and onset of substance use disorders have been difficult to characterize in relationship to chronic pain. During the first 5 years after the onset of chronic pain, patients are at increased risk for developing new substance use disorders (Brown et al. 1996). This risk is highest in patients with a history of substance abuse or dependence, childhood physical or sexual abuse, and psychiatric comorbidity (Aronoff 2000; Fishbain et al. 1998). In a study of chronic LBP patients, 34% had a substance use disorder, yet in 77% of cases the substance abuse was present before the onset of the chronic pain (Brown et al. 1996; Polatin et al. 1993). A cycle of pain followed by relief *after* taking medications is a classic example

of operant reinforcement of *future* medication use that eventually becomes abuse (Fordyce et al. 1973). Patients with substance abuse exhibit abnormalities in pain perception and tolerance. An increased sensitivity to pain and the reinforcing effects of relieving pain with substance use may lead to the development of substance abuse in patients with chronic pain.

Reliance on medications that provide pain relief can result in a number of stereotyped patient behaviors that can either represent or be mistaken for addiction. Persistent pain can lead to increased focus on opioid medications. Patients may take extraordinary measures to ensure an adequate medication supply even in the absence of addiction. This may be manifested as requests for premature refills, higher doses, or extra quantities of medication, or as seeking medication from additional sources. Patients understandably fear the reemergence of pain and withdrawal symptoms if they run out of medication. Drug-seeking behavior may be the result of an anxious patient trying to maintain a previous level of pain control. The patient's actions may represent pseudoaddiction that results from therapeutic dependence and undertreatment but not addiction (Kirsh et al. 2002; Weaver and Schnoll 2002). Since these behaviors occur in both pseudo- and true addiction, the distinction is based in part on whether the behaviors are infrequent and isolated versus repetitive and persistent, and whether they abate with adequate opioid therapy.

In patients with higher risk of addiction, prevention should begin with a treatment contract to clarify the conditions under which opioids will be provided. The contract emphasizes a single physician being responsible for prescriptions and explicitly describes all the conditions under which use of opioids will be considered inappropriate and which may lead to discontinuation. Under optimal circumstances, opioid contracts attempt to improve compliance by distributing information and using a mutually agreed-upon treatment plan that includes consequences for aberrant behaviors and incorporates the primary care physician to form a "trilateral" agreement with the patient and pain specialist (Fishman et al. 2002). When there is concern that a patient will have difficulty taking medications as directed, a policy of prescribing small quantities, performing random pill counts, and not refilling lost supplies should be explicitly discussed and then followed. External sources of information, such as urine toxicology testing, interviews with significant others, direct contact with pharmacists, data from prescription monitoring programs, and review of medical records, can improve detection of substance use disorders. In one study, patients who denied using illicit substances that were detected on urine toxicology were more likely to be younger, to be receiving worker's compensation benefits, and to have a previous diagnosis of polysubstance abuse (Katz and Fanciullo 2002).

Patients with substance use disorders have increased rates of chronic pain and are at the greatest risk for stigmatization and undertreatment with appropriate medications (Gilson and Joranson 2002; Rosenblum et al. 2003). Ironically, this places them at additional risk of drug-seeking behaviors, including self-medication with illicit drugs. Almost one-quarter of patients admitted to inpatient residential substance abuse treatment and more than one-third of patients in methadone maintenance treatment programs reported severe chronic pain, with almost half of the inpatients and two-thirds of the methadone maintenance patients experiencing pain-related interference in functioning (Rosenblum et al. 2003). In another study of methadone maintenance therapy, patients with pain were more likely to overuse both prescribed and nonprescribed medications

(Jamison et al. 2000). Patients with substance abuse and back pain were less likely to complete a substance abuse treatment program compared with those without pain (Stack et al. 2000).

Depression and Distress

Pain in Patients With Depression

Approximately 60% of patients with depression report pain symptoms at the time of diagnosis (Magni et al. 1985; Von Knorring et al. 1983). In WHO data from 14 countries on five continents, 69% (range= 45%–95%) of patients with depression presented with only somatic symptoms, of which pain complaints were most common (Simon et al. 1999). A survey of almost 19,000 Europeans found a fourfold increase in the prevalence of chronic painful conditions in respondents with major depression (Ohayon and Schatzberg 2003).

Depressive disorder increased the risk of developing chronic musculoskeletal pain, headache, and chest pain up to 3 years later (Leino and Magni 1993; Magni et al. 1993, 1994; Von Korff et al. 1993). Even after 8 years, depressed patients remained twice as likely to develop chronic pain. Five years later, depression at baseline was a significant predictor in the 25% of at-risk women who developed fibromyalgia (Forseth et al. 1999).

Depression in Patients With Chronic Pain

In 1,016 health maintenance organization (HMO) members, the prevalence of depression was 12% in individuals with three or more pain complaints, compared with only 1% in those with one or no pain complaints (Dworkin et al. 1990). The Canadian National Population Health Survey found that the incidence of major depression was approximately doubled in subjects who reported a long-term medical condition such as back problems, migraine, and sinusitis (Livingston et al. 2000; Patten 2001). In a study of late-onset depression in the elderly, joint pain was one of the most important predictors of incident depression 5 years later (Hein et al. 2003).

One-third to over half of patients presenting to clinics specializing in the evaluation of chronic pain have a current major depression (Dersh et al. 2002; Fishbain et al. 1997a; Smith 1992). In groups of patients with medically unexplained symptoms such as back pain, two-thirds of patients have a history of recurrent major depression, compared with less than 20% of medically ill control groups (Atkinson et al. 1991; Katon and Sullivan 1990; Sullivan and Katon 1993).

Affective Distress Versus Affective Disorder

Diagnostic criteria, structured interviews, and self-report questionnaires might measure different constructs than major depression when applied to patients with chronic pain (Lebovits 2000). Self-report measures of depression are reliable and have predictive validity in patients with chronic pain (Turk and Okifuji 1994). Principal components analyses of the responses of patients with chronic pain on the Beck Depression Inventory find three factors consistent with the core criteria of major depression: low mood, impaired self attitude, poor vital sense. One study described the three factors as sadness, self-reproach, and somatic symptoms, and another as negative attitudes/suicide, physiological manifestations, and performance difficulty (Novy et al. 1995).

In a study comparing separate measures of affective distress, self-reported depressive symptoms, and major depression in patients with chronic pain, the relationship between pain and depression remained significant even when the somatic items of depressive symptoms were excluded (Geisser et al. 2000). Self-reported depressive symptoms were related to the evaluative or cognitive component of pain. In contrast, symptoms of affective distress were uniquely related to the sensory or emotional component of pain. Self-reported symptoms of affective distress and depressive symptoms were independently associated with increased pain, greater disability, and more negative thoughts about pain. A diagnosis of major depression was found only to make unique contributions to measures of negative thoughts about pain and self-reported disability.

Consequences of Depression

Depression in patients with chronic pain is associated with greater pain intensity, more pain persistence, less life control, more use of passive-avoidant coping strategies, noncompliance with treatment, application for early retirement, and greater interference from pain, including more pain behaviors observed by others (Hasenbring et al. 1994; Haythornthwaite et al. 1991; Magni et al. 1993; Weickgenant et al. 1993). Primary care patients with musculoskeletal pain complicated by depression are significantly more likely to use medications daily, including sedative-hypnotics, and in combinations (Mantyselka et al. 2002). In a study of more than 15,000 employees who filed health claims, the cost of managing chronic conditions such as back problems was multiplied by 1.7 when comorbid depression was present (Druss et al. 2000). Depressed patients with chronic facial pain were more likely to be noncompliant (Riley et al. 1999).

Depression is a better predictor of disability than pain intensity and duration (Rudy et al. 1988). For example, fibromyalgia patients with depression were significantly more likely to live alone, report functional disability, and describe maladaptive thoughts (Okifuji et al. 2000). The presence of depression in whiplash patients reduced the insurance claim closure rate by 37% (Cote et al. 2001). This rate was unaffected even after the insurance system eliminated compensation for pain and suffering. The presence of preoperative depression in patients undergoing lumbar diskectomy predicted poorer surgical outcome at 1-year follow-up (Junge et al. 1995). In patients with rheumatoid arthritis, depressive symptoms were significantly associated with negative health and functional outcomes, as well as increased health services utilization (Katz and Yelin 1993). Depression consistently predicted level of functioning, pain severity, pain-related disability, and more use of passive coping (Fisher et al. 2001). In a clinical trial of 1,001 depressed patients older than 60 years with arthritis, antidepressants and/or problem-solving-oriented psychotherapy not only reduced depressive symptoms but also improved pain, functional status, and quality of life (Lin et al. 2003).

Patients suffering from chronic pain syndromes, including migraine, chronic abdominal pain, and orthopedic pain syndromes, report increased rates of suicidal ideation, suicide attempts, and suicide completion (Fishbain et al. 1991; Magni et al. 1998). Patients with chronic pain completed suicide at two to three times the rate in the general population (Fishbain et al. 1991). Cancer patients with pain and depression, but not pain alone, were significantly more likely to take steps to end their lives (Emanuel et al. 1996).

Relationship Between Pain and Depression

The existing models of the relationship between pain and depression were recently detailed (Bair et al. 2003; Pincus and Williams 1999). In addition to depression being a consequence of chronic pain, there are mediating biopsychosocial factors in the interaction between depression and chronic pain (Fishbain et al. 1997a; Pincus and Williams 1999). The diathe-

sis–stress model postulates an interaction between personal premorbid vulnerabilities activated and exacerbated by life stressors such as chronic pain and the subsequent outcome of depression or other psychopathology. In a study of patients with chronic LBP, regression models that included all cognitive-behavioral variables (self-control, cognitive distortion, interference with instrumental activities of daily living) produced the strongest association with self-reported depression (Maxwell et al. 1998). Without these cognitive factors, there was no significant association of pain and disability with depression—a finding consistent with the diathesis–stress model. Other intervening factors have also been identified. A study of nearly 4,000 twin pairs found that genetic factors accounted for 60% of the association between back and neck pain and symptoms of depression and anxiety (Reichborn-Kjennerud et al. 2002).

More sophisticated models add the component of illness behaviors/disability, which functions both as a response of the vulnerable individual to a significant stressor and, later, as a stressor itself (Revenson and Felton 1989). The severity of depression was unaffected by pain intensity when pain-related disability was controlled for (Von Korff et al. 1992). If pain causes disability that decreases an individual's participation in activities, the risk of depression is significantly increased (Williamson and Schulz 1992). In patients with chronic LBP, the association between pain and depression was found to be attributable to disability and illness attitudes (Dickens et al. 2000). A study of patients in primary care found that after a variety of factors, such as disability and perceived health, were controlled for, anxiety and depression were no longer associated with the diagnoses of headache, osteoarthritis, and abdominal pain (Wu et al. 2002).

The neurobiology of pain and that of depression overlap (Bair et al. 2003; Bolay and Moskowitz 2002; Hunt and Mantyh 2001; Price 2000; Riedel and Neeck 2001). In particular, the descending pathways of pain modulation in the central nervous system that utilize monoamine neurotransmitters in the limbic system, periaqueductal gray, rostral-ventromedial medulla, and dorsolateral pontine tegmentum influence aspects of affect and attention (Millan 2002). Pain can be decreased by descending inhibition as first postulated by the gate theory of Melzack and Wall (1965). Increased levels of serotonin and norepinephrine diminish peripheral nociceptive inputs and augment descending central inhibition. The functional deficiency of monoamine neurotransmitters or related neurochemical dysfunctions in affective disorder could partially explain the linkages between pain and depression.

Anxiety, Fear, Catastrophizing, and Anger

Patients with a variety of chronic pain syndromes have increased rates of both anxiety symptoms and current anxiety disorders (Dersh et al. 2002; Fishbain et al. 1986; Juang et al. 2000; Polatin et al. 1993; Weissman and Merikangas 1986). Almost 50% of patients with chronic pain report anxiety symptoms, and up to 30% of patients have an anxiety disorder such as panic disorder and generalized anxiety disorder (Fishbain et al. 1998; Katon et al. 1985). One prospective study of 1,007 young adults found that a baseline history of migraine was significantly associated with an increased risk (OR=12.8) of first-incidence panic disorder (Breslau and Davis 1993). In a study of patients with fibromyalgia, more than half of the patients reported clinically relevant posttraumatic stress disorder (PTSD)–like symptoms that were significantly associated with greater levels of pain,

emotional distress, interference, and disability (Sherman et al. 2000).

Conversely, anxiety symptoms and disorders are associated with high levels of somatic preoccupation and physical symptoms. Pain intensity in rheumatoid arthritis patients was found to be significantly influenced by the presence of anxiety and depression even after disease activity had been controlled for (Smedstad et al. 1995). Men with high levels of anxiety experienced greater pain severity, interference from pain, and limitations in daily activities (Edwards et al. 2000). Almost two-thirds of patients with panic disorder reported at least one current pain symptom (Schmidt et al. 2002). Pain was related to higher levels of anxiety symptoms, panic frequency, and cognitive features of anxiety.

The fear–avoidance model and expectancy model of fear provide explanations for the initiation and maintenance of chronic pain disability (Greenberg and Burns 2003; Reis 1991; Vlaeyen and Linton 2000). Fear of pain, movement, or reinjury and other negative consequences that result in the avoidance of activities promote the transition to and sustaining of chronic pain and its associated disabilities (Asmundson et al. 1999). Patients with chronic LBP who restricted their activities developed physiological changes (muscle atrophy, weight gain) and functional deterioration attributed to deconditioning (Verbunt et al. 2003). This process is reinforced by low self-efficacy, catastrophic interpretations, and increased expectations of failure regarding attempts to engage in rehabilitation.

Fear–avoidance beliefs were one of the most significant predictors of failure to return to work in patients with chronic LBP (Waddell et al. 1993). Operant conditioning reinforces disability if the avoidance provides any short-term benefits, such as reducing anticipatory anxiety or relieving the individual of unwanted responsibilities. In patients with chronic LBP, improvements in disability following physical therapy were associated with decreases in pain, psychological distress, and fear–avoidance beliefs but not in specific physical deficits (Mannion et al. 2001). Decreasing work-specific fears was a more important outcome than addressing general fears of physical activity in predicting improved physical capability for work (Vowles and Gross 2003).

Catastrophic thinking about pain has been attributed to the amplification of threatening information, and it interferes with patients' remaining involved with productive instead of pain-related activities (Crombez et al. 1998). Catastrophizing intensifies the experience of pain and increases emotional distress as well as self-perceived disability (Severeijns et al. 2001; Sullivan et al. 2001). This multidimensional construct includes elements of cognitive rumination, symptom magnification, and feelings of helplessness (Van Damme et al. 2002). Changing negative cognitions improves treatment outcome. Early treatment catastrophizing and helplessness of patients in a 4-week multidisciplinary pain program predicted late-treatment outcomes (Burns et al. 2003).

Pain-related cognitions such as catastrophizing and fear–avoidance beliefs predict poor adjustment to chronic pain better than objective factors such as disease status, physical impairment, or occupational descriptions (Hasenbring et al. 2001). High levels of catastrophizing and fear of injury prospectively predicted disability due to new-onset LBP 6 months later (Picavet et al. 2002). Catastrophizing was the only form of coping significantly associated with poor adjustment to spinal cord injury (Turner et al. 2002).

Anger is distinguished from the trait of hostility and the goal-oriented behavior of aggression (Fernandez and Turk 1995). In a sample of patients with chronic pain, 70%

reported anger that was most commonly directed at themselves (74%) and health care professionals (62%) (Okifuji et al. 1999). Patients have different anger management styles that range from suppression (anger-in) to expression or engagement (anger-out). Women with chronic pain who were low in hostility and high on anger expression were more likely to report lower pain intensity and higher levels of activity (Burns et al. 1996). In contrast, patients who reported the highest levels of pain and associated interference were men with high hostility and suppression of anger.

Pharmacological Treatment

Unfortunately, medications are often underutilized and underdosed. In one study of patients with neuropathic pain, 73% complained of inadequate pain control, but 72% had never received anticonvulsants, 60% TCAs, or 41% opioids, and 25% had never received any of the above (Gilron et al. 2002). Physicians still attempt to alleviate pain with simple analgesics and fail to appreciate the subtleties of the "adjuvant" medications, which possess multiple pharmacological actions.

Opioids

Comprehensive reviews describe opioid pharmacology and opioid peptide systems (Ballantyne and Mao 2003; Bodnar and Hadjimarkou 2002; Inturrisi 2002; Kieffer and Gaveriaux-Ruff 2002; Riedel and Neeck 2001; Vaccarino and Kastin 2001). The analgesic effects of opioids typically decrease the distressing affective component of pain more than the sensation of pain. The treatment of nonmalignant chronic pain with opioids remains a subject of considerable debate, with fears of regulatory pressure, medication abuse, and criminal prosecution creating reluctance to prescribe opioids (Potter et al. 2001; Schug et al. 1991). The prescription of long-term opioids for the treatment of chronic nonmalignant pain has increased (J.D. Clark 2002; Fanciullo et al. 2002).

In the treatment of chronic nonmalignant pain, opioids reduce pain, pain-related disability, depression, insomnia, and physical dysfunction (M.R. Clark 2000b; Moulin et al. 1996; Roth et al. 2000; Sittl et al. 2003). Studies of neuropathic pain show that opioids provide direct analgesic benefits and do not just counteract the unpleasantness of pain (Dellemijn and Vanneste 1997; Watt et al. 1996). Levorphanol reduced pain, affective distress, and interference with function from neuropathic pain (Rowbotham et al. 2003). Continuous-release morphine decreased pain in patients with postherpetic neuralgia significantly more than did TCAs (Raja et al. 2002).

Successful treatment with opioids requires the assessment and documentation of improvements in function and analgesia without accompanying adverse side effects and aberrant behaviors (Nedeljkovic et al. 2002; Passik and Weinreb 2000). The Federation of State Medical Boards, American Academy of Pain Medicine, American Pain Society, and American Geriatrics Society have all produced guidelines for the treatment of chronic pain (American Geriatrics Society Panel on Chronic Pain in Older Persons 1998). With legislation to support these educational and governmental initiatives, attitudes toward, acceptance of, and access to chronic opioid therapy are improving (Joranson et al. 2002). If opioid therapy is unsuccessful, the medication should be gradually tapered and discontinued.

Most long-acting opioids are expensive. Methadone offers a low-cost alternative with the unique advantage of suppressing withdrawal symptoms for more than 24 hours. Unfortunately, the analgesic properties of methadone are similar to those of immediate-release morphine, necessitating a 6-hour dosing schedule for the treatment of chronic pain. Generic formulations of continuous-release morphine and oxycodone offer affordable options. In a randomized, open-label crossover trial in patients with chronic non-cancer pain treated with opioids, transdermal fentanyl was preferred to sustained-release oral morphine (65% vs. 28%), with the greater preference attributed to better pain relief, an enhanced quality of life, and less constipation (Allan et al. 2001). Transdermal fentanyl produced significantly better cost–utility ratios than continuous-release formulations of morphine and oxycodone for each quality-adjusted life year gained despite higher costs of therapy (Neighbors et al. 2001).

Long-term administration of opioids predisposes one to tolerance, but chronic pain may actually facilitate its development (Christensen and Kayser 2000). While several physiological mechanisms have been described to explain this phenomenon, tolerance is uncommon in clinical practice (Borgland 2001; Cahill et al. 2001; Dogrul et al. 2002; Freye and Latasch 2003; Mao et al. 2002; Portenoy 1990). The incidence of analgesic tolerance is lower with more potent opioids such as fentanyl, presumably because they are more receptor specific and fewer receptors are needed to induce an analgesic effect. Although constipation is likely to persist, tolerance to most opioid side effects usually occurs. The loss of preexisting analgesia can have many causes besides tolerance and should be carefully evaluated so as to determine its etiology. Disease progression or other changes in the patient's chronic pain condition should be considered before this loss is attributed to tolerance. A return of, or even an increase in, pain can be the result of new injury, worsening neurological damage, comorbid psychiatric disorders, or medication effects such as toxicity, withdrawal, or opioid-induced hyperalgesia (Liu and Anand 2001).

When tolerance to an analgesic agent develops, suggested strategies have included simultaneous administration of other agents (opioid agonists with differing receptor affinities; ultra-low-dose opioid antagonists; calcium channel blockers; α_2-adrenergic agonists; COX-2 inhibitors; NMDA receptor antagonists such as ketamine, dextromethorphan, memantine, and amantadine); opioid rotation to a more potent agonist; and intermittent cessation of certain agents (e.g., opioids, benzodiazepines) (Bolan et al. 2002; Pasternak 2001). Augmentation of analgesia may occur by using opioids that possess NMDA antagonist action, such as methadone, or those that inhibit monoamine reuptake, such as methadone, tramadol, and levorphanol (Rojas-Corrales et al. 2002; Sang 2000).

Antidepressants

The neurobiology of pain suggests potential efficacy for all antidepressants in the treatment of chronic pain (Ansari 2000; Lynch 2001; Mattia et al. 2002). The analgesic effect of antidepressants is thought to be primarily mediated by the blockade of reuptake of norepinephrine and serotonin, increasing their levels to enhance the activation of descending inhibitory neurons (Ollat and Cesaro 1995). However, antidepressants may produce antinociceptive effects through a variety of other pharmacological mechanisms (Ansari 2000; Carter and Sullivan 2002).

Tricyclic Antidepressants

In 1960, the first report of imipramine use for trigeminal neuralgia was published (Paoli et al. 1960). Since then, antidepressants, particularly the TCAs, have been commonly prescribed for many chronic pain syndromes, including diabetic neuropathy, postherpetic neuralgia, central pain, post-stroke pain, tension-type headache, migraine, and orofacial pain (Ansari 2000; M.R. Clark 2000b; Collins et al. 2000; Lynch 2001). TCAs have been most effective in relieving neuropathic pain and headache syndromes (Gruber et al. 1996; MacFarlane et al. 1997; Max et al. 1987; McQuay et al. 1996; Volmink et al. 1996; Vrethem et al. 1997; Wesselmann and Reich 1996). Meta-analyses of randomized, controlled trials concluded that TCAs are the most effective agents for the treatment of postherpetic neuralgia and that nortriptyline is better tolerated than amitriptyline with equivalent efficacy (Dworkin and Schmader 2003; Lynch 2001; Roose et al. 1981; Volmink et al. 1996; Watson et al. 1988).

Only 25% of patients in one multidisciplinary pain center were prescribed TCAs, and 73% of treated patients were prescribed only the equivalent of 50 mg or less of amitriptyline (Richeimer et al. 1997). The cost of TCAs for pain treatment is much lower than the cost of other antidepressants and most analgesics (Adelman and Von Seggern 1995). A number of treatment studies of postherpetic neuralgia and painful diabetic peripheral neuropathy have used TCAs, with over 60% of patients reporting improvement (Max 1994; Onghena and Van Houdenhove 1992). Typically, the analgesic effects of antidepressants are independent of improvement in mood. Analgesia usually occurs at lower doses and with earlier onset of action than expected for the treatment of depression. The results of investigations to determine drug concentrations needed for pain relief support higher serum levels but remain contradictory (Kishore-Kumar et al. 1990; Sindrup et al. 1989).

Noradrenergic activity is often associated with better analgesic effects than serotonergic activity alone. The relatively noradrenergic antidepressants (i.e., with a serotonin/norepinephrine ratio of less than 1.0) include amitriptyline, imipramine, doxepin, nortriptyline, desipramine, and maprotiline (Richelson 1994). While tertiary amines have been used most commonly, the secondary amines have fewer side effects and are less likely to be discontinued. Randomized, controlled trials have not demonstrated consistent differences in efficacy between the TCAs (Bryson and Wilde 1996; Collins et al. 2000; Sindrup and Jensen 1999, 2000).

Selective Serotonin Reuptake Inhibitors

The selective serotonin reuptake inhibitors (SSRIs) produce weak antinociceptive effects in animal models of acute pain (Gatch et al. 1998; Paul and Hornby 1995; Schreiber et al. 1996). This antinociception is blocked by serotonin receptor antagonists and is enhanced by opioid receptor agonists. In human clinical trials, the efficacy of SSRIs in chronic pain syndromes has been variable and inconsistent (Belcheva et al. 1995; Jung et al. 1997; Tokunaga et al. 1998). Desipramine was superior to fluoxetine in the treatment of painful diabetic peripheral neuropathy (Max et al. 1992). On the other hand, paroxetine and citalopram were beneficial in studies of patients with diabetic neuropathy (Sindrup et al. 1990, 1992). A 12-week course of fluoxetine improved outcome measures in women with fibromyalgia (Arnold et al. 2002). The SSRIs may be effective in the treatment of some headaches, especially migraine (Bank 1994; Foster and Bafaloukos 1994; Saper et al. 1994). Fluvoxamine, but not fluoxetine, improved neuropathic pain independently of antidepressant effects (Ciaramella et al. 2000).

Serotonin-Norepinephrine Reuptake Inhibitors and Other Antidepressants

Venlafaxine and duloxetine inhibit the presynaptic reuptake of both serotonin and norepinephrine. Duloxetine more potently blocks serotonin and norepinephrine transporters (Bymaster et al. 2001). There is evidence of its analgesic efficacy in preclinical models and in clinical populations (Enggaard et al. 2001; Lang et al. 1996). Duloxetine is an effective treatment for major depression and significantly reduced pain complaints in these patients (Detke et al. 2002). Controlled trials have shown duloxetine to be effective in fibromyalgia and painful diabetic neuropathy (Arnold et al. 2005; Goldstein et al. 2005; Raskin et al. 2005). Patients with neuropathic pain following treatment of breast cancer showed pain relief with venlafaxine and improved response at higher doses that may be attributable to increased reuptake inhibition of norepinephrine (Tasmuth et al. 2002). Venlafaxine has also been effective in the treatment of painful diabetic neuropathy and in prophylaxis of migraine (Ozyalcin et al. 2005; Rowbotham et al. 2004). In patients with neuropathic pain but without depression, bupropion decreased pain intensity and interference of pain with quality of life (Semenchuk et al. 2001). In a small open-label trial of diabetic neuropathy, nefazodone significantly reduced pain, paresthesias, and numbness (Goodnick et al. 2000). Monoamine oxidase inhibitors decrease the frequency and severity of migraine headaches (Merikangas and Merikangas 1995). Trazodone is commonly prescribed for insomnia, and several reports suggested efficacy for chronic pain. However, in higher-quality studies, trazodone was ineffective in decreasing pain (Goodkin et al. 1990; Marek et al. 1992).

Anticonvulsants

Phenytoin was first reported as a successful treatment for trigeminal neuralgia in 1942 (Bergouignan 1942). Carbamazepine is the most widely studied anticonvulsant effective for neuropathic pain (Tanelian and Victory 1995). Anticonvulsants are effective for trigeminal neuralgia, diabetic neuropathy, postherpetic neuralgia, and migraine recurrence (McQuay et al. 1995; Tremont-Lukats et al. 2000; Wiffen et al. 2000). Therapeutic serum levels have not been clearly established, but some evidence suggests lower levels than for seizures may be effective in decreasing pain (Moosa et al. 1993).

Valproic acid is most commonly used in the prophylaxis of migraine but is also effective in the treatment of neuropathic pain (R. Jensen et al. 1994). Valproate was an effective prophylactic treatment in over two-thirds of patients with migraine and almost three-quarters of those with cluster headache (Gallagher et al. 2002; Kaniecki 1997; Klapper 1997; Rothrock 1997).

Gabapentin has been reported to reduce neuropathic pain in multiple sclerosis, migraine, postherpetic neuralgia, spinal cord injury, HIV-related neuropathy, and reflex sympathetic dystrophy (Houtchens et al. 1997; La Spina et al. 2001; To et al. 2002; Wetzel and Connelly 1997). Randomized, double-blind, placebo-controlled clinical trials have confirmed the efficacy of gabapentin in the treatment of diabetic peripheral neuropathy, postherpetic neuralgia, and postamputation phantom limb pain (Backonja et al. 1998; Bone et al. 2002; Mellegers et al. 2001; Rice et al. 2001; Rowbotham et al. 1998; Serpell 2002). A retrospective analysis found that patients were more likely to benefit from gabapentin if they had experienced allodynia as a feature of their neuropathic pain (Gustorff et al. 2002).

Lamotrigine may be effective in reducing poststroke pain and the pain of HIV neuropathies, phantom limbs, neuroma hypersensitivity, trigeminal neuralgia, causalgia, and postherpetic neuralgia (T. S. Jensen 2002; Simpson et al. 2003). Lamotrigine decreased the pain of diabetic neuropathy without associated improvements in mood or pain-related disability (Eisen-berg et al. 2001). Lamotrigine produced analgesia that was correlated with serum drug concentrations and comparable to that obtained with phenytoin and dihydrocodeine (Webb and Kamali 1998).

Topiramate, tiagabine, pregabalin, vigabatrin, retigabine, levetiracetam, and zonisamide are new anticonvulsants with a spectrum of pharmacological actions and antinociceptive effects in animal models (Cutrer 2001; Marson et al. 1997). Pregabalin is similar to gabapentin but has greater potency (Bryans and Wustrow 1999; Chen et al. 2001). Pregabalin has been efficacious for the treatment of painful diabetic neuropathy, postherpetic neuralgia, and fibromyalgia (Crofford et al. 2005; Freyn-hagen et al. 2005; Richter et al. 2005; Sabatowski et al. 2004). Topiramate offers the advantages of low protein binding, minimal hepatic metabolism and unchanged renal excretion, few drug interactions, long half-life, and the unusual side effect of weight loss. A pilot study found that tiagabine improved pain symptoms and neuronal function assessed with quantitative sensory testing in patients with painful neuropathy (Novak et al. 2001).

Local Anesthetics

Topical lidocaine has been approved for the treatment of postherpetic neuralgia and does not produce significant serum levels (Argoff 2000). Oral mexiletine has been an effective treatment for neuropathic pain in painful diabetic neuropathy, peripheral nerve injury, alcoholic neuropathy, and phantom limb, but not cancer-related pain (Chabal et al. 1992; Davis 1993; Kalso et al. 1998; Nishiyama and Sakuta 1995). Mexiletine decreased reports not only of pain but also of the accompanying paresthesias and dysesthesias (Dejgard et al. 1988). Mexiletine also has been shown to decrease pain and sleep disturbances associated with painful diabetic neuropathy (Oskarsson et al. 1997).

Calcium Channel Blockers

Verapamil is the most commonly prescribed calcium channel blocker for chronic pain and has proven to be effective in the treatment of migraine and cluster headaches (Lewis and Solomon 1996; Markley 1991). The calcium channel blockers diltiazem and verapamil have also been found to potentiate morphine analgesia (Hodoglugil et al. 1996; Taniguchi et al. 1995). Now in clinical trials, the experimental neuron-specific calcium channel blockers ziconotide and related omega-conopeptides possess potent analgesic, antihyperesthetic, and antiallodynic activity, as well as synergistic analgesic effects with morphine without producing tolerance (Jain 2000; M.T. Smith et al. 2002; Wang et al. 2000).

Benzodiazepines

Benzodiazepines are commonly prescribed for insomnia and anxiety in patients with chronic pain; however, there is little evidence of their utility, and they may be counterproductive (Holister et al. 1981; King and Strain 1990). Only a limited number of chronic pain conditions, such as trigeminal neuralgia, tension headache, and temporomandibular disorder, were found to improve when treated with benzodiazepines (Dellemijn and Fields 1994). Clonazepam has been reported to provide long-term relief of the episodic lancinating variety of phantom limb pain (Bartusch et al. 1996). A recent extensive review failed to conclude that benzodiazepines significantly improve spasticity following spinal cord injury (Taricco et al. 2000).

Benzodiazepines also cause cognitive impairment (Buffett-Jerrott and Stewart 2002; Hendler et al. 1980). In patients with chronic pain, benzodiazepines, but not opioids, were associated with decreased activity levels, higher rates of health care visits, increased domestic instability, depression, and more disability days (Ciccone et al. 2000). Combining benzodiazepines with opioids may cause several problems. In methadone-related mortality, almost 75% of deaths were attributable to a combination of drug effects, and benzodiazepines were present in 74% of the deceased (Caplehorn and Drummer 2002; Ernst et al. 2002). Benzodiazepines have been associated with exacerbation of pain and interference with opioid analgesia (Nemmani and Mogil 2003; Sawynok 1985). They also increase the rate of developing tolerance to opioids (Freye and Latasch 2003).

Psychological Treatment

The biopsychosocial model of chronic pain recognizes the importance of a large number of factors, their interrelationships, and their contributions to ongoing suffering and eventually successful treatment (Keefe et al. 1996; Turk and Okifuji 2002). Controversy persists over which type of psychological treatment is most effective in the treatment of chronic pain. No differences were found between the treatment effects of cognitive versus behavioral therapies in patients mildly disabled by chronic LBP (Turner and Jensen 1993). Cognitive-behavioral therapy (CBT) provided as part of an individual therapy program offered no advantage over a group-based multidisciplinary program over 1 year (Turner-Stokes et al. 2003). Patients who are oriented toward self-management, with decreased perceptions of disability and less negative emotional responses to pain, are those most likely to improve (McCracken and Turk 2002). If treatment effects are to be optimized, more specific psychotherapies need to be designed for different types of pain patients.

Cognitive-Behavioral Therapy

Psychological treatment for chronic pain was pioneered by Fordyce, who used an operant conditioning behavioral model (Fordyce et al. 1973). Pain behaviors such as grimacing, guarding, and taking pain medication are indicators of perceived pain severity and functional disability, and such behaviors predict whether patients receive opioids (Chapman et al. 1985; Romano et al. 1988; Turk and Matyas 1992; Turk and Okifuji 1997). In treatment, productive behaviors are targeted for reinforcement and pain behaviors are targeted for extinction. For patients with chronic LBP, behavioral treatment decreased pain intensity and improved behavioral outcomes, including functional status (van Tulder et al. 2001).

The cognitive-behavioral model of chronic pain assumes that individual perceptions and evaluations of life experiences affect emotional and behavioral reactions to these experiences. If patients believe pain, depression, and disability are inevitable and uncontrollable, they will experience more negative affective responses, increased pain, and even more impaired physical and psychosocial functioning. The components of CBT, such as relaxation, cognitive restructuring, and coping self-statement training, interrupt this cycle of disability and enhance operant-behavioral treatment (Turner 1982; Turner and Chapman 1982). Patients are taught to become active participants in the management of their pain by using methods that minimize distressing thoughts and feelings.

Outcome studies of CBT in patients with syndromes ranging from specific painful diseases to vague functional somatoform symptoms have demonstrated significant improvements in pain intensity, pain behaviors, physical symptoms, affective distress, depression, coping, physical functioning, treatment-related and indirect socioeconomic costs, and return to work (Hiller et al. 2003; Kroenke and Swindle 2000; McCracken and Turk 2002; Morley et al. 1999). Pain reduction and improved physical function have been found to continue up to 12 months after the completion of active CBT (Gardea et al. 2001; Keefe et al. 1990; Nielson and Weir 2001). Patients on sick leave with nonspecific LBP treated with the addition of problem-solving therapy to behavioral graded activity had significantly fewer future sick leave days, higher rates of returning to work, and lower rates of receiving disability pensions (van den Hout et al. 2003). The risk for long-term sick absence of patients with spinal pain was lowered by a factor of 9.3 at 1-year follow-up with a 6-session CBT group intervention (Linton and Andersson 2000). Pain-related fear and catastrophizing of patients were more likely to improve with individually tailored, fear-eliciting, and hierarchically ordered physical movements instead of following a general graded activity treatment program for back pain (Vlaeyen et al. 2002). A CBT program in a military population with nonmalignant chronic pain reduced outpatient visits by 87% in the first 3 months after treatment (Peters et al. 2000).

Mediators of Treatment Effects

The success of CBT has focused attention on many elements of the chronic pain experience to improve outcome. *Adjustment* is defined as the ability to carry out normal physical and psychosocial activities. The three dimensions of adjustment are social functioning (e.g., employment, functional ability), morale (e.g., depression, anxiety), and somatic health (e.g., pain intensity, medication use, health care utilization) (M.P. Jensen et al. 1991; Lazarus and Folkman 1984). These concepts address resilience to the effects of chronic illness, the alleviation of suffering, and the development of a more positive concept of self or identity for the patient (Buchi et al. 2002).

Acceptance of chronic pain is a factor reported to influence patient adjustment. An analysis of patient accounts of their acceptance of chronic pain involved themes such as taking control, living day to day, acknowledging limitations, being empowered, accepting loss of self, believing that there is more to life than pain, not fighting battles that cannot be won, and relying on spiritual strength (Risdon et al. 2003). Acceptance is a realistic approach to living with pain that incorporates both disengagement from struggling against pain and engagement in productive everyday activities with achievable goals. Acceptance of pain is associated with reports of lower pain intensity, less pain-related anxiety and avoidance, less depression, less physical and psychosocial disability, more daily uptime, and better work status (McCracken 1998).

The effectiveness of particular coping strategies is dependent on many aspects of a patient's experience. In a 6-month follow-up study of patients completing an inpatient pain program, improvement was associated with decreases in the use of passive coping strategies such as taking medications or hoping pain will decrease (M.P. Jensen et al. 1994). Some types of emotion-focused coping are adaptive for some patients. For example, patients with myofascial pain were significantly more likely to report pain, impairment, and depression if they used passive coping strategies in contrast to emotion-focused coping, which was associated with significantly better adjustment (J.A. Smith et al. 2002). The active coping strategies concept is consistent with the cognitive-behavioral model of chronic pain, although it still remains unclear how many unique coping strategies exist and whether changes in coping lead to or are the result of changes in patient adjustment (Hadjistavropoulos et al. 1999; M.P. Jensen et al. 1991; Tan et al. 2001).

Placebo Response

Placebo effects are complex phenomena but similar to the effects of active treatments (Turner et al. 1994). The literature supporting the placebo effect has been criticized as flawed, misinterpreted, and overrated (Kienle and Kienle 1997). In a clinical setting it is difficult to separate "true" improvements from placebo responses to treatment as well as other factors such as regression to the mean and the natural history of the condition. Multiple patient and practitioner characteristics, such as expectancy, conditioning, and learning, affect the placebo response, and most are almost impossible to control for (Ploghaus et al. 2003; Price et al. 1999). Evidence supports a role of the endogenous opioid and sympathetic nervous systems in placebo-induced analgesia that can be reversed with opioid antagonists (Pollo et al. 2003; ter Riet et al. 1998).

Multidisciplinary Treatment

Methodology

Patients with chronic pain suffer dramatic reductions in physical, psychological, and social well-being with lower-rated health-related quality of life than those with almost all other medical conditions (Becker et al. 1997; Skevington 1998). The multidisciplinary pain center offers the full range of treatments for the most difficult pain syndromes in a setting that encourages patients to take an active role in improving their functional status and reinforces positive changes in behavior (Gibson et al. 1996; Helme et al. 1996). Specifically, interventions are designed to change maladaptive behavior such as inactivity and social withdrawal; alter maladaptive cognitions such as somatization, catastrophizing, and passive expectations of medical care; adopt active and positive coping skills; identify and stop operant conditioned behavior; and increase emotional control and stability while decreasing affective distress and depression.

Effectiveness

Multidisciplinary pain programs improve patient functioning globally and in a number of specific areas, especially pain intensity, depression, disability, pain-related cognitions, and coping responses (Cutler et al. 1994; Fishbain et al. 1993; Flavell et al. 1996; M.P. Jensen et al. 2001). Multidisciplinary rehabilitation programs that include psychological and cognitive treatment are known to be effective for the treatment of chronic pain (Cutler et al. 1994; Fishbain et al. 1993; Flavell et al. 1996; Flor et al. 1992). Quality of life improves with multidisciplinary pain treatment, and good quality of life is associated with low levels of pain, distress, and interference with performing daily activities (Skevington et al. 2001). A meta-analysis of 65 studies evaluated the efficacy of treatments in patients who attended multidisciplinary pain clinics (Flor et al. 1992). Combination treatments were superior to unimodal treatments, treatment effects were maintained over a period of up to 7 years, and improvements were found not only on subjective but also on objective measures such as return to work and decreased health care utilization.

Ultimately, the goal of treating patients with chronic pain is to end disability and return them to work or other productive activities. Patients with chronic pain encounter many obstacles to returning to work, including their own negative perceptions and beliefs about work, such as poor self-efficacy and use of maladaptive coping strategies (Grossi et al. 1999; Marhold et al. 2002; Schult et al. 2000). In a longitudinal follow-up study of chronic back pain, patients who were not working and involved in litigation had the highest scores on measures of pain, depression, and disability (Suter 2002). One of the most important predictors is the patient's own intention of returning to work (Fishbain et al. 1997b). For example, job availability, satisfaction, dangerousness, physical demands, and litigation status are more likely to influence a patient's return to work (Fishbain et al. 1995, 1999a; Hildebrandt et al. 1997). In the longest follow-up study (13 years) of an inpatient pain management program, only half of the patients were unemployed, compared with almost 90% of the patients at the time of their admission (Maruta et al. 1998).

References

Adams MA, Mannion AF, Nolan P: Personal risk factors for first time low back pain. Spine 24:2497–2505, 1999

Adelman JU, Von Seggern R: Cost considerations in headache treatment, part 1: prophylactic migraine treatment. Headache 35:479–487, 1995

Allan L, Hays H, Jensen NH, et al: Randomised crossover trial of transdermal fentanyl and sustained release oral morphine for treating chronic non-cancer pain. BMJ 322:1154–1158, 2001

American Academy of Pain Medicine, the American Pain Society, and the American Society of Addiction Medicine: Definitions related to the use of opioids for the treatment of pain. WMJ 100:28–29, 2001

American Geriatrics Society Panel on Chronic Pain in Older Persons: The management of chronic pain in older persons. J Am Geriatr Soc 46:635–651, 1998

American Psychiatric Association: Diagnostic and Statistical Manual of Mental Disorders, 2nd Edition. Washington, DC, American Psychiatric Press, 1968

American Psychiatric Association: Diagnostic and Statistical Manual of Mental Disorders, 3rd Edition. Washington, DC, American Psychiatric Press, 1980

American Psychiatric Association: Diagnostic and Statistical Manual of Mental Disorders, 3rd Edition, Revised. Washington, DC, American Psychiatric Press, 1987

American Psychiatric Association: Diagnostic and Statistical Manual of Mental Disorders, 4th Edition. Washington, DC, American Psychiatric Press, 1994

American Psychiatric Association: Diagnostic and Statistical Manual of Mental Disorders, 4th Edition, Text Revision. Washington, DC, American Psychiatric Press, 2000

Ansari A: The efficacy of newer antidepressants in the treatment of chronic pain: a review of current literature. Harv Rev Psychiatry 7:257–277, 2000

Argoff CE: New analgesics for neuropathic pain: the lidocaine patch. Clin J Pain 16:S62–S66, 2000

Arnold LM, Hess EV, Hudson JI, et al: A randomized, placebo-controlled, double-blind, flexible-dose study of fluoxetine in the treatment of women with fibromyalgia. Am J Med 112:191–197, 2002

Arnold LM, Rosen A, Pritchett YL, et al: A randomized, double-blind, placebo-controlled trial of duloxetine in the treatment of women with fibromyalgia with or without major depressive disorder. Pain 119:5–15, 2005

Aronoff GM: Opioids in chronic pain management: is there a significant risk of addiction? Curr Rev Pain 4:112–121, 2000

Aronoff GM, Tota-Faucette M, Phillips L, et al: Are pain disorder and somatization disorder valid diagnostic entities? Curr Rev Pain 4:309–312, 2000

Asmundson GJG, Norton PJ, Norton GR: Beyond pain: the role of fear and avoidance in chronicity. Clin Psychol Rev 19:97–119, 1999

Atkinson JH, Slater MA, Patterson TL, et al: Prevalence, onset and risk of psychiatric disorders in men with chronic low back pain: a controlled study. Pain 45:111–121, 1991

Auerbach SM, Laskin DM, Frantsve LM, et al: Depression, pain, exposure to stressful life events, and long-term outcomes in temporomandibular disorder patients. J Oral Maxillofac Surg 59:628–633, 2001

Backonja M, Beydoun A, Edwards KR, et al: Gabapentin for the symptomatic treatment of painful neuropathy in patients with diabetes mellitus: a randomized controlled trial. JAMA 280:1831–1836, 1998

Bair MJ, Robinson RL, Katon W, et al: Depression and pain comorbidity: a literature review. Arch Intern Med 163:2433–2445, 2003

Ballantyne JC, Mao J: Opioid therapy for chronic pain. N Engl J Med 349:1943–1953, 2003

Bank J: A comparative study of amitriptyline and fluvoxamine in migraine prophylaxis. Headache 34:476–478, 1994

Bartusch SL, Sanders BJ, D'Alessio JG, et al: Clonazepam for the treatment of lacinating phantom limb pain. Clin J Pain 12:59–62, 1996

Becker N, Bondegaard Thomsen A, Olsen AK, et al: Pain epidemiology and health related quality of life in chronic non-malignant pain patients referred to a Danish multidisciplinary pain center. Pain 73:393–400, 1997

Belcheva S, Petkov VD, Konstantinova E, et al: Effects on nociception of the Ca2+ and 5-HT antagonist dotarizine and other 5-HT receptor agonists and antagonists. Acta Physiol Pharmacol Bulg 21:93–98, 1995

Bergouignan M: Cures heureuses de nevralgies faciales essentielles par le diphenyl-hydantoinate de soude. Rev Laryngol Otol Rhinol 63:34–41, 1942

Bodnar RJ, Hadjimarkou MM: Endogenous opiates and behavior: 2001. Peptides 23:2307–2365, 2002

Bogetto F, Maina G, Ferro G, et al: Psychiatric comorbidity in patients with burning mouth syndrome. Psychosom Med 60:378–385, 1998

Bolan EA, Tallarida RJ, Pasternak GW: Synergy between mu opioid ligands: evidence for functional interactions among mu opioid receptor subtypes. J Pharmacol Exp Ther 303:557–562, 2002

Bolay H, Moskowitz MA: Mechanisms of pain modulation in chronic syndromes. Neurology 59 (suppl 2):S2–S7, 2002

Bone M, Critchley P, Buggy DJ: Gabapentin in postamputation phantom limb pain: a randomized, double-blind, placebo-controlled, cross-over study. Reg Anesth Pain Med 27:481–516, 2002

Bonica JJ: Definitions and taxonomy of pain, in The Management of Pain. Edited by Bonica JJ. Philadelphia, PA, Lea & Febiger, 1990, pp 18–27

Borgland SL: Acute opioid receptor desensitization and tolerance: is there a link? Clin Exp Pharmacol Physiol 28:147–154, 2001

Bowsher D: The management of central post-stroke pain. Postgrad Med J 71:598–604, 1995

Bowsher D: Postherpetic neuralgia and its treatment: a retrospective survey of 191 patients. J Pain Symptom Manage 12:290–299, 1996

Bowsher D: The effects of pre-emptive treatment of postherpetic neuralgia with amitriptyline: a randomized, double-blind, placebo-controlled trial. J Pain Symptom Manage 13:327–331, 1997a

Bowsher D: The management of postherpetic neuralgia. Postgrad Med J 73:623–629, 1997b

Breslau N, Davis GC: Migraine, physical health and psychiatric disorder: a prospective epidemiologic study in young adults. J Psychiatr Res 27:211–221, 1993

Brown RL, Patterson JJ, Rounds LA, et al: Substance use among patients with chronic pain. J Fam Pract 43:152–160, 1996

Bruehl S, Carlson CR: Predisposing psychological factors in the development of reflex sympathetic dystrophy: a review of the empiric evidence. Clin J Pain 8:287–299, 1992

Bryans JS, Wustrow DJ: 3-substituted GABA analogs with central nervous system activity: a review. Med Res Rev 19:149–177, 1999

Bryson HM, Wilde MI: Amitriptyline: a review of its pharmacological properties and therapeutic use in chronic pain states. Drugs Aging 8:459–476, 1996

Buchi S, Buddeberg C, Klaghofer R, et al: Preliminary validation of PRISM (Pictorial Representation of Illness and Self Measure): a brief method to assess suffering. Psychother Psychosom 71:333–341, 2002

Buffett-Jerrott SE, Stewart SH: Cognitive and sedative effects of benzodiazepine use. Curr Pharm Des 8:45–58, 2002

Burkey AR, Carstens E, Wenniger JJ, et al: An opioidergic cortical antinociception triggering site in the agranular insular cortex of the rat that contributes to morphine antinociception. J Neurosci 16:6612–6623, 1996

Burns JW, Johnson BJ, Mahoney N, et al: Anger management style, hostility and spouse responses: gender differences in predictors of adjustment among chronic pain patients. Pain 64:445–453, 1996

Burns JW, Kubilus A, Bruehl S, et al: Do changes in cognitive factors influence outcome following multidisciplinary treatment for chronic pain? A cross-lagged panel analysis. J Consult Clin Psychol 71:81–91, 2003

Bymaster FP, Dreshfield-Ahmad LJ, Threlkeld PG, et al: Comparative affinity of duloxetine and venlafaxine for serotonin and norepinephrine transporters in vitro and in vivo, human serotonin receptor subtypes, and other neuronal receptors. Neuropsychopharmacology 25:871–880, 2001

Cahill CM, Morinville A, Lee MC, et al: Prolonged morphine treatment targets delta opioid receptors to neuronal plasma membranes and enhances delta-mediated antinociception. J Neurosci 21:7598–7607, 2001

Caplehorn JR, Drummer OH: Fatal methadone toxicity: signs and circumstances, and the role of benzodiazepines. Aust N Z J Public Health 26:358–362, 2002

Carey TS, Garrett JM, Jackman AM: Beyond the good prognosis: examination of an inception cohort of patients with chronic low back pain. Spine 25:115–120, 2000

Carter GT, Sullivan MD: Antidepressants in pain management. Curr Opin Invest Drugs 3:454–458, 2002

Chabal C, Jacobson L, Mariano AJ, et al: The use of oral mexiletine for the treatment of pain after peripheral nerve injury. Anesthesiology 76:513–517, 1992

Chabal C, Erjavec MK, Jacobson L, et al: Prescription opiate abuse in chronic pain patients: clinical criteria, incidence, and predictors. Clin J Pain 13:150–155, 1997

Chapman CR, Casey KL, Dubner R, et al: Pain measurement: an overview. Pain 22:1–31, 1985

Chen SR, Xu Z, Pan HL: Stereospecific effect of pregabalin on ectopic afferent discharges and neuropathic pain induced by sciatic nerve ligation in rats. Anesthesiology 95:1473–1479, 2001

Cheshire WP: Defining the role for gabapentin in the treatment of trigeminal neuralgia: a retrospective study. J Pain 3:137–142, 2002

Christensen D, Kayser V: The development of pain-related behaviour and opioid tolerance after neuropathy-inducing surgery and sham surgery. Pain 88:231–238, 2000

Ciaramella A, Grosso S, Poli P: Fluoxetine versus fluvoxamine for treatment of chronic pain. Minerva Anestesiol 66:55–61, 2000

Ciccone DS, Just N, Bandilla EB: A comparison of economic and social reward in patients with chronic nonmalignant back pain. Psychosom Med 61:552–563, 1999

Ciccone DS, Just N, Bandilla EB, et al: Psychological correlates of opioid use in patients with chronic nonmalignant pain: a preliminary test of the downhill spiral hypothesis. J Pain Symptom Manage 20:180–192, 2000

Clark JD: Chronic pain prevalence and analgesic prescribing in a general medical population. J Pain Symptom Manage 23: 131–137, 2002

Clark MR: Pain, in Textbook of Geriatric Neuropsychiatry. Edited by Coffey CE, Cummings JL. Washington, DC, American Psychiatric Press, 2000a, pp 415–440

Clark MR: Pharmacological treatments for chronic nonmalignant pain. Int Rev Psychiatry 12:148–156, 2000b

Clark MR, Cox TS: Refractory Chronic Pain. Psychiatr Clin North Am 25:71–88, 2002

Clark WC, Yang JC, Tsui SL, et al: Unidimensional pain rating scales: a multidimensional affect and pain survey (MAPS) analysis of what they really measure. Pain 98:241–247, 2002

Collins SL, Moore RA, McQuay HJ, et al: Antidepressants and anticonvulsants for diabetic neuropathy and postherpetic neuralgia: a quantitative systematic review. J Pain Symptom Manage 20:449–458, 2000

Compton P, Darakjian J, Miotto K: Screening for addiction in patients with chronic pain and "problematic" substance use: evaluation of a pilot assessment tool. J Pain Symptom Manage 16:355–363, 1998

Cote P, Hogg-Johnson S, Cassidy JD, et al: The association between neck pain intensity, physical functioning, depressive symptomatology and time-to-claim-closure after whiplash. J Clin Epidemiol 54:275–286, 2001

Crofford LJ, Rowbotham MC, Mease PJ, et al: Pregabalin for the treatment of fibromyalgia syndrome: results of a randomized, double-blind, placebo-controlled trial. Arthritis Rheum 52:1264–1273, 2005

Croft PR, Papageorgiou AC, Ferry S, et al: Psychological distress and low back pain: evidence from a prospective study in the general population. Spine 20:2731–2737, 1996

Crombez G, Eccleston C, Baeyens F, et al: When somatic information threatens, catastrophic thinking enhances attentional interference. Pain 75:187–198, 1998

Cutler BR, Fishbain DA, Rosomoff HL, et al: Does nonsurgical pain center treatment of chronic pain return patients to work? A review and meta-analysis of the literature. Spine 19:643–652, 1994

Cutrer FM: Antiepileptic drugs: how they work in headache. Headache 41:S3–S10, 2001

Davis RW: Successful treatment for phantom pain. Orthopaedics 16:691–695, 1993

DeBerard MS, Masters KS, Colledge AL, et al: Outcomes of posterolateral lumbar fusion in Utah patients receiving workers' compensation: a retrospective cohort study. Spine 26:738–746, 2001

Dejgard A, Petersen P, Kastrup J: Mexiletine for treatment of chronic painful diabetic neuropathy. Lancet 1:9–11, 1988

Dellemijn PL, Fields HL: Do benzodiazepines have a role in chronic pain management? Pain 57:137–152, 1994

Dellemijn PL, Vanneste JA: Randomised double-blind active-placebo-controlled crossover trial of intravenous fentanyl in neuropathic pain. Lancet 349:753–758, 1997

Dersh J, Polatin PB, Gatchel RJ: Chronic pain and psychopathology: research findings and theoretical considerations. Psychosom Med 64:773–786, 2002

Detke MJ, Lu Y, Goldstein DJ, et al: Duloxetine 60 mg once daily dosing versus placebo in the acute treatment of major depression. J Psychiatr Res 36:383–390, 2002

Devor M, Amir R, Rappaport ZH: Pathophysiology of trigeminal neuralgia: the ignition hypothesis. Clin J Pain 18:4–13, 2002

Deyo RA, Weinstein JN: Low back pain. N Engl J Med 344:363–370, 2001

Dickens C, Jayson M, Sutton C, et al: The relationship between pain and depression in a trial using paroxetine in sufferers of chronic low back pain. Psychosomatics 41:490–499, 2000

Dickinson WP, Dickinson LM, deGruy FV, et al: The somatization in primary care study: a tale of three diagnoses. Gen Hosp Psychiatry 25:1–7, 2003

Dogrul A, Zagli U, Tulunay FC: The role of T-type calcium channels in morphine analgesia, development of antinociceptive tolerance and dependence to morphine, and morphine abstinence syndrome. Life Sci 71:725–734, 2002

Drage LA, Rogers RS 3rd: Burning mouth syndrome. Dermatol Clin 21:135–145, 2003

Druss BG, Rosenheck RA, Sledge WH: Health and disability costs of depressive illness in a major U.S. corporation. Am J Psychiatry 157:1274–1278, 2000

Dworkin RH, Schmader KE: Treatment and prevention of postherpetic neuralgia. Clin Infect Dis 36:877–882, 2003

Dworkin SF, Von Korff M, LeResche L: Multiple pains and psychiatric disturbance: an epidemiologic investigation. Arch Gen Psychiatry 47:239–244, 1990

Dworkin SF, Huggins KH, Wilson L, et al: A randomized clinical trial using research diagnostic criteria for temporomandibular disorders-axis II to target clinic cases for a tailored self-care TMD treatment program. J Orofac Pain 16:48–63, 2002

Edwards R, Augustson EM, Fillingim R: Sex-specific effects of pain-related anxiety on adjustment to chronic pain. Clin J Pain 16:46–53, 2000

Ehde DM, Jensen MP, Engel JM, et al: Chronic pain secondary to disability: a review. Clin J Pain 19:3–17, 2003

Eide PK, Stubhaug A, Stenehjem AE: Central dysesthesia pain after traumatic spinal cord injury is dependent on N-methyl-D-aspartate receptor activation. Neurosurgery 37:1080–1087, 1995

Eisenberg E, Lurie Y, Braker C, et al: Lamotrigine reduces painful diabetic neuropathy: a randomized controlled study. Neurology 57:505–509, 2001

Elias WJ, Burchiel KJ: Trigeminal neuralgia and other neuropathic pain syndromes of the head and face. Curr Pain Headache Rep 6:115–124, 2002

Emanuel EJ, Fairclough DL, Daniels ER, et al: Euthanasia and physician-assisted suicide: attitudes and experiences of oncology patients, oncologists, and the public. Lancet 347:1805–1810, 1996

Enggaard TP, Klitgaard NA, Gram LF, et al: Specific effect of venlafaxine on single and repetitive experimental painful stimuli in humans. Clin Pharmacol Ther 69:245–251, 2001

Epker J, Gatchel RJ: Coping profile differences in the biopsychosocial functioning of patients with temporomandibular disorder. Psychosom Med 62:69–75, 2000

Ernst E, Bartu A, Popescu A, et al: Methadone-related deaths in Western Australia 1993–99. Aust NZ J Public Health 26:364–370, 2002

Fanciullo GJ, Ball PA, Girault G, et al: An observational study on the prevalence and pattern of opioid use in 25,479 patients with spine and radicular pain. Spine 27:201–205, 2002

Feldman SI, Downey G, Schaffer-Neitz R: Pain, negative mood, and perceived support in chronic pain patients: a daily diary study of people with reflex sympathetic dystrophy syndrome. J Consult Clin Psychol 67:776–785, 1999

Fernandez E, Turk DC: The scope and significance of anger in the experience of chronic pain. Pain 61:165–175, 1995

Fields HL, Rowbotham M, Baron R: Postherpetic neuralgia: irritable nociceptors and deafferentation. Neurobiol Dis 5:209–227, 1998

Fishbain DA, Goldberg M, Meagher BR, et al: Male and female chronic pain patients characterized by DSM-III diagnostic criteria. Pain 26:181–187, 1986

Fishbain DA, Goldberg M, Rosomoff RS, et al: Completed suicide in chronic pain. Clin J Pain 7:29–36, 1991

Fishbain DA, Rosomoff HL, Rosomoff RS: Drug abuse, dependence: addiction in chronic pain patients. Clin J Pain 8:77–85, 1992

Fishbain DA, Rosomoff HL, Goldberg M, et al: The prediction of return to the workplace after multidisciplinary pain center treatment. Clin J Pain 9:3–15, 1993

Fishbain DA, Rosomoff HL, Cutler RB, et al: Do chronic pain patients' perceptions about their preinjury jobs determine their intent to return to the same type of job post-pain facility treatment? Clin J Pain 11:267–278, 1995

Fishbain DA, Cutler R, Rosomoff HL, et al: Chronic pain-associated depression: antecedent or consequence of chronic pain? A review. Clin J Pain 13:116–137, 1997a

Fishbain DA, Cutler RB, Rosomoff HL, et al: Impact of chronic pain patients' job perception variables on actual return to work. Clin J Pain 13:197–206, 1997b

Fishbain D, Cutler R, Rosomoff H: Comorbid psychiatric disorders in chronic pain patients. Pain Clin 11:79–87, 1998

Fishbain DA, Cutler RB, Rosomoff HL, et al: Prediction of "intent," "discrepancy with intent," and "discrepancy with nonintent" for the patient with chronic pain to return to work after treatment at a pain facility. Clin J Pain 15:141–150, 1999a

Fishbain DA, Cutler RB, Rosomoff HL, et al: Validity of self-report drug use in chronic pain patients. Clin J Pain 15:184–191, 1999b

Fisher BJ, Haythornthwaite JA, Heinberg LJ, et al: Suicidal intent in patients with chronic pain. Pain 89:199–206, 2001

Fishman SM, Mahajan G, Jung S, et al: The trilateral opioid contract: bridging the pain clinic and the primary care physician through the opioid contract. J Pain Symptom Manage 24:335–344, 2002

Flavell HA, Carrafa GP, Thomas CH, et al: Managing chronic back pain: impact of an interdisciplinary team approach. Med J Aust 165:253–255, 1996

Flor H, Fydrich T, Turk DC: Efficacy of multidisciplinary pain treatment centers: a meta-analytic review. Pain 49:221–230, 1992

Foley K: Pain in the elderly, in Principles of Geriatric Medicine and Gerontology. Edited by Hazzard WR, Bierman EL, Blass JP, et al. New York, McGraw-Hill, 1994, pp 317–331

Fordyce W, Fowler R, Lehmann J, et al: Operant conditioning in the treatment of chronic pain. Arch Phys Med Rehabil 54:399–408, 1973

Forseth KO, Husby G, Gran JT, et al: Prognostic factors for the development of fibromyalgia in women with self-reported musculoskeletal pain: a prospective study. J Rheumatol 26: 2458–2467, 1999

Foster CA, Bafaloukos J: Paroxetine in the treatment of chronic daily headache. Headache 34:587–589, 1994

Freye E, Latasch L: Development of opioid tolerance: molecular mechanisms and clinical consequences. Anasthesiol Intensivmed Notfallmed Schmerzther 38:14–26, 2003

Freynhagen R, Strojek K, Griesing T, et al: Efficacy of pregabalin in neuropathic pain evaluated in a 12-week, randomised, double-blind, multicentre, placebo-controlled trial of flexible- and fixed-dose regimens. Pain 115:254–263, 2005

Gallagher RM, Mueller LL, Freitag FG: Divalproex sodium in the treatment of migraine and cluster headache. J Am Osteopath Assoc 102:92–94, 2002

Gardea MA, Gatchel RJ, Mishra KD: Long-term efficacy of biobehavioral treatment of temporomandibular disorders. J Behav Med 24:341–359, 2001

Gatch MB, Negus SS, Mello NK: Antinociceptive effects of monoamine reuptake inhibitors administered alone or in combination with mu opioid agonists in rhesus monkeys. Psychopharmacology 135:99–106, 1998

Geisser ME, Roth RS, Theisen ME, et al: Negative affect, self-report of depressive symptoms, and clinical depression: relation to the experience of chronic pain. Clin J Pain 16:110–120, 2000

Gibson SJ, Farrell MJ, Katz B, et al: Multidisciplinary management of chronic nonmalignant pain in older adults, in Pain in the Elderly. Edited by Ferrell BR, Ferrell BA. Seattle, WA, IASP Press, 1996, pp 91–99

Gilron I, Bailey J, Weaver DF, et al: Patients' attitudes and prior treatments in neuropathic pain: a pilot study. Pain Res Manag 7:199–203, 2002

Gilson AM, Joranson DE: U.S. policies relevant to the prescribing of opioid analgesics for the treatment of pain in patients with addictive disease. Clin J Pain 18:S91–S98, 2002

Goadsby PJ: How do the currently used prophylactic agents work in migraine? Cephalalgia 17:85–92, 1997

Goldstein DJ, Lu Y, Detke MJ, et al: Duloxetine vs. placebo in patients with painful diabetic neuropathy. Pain 116:109–118, 2005

Goodkin K, Gullion C, Agras WS: A randomized, double-blind, placebo-controlled trial of trazodone hydrochloride in chronic low back pain syndrome. J Clin Psychopharmacol 10:269–278, 1990

Goodnick PJ, Breakstone K, Kumar A, et al: Nefazodone in diabetic neuropathy: response and biology. Psychosom Med 62:599–600, 2000

Grabe HJ, Meyer C, Hapke U, et al: Somatoform pain disorder in the general population. Psychother Psychosom 72:88–94, 2003

Greenberg J, Burns JW: Pain anxiety among chronic pain patients: specific phobia or manifestation of anxiety sensitivity? Behav Res Ther 41:223–240, 2003

Grossi G, Soares JJ, Angesleva J, et al: Psychosocial correlates of long-term sick-leave among patients with musculoskeletal pain. Pain 80:607–619, 1999

Gruber AJ, Hudson JI, Pope HG Jr: The management of treatment-resistant depression in disorders on the interface of psychiatry and medicine: fibromyalgia, chronic fatigue syndrome, migraine, irritable bowel syndrome, atypical facial pain, and premenstrual dysphoric disorder. Psychiatr Clin North Am 19:351–369, 1996

Gureje O, Von Korff M, Simon GE, et al: Persistent pain and well-being: a World Health Organization study in primary care. JAMA 280:147–151, 1998

Gustorff B, Nahlik G, Spacek A, et al: Gabapentin in the treatment of chronic intractable pain. Schmerz 16:9–14, 2002

Hadjistavropoulos HD, MacLeod FK, Asmundson GJ: Validation of the Chronic Pain Coping Inventory. Pain 80:471–481, 1999

Hasenbring M, Marienfeld G, Kuhlendahl D, et al: Risk factors of chronicity in lumbar disc patients: a prospective investigation of biologic, psychologic, and social predictors of therapy outcome. Spine 19:2759–2765, 1994

Hasenbring M, Hallner D, Klasen B: Psychological mechanisms in the transition from acute to chronic pain: over- or underrated? Schmerz 15:442–447, 2001

Hasselstrom J, Liu-Palmgren J, Rasjo-Wraak G: Prevalence of pain in general practice. Eur J Pain 6:375–385, 2002

Haythornthwaite JA, Sieber WJ, Kerns RD: Depression and the chronic pain experience. Pain 46:177–184, 1991

Hein S, Bonsignore M, Barkow K, et al: Lifetime depressive and somatic symptoms as preclinical markers of late-onset depression. Eur Arch Psychiatry Clin Neurosci 253:16–21, 2003

Helme RD, Katz B, Gibson SJ, et al: Multidisciplinary pain clinics for older people: do they serve a role? Clin Geriatr Med 12:563–582, 1996

Hendler N, Cimini C, Ma T, et al: A comparison of cognitive impairment due to benzodiazepines and to narcotics. Am J Psychiatry 137:828–830, 1980

Hildebrandt J, Pfingsten M, Saur P, et al: Prediction of success from a multidisciplinary treatment program for chronic low back pain. Spine 22:990–1001, 1997

Hiller W, Fichter MM, Rief W: A controlled treatment study of somatoform disorders including analysis of healthcare utilization and cost-effectiveness. J Psychosom Res 54:369–380, 2003

Hodoglugil U, Guney HZ, Savran B, et al: Temporal variation in the interaction between calcium channel blockers and morphine-induced analgesia. Chronobiol Int 13:227–234, 1996

Hoffman NG, Olofsson O, Salen B, et al: Prevalence of abuse and dependency in chronic pain patients. Int J Addict 30:919–927, 1995

Holister LE, Conley FK, Britt R, et al: Longterm use of diazepam. JAMA 246:1568–1570, 1981

Holroyd KA, O'Donnell FJ, Stensland M, et al: Management of chronic tension-type headache with tricyclic antidepressant medication, stress management therapy, and their combination: a randomized controlled trial. JAMA 285:2208–2215, 2001

Houtchens MK, Richert JR, Sami A, et al: Open label gabapentin treatment for pain in multiple sclerosis. Mult Scler 3:250–253, 1997

Hunt SP, Mantyh PW: The molecular dynamics of pain control. Nat Rev Neurosci 2:83–91, 2001

Huppe A, Raspe H: Efficacy of inpatient rehabilitation for chronic back pain in Germany: a systematic review 1980–2001. Rehabilitation 42:143–154, 2003

Inturrisi CE: Clinical pharmacology of opioids for pain. Clin J Pain 18:S3–S13, 2002

Jain KK: An evaluation of intrathecal ziconotide for the treatment of chronic pain. Expert Opin Investig Drugs 9:2403–2410, 2000

Jamison RN, Kauffman J, Katz NP: Characteristics of methadone maintenance patients with chronic pain. J Pain Symptom Manage 19:53–62, 2000

Jensen MP, Turner JA, Romano JM, et al: Coping with chronic pain: a critical review of the literature. Pain 47:249–283, 1991

Jensen MP, Turner JA, Romano JM: Correlates of improvement in multidisciplinary treatment of chronic pain. J Consult Clin Psychol 62:172–179, 1994

Jensen MP, Turner JA, Romano JM: Changes in beliefs, catastrophizing, and coping are associated with improvement in multidisciplinary pain treatment. J Consult Clin Psychol 69:655–662, 2001

Jensen R, Brinck T, Olesen J: Sodium valproate has a prophylactic effect in migraine without aura: a triple-blind, placebo-controlled crossover study. Neurology 44:647–651, 1994

Jensen TS: Anticonvulsants in neuropathic pain: rationale and clinical evidence. Eur J Pain 6 (suppl A):61–68, 2002

Johnson RW, Dworkin RH: Treatment of herpes zoster and postherpetic neuralgia. BMJ 326:748–750, 2003

Joranson DE, Gilson AM, Dahl JL, et al: Pain management, controlled substances, and state medical board policy: a decade of change. J Pain Symptom Manage 23:138–147, 2002

Juang KD, Wang SJ, Fuh JL, et al: Comorbidity of depressive and anxiety disorders in chronic daily headache and its subtypes. Headache 40:818–823, 2000

Jung AC, Staiger T, Sullivan M: The efficacy of selective serotonin reuptake inhibitors for the management of chronic pain. J Gen Intern Med 12:384–389, 1997

Junge A, Dvorak J, Ahrens S: Predictors of bad and good outcomes of lumbar disc surgery: a prospective clinical study with recommendations for screening to avoid bad outcomes. Spine 20:460–468, 1995

Kalso E, Tramer MR, McQuay HJ, et al: Systemic local-anaesthetic-type drugs in chronic pain: a systematic review. Eur J Pain 2:3–14, 1998

Kaniecki RG: A comparison of divalproex with propranolol and placebo for the prophylaxis of migraine without aura. Arch Neurol 54:1141–1145, 1997

Kapur N, Kamel IR, Herlich A: Oral and craniofacial pain: diagnosis, pathophysiology, and treatment. Int Anesthesiol Clin 41:115–150, 2003

Karjalainen K, Malmivaara A, van Tulder M, et al: Multidisciplinary biopsychosocial rehabilitation for subacute low back pain among working age adults. Cochrane Database Syst Rev 1:CD002193, 2003

Katon W, Sullivan M: Depression and a chronic medical illness. J Clin Psychiatry 150 (suppl):3–11, 1990

Katon W, Egan K, Miller D: Chronic pain: lifetime psychiatric diagnoses and family history. Am J Psychiatry 142:1156–1160, 1985

Katz N, Fanciullo GJ: Role of urine toxicology testing in the management of chronic opioid therapy. Clin J Pain 18:S76–S82, 2002

Katz PP, Yelin EH: Prevalence and correlates of depressive symptoms among persons with rheumatoid arthritis. J Rheumatol 20:790–796, 1993

Keefe FJ, Caldwell DS, Williams DA, et al: Pain coping skills training in the management of osteoarthritic knee pain, II: follow-up results. Behav Ther 21:435–447, 1990

Keefe FJ, Beaupre PM, Weiner DK, et al: Pain in older adults: a cognitive-behavioral perspective, in Pain in the Elderly. Edited by Ferrell BR, Ferrell BA. Seattle, WA, IASP Press, 1996, pp 11–19

Kieffer BL, Gaveriaux-Ruff C: Exploring the opioid system by gene knockout. Prog Neurobiol 66:285–306, 2002

Kienle GS, Kienle H: The powerful placebo effect: fact or fiction? J Clin Epidemiol 50:1311–1318, 1997

King SA: The classification and assessment of pain. Int Rev Psychiatry 12:86–90, 2000

King SA, Strain JJ: Benzodiazepine use by chronic pain patients. Clin J Pain 6:143–147, 1990

Kirsh KL, Whitcomb LA, Donaghy K, et al: Abuse and addiction issues in medically ill patients with pain: attempts at clarification of terms and empirical study. Clin J Pain 18: S52–S60, 2002

Kishore-Kumar R, Max MB, Schafer SC, et al: Desipramine relieves post-herpetic neuralgia. Clin Pharm Ther 47:305–312, 1990

Klapper J: Divalproex sodium in migraine prophylaxis: a dose-controlled study. Cephalalgia 17:103–108, 1997

Kouyanou K, Pither CE, Wessely S: Medication misuse, abuse and dependence in chronic pain patients. J Psychosom Res 43:497–504, 1997

Kroenke K: Patients presenting with somatic complaints: epidemiology, psychiatric comorbidity and management. Int J Methods Psychiatr Res 12:34–43, 2003

Kroenke K, Mangelsdorff A: Common symptoms in ambulatory care: incidence, evaluation, therapy, and outcome. Am J Med 86:262–266, 1989

Kroenke K, Swindle R: Cognitive-behavioral therapy for somatization and symptom syndromes: a critical review of controlled clinical trials. Psychother Psychosom 69:205–215, 2000

Kroenke K, Spitzer RL, deGruy FV, et al: Multisomatoform disorder: an alternative to undifferentiated somatoform disorder for the somatizing patient in primary care. Arch Gen Psychiatry 54:352–358, 1997

La Spina I, Porazzi D, Maggiolo F, et al: Gabapentin in painful HIV-related neuropathy: a report of 19 patients, preliminary observations. Eur J Neurol 8:71–75, 2001

Lake AE 3rd: Behavioral and nonpharmacologic treatments of headache. Med Clin North Am 85:1055–1075, 2001

Lake AE 3rd, Saper JR: Chronic headache: new advances in treatment strategies. Neurology 59 (suppl 2):S8–S13, 2002

Lang E, Hord AH, Denson D: Venlafaxine hydrochloride (Effexor) relieves thermal hyperalgesia in rats with an experimental mononeuropathy. Pain 68:151–155, 1996

Lang E, Liebig K, Kastner S, et al: Multidisciplinary rehabilitation versus usual care for chronic low back pain in the community: effects on quality of life. Spine 3:270–276, 2003

Larson SL, Clark MR, Eaton WW: Depressive disorder as a long-term antecedent risk factor for incident back pain: a thirteen year follow-up study from the Baltimore Epidemiological Catchment Area sample. Psychol Med 34:1–9, 2004

Lazarus RA, Folkman S: Stress, Appraisal, and Coping. New York, Springer, 1984

Lebovits AH: The psychological assessment of patients with chronic pain. Curr Rev Pain 4:122–126, 2000

Lee DJ, Benzon HT: Anesthesiologic treatments for complex regional pain syndrome, in Essentials of Pain Medicine. Edited by Benzon HT, Raja SN. Philadelphia, Churchill-Livingstone, 1999, pp 255–258

Leino P, Magni G: Depressive and distress symptoms as predictors of low back pain, neck-shoulder pain, and other musculoskeletal morbidity: a 10 year follow-up of metal industry employees. Pain 53:89–94, 1993

Lemstra M, Stewart B, Olszynski WP: Effectiveness of multidisciplinary intervention in the treatment of migraine: a randomized clinical trial. Headache 42:845–854, 2002

Lewis TA, Solomon GD: Advances in cluster headache management. Cleve Clin J Med 63:237–244, 1996

Lin EH, Katon W, Von Korff M, et al: Effect of improving depression care on pain and functional outcomes among older adults with arthritis: a randomized controlled trial. JAMA 290:2428–2439, 2003

Linton SJ, Andersson T: Can chronic disability be prevented? A randomized trial of a cognitive-behavior intervention and two forms of information for patients with spinal pain. Spine 25:2825–2831, 2000

Lipchik GL, Nash JM: Cognitive-behavioral issues in the treatment and management of chronic daily headache. Curr Pain Headache Rep 6:473–479, 2002

Lipton RB, Stewart WF, von Korff M: Burden of migraine: societal costs and therapeutic opportunities. Neurology 48 (suppl 3):S4–S9, 1997

Liu JG, Anand KJ: Protein kinases modulate the cellular adaptations associated with opioid tolerance and dependence. Brain Res Brain Res Rev 38:1–19, 2001

Livingston G, Watkin V, Milne B, et al: Who becomes depressed? The Islington community study of old people. J Affect Disord 58:125–133, 2000

Long DM, Filtzer DL, BenDebba M, et al: Clinical features of the failed-back syndrome. J Neurosurg 69:61–71, 1988

Love S, Coakham HB: Trigeminal neuralgia: pathology and pathogenesis. Brain 124:2347–2360, 2001

Lynch ME: Psychological aspects of reflex sympathetic dystrophy: a review of the adult and paediatric literature. Pain 49:337–347, 1992

Lynch ME: Antidepressants as analgesics: a review of randomized controlled trials. J Psychiatry Neurosci 26:30–36, 2001

MacFarlane BV, Wright A, O'Callaghan J, et al: Chronic neuropathic pain and its control by drugs. Pharmacol Ther 75:1–19, 1997

Magni G, Schifano F, DeLeo D: Pain as a symptom in elderly depressed patients: relationship to diagnostic subgroups. Eur Arch Psychiatry Neurol Sci 235:143–145, 1985

Magni G, Marchetti M, Moreschi C, et al: Chronic musculoskeletal pain and depressive symptoms in the National Health and Nutrition Examination, I: epidemiologic follow-up study. Pain 53:163–168, 1993

Magni G, Moreschi C, Rigatti-Luchini S, et al: Prospective study on the relationship between depressive symptoms and chronic musculoskeletal pain. Pain 56:289–297, 1994

Magni G, Rigatti-Luchini S, Fracca F, et al: Suicidality in chronic abdominal pain: an analysis of the Hispanic Health and Nutrition Examination Survey (HHANES). Pain 76:137–144, 1998

Mannion AF, Junge A, Taimela S, et al: Active therapy for chronic low back pain, part 3: factors influencing self-rated disability and its change following therapy. Spine 26:920–929, 2001

Mantyselka P, Ahonen R, Viinamaki H, et al: Drug use by patients visiting primary care physicians due to nonacute musculoskeletal pain. Eur J Pharm Sci 17:210–216, 2002

Mantyselka PT, Turunen JH, Ahonen RS, et al: Chronic pain and poor self-rated health. JAMA 290:2435–2442, 2003

Mao J, Sung B, Ji RR, et al: Chronic morphine induces downregulation of spinal glutamate transporters: implications in morphine tolerance and abnormal pain sensitivity. J Neurosci 22:8312–8323, 2002

Marek GJ, McDougle CJ, Price LH, et al: A comparison of trazodone and fluoxetine: implications for a serotonergic mechanism of antidepressant action. Psychopharmacology 109:2–11, 1992

Marhold C, Linton SJ, Melin L: Identification of obstacles for chronic pain patients to return to work: evaluation of a questionnaire. J Occup Rehabil 12:65–75, 2002

Markley HG: Verapamil and migraine prophylaxis: mechanisms and efficacy. Am J Med 90:48S–53S, 1991

Marson AG, Kadir ZA, Hutton JL, et al: The new antiepileptic drugs: a systematic review of their efficacy and tolerability. Epilepsia 38:859–880, 1997

Maruta T, Malinchoc M, Offord KP, et al: Status of patients with chronic pain 13 years after treatment in a pain management center. Pain 74:199–204, 1998

Mathew NT: Antiepileptic drugs in migraine prevention. Headache 41 (suppl 1):S18–S24, 2001

Mathew NT, Kailasam J, Meadors L: Prophylaxis of migraine, transformed migraine, and cluster headache with topiramate. Headache 42:796–803, 2002

Mattia C, Paoletti F, Coluzzi F, et al: New antidepressants in the treatment of neuropathic pain: a review. Minerva Anestesiol 68:105–114, 2002

Max MB: Treatment of post-herpetic neuralgia: antidepressants. Ann Neurol 35:850–853, 1994

Max MB, Culnane M, Schafer SC, et al: Amitriptyline relieves diabetic neuropathy pain in patients with normal or depressed mood. Neurology 37:589–596, 1987

Max M, Lynch S, Muir J, et al: Effects of desipramine, amitriptyline and fluoxetine on pain in diabetic neuropathy. N Engl J Med 326:1250–1256, 1992

Maxwell TD, Gatchel RJ, Mayer TG: Cognitive predictors of depression in chronic low back pain: toward an inclusive model. J Behav Med 21:131–143, 1998

McCracken LM: Learning to live with the pain: acceptance of pain predicts adjustment in persons with chronic pain. Pain 74:21–27, 1998

McCracken LM, Turk DC: Behavioral and cognitive-behavioral treatment for chronic pain: outcome, predictors of outcome, and treatment process. Spine 27:2564–2573, 2002

McCreary CP, Clark GT, Merril RI, et al: Psychological distress and diagnostic subgroups of temporomandibular disorder patients. Pain 44:29–34, 1991

McQuay H, Carroll D, Jadad AR, et al: Anticonvulsant drugs for management of pain: a systematic review. BMJ 311:1047–1052, 1995

McQuay HJ, Tramer M, Nye BA, et al: A systematic review of antidepressants in neuropathic pain. Pain 68:217–227, 1996

Meldrum ML: A capsule history of pain management. JAMA 290:2470–2475, 2003

Mellegers MA, Furlan AD, Mailis A: Gabapentin for neuropathic pain: systematic review of controlled and uncontrolled literature. Clin J Pain 17:284–295, 2001

Melzack R, Wall PD: Pain mechanisms: a new theory. Science 150:971–979, 1965

Mendell JR, Sahenk Z: Clinical practice: painful sensory neuropathy. N Engl J Med 348:1243–1255, 2003

Merikangas KR, Merikangas JR: Combination monoamine oxidase inhibitor and beta-blocker treatment of migraine, with anxiety and depression. Biol Psychiatry 38:603–610, 1995

Merskey H, Lindblom U, Mumford JM, et al: Pain terms: a current list with definitions and notes on usage. Pain Suppl 3:S215–S221, 1986

Millan MJ: Descending control of pain. Prog Neurobiol 66:355–474, 2002

Moosa RS, McFayden ML, Miller R, et al: Carbamazepine and its metabolites in neuralgias: concentration-effect relations. Eur J Clin Pharm 45:297–301, 1993

Morley S, Eccleston C, Williams A: Systematic review and meta-analysis of randomized controlled trials of cognitive behaviour therapy and behaviour therapy for chronic pain in adults, excluding headache. Pain 80:1–13, 1999

Moulin DE, Iezzi A, Amireh R, et al: Randomised trial of oral morphine for chronic non-cancer pain. Lancet 347:143–147, 1996

Nedeljkovic SS, Wasan A, Jamison RN: Assessment of efficacy of long-term opioid therapy in pain patients with substance abuse potential. Clin J Pain 18:S39–S51, 2002

Neighbors DM, Bell TJ, Wilson J, et al: Economic evaluation of the fentanyl transdermal system for the treatment of chronic moderate to severe pain. J Pain Symptom Manage 21:129–143, 2001

Nemmani KV, Mogil JS: Serotonin-GABA interactions in the modulation of mu- and kappa-opioid analgesia. Neuropharmacology 44:304–310, 2003

Nicholson B: Responsible prescribing of opioids for the management of chronic pain. Drugs 63:17–32, 2003

Nickel R, Raspe HH: Chronic pain: epidemiology and health care utilization. Nervenarzt 72:897–906, 2001

Nielson WR, Weir R: Biopsychosocial approaches to the treatment of chronic pain. Clin J Pain 17 (suppl):S114–S127, 2001

Nishiyama K, Sakuta M: Mexiletine for painful alcoholic neuropathy. Intern Med 34:577–579, 1995

Novak V, Kanard R, Kissel JT, et al: Treatment of painful sensory neuropathy with tiagabine: a pilot study. Clin Auton Res 11:357–361, 2001

Novy DM, Nelson DV, Berry LA, et al: What does the Beck Depression Inventory measure in chronic pain? A reappraisal. Pain 61:261–270, 1995

Ohayon MM, Schatzberg AF: Using chronic pain to predict depressive morbidity in the general population. Arch Gen Psychiatry 60:39–47, 2003

Okifuji A, Turk DC, Curran SL: Anger in chronic pain: investigations of anger targets and intensity. J Psychosom Res 47: 1–12, 1999

Okifuji A, Turk DC, Sherman JJ: Evaluation of the relationship between depression and fibromyalgia syndrome: why aren't all patients depressed? J Rheumatol 27:212–219, 2000

Ollat H, Cesaro P: Pharmacology of neuropathic pain. Clin Neuropharmacol 18:391–404, 1995

Onghena P, Van Houdenhove B: Antidepressant-induced analgesia in chronic non-malignant pain: a meta-analysis of 39 placebo-controlled studies. Pain 49:205–219, 1992

Oskarsson P, Ljunggren JG, Lins PE: Efficacy and safety of mexiletine in the treatment of painful diabetic neuropathy. Diabetes Care 20:1594–1597, 1997

Ospina M, Harstall C: Prevalence of Chronic Pain: An Overview (Report No. 28). Edmonton, Alberta, Alberta Heritage Foundation for Medical Research, Health Technology Assessment 2002

Ozyalcin SN, Talu GK, Kiziltan E, et al: The efficacy and safety of venlafaxine in the prophylaxis of migraine. Headache 45:144–152, 2005

Paoli F, Darcourt G, Corsa P: Note prelimi- naire su l'action de l'impramine dans les etats douloureux. Revue de Neurologie 2:503–504, 1960

Parmelee PA: Pain in cognitively impaired older persons. Clin Geriatr Med 12:473– 487, 1996

Passik SD, Weinreb HJ: Managing chronic non- malignant pain: overcoming obstacles to the use of opioids. Adv Ther 17:70–83, 2000

Pasternak GW: The pharmacology of mu anal- gesics: from patients to genes. Neurosci- entist 7:220–231, 2001

Patten SB: Long-term medical conditions and major depression in a Canadian popula- tion study at waves 1 and 2. J Affect Disord 63:35–41, 2001

Paul D, Hornby PJ: Potentiation of intrathe- cal DAMGO antinociception, but not gastrointenstinal transit inhibition, by 5- hydroxytryptamine and norepinephrine uptake blockade. Life Sci 56:PL83–PL87, 1995

Pengel HM, Maher CG, Refshauge KM: Sys- tematic review of conservative interven- tions for subacute low back pain. Clin Re- habil 16:811–820, 2002

Peters L, Simon EP, Folen RA, et al: The COPE program: treatment efficacy and medical utilization outcome of a chronic pain management program at a major mil- itary hospital. Mil Med 165:954–960, 2000

Pfingsten M, Hildebrandt J, Saur P, et al: Mul- tidisciplinary treatment program for chronic low back pain, part 4: prognosis of treatment outcomes and final conclusions. Schmerz 11:30–41, 1997

Picavet HS, Vlaeyen JW, Schouten JS: Pain catastrophizing and kinesiophobia: pre- dictors of chronic low back pain. Am J Ep- idemiol 156:1028–1034, 2002

Pincus T, Williams A: Models and measure- ments of depression in chronic pain. J Psy- chosom Res 47:211–219, 1999

Pincus T, Burton AK, Vogel S, et al: A system- atic review of psychological factors as pre- dictors of chronicity/disability in prospec- tive cohorts of low back pain. Spine 27:E109–E120, 2002

Pinto A, Sollecito TP, DeRossi SS: Burning mouth syndrome: a retrospective analysis of clinical characteristics and treatment out- comes. N Y State Dent J 69:18–24, 2003

Ploghaus A, Becerra L, Borras C, et al: Neural circuitry underlying pain modulation: ex- pectation, hypnosis, placebo. Trends Cogn Sci 7:197–200, 2003

Polatin PB, Kinney RK, Gatchel RJ, et al: Psy- chiatric illness and chronic low back pain. Spine 18:66–71, 1993

Pollo A, Vighetti S, Rainero I, et al: Placebo analgesia and the heart. Pain 102:125– 133, 2003

Portenoy RK: Chronic opioid therapy in non- malignant pain. J Pain Symptom Manage 5 (suppl 1):S46–S62, 1990

Portenoy RK, Foley KM: Chronic use of opi- oid analgesics in non-malignant pain: re- port of 38 cases. Pain 25:171–186, 1986

Potter M, Schafer S, Gonzalez-Mendez E, et al: Opioids for chronic nonmalignant pain: atti- tudes and practices of primary care physi- cians in the UCSF/Stanford Collaborative Research Network. University of California, San Francisco. J Fam Pract 50:145–151, 2001

Price DD: Psychological and neural mecha- nisms of the affective dimension of pain. Science 288:1769–1772, 2000

Price DD, Milling LS, Kirsch I, et al: An anal- ysis of factors that contribute to the mag- nitude of placebo analgesia in an experi- mental paradigm. Pain 83:147–156, 1999

Raja SN, Haythornthwaite JA, Pappagallo M, et al: Opioids versus antidepressants in postherpetic neuralgia: a randomized, pla- cebo-controlled trial. Neurology 59:1015– 1021, 2002

Raskin J, Pritchett YL, Wang F, et al: A dou- ble-blind, randomized multicenter trial comparing duloxetine with placebo in the management of diabetic peripheral neuropathic pain. Pain Med 6:346–356, 2005

Reichborn-Kjennerud T, Stoltenberg C, Tambs K, et al: Back-neck pain and symp- toms of anxiety and depression: a popula- tion-based twin study. Psychol Med 32:1009–1020, 2002

Reid MC, Engles-Horton LL, Weber MB, et al: Use of opioid medications for chronic noncancer pain syndromes in primary care. J Gen Intern Med 17:238–240, 2002

Reis S: Expectancy theory of fear, anxiety, and panic. Clin Psychol Rev 11:141–153, 1991

Revenson TA, Felton BT: Disability and coping as predictors of psychological adjustment to rheumatoid arthritis. J Consult Clin Psychol 57:344–348, 1989

Rice AS, Maton S, Postherpetic Neuralgia Study Group: Gabapentin in postherpetic neuralgia: a randomised, double blind, placebo controlled study. Pain 94:215–224, 2001

Richeimer SH, Bajwa ZH, Kahraman SS, et al: Utilization patterns of tricyclic antidepressants in a multidisciplinary pain clinic: a survey. Clin J Pain 13:324–329, 1997

Richelson E: Pharmacology of antidepressants: characteristics of the ideal drug. Mayo Clin Proc 69:1069–1081, 1994

Richter RW, Portenoy R, Sharma U, et al: Relief of painful diabetic peripheral neuropathy with pregabalin: a randomized, placebo-controlled trial. Pain 6:253–260, 2005

Riedel W, Neeck G: Nociception, pain, and antinociception: current concepts. Z Rheumatol 60:404–415, 2001

Riley JL 3rd, Robinson ME, Wise EA, et al: Predicting treatment compliance following facial pain evaluation. Cranio 17:9–16, 1999

Risdon A, Eccleston C, Crombez G, et al: How can we learn to live with pain? A Q-methodological analysis of the diverse understandings of acceptance of chronic pain. Soc Sci Med 56:375–386, 2003

Rizzo MA: Successful treatment of painful traumatic mononeuropathy with carbamazepine: insights into a possible molecular pain mechanism. J Neurol Sci 152:103–106, 1997

Rojas-Corrales MO, Berrocoso E, Gibert-Rahola J, et al: Antidepressant-like effects of tramadol and other central analgesics with activity on monoamines reuptake, in helpless rats. Life Sci 72:143–152, 2002

Romano JM, Syrjala KL, Levy RL, et al: Overt pain behaviors: relationship to patient functioning and treatment outcome. Behav Ther 19:191–201, 1988

Rommel O, Malin JP, Zenz M, et al: Quantitative sensory testing, neurophysiological and psychological examination in patients with complex regional pain syndrome and hemisensory deficits. Pain 93:279–293, 2001

Roose SP, Glassman AH, Siris S: Comparison of imipramine and nortriptyline-induced orthostatic hypotension: a meaningful difference. J Clin Psychopharmacol 1:316–319, 1981

Rosenblum A, Joseph H, Fong C, et al: Prevalence and characteristics of chronic pain among chemically dependent patients in methadone maintenance and residential treatment facilities. JAMA 289:2370–2378, 2003

Roth SH, Fleischmann RM, Burch FX, et al: Around-the-clock, controlled-release oxycodone therapy for osteoarthritis-related pain: placebo-controlled trial and long-term evaluation. Arch Intern Med 160:853–860, 2000

Rothrock JF: Clinical studies of valproate for migraine prophylaxis. Cephalalgia 17:81–83, 1997

Rowbotham M, Harden N, Stacey B, et al: Gabapentin for the treatment of postherpetic neuralgia: a randomized controlled trial. JAMA 280:1837–1842, 1998

Rowbotham MC, Twilling L, Davies PS, et al: Oral opioid therapy for chronic peripheral and central neuropathic pain. N Engl J Med 348:1279–1281, 2003

Rowbotham MC, Goli V, Kunz NR, et al: Venlafaxin extended release in the treatment of painful diabetic neuropathy: a double-blind, placebo-conrolled study. Pain 110:697–706, 2004 [erratum: 113:248, 2005]

Rudy TE, Kerns RD, Turk DC: Chronic pain and depression: toward a cognitive-behavioral mediation model. Pain 35:129–140, 1988

Rudy TE, Turk DC, Kubinski JA, et al: Differential treatment responses of TMD patients as a function of psychological characteristics. Pain 61:103–112, 1995

Sabatowski R, Galvez R, Cherry DA, et al: Pregabalin reduces pain and improves sleep and mood disturbances in patients with post-herpetic neuralgia: results of a randomised, placebo-controlled trial. Pain 109:26–35, 2004

Sang CN: NMDA-receptor antagonists in neuropathic pain: experimental methods to clinical trials. J Pain Symptom Manage 19 (suppl):S21–S25, 2000

Saper JR, Silberstein SD, Lake AE 3rd, et al: Double-blind trial of fluoxetine: chronic daily headache and migraine. Headache 34:497–502, 1994

Savage SR: Assessment for addiction in pain-treatment settings. Clin J Pain 18:S28–S38, 2002

Savage SR, Joranson DE, Covington EC, et al: Definitions related to the medical use of opioids: evolution towards universal agreement. J Pain Symptom Manage 26:655–667, 2003

Sawynok J: GABAergic mechanisms of analgesia: an update. Pharmacol Biochem Behav 26:463–474, 1985

Scadding FW: Peripheral neuropathies, in Textbook of Pain, 3rd Edition. Edited by Wall PD, Melzack R. Edinburgh, Churchill Livingstone, 1994, pp 667–683

Schade V, Semmer N, Main CJ, et al: The impact of clinical, morphological, psychosocial and work-related factors on the outcome of lumbar diskectomy. Pain 80:239–249, 1999

Schmader KE: Epidemiology and impact on quality of life of postherpetic neuralgia and painful diabetic neuropathy. Clin J Pain 18:350–354, 2002

Schmidt NB, Santiago HT, Trakowski JH, et al: Pain in patients with panic disorder: relation to symptoms, cognitive characteristics and treatment outcome. Pain Res Manag 7:134–141, 2002

Schreiber S, Backer MM, Yanai J, et al: The antinociceptive effect of fluvoxamine. Eur Neuropsychopharmacol 6:281–284, 1996

Schug SA, Merry AF, Acland RH: Treatment principles for the use of opioids in pain of nonmalignant origin. Drugs 42:228–239, 1991

Schult ML, Soderback I, Jacobs K: Multidimensional aspects of work capability. Work 15:41–53, 2000

Semenchuk MR, Sherman S, Davis B: Double-blind, randomized trial of buproprion SR for the treatment of neuropathic pain. Neurology 57:1583–1588, 2001

Serpell MG: Neuropathic pain study group: gabapentin in neuropathic pain syndromes. A randomised, double-blind, placebo-controlled trial. Pain 99:557–566, 2002

Severeijns R, Vlaeyen JW, van den Hout MA, et al: Pain catastrophizing predicts pain intensity, disability, and psychological distress independent of the level of physical impairment. Clin J Pain 17:165–172, 2001

Sherman JJ, Turk DC, Okifuji A: Prevalence and impact of posttraumatic stress disorder-like symptoms on patients with fibromyalgia syndrome. Clin J Pain 16:127–134, 2000

Silberstein SD, Peres MF, Hopkins MM, et al: Olanzapine in the treatment of refractory migraine and chronic daily headache. Headache 42:515–518, 2002

Simon GE, VonKorff M, Piccinelli M, et al: An international study of the relation between somatic symptoms and depression. N Engl J Med 341:1329–1335, 1999

Simpson DM, McArthur JC, Olney R, et al: Lamotrigine for HIV-associated painful sensory neuropathies: a placebo-controlled trial. Neurology 60:1508–1514, 2003

Sindrup SH, Jensen TS: Efficacy of pharmacological treatments of neuropathic pain: an update and effect related to mechanism of drug action. Pain 83:389–400, 1999

Sindrup SH, Jensen TS: Pharmacologic treatment of pain in polyneuropathy. Neurology 55:915–920, 2000

Sindrup SH, Jensen TS: Pharmacotherapy of trigeminal neuralgia. Clin J Pain 18:22–27, 2002

Sindrup SH, Ejlertsen B, Froland A, et al: Imipramine treatment in diabetic neuropathy: relief of subjective symptoms without changes in peripheral and autonomic nerve function. Eur J Clin Pharmacol 37:151–153, 1989

Sindrup SH, Gram LF, Brosen K, et al: The SSRI paroxetine is effective in the treatment of diabetic neuropathy symptoms. Pain 42:135–144, 1990

Sindrup SH, Bjerre U, Dejaard A, et al: The SSRI citalopram relieves the symptoms of diabetic neuropathy. Clin Pharmacol Ther 52:547–552, 1992

Sittl R, Griessinger N, Likar R: Analgesic efficacy and tolerability of transdermal buprenorphine in patients with inadequately controlled chronic pain related to cancer and other disorders: a multicenter, randomized, double-blind, placebo-controlled trial. Clin Ther 25:150–168, 2003

Skevington SM: Investigating the relationship between pain and discomfort and quality of life, using the WHOQOL. Pain 76:395–406, 1998

Skevington SM, Carse MS, Williams AC: Validation of the WHOQOL-100: pain management improves quality of life for chronic pain patients. Clin J Pain 17:264–275, 2001

Smedstad LM, Vaglum P, Kvien TK, et al: The relationship between self-reported pain and sociodemographic variables, anxiety, and depressive symptoms in rheumatoid arthritis. J Rheumatol 22:514–520, 1995

Smith GR: The epidemiology and treatment of depression when it coexists with somatoform disorders, somatization, or pain. Gen Hosp Psychiatry 14:265–272, 1992

Smith JA, Lumley MA, Longo DJ: Contrasting emotional approach coping with passive coping for chronic myofascial pain. Ann Behav Med 24:326–335, 2002

Smith MT, Cabot PJ, Ross FB, et al: The novel N-type calcium channel blocker, AM336, produces potent dose-dependent antinociception after intrathecal dosing in rats and inhibits substance P release in rat spinal cord slices. Pain 96:119–127, 2002

Stack K, Cortina J, Samples C, et al: Race, age, and back pain as factors in completion of residential substance abuse treatment by veterans. Psychiatr Serv 51:1157–1161, 2000

Staiger TO, Gaster B, Sullivan MD, et al: Systematic review of antidepressants in the treatment of chronic low back pain. Spine 28:2540–2545, 2003

Stanton-Hicks M, Janig W, Hassenbusch S, et al: Reflex sympathetic dystrophy: changing concepts and taxonomy. Pain 63:127–133, 1995

Starkstein SE, Preziosi TJ, Robinson RG: Sleep disorders, pain, and depression in Parkinson's disease. Eur Neurol 31:352–355, 1991

Stewart WF, Ricci JA, Chee E, et al: Lost productive time and cost due to common pain conditions in the US workforce. JAMA 290:2443–2454, 2003

Stone AA, Shiffman S, Schwartz JE, et al: Patient non-compliance with paper diaries. BMJ 324:1193–1194, 2002

Streltzer J, Eliashof BA, Kline AE, et al: Chronic pain disorder following physical injury. Psychosomatics 41:227–234, 2000

Sullivan M: DSM-IV pain disorder: a case against the diagnosis. Int Rev Psychiatry 12:91–98, 2000

Sullivan M, Katon W: Somatization: the path between distress and somatic symptoms. Am Pain Soc J 2:141–149, 1993

Sullivan MJ, Thorn B, Haythornthwaite JA, et al: Theoretical perspectives on the relation between catastrophizing and pain. Clin J Pain 17:52–64, 2001

Suter PB: Employment and litigation: improved by work, assisted by verdict. Pain 100:249–257, 2002

Szirmai A: Vestibular disorders in patients with migraine. Eur Arch Otorhinolaryngol Suppl 1:S55–S57, 1997

Tan G, Jensen MP, Robinson-Whelen S, et al: Coping with chronic pain: a comparison of two measures. Pain 90:127–133, 2001

Tanelian DL, Victory RA: Sodium channel-blocking agents: their use in neuropathic pain conditions. Pain Forum 4:75–80, 1995

Taniguchi K, Miyagawa A, Mizutani A, et al: The effect of calcium channel antagonist administered by iontophoresis on the pain threshold. Acta Anaesthesiol Belg 46:69–73, 1995

Taricco M, Adone R, Pagliacci C, et al: Pharmacological interventions for spasticity following spinal cord injury. Cochrane Database Syst Rev 2:CD001131, 2000

Tasmuth T, Hartel B, Kalso E: Venlafaxine in neuropathic pain following treatment of breast cancer. Eur J Pain 6:17–24, 2002

ter Riet G, de Craen AJ, de Boer A, et al: Is placebo analgesia mediated by endogenous opioids? A systematic review. Pain 76:273–275, 1998

To TP, Lim TC, Hill ST, et al: Gabapentin for neuropathic pain following spinal cord injury. Spinal Cord 40:282–285, 2002

Tokunaga A, Saika M, Senba E: 5-HT2A receptor subtype is involved in the thermal hyperalgesic mechanism of serotonin in the periphery. Pain 76:349–355, 1998

Tremont-Lukats IW, Megeff C, Backonja MM: Anticonvulsants for neuropathic pain syndromes: mechanisms of action and place in therapy. Drugs 60:1029–1052, 2000

Trief PM, Grant W, Fredrickson B: A prospective study of psychological predictors of lumbar surgery outcome. Spine 25:2616–2621, 2000

Turk DC: The role of psychological factors in chronic pain. Acta Anaesthesiol Scand 43:885–888, 1999

Turk DC, Matyas TA: Pain-related behaviors: communication of pain. Am Pain Soc J 1:109–111, 1992

Turk DC, Okifuji A: Detecting depression in chronic pain patients: adequacy of self reports. Behav Res Ther 32:9–16, 1994

Turk DC, Okifuji A: What features affect physicians' decisions to prescribe opioids for chronic noncancer pain patients? Clin J Pain 13:330–336, 1997

Turk DC, Okifuji A: Psychological factors in chronic pain: evolution and revolution. J Consult Clin Psychol 70:678–690, 2002

Turner JA: Psychological interventions for chronic pain: a critical review, II: operant conditioning, hypnosis, and cognitive-behavioral therapy. Pain 12:23–46, 1982

Turner JA, Chapman CR: Psychological interventions for chronic pain: a critical review, I: relaxation training and biofeedback. Pain 12:1–21, 1982

Turner JA, Jensen MP: Efficacy of cognitive therapy for chronic low back pain. Pain 52:169–177, 1993

Turner JA, Deyo RA, Loeser JD, et al: The importance of placebo effects in pain treatment and research. JAMA 271:1609–1614, 1994

Turner JA, Jensen MP, Warms CA, et al: Catastrophizing is associated with pain intensity, psychological distress, and pain-related disability among individuals with chronic pain after spinal cord injury. Pain 98:127–134, 2002

Turner-Stokes L, Erkeller-Yuksel F, Miles A, et al: Outpatient cognitive behavioral pain management programs: a randomized comparison of a group-based multidisciplinary versus an individual therapy model. Arch Phys Med Rehabil 84:781–788, 2003

Vaccarino AL, Kastin AJ: Endogenous opiates: 2000. Peptides 22:2257–2328, 2001

Van Damme S, Crombez G, Bijttebier P, et al: A confirmatory factor analysis of the Pain Catastrophizing Scale: invariant factor structure across clinical and non-clinical populations. Pain 96:319–324, 2002

van den Hout JH, Vlaeyen JW, Heuts PH, et al: Secondary prevention of work-related disability in nonspecific low back pain: does problem-solving therapy help? A randomized clinical trial. Clin J Pain 19:87–96, 2003

van Tulder MW, Ostelo R, Vlaeyen JW, et al: Behavioral treatment for chronic low back pain: a systematic review within the framework of the Cochrane Back Review Group. Spine 26:270–281, 2001

Verbunt JA, Seelen HA, Vlaeyen JW, et al: Disuse and deconditioning in chronic low back pain: concepts and hypotheses on contributing mechanisms. Eur J Pain 7:9–21, 2003

Verdugo RJ, Ochoa JL: Abnormal movements in complex regional pain syndrome: assessment of their nature. Muscle Nerve 23:198–205, 2000

Verhaak PF, Kerssens JJ, Dekker J, et al: Prevalence of chronic benign pain disorder among adults: a review of the literature. Pain 77:231–239, 1998

Vlaeyen JW, Linton SJ: Fear-avoidance and its consequences in chronic musculoskeletal pain: a state of the art. Pain 85: 317–332, 2000

Vlaeyen JW, de Jong J, Geilen M, et al: The treatment of fear of movement/(re)injury in chronic low back pain: further evidence on the effectiveness of exposure in vivo. Clin J Pain 18:251–261, 2002

Volmink J, Lancaster T, Gray S, et al: Treatments for postherpetic neuralgia: a systematic review of randomized controlled trials. Fam Pract 13:84–91, 1996

Von Knorring L, Perris C, Eisemann M, et al: Pain as a symptom in depressive disorders, I: relationship to diagnostic subgroup and depressive symptomatology. Pain 15:19–26, 1983

Von Korff M, Ormel J, Katon W, et al: Disability and depression among high utilizers of health care: a longitudinal analysis. Arch Gen Psychiatry 49:91–100, 1992

Von Korff M, LeResche L, Dworkin SF: First onset of common pain symptoms: a prospective study of depression as a risk factor. Pain 55:251–258, 1993

Vowles KE, Gross RT: Work-related beliefs about injury and physical capability for work in individuals with chronic pain. Pain 101:291–298, 2003

Vrethem M, Boivie J, Arnqvist H, et al: A comparison of amitriptyline and maprotiline in the treatment of painful polyneuropathy in diabetics and nondiabetics. Clin J Pain 13: 313–323, 1997

Waddell G, Newton M, Henderson I, et al: A fear-avoidance beliefs questionnaire (FABQ) and the role of fear-avoidance beliefs in chronic low back pain and disability. Pain 52:157–168, 1993

Wang YX, Gao D, Pettus M, et al: Interactions of intrathecally administered ziconotide, a selective blocker of neuronal N-type voltage-sensitive calcium channels, with morphine on nociception in rats. Pain 84:271–281, 2000

Watson CP, Evans RJ, Watt VR, et al: Postherpetic neuralgia: 208 causes. Pain 35:289–298, 1988

Watt JW, Wiles JR, Bowsher DR: Epidural morphine for postherpetic neuralgia. Anaesthesia 51:647–651, 1996

Waxman R, Tennant A, Helliwell P: Community survey of factors associated with consultation for low back pain. BMJ 317:1564–1567, 1998

Weaver M, Schnoll S: Abuse liability in opioid therapy for pain treatment in patients with an addiction history. Clin J Pain 18:S61–S69, 2002

Webb J, Kamali F: Analgesic effects of lamotrigine and phenytoin on cold-induced pain: a crossover placebo-controlled study in healthy volunteers. Pain 76:357–363, 1998

Weickgenant AL, Slater MA, Patterson TL, et al: Coping activities in chronic low back pain: relationship with depression. Pain 53:95–103, 1993

Weissman MM, Merikangas KR: The epidemiology of anxiety and panic disorders: an update. J Clin Psychiatry 47(suppl): 11–17, 1986

Wesselmann U, Raja SN: Reflex sympathetic dystrophy/causalgia. Anesthesiol Clin North Am 15:407–427, 1997

Wesselmann U, Reich SG: The dynias. Semin Neurol 16:63–74, 1996

Wetzel CH, Connelly JF: Use of gabapentin in pain management. Ann Pharmacother 31:1082–1083, 1997

Wiffen P, Collins S, McQuay H, et al: Anticonvulsant drugs for acute and chronic pain. Cochrane Database Syst Rev 3:CD001133, 2000

Williamson GM, Schulz R: Pain, activity restriction and symptoms of depression among community-residing elderly adults. J Gerontol 47:367–372, 1992

Wu LR, Parkerson GR Jr, Doraiswamy PM: Health perception, pain, and disability as correlates of anxiety and depression symptoms in primary care patients. J Am Board Fam Pract 15:183–190, 2002

Yamamoto T, Katayama Y, Hirayama T, et al: Pharmacological classification of central post-stroke pain: comparison with the results of chronic motor cortex stimulation therapy. Pain 72:5–12, 1997

Zakrzewska JM: Diagnosis and differential diagnosis of trigeminal neuralgia. Clin J Pain 18:14–21, 2002

Zakrzewska JM, Glenny AM, Forssell H: Interventions for the treatment of burning mouth syndrome. Cochrane Database Syst Rev 3:CD002779, 2001

Self-Assessment Questions

Select the single best response for each question.

1. The International Association for the Study of Pain (IASP) has defined *pain* as

    A. An unpleasant, abnormal sensation that can be spontaneous or evoked.
    B. An increased response to a stimulus that is normally painful.
    C. An unpleasant sensory and emotional experience associated with actual or potential tissue damage.
    D. An abnormal sensation, spontaneous or evoked, that is not unpleasant.
    E. None of the above.

2. Visual prodromal symptoms, such as scintillating scotomata, are indicative of what type of headache?

    A. Classic migraine.
    B. Complicated migraine.
    C. Chronic daily headache.
    D. Common migraine.
    E. Hemicrania continua.

3. Which of the following statements concerning low back pain is *true?*

    A. Nearly 25% percent of patients with acute low back pain will go on to develop chronic symptoms.
    B. The least powerful predictor of chronicity is poor functional status 4 weeks after seeking treatment.
    C. Economic and social rewards are not associated with higher levels of disability and depression in patients with chronic back pain.
    D. Psychological factors highly correlated with low back pain include distress, depressed mood, and somatization.
    E. The presence of an anxiety disorder has been demonstrated to increase the risk of developing chronic musculoskeletal pain 3 years later.

4. Using DSM-IV diagnostic criteria for pain disorder, researchers have estimated the lifetime prevalence of somatoform pain disorder to be

    A. 5%.
    B. 12%.
    C. 17%.
    D. 22%.
    E. 34%.

5. During the first 5 years after the onset of chronic pain, patients are at increased risk of developing new substance use disorders and experiencing additional physical injuries. This risk is highest in patients with a history of

    A. Substance abuse or dependence.
    B. Childhood physical abuse.
    C. Psychiatric comorbidity.
    D. Childhood sexual abuse.
    E. All of the above.

Appendix

Answer Guide to Self-Assessment Questions

The self-assessment questions in this Appendix, as well as additional questions covering all topics in *The American Psychiatric Publishing Textbook of Psychosomatic Medicine*, are available for purchase online at cme.psychiatryonline.org. Purchase the online version and receive instant scoring and CME credits.

Chapter 1—Psychiatric Assessment and Consultation

Select the single best response for each question.

1. Clinical assessment of memory and executive functions is an important component in the diagnosis and management of cognitive disorders. Regarding clinical assessment of cognitive function, all of the following are true *except*

   A. Having the patient register and then later recall specific information (e.g., three objects) is a test of episodic memory.
   B. Semantic memory is assessed by questions of general knowledge and naming of common objects.
   C. Executive function refers to the abilities that allow one to plan, initiate, organize, and monitor thought and behavior.
   D. Having the patient name as many objects in a category (e.g., names of animals) as he or she can within 1 minute assesses frontal lobe function.
   E. The go/no-go test of ability to inhibit a response assesses frontal lobe inhibitory function.

   The correct response is option A.

   Having the patient register and then later recall specific information (e.g., three objects) is a test of working memory. Episodic memory is assessed by the patient's ability to recall aspects of his or her own history. Semantic memory is assessed by general-knowledge questions. Procedural memory deficits can be observed in patient behavior in interview. Tasks that can be used to gain some insight into frontal lobe function include verbal fluency, such as listing as many animals as possible in 1 minute; motor sequencing, such as asking the patient to replicate a sequence of three hand positions; and the "go/no go" task, which requires the patient to tap the desk once if the examiner taps once, but not to tap if the examiner taps twice. **(p. 3)**

2. Language disorders involve the dominant cortical hemisphere and are important in neuropsychiatric illness encountered in psychosomatic medicine practice. Which of the following is *not* true regarding clinical presentation and assessment of the aphasias?

   A. Naming of objects is affected in Broca's (expressive) aphasia.
   B. Naming of objects is affected in Wernicke's (receptive) aphasia.
   C. Wernicke's aphasia overlaps with psychotic disorders in that both conditions feature poor insight and incoherent speech.
   D. Conduction aphasia features impaired naming with preserved repetition.
   E. Global dysphasia combines features of both Broca's and Wernicke's aphasias.

   The correct response is option D.

   Conduction aphasia features selective impairment of repetition. Global dysphasia combines features of Broca's and Wernicke's aphasias. **(p. 4)**

3. In the task of differentiating primary psychiatric from secondary medical etiologies of hallucinatory experiences, the affected sensory modality may guide the clinician to the more likely etiology. Which of the following types of hallucinations is often seen in substance abuse?

A. Tactile.
B. Auditory.
C. Visual.
D. Gustatory.
E. Olfactory.

The correct response is option A.

Tactile hallucinations are often seen in substance abuse. Prominent visual, olfactory, gustatory, or tactile hallucinations suggest a secondary medical etiology, whereas olfactory and gustatory hallucination may be manifestations of seizures. **(p. 4)**

4. The adjunctive use of neuroimaging is an important part of psychosomatic medicine practice. The consultant often must determine which imaging modality is most appropriate for the clinical problem at hand. Which of the following pathological entities is better visualized by computed tomography (CT) than by magnetic resonance imaging (MRI)?

A. Basal ganglia lesion (e.g., Parkinson's disease).
B. Brain stem lesion with motor signs.
C. Cerebellar tumor.
D. Acute intracranial hemorrhage.
E. Vascular dementia with frontal lobe signs.

The correct response is option D.

CT is most useful in cases of suspected acute intracranial hemorrhage and when MRI is contraindicated, as in patients with metallic implants. MRI provides better resolution of lesions of the basal ganglia, amygdala, and other limbic structures and abnormalities of the brain stem and posterior fossa. **(p. 5)**

5. The electroencephalogram (EEG) may be a useful diagnostic tool in psychosomatic medicine, but it is subject to some important limitations. Which of the following clinical situations is most likely to be clarified by the use of an EEG?

A. The search for a specific etiology of an established case of delirium.
B. An insidious onset and slowly progressive dementia.
C. Cognitive and motor deficits suggesting cerebral infarction.
D. Distinguishing between neurological and psychiatric etiologies for a mute, uncommunicative patient.
E. Localization of cerebral injury in traumatic brain injury.

The correct response is option D.

An EEG may be helpful in distinguishing between neurological and psychiatric etiologies for a mute, uncommunicative patient. It may also facilitate the evaluation of rapidly progressive dementia or profound coma. However, the EEG is often not helpful in the evaluation of space-occupying lesions, cerebral infarctions, or head injury. Also, the EEG rarely indicates a specific etiology of delirium and is not indicated in every delirious patient. **(p. 7)**

Chapter 2—Heart Disease

Select the single best response for each question.

1. Depression and anxiety in heart disease patients may significantly affect quality of life and may complicate medical management. All of the following statements are true *except*

   A. Depression is the most common comorbid psychiatric illness in coronary artery disease patients.
   B. The prevalence of major depression following coronary artery bypass graft (CABG) is 20%–30%.
   C. The point prevalence of major depression in congestive heart failure (CHF) approaches 20%.
   D. Panic disorder occurs at a much higher rate in patients with mitral valve prolapse confirmed by echocardiography than in healthy control subjects.
   E. Subsyndromal posttraumatic stress disorder (PTSD) is common in patients with automatic implantable cardioverter-defibrillators (AICDs).

   The correct response is option D.

   Panic disorder does not occur at higher-than-expected rates in patients with echocardiographically confirmed mitral valve prolapse. Depression in coronary artery disease patients is in the 15%–20% range. Studies of depression following CABG demonstrate a prevalence of 20%–30%. Other studies have estimated a prevalence of significant depressive symptoms in 20%–30% of CHF patients. **(pp. 14–15)**

2. A cardiac patient presents to a psychiatrist with a complaint of mood symptoms and of seeing yellow rings around objects in the visual field. The medication most likely responsible for these symptoms is

   A. Reserpine.
   B. Digoxin.
   C. Clonidine.
   D. Beta-blocker.
   E. Alpha-blocker.

   The correct response is option B.

   Common side effects of digoxin include visual hallucinations (classically, yellow rings around objects), delirium, and depression. **(p. 16, Table 2–1)**

3. Regarding cardiac transplantation surgery for end-stage cardiac disease and its psychiatric implications, all of the following are true *except*

   A. Patients awaiting transplantation commonly experience depression secondary to their helplessness to influence their own chances of survival.
   B. Patients on transplant waiting lists often experience guilt about the need for another patient to die to give them a heart.
   C. Patients on transplant waiting lists tend to minimize and/or deny their illness and to display ambivalence about the surgery.
   D. Most patients experience an initial depression at awakening from transplant surgery.

E. Steroid-induced mood disorder and other types of depression are seen in 20%–40% of patients during the first postoperative year.

The correct response is option D.

Most patients experience an initial euphoria at awakening from transplant surgery, knowing that they have now been delivered from end-stage heart failure. Positive feelings tend to subside as complications occur and as the patient settles into the work of rehabilitation. **(pp. 21–22)**

4. Regarding cardiac implications of antidepressants and antipsychotics, all of the following are true *except*

    A. Tricyclic antidepressants (TCAs) can increase mortality in post–myocardial infarction (MI) patients with premature ventricular contractions (PVCs).
    B. Selective serotonin reuptake inhibitors (SSRIs) plus concurrent use of beta-blockers have been shown to lead to symptomatic bradycardia.
    C. Ziprasidone increases the QTc interval and has been associated with an increased risk of sudden death.
    D. A QTc interval greater than 500 msec contraindicates the use of haloperidol and thioridazine.
    E. Among the antipsychotics, thioridazine carries the highest risk of torsades de pointes.

The correct response is option C.

Ziprasidone increases the QTc interval but has not been associated with sudden death. TCAs have quinidine-like effects on cardiac conduction and can increase mortality in post-MI patients with PVCs. Occasional cases of symptomatic bradycardia have been associated with concurrent use of SSRIs with beta-blockers. A QTc interval greater than 500 msec is considered a contraindication for haloperidol and thioridazine. Thioridazine is the antipsychotic most strongly associated with torsades de pointes. **(pp. 24–25)**

5. Which of the following psychotropic medications is associated with a quinidine-like type IA antiarrhythmic effect?

    A. Carbamazepine.
    B. Valproate.
    C. Lithium carbonate.
    D. Lamotrigine.
    E. Buspirone.

The correct response is option A.

Carbamazepine resembles the TCAs in having a quinidine-like type IA antiarrhythmic effect and may cause atrioventricular conduction disturbances. **(p. 26)**

Chapter 3—Lung Disease

Select the single best response for each question.

1. Which of the following statements concerning psychological factors in asthma is *false?*
   A. People with Cluster B personality disorders are more likely to have asthma.
   B. Psychological factors may influence asthma through behavioral mechanisms.
   C. Poor adherence with follow-up visits and poor inhaler technique may be associated with asthma deaths.
   D. Patients with asthma are more likely to hold catastrophic beliefs or cognitions.
   E. Asthma attacks may be provoked by psychological distress.

   The correct response is option A.

   No particular personality type is more susceptible to the development of asthma. Psychological factors may influence asthma through behavioral mechanisms. Psychological morbidity is associated with high levels of denial and delays in seeking medical care. Several psychological factors in asthma patients may be associated with asthma deaths; these factors include poor adherence with follow-up visits, poor inhaler technique, psychosis, financial problems, and learning difficulties. Similar to patients with panic disorder, patients with asthma have a tendency to hold catastrophic beliefs. Asthma attacks have long been thought to be provoked by psychological distress. **(p. 36)**

2. In patients with chronic obstructive pulmonary disease (COPD), anxiety and depression have been found to be associated with
   A. Higher relapse after emergency treatment.
   B. Increased disability.
   C. Lower exercise tolerance.
   D. Noncompliance with treatment.
   E. All of the above.

   The correct response is option E.

   Depression and anxiety in COPD patients have led to lower exercise tolerance (Withers et al. 1999), noncompliance with treatment (Bosley et al. 1996), and increased disability (Aydin and Ulusahin 2001). Psychological factors may predict whether a patient with COPD is at higher risk of relapse after emergency treatment. In one study, COPD patients with anxiety or depression had a higher rate of relapse within 1 month (53%) compared with those in the group without anxiety or depression (19%) (Dahlen and Janson 2002). **(p. 38)**

3. Regarding sarcoidosis, which of the following statements is *true?*
   A. Sarcoidosis affects white patients more than African American patients.
   B. In Europe, Italians have high prevalence rates.
   C. Onset of the illness usually occurs between the ages of 20 and 40 years.
   D. The disease follows a progressive downhill course, with nearly 25% of patients dying from it.
   E. All of the above.

The correct response is option C.

Onset of sarcoidosis is usually between the ages of 20 and 40 years. Sarcoidosis affects black patients more than white patients in the United States (40 per 100,000 vs. 5 per 100,000). In Europe, Swedes and Danes have high prevalence rates. Diagnosis may be delayed by failure to recognize the slowly progressive symptoms until characteristic findings are detected on a chest X ray. The disease often follows a relapsing and remitting course, with recovery in 80% of patients, but about 5% die from sarcoidosis. **(p. 39)**

4. Psychiatric factors that are considered to be absolute contraindications to lung transplantation include all of the following *except*

    A. Active alcoholism.
    B. Anxiety disorders.
    C. Noncompliance with treatment.
    D. Drug abuse.
    E. Cigarette use.

The correct response is option B.

Anxiety is not an absolute contraindication to lung transplantation. Psychiatric factors considered to be absolute contraindications include active alcoholism, drug abuse or cigarette use, severe psychiatric illness, and noncompliance with treatment (Aris et al. 1997; Paradowski 1997; Snell et al. 1993). **(p. 42)**

5. In the treatment of anxiety disorders in pulmonary disease, which of the following classes of psychotropic medications are contraindicated due to the risk of inducing vasospasm?

    A. Buspirone.
    B. Short-acting benzodiazepines.
    C. Long-acting benzodiazepines.
    D. SSRIs.
    E. Beta-blockers.

The correct response is option E.

Beta-blockers should not be used for anxiety in asthma patients, because of resulting bronchoconstriction. **(p. 44)**

References

Aris RM, Gilligan PH, Neuring IP, et al: The effect of panresistant bacteria in cystic fibrosis patients on lung transplant outcome. Am J Respir Crit Care Med 155:1699–1704, 1997

Aydin IO, Ulusahin A: Depression, anxiety comorbidity, and disability in tuberculosis and chronic obstructive pulmonary disease patients: applicability of GHQ-12. Gen Hosp Psychiatry 23:77–83, 2001

Bosley CM, Corden ZM, Rees PJ, et al: Psychological factors associated with use of home nebulized therapy for COPD. Eur Respir J 9:2346–2350, 1996

Dahlen I, Janson C: Anxiety and depression are related to the outcome of emergency treatment in patients with obstructive pulmonary disease. Chest 122:1633–1637, 2002

Paradowski LJ: Saprophytic fungal infections and lung transplantation revisited. J Heart Lung Transplant 16:524–531, 1997

Snell G, deHoyos A, Krajden M, et al: Pseudomonas capacia in lung transplantation recipients with cystic fibrosis. Chest 103:466–471, 1993

Withers NJ, Rudkin ST, White RJ: Anxiety and depression in severe chronic obstructive pulmonary disease: the effects of pulmonary rehabilitation. J Cardiopulm Rehabil 19:362–365, 1999

Chapter 4—Gastrointestinal Disorders

Select the single best response for each question.

1. Peptic ulcer disease is a common gastrointestinal illness, with a substantial psychiatric component in many cases. All of the following statements are true *except*

   A. The clinical use of nonsteroidal anti-inflammatory drugs (NSAIDs) has been identified as a major risk factor for the development of peptic ulcer disease.
   B. The presence of gut infection with *Helicobacter pylori* is associated with the development of peptic ulcer disease.
   C. It has been estimated that approximately 25% of individuals in Western countries will develop peptic ulcer disease.
   D. The prevalence of anxiety and depressive disorders appears increased in patients with peptic ulcer disease.
   E. Stressful life events have been associated with the onset, perpetuation, and recurrence of peptic ulcers.

   The correct response is option C.

   It has been estimated that approximately 10% of individuals in Western countries will develop a peptic ulcer sometime during their lifetime. *H. pylori* infection and use of NSAIDs are major risk factors for peptic ulcer disease. The prevalence of anxiety and depressive disorders appears increased in patients with peptic ulcer disease. The onset, perpetuation, and recurrence of peptic ulcers are associated with stressful life events such as earthquakes. **(p. 56)**

2. Inflammatory bowel disease (IBD), which includes Crohn's disease and ulcerative colitis, is commonly associated with behavioral and emotional factors, which may lead to involvement of the psychosomatic medicine physician. Which of the following statements is *true?*

   A. The prevalence rate of psychiatric disorders is much higher in IBD (40%–50%) than in other chronic physical illnesses.
   B. The relationship between psychiatric disorders and stress and IBD has been clearly delineated.
   C. There is no clear evidence to suggest that anxiety and depression impair health-related quality of life in patients with IBD.
   D. Because of the seriousness of medical complications, IBD patients have a higher risk of comorbid psychiatric illness compared with patients with functional bowel disorder.
   E. Among IBD patients, mood disorders are more common in older patients and in those with a history of previously diagnosed psychiatric illness.

The correct response is option E.

The prevalence rate of psychiatric disorders in IBD patients (21%–35%) is similar to that found in patients with other chronic physical illnesses. Among IBD patients, mood disorders are more common in older patients and in those with a previous history of psychiatric disorders. The relationship between psychiatric disorders and IBD is unclear. Patients may develop a psychiatric disorder because of experiences independent of the disease process. There is clear evidence that anxiety and depression impair health-related quality of life in patients with IBD. Patients with IBD show a higher prevalence of psychological disorder than the general population but a lower prevalence than patients with IBS or other functional bowel disorders. **(pp. 57–58)**

3. Irritable bowel syndrome (IBS) and functional dyspepsia are considered to be functional gastrointestinal disorders. Which of the following statements is *true?*

   A. The most common functional gastrointestinal disorder is functional dyspepsia.
   B. The prevalence of anxiety and mood disorders in patients with functional gastrointestinal illness is between 30% and 40%.
   C. Patients with chronic functional gastrointestinal disorders are more likely to present with anxiety, whereas first-time clinic patients usually present with depression.
   D. Psychiatric treatment of anxiety and mood disorders in these patients is associated with improved health-related quality of life.
   E. Patients with functional dyspepsia or IBS who consult physicians are less likely to have depression than equivalent patients who do not seek medical care.

The correct response is option D.

Psychiatric treatment of anxiety and depression has been demonstrated to improve health-related quality of life. The most common functional gastrointestinal disorder is IBS. The prevalence of anxiety and mood disorders in patients with functional gastrointestinal disorders is between 50% and 60%. Anxiety is more prominent in first-time clinic attenders, whereas depression seems more prominent in those who have chronic symptoms. Compared with nonconsulting patients, patients with functional dyspepsia and IBS patients who consult physicians have more anxiety and depression and more worries about their health, especially fears of cancer. **(pp. 60–61)**

4. Speech therapy has been found to be useful for symptomatic relief of which of the following functional gastrointestinal illnesses?

   A. Globus.
   B. Gastroesophageal reflux.
   C. Functional abdominal pain.
   D. Cyclic vomiting.
   E. IBS.

The correct response is option A.

Speech therapy may be helpful for globus. **(p. 62)**

5. Antidepressant therapy may be helpful in managing IBS patients. Among the following classes, which has been clearly shown to be of benefit in IBS?

A. Tricyclic antidepressants (TCAs).
B. Monoamine oxidase inhibitors (MAOIs).
C. Selective serotonin reuptake inhibitors (SSRIs).
D. Selective norepinephrine reuptake inhibitors (SNRIs).
E. Trazodone and nefazodone.

The correct response is option A.

There is clear evidence of the effectiveness of TCAs, which are effective in low doses and have rapid onset. SSRIs are active at higher doses and have a slower onset of action. **(p. 65)**

Chapter 5—Renal Disease

Select the single best response for each question.

1. Regarding end-stage renal disease (ESRD) in the United States, which of the following statements is *true?*

   A. Each year nearly 80,000 Americans develop ESRD.
   B. More than 340,000 patients are being treated for kidney failure.
   C. Nearly 240,000 individuals are receiving maintenance dialysis.
   D. Approximately 100,000 people have a functioning kidney transplant.
   E. All of the above.

   The correct response is option E.

   Each year, approximately 80,000 Americans develop ESRD. More than 340,000 patients are being treated for kidney failure. Nearly 240,000 individuals are receiving maintenance dialysis, and approximately 100,000 people have a functioning kidney transplant. **(p. 75)**

2. In a review of psychiatric illness involving 200,000 U.S. dialysis patients, it was reported that

   A. Nearly 10% had been hospitalized with a psychiatric diagnosis.
   B. Dementia was the most common psychiatric illness.
   C. Compared with other medical illnesses, the primary diagnosis of depression was higher in patients with ischemic heart disease than in patients with renal failure.
   D. A and C.
   E. A, B, and C.

   The correct response is option A.

   Among these dialysis patients, almost 10% had previously been hospitalized with a psychiatric diagnosis, and for 25% of this subgroup the psychiatric diagnosis was the primary reason for hospitalization (Kimmel et al. 1993). Depression and other affective disorders were the most common diagnoses, followed by delirium and dementia. The primary diagnosis of depression was more frequent in renal failure patients than in those with ischemic heart disease or cerebrovascular disease (Kimmel et al. 1993). **(p. 76)**

3. Noncompliance with dialysis treatment is associated with all of the following variables *except*

    A. Hostility toward authority.
    B. Memory impairment.
    C. Ethnic barriers.
    D. Financial problems.
    E. Anxiety.

    The correct response is option E.

    Among the factors associated with noncompliance with dialysis treatment are depression, hostility toward authority, memory impairment, ethnic barriers, and financial problems (Anderson and Kirk 1982). **(p. 78)**

4. According to recently published U.S. guidelines (Moss et al. 2000), which of the following conditions is *not* an appropriate reason to withhold dialysis?

    A. End-stage cancer.
    B. Permanent unconsciousness (as in a persistent vegetative state).
    C. Severe delirium.
    D. Severe, continued, and unrelenting pain.
    E. Multiple organ system failure in a hospitalized patient.

    The correct response is option C.

    Severe delirium is not an appropriate reason to withhold dialysis. Valid rationales for withholding dialysis include severe/irreversible dementia, permanent unconsciousness, severe/continued/unrelenting pain, and multiple organ system failure. **(p. 80)**

5. Which of the following forms of psychotherapy has been shown to be helpful in treating patients with end-stage renal disease?

    A. Behavioral contracting and weekly telephone contacts.
    B. Hypnosis.
    C. Behavioral interventions.
    D. Group therapy.
    E. All of the above.

    The correct response is option E.

    In a study of five Boston patients (Surman and Tolkoff-Rubin 1984), hypnosis was successful in curtailing psychiatric symptoms. In a study of 116 patients, Cummings et al. (1981) demonstrated that behavioral contracting and weekly telephone contacts were effective in the short term in improving compliance with medical regimens. Behavioral interventions were shown to improve compliance with fluid retention in both a small quasi-experimental study (Sagawa et al. 2003) and a controlled trial (Christensen et al. 2002). A controlled trial of group therapy in Israeli dialysis patients showed a significant decrease in psychological distress and interdialytic weight gain in those who received group therapy (Auslander and Buchs 2002). Any form of psychotherapy stands the best chance of success if conducted during dialysis treatment sessions (Levy 1999). **(p. 81)**

References

Anderson RJ, Kirk LM: Methods of improving compliance in chronic disease states. Arch Intern Med 142:1673–1675, 1982

Auslander GK, Buchs A: Evaluating an activity intervention with hemodialysis patients in Israel. Soc Work Health Care 35:407–423, 2002

Christensen AJ, Moran PJ, Wiebe JS, et al: Effect of a behavioral self-regulation intervention on patient adherence in hemodialysis. Health Psychol 21:393–397, 2002

Cummings KB, Becker M, Kirscht JP, et al: Intervention strategies to improve compliance with medical regimens by ambulatory hemodialysis patients. J Behav Med 4:111–127, 1981

Kimmel PL, Weihs K, Peterson RA: Survival in hemodialysis patients: the role of depression. J Am Soc Nephrol 3:12–27, 1993

Levy NB: Renal failure, dialysis and transplantation, in Psychiatric Treatment of the Medically Ill. Edited by Robinson RG. New York, Marcel Dekker, 1999, pp 141–153

Moss AH, Renal Physicians Association, American Society of Nephrology Working Group: a new clinical practice guideline on initiation and withdrawal of dialysis that makes explicit the role of palliative medicine. J Palliat Med 3:253–260, 2000

Robertson S, Newbigging K, Isles CG, et al: High incidence of renal failure requiring short-term dialysis: a prospective observational study. Q J Med 95:585–590, 2002

Sagawa M, Oka M, Chaboyer W: The utility of cognitive behavioural therapy on chronic haemodialysis patients' fluid intake: a preliminary examination. Int J Nurs Stud 40:367–373, 2003

Surman OS, Tolkoff-Rubin N: Use of hypnosis in patients receiving hemodialysis for end stage renal disease. Gen Hosp Psychiatry 6:31–35, 1984

Chapter 6—Endocrine Disorders

Select the single best response for each question.

1. The psychiatric care of diabetes mellitus (DM) poses several challenges for both psychiatric illness management and patients' global levels of health and functioning. Specifically, mood disorders are a significant problem in this population. All of the following are true *except*

   A. Psychiatric disorders are associated with treatment noncompliance and vascular complications in type 1, but not type 2, diabetes.

   B. The prevalence of depression in diabetic patients is two to three times higher than that in the general population.

   C. Lustman et al. (2000) have postulated that depression and poor glycemic control are reciprocally linked.

   D. Depression in diabetes mellitus typically antedates the development of vascular complications.

   E. It does not appear that the increased rate of depression in diabetes can be explained solely by emotional reactions to a chronic disease with complications.

The correct response is option A.

In both type 1 and type 2 diabetes, psychiatric disorders are associated with treatment noncompliance and vascular complications. The prevalence of depression in diabetes mellitus is two to three times higher than that in the general population. Although depression may also result from complications of diabetes and disease duration, it has been found to occur relatively early in the course of illness, before the onset of complications (Jacobson et al. 2002). Therefore, it does not appear that the increased rate of depression in diabetes can be explained solely by emotional reactions to a chronic disease with complications. **(pp. 90–91)**

2. Besides depressive disorders, other psychiatric illnesses are of clinical importance in diabetes. Which of the following statements is *true*?

   A. The high risk of diabetes in bipolar disorder patients primarily relates to type 1 diabetes.
   B. In bipolar disorder patients with type 2 diabetes, any excess weight is accounted for by weight gain from psychotropic medications.
   C. The onset of diabetes rarely occurs suddenly or dramatically with several of the atypical antipsychotics.
   D. It is believed that antagonism of 5-HT$_{1A}$ receptors may lead to decreased levels of insulin and increased blood glucose in schizophrenic patients treated with atypical antipsychotics.
   E. Atypical antipsychotics least likely to cause weight gain and glucose intolerance include risperidone and quetiapine.

The correct response is option D.

Antagonism of 5-HT$_{1A}$ receptors may play a role in decreasing levels of insulin and increasing hyperglycemia. In patients with known diabetes, atypical antipsychotic agents least likely to cause weight gain and glucose intolerance (e.g., aripiprazole and ziprasidone) should be favored. The high risk of diabetes in bipolar patients is associated with but not *fully* accounted for by weight gain–associated psychotropic drugs. The increased risk of diabetes in bipolar disorder and schizophrenia precedes the use of atypical agents. With several of the atypical antipsychotics, the onset of diabetes may occur suddenly and dramatically, with emergent ketoacidosis or hyperosmolar coma. **(pp. 91–92)**

3. Hyperthyroidism is a useful clinical model for psychiatric illness arising from metabolic disturbance. The symptoms of hyperthyroidism converge with those of several psychiatric illness groups. All of the following are true *except*

   A. Presence and severity of psychiatric symptoms in Graves' disease correlate directly with thyroid hormone levels.
   B. The most common cause of hyperthyroidism is Graves' disease.
   C. Patients with Graves' disease often present with anxiety, hypomania, irritability, depression, and/or cognitive difficulties.
   D. Antithyroid therapy is associated with improvement in psychiatric symptoms.
   E. Hyperthyroidism with anxious dysphoria is more common in younger, rather than older, patients.

The correct response is option A.

Physiological and psychiatric symptoms correlated poorly with thyroid hormone levels in Graves' disease patients (Trzepacz et al. 1989). Graves' disease is associated with anxiety, hypomania, depression, and cognitive difficulties, which may improve with antithyroid treatment. Anxious dysphoria is more common in younger patients. **(pp. 93–94)**

4. Hypothyroidism offers another model of an endocrinologically based psychiatric illness. Regarding hypothyroidism and psychiatric illness, which of the following statements is *true?*

   A. An elevated serum thyroid-stimulating hormone (TSH) concentration serves both to screen for and to confirm hypothyroidism.
   B. Grade 1 hypothyroidism involves overt clinical symptoms, elevated TSH, and low serum thyroxine (T_4) concentrations.
   C. Subclinical hypothyroidism is equally common in men and women.
   D. The most common cause of hypothyroidism is from lithium treatment.
   E. Subclinical hypothyroidism infrequently occurs in elderly women.

   The correct response is option B.

   The best screening test for hypothyroidism is an elevated serum TSH level, but an elevated TSH level should be followed by a free T_4 determination to confirm the diagnosis. Subclinical hypothyroidism affects mainly women and is particularly common in elderly women. The most common cause of hypothyroidism is autoimmune thyroiditis (Hashimoto's thyroiditis). **(p. 94)**

5. Various antipsychotic agents are associated with increased serum prolactin and resultant systemic complications. Which of the following atypical antipsychotic agents carries the highest risk of increased prolactin?

   A. Clozapine.
   B. Olanzapine.
   C. Ziprasidone.
   D. Risperidone.
   E. Quetiapine.

   The correct response is option D.

   Risperidone raises the serum prolactin concentration by an average of 45–80 ng/mL, with larger increases in women than in men. Clozapine, quetiapine, and olanzapine either cause no increase in prolactin secretion or increase prolactin transiently. **(p. 99)**

References

Jacobson AM, Samson JA, Weinger K, et al: Diabetes, the brain, and behavior: is there a biological mechanism underlying the association between diabetes and depression? Int Rev Neurobiol 51:455–479, 2002

Lustman PJ, Anderson RJ, Freedland KE, et al: Depression and poor glycemic control: a meta-analytic review of the literature. Diabetes Care 23:934–942, 2000

Trzepacz PT, Klein I, Roberts M, et al: Graves' disease: an analysis of thyroid hormone levels and hyperthyroid signs and symptoms. Am J Med 87:558–561, 1989

Chapter 7—Oncology

Select the single best response for each question.

1. Many research groups have assessed depression in cancer patients. Cancer types highly associated with depression include all of the following *except*

   A. Breast cancer.
   B. Lymphoma.
   C. Lung cancer.
   D. Oropharyngeal cancer.
   E. Pancreatic cancer.

   The correct response is option B.

   Cancer types highly associated with depression include oropharyngeal (22%–57%), pancreatic (33%–50%), breast (1.5%–46%), and lung (11%–44%). **(p. 110)**

2. An increased risk of suicide in cancer patients is associated with all of the following *except*

   A. Advanced stage of disease.
   B. Inadequately controlled pain.
   C. Social isolation.
   D. Female gender.
   E. History of psychiatric illness.

   The correct response is option D.

   An increased risk of suicide in cancer patients is associated with male gender, advanced stage of disease, poor prognosis, delirium with poor impulse control, inadequately controlled pain, depression, history of psychiatric illness, current or previous alcohol or substance abuse, previous suicide attempts, physical and emotional exhaustion, social isolation, and extreme need for control. Recognition of suicidal thoughts should lead to emergent psychiatric evaluation with frank discussion. **(p. 111)**

3. Common causes of cancer-related fatigue include which of the following cancer treatments?

   A. Interferon.
   B. Chemotherapy.
   C. Irradiation.
   D. All of the above.
   E. None of the above.

   The correct response is option D.

   Cancer-related fatigue is caused by interferon, chemotherapy, and radiation therapy, in addition to pain, hormonal imbalances, drug effects of opioids and sedatives, and psychiatric disorders such as depression and sleep disruption. **(p. 114, Table 7–2)**

4. In general, which of the following variables is associated with *less* mental distress in men with prostate cancer?

   A. More serious disease.
   B. Undergoing radiation treatment.

C. Younger age.

D. Undergoing surgery.

E. None of the above.

The correct response is option D.

In general, men undergoing surgery, older men, and men with less serious disease have less mental distress (Litwin et al. 2002). **(p. 116)**

5. Neuropsychiatric side effects of chemotherapeutic agents are common and need to be addressed by the clinician. Which of the following is associated with the triad of depression, fatigue, and encephalopathy:

A. Cisplatin.

B. 5-Fluorouacil.

C. Taxanes.

D. Thalidomide.

E. Vincristine.

The correct response is option E.

Vincristine's side effects include depression, fatigue, and encephalopathy. Cisplatin may rarely cause encephalopathy and sensory neuropathy. Side effects of 5-fluorouracil include fatigue, rare seizure or confusion, and cerebellar syndrome. Thalidomide may cause fatigue, and taxanes sensory neuropathy and fatigue. **(p. 113, Table 7–1)**

References

Litwin MS, Lubeck DP, Spitalny GM, et al: Mental health in men treated for early stage prostate carcinoma. Cancer 95:54–60, 2002

Massie MJ: Prevalence of depression in patients with cancer. J Natl Cancer Inst Monogr 32:57–71, 2004

Chapter 8—Rheumatology

Select the single best response for each question.

1. Depression is a common problem in rheumatoid arthritis. However, consideration of the specific needs and complexity of these patients is important. Which is the recommended first-line pharmacological management strategy for depression in rheumatoid arthritis?

A. Selective serotonin reuptake inhibitors (SSRIs), with doses limited to one-half the usual adult dose.

B. SSRIs, in typical adult doses.

C. Tricyclic antidepressants (TCAs), limited to low doses only.

D. TCAs in low doses, routinely combined with SSRIs.

E. Full-dose TCAs.

The correct response is option B.

SSRIs, such as fluoxetine or citalopram, in doses to recommended maxima should be considered as first-line treatment for depression in rheumatoid arthritis. TCAs in low doses are useful only for pain relief. Combined use of TCAs and SSRIs greatly increases the risk of adverse events and should be avoided unless done under expert guidance. **(p. 135)**

2. Regarding central nervous system (CNS) or psychiatric complications in rheumatoid arthritis, which of the following statements is *not* true?

    A. Neurological complications are common in rheumatoid arthritis due to direct CNS involvement.
    B. Psychiatric illness in rheumatoid arthritis most commonly occurs as emotional reactions to having a serious systemic illness.
    C. Depressive symptoms correlate with levels of physical pain in rheumatoid arthritis.
    D. Social stresses independent of those of rheumatoid arthritis are likely to contribute to the development of depression.
    E. Neuroticism in rheumatoid arthritis patients is associated with more distress, regardless of pain levels.

The correct response is option A.

Neurological complications in rheumatoid arthritis are not common, and direct involvement of the CNS is rare. **(pp. 136–137)**

3. Which of the following is *not* associated with greater risk of depression in osteoarthritis?

    A. Older age.
    B. Lower level of education.
    C. Greater self-reported impact of osteoarthritis on patient's life.
    D. More pain.
    E. Objective measures of functional disability.

The correct response is option A.

When depression occurs in patients with osteoarthritis, it has been shown to be associated with a number of factors: younger age, less education, higher pain, and greater self-reported impact of the disease. **(p. 138)**

4. Among the neuropsychiatric syndromes in systemic lupus erythematosus (SLE) specified by the American College of Rheumatology (1999), which of the following is the most common?

    A. Mood disorders.
    B. Anxiety disorders.
    C. Psychosis.
    D. Cognitive dysfunction.
    E. Acute confusional state/delirium.

The correct response is option D.

Cognitive dysfunction is the most common neuropsychiatric disorder in patients with SLE, affecting up to 80% of SLE patients. Depression is the second most common disorder, present in approximately 50% of patients. It is unclear whether anxiety is attributable to direct CNS involvement or simply a reaction to chronic illness. Distinguishing psychosis caused by CNS lupus from corticosteroid-induced psychosis presents a major diagnostic challenge. Delirium is common in severe SLE. **(p. 140)**

5. Confusion, psychosis, mania, aggression, depression, nightmares, anxiety, and delirium have all been associated with which of the following medications for SLE?

    A. Gold salts.
    B. Penicillamine.
    C. Azathioprine.
    D. Leflunomide.
    E. Hydroxychloroquine.

The correct response is option E.

Hydroxychloroquine produces many psychiatric side effects. Gold salts and penicillamine do not appear to produce psychiatric side effects; azathioprine may cause delirium. **(p. 145, Table 8–2)**

Reference

American College of Rheumatology Ad Hoc Committee on Neuropsychiatric Lupus Nomenclature: Nomenclature and case definitions for neuropsychiatric lupus syndromes. Arthritis Rheum 42:599–608, 1999

Chapter 9—Chronic Fatigue and Fibromyalgia Syndromes

Select the single best response for each question.

1. All of the following psychiatric disorders are among the exclusion criteria for chronic fatigue syndrome *except*

    A. Dementia.
    B. Anorexia or bulimia nervosa.
    C. Unipolar depression without melancholia.
    D. Alcohol or substance misuse.
    E. Bipolar depression.

The correct response is option C.

Unipolar depression without melancholia is *not* an exclusion criterion for chronic fatigue syndrome. **(p. 155, Table 9–1)**

2. The American College of Rheumatology (ACR) has developed diagnostic criteria for fibromyalgia. Which of the following is/are included in the criteria?

    A. Widespread pain.
    B. Symptom duration of at least 1 year.
    C. Pain at 11 or more of 18 specific sites on the body.
    D. A and C.
    E. A, B, and C.

The correct response is option D.

The ACR criteria published in 1990 are the most widely accepted (Wolfe et al. 1990). These specify widespread pain of at least 3 months' duration and tenderness at 11 or more of 18 specific sites on the body. **(p. 156, Table 9–2)**

3. Which of the following psychiatric disorders is most commonly found in patients with chronic fatigue syndrome or fibromyalgia syndrome?

    A. Depression.
    B. Psychosis.
    C. Anxiety.
    D. A and C.
    E. A, B, and C.

The correct response is option D.

In clinical practice, many but not all patients with chronic fatigue syndrome or fibromyalgia syndrome can be given a psychiatric diagnosis. Most will meet criteria for depression or an anxiety syndrome. **(p. 157)**

4. Which of the following is one of the best-supported biological abnormalities reported to be associated with both chronic fatigue syndrome and fibromyalgia syndrome?

    A. Low blood levels of cortisol.
    B. High blood levels of cortisol.
    C. Low cerebrospinal fluid (CSF) levels of substance P.
    D. Elevated blood pressure.
    E. Abnormalities of muscle metabolism.

The correct response is option A.

One of the best-supported biological abnormalities reported to be associated with both chronic fatigue syndrome and fibromyalgia syndrome is changes in neuroendocrine stress hormones. A repeated observation has been a tendency toward low blood levels of cortisol and a poor cortisol response to stress (Parker et al. 2001). This finding differs from what would be expected in depression (in which blood levels of cortisol are typically elevated) but is similar to effects reported in other stress-induced and anxiety states. It is not known whether these changes in neuroendocrine stress hormones represent a primary abnormality or merely a consequence of inactivity or sleep disruption, however. Patients with fibromyalgia syndrome also show elevated cerebrospinal fluid levels of substance P (Russell et al. 1994). However, elevated substance P has not been found in chronic fatigue syndrome patients (Evengard et al. 1998). Failure to maintain blood pressure when assuming erect posture (orthostatic intolerance)—and particularly a pattern in which the heart rate increases abnormally (postural orthostatic tachycardia syndrome)—has been reported in both chronic fatigue syndrome (Rowe et al. 1995) and fibromyalgia syndrome (Bou-Holaigah et al. 1997). **(p. 162)**

5. All of the following medical disorders are commonly found in patients evaluated for either chronic fatigue syndrome or fibromyalgia syndrome *except*

    A. Sleep apnea.

B. Rheumatoid arthritis.
C. Spinal stenosis.
D. Anemia.
E. Thyroid disorders.

The correct response is option B.

Rheumatoid arthritis is uncommon (~1 per 2,500–1,000,000 cases) in fibromyalgia syndrome; the incidence of sleep apnea, spinal stenosis, anemia, and thyroid disorders is approximately 1 per 100 cases. **(pp. 166–167, Table 9–4)**

References

Bou-Holaigah I, Calkins H, Flynn JA, et al: Provocation of hypotension and pain during upright tilt table testing in adults with fibromyalgia. Clin Exp Rheumatol 15:239–246, 1997

Evengard B, Nilsson CG, Lindh G, et al: Chronic fatigue syndrome differs from fibromyalgia: no evidence for elevated substance P levels in cerebrospinal fluid of patients with chronic fatigue syndrome. Pain 78:153–155, 1998

Parker AJ, Wessely S, Cleare AJ: The neuroendocrinology of chronic fatigue syndrome and fibromyalgia. Psychol Med 31:1331–1345, 2001

Rowe PC, Bou Holaigah I, Kan JS, et al: Is neurally mediated hypotension an unrecognised cause of chronic fatigue? Lancet 345:623–624, 1995

Russell IJ, Orr MD, Littman B, et al: Elevated cerebrospinal fluid levels of substance P in patients with the fibromyalgia syndrome. Arthritis Rheum 37:1593–1601, 1994

Wolfe F, Smythe HA, Yunus MB, et al: The American College of Rheumatology 1990 criteria for the classification of fibromyalgia: report of the Multicenter Criteria Committee. Arthritis Rheum 33:160–172, 1990

Chapter 10—Infectious Diseases

Select the single best response for each question.

1. Pediatric autoimmune neuropsychiatric disorder associated with streptococcal infection (PANDAS) offers a compelling model for infectious disease–induced psychiatric illness. All of the following are true regarding PANDAS *except*

    A. PANDAS frequently has an episodic course characterized by abrupt onset of symptoms with frequent relapses and remissions.
    B. PANDAS consists of obsessive-compulsive and tic symptoms that occur following group A beta-hemolytic streptococcus (GABHS) infection.
    C. The infection most commonly implicated is pharyngitis.
    D. Antistreptolysin-O (ASO) titers rise with GABHS infections, and levels covary with symptoms.
    E. Because of the high specificity of ASO titers in evaluation, throat cultures are not necessary.

The correct response is option E.

Throat cultures are recommended in addition to ASO titers (Swedo et al. 1998). Prompt antibiotic treatment may prevent the expected rise in ASO titers. **(p. 183)**

2. Rocky Mountain spotted fever (RMSF) is another infectious disease that is associated with neuropsychiatric complications. Which of the following statements is *true?*

A. The incidence of RMSF peaks in October through April.
B. Central nervous system (CNS) involvement is seen in 25% of RMSF cases and includes lethargy, confusion, and delirium.
C. Irritability, personality changes, and apathy may occur commonly in elderly individuals before the rash in RMSF.
D. Encephalopathy in RMSF is rare unless computed tomography (CT) or magnetic resonance imaging (MRI) scans are abnormal.
E. Over 50% of U.S. RMSF cases occur in the mountainous west.

The correct response is option B.

The incidence of RMSF peaks in May through September. CNS involvement occurs in 25% of RMSF cases and includes lethargy, confusion, and occasionally fulminant delirium. Irritability, personality changes, and apathy may occur before the rash, particularly in children. Encephalopathy is seen in 80% of patients with normal scans. Half of U.S. cases occur in the South Atlantic region. **(p. 184)**

3. Viral hepatitis is a common clinical problem with psychiatric implications. Which of the following statements is *true?*

A. Depression is a contraindication to interferon therapy.
B. Fatigue in chronic hepatitis is more closely related to disease severity than to depression or social factors.
C. Depression is uncommon in hepatitis C and B infections.
D. Depression is induced in 20%–40% of patients treated with interferon.
E. Depression induced by interferon is not responsive to selective serotonin reuptake inhibitors (SSRIs).

The correct response is option D.

Treatment with interferon causes depression in 20%–40% of patients. Depression associated with hepatitis or interferon is amenable to treatment with antidepressants; therefore, depression should not be considered a contraindication to interferon therapy. Dosing should be adjusted downward for patients with impaired liver function. Fatigue in chronic hepatitis is more closely correlated with depression and other psychological factors than with severity of hepatitis. Depression is frequently comorbid, especially in the chronic forms of hepatitis B and C infection. **(p. 191)**

4. Meningoencephalitis with prominent somnolence, colloquially known as sleeping sickness, is associated with which of the following infections?

A. Neurocysticercosis.
B. Toxoplasmosis.
C. Trypanosomiasis.
D. Malaria.
E. Schistosomiasis.

The correct response is option C.

Trypanosomiasis, caused by a subspecies of *Trypanosoma brucei,* is transmitted to humans and animals by the bite of the blood-sucking tsetse fly. Toxoplasmosis is caused by the parasite *Toxoplasma gondii;* latent infection is common, but psychosis has been reported as a presenting symptom in CNS infection. Neurocysticercosis, an infection of the CNS caused by the larval form of *Taenia solium*, is the leading cause of seizures in adults in endemic areas. Other psychiatric symptoms include depression, psychosis, and cognitive decline. Malaria, caused by *Plasmodium falciparum*, begins with disorientation, mild stupor, and psychosis and rapidly progresses to seizures and coma with decerebrate posturing. Schistosomiasis, caused by trematodes of the genus *Schistosoma*, has few CNS symptoms. **(pp. 193–194)**

5. Which of the following drugs has been associated with irritability and depression?

    A. Procaine penicillin.
    B. Quinolones.
    C. Acyclovir.
    D. Interferon-alpha.
    E. Interleukin-2.

    The correct response is option D.

    Procaine penicillin can cause anxiety and psychosis; quinolones may produce psychosis and agitation; acyclovir may produce psychosis and delirium; interleukin-2 may produce psychosis; and interferon-alpha may produce irritability and depression. **(p. 194, Table 10–2)**

Reference

Swedo SE, Susan E, Leonard HL, et al: Pediatric autoimmune neuropsychiatric disorders associated with streptococcal infections: clinical description of the first 50 cases. Am J Psychiatry 155:264–271, 1998

Chapter 11—HIV/AIDS

Select the single best response for each question.

1. The most common neoplasm seen in AIDS patients is

    A. Sarcoma.
    B. Lung cancer.
    C. Pancreatic cancer.
    D. Colon cancer.
    E. Lymphoma.

    The correct response is option E.

    Lymphoma is the most common central nervous system (CNS) neoplasm seen in AIDS patients, affecting between 0.6% and 3.0%. The patient is generally afebrile; may develop a single lesion with focal neurological signs or small multifocal lesions; and most commonly presents with mental status change. Seizures occur in about 15% of these patients. **(p. 207)**

2. The addition of zidovudine to antiviral treatment regimens for HIV infection has resulted in

    A. Worsening of cognitive functioning.
    B. Improvement in cognitive functioning.
    C. Onset of parkinsonian symptoms.
    D. Increased risk for psychosis.
    E. Increased delirium.

The correct response is option B.

The AIDS Clinical Trials Group trial compared high doses of zidovudine with placebo but was stopped prematurely after preliminary data showed dramatic cognitive improvement in those receiving zidovudine (Sidtis et al. 1993). A sharp decline in the incidence of HIV-associated dementia was observed following widespread use of zidovudine (Chiesi et al. 1990, 1996; Portegies et al. 1989), and HIV-associated dementia became rare in patients receiving continued zidovudine treatment (Portegies et al. 1989). **(p. 210)**

3. HIV is believed to increase the risk of developing major depression through which of the following mechanisms?

    A. Chronic stress.
    B. Worsening social isolation.
    C. Demoralization.
    D. Direct injury to subcortical brain areas.
    E. All of the above.

The correct response is option E.

HIV increases the risk of developing major depression through a variety of mechanisms, including direct injury to subcortical areas of brain, chronic stress, worsening social isolation, and intense demoralization. Direct evidence for a relationship between worsening HIV disease and the development of major depression is limited, but several studies have supported this link, particularly the Multicenter AIDS Cohort Study (Lyketsos et al. 1996). This study showed that rates of depression increased 2.5-fold as CD4 cells declined to fewer than 200/mm^3 just before patients developed AIDS, suggesting that lower CD4 cell counts predict increased rates of depression. **(p. 212)**

4. AIDS mania often has a clinical profile different from that of primary mania. All of the following are characteristics of AIDS mania *except*

    A. Irritable mood.
    B. Infrequent spontaneous remissions.
    C. Psychomotor agitation.
    D. More chronic than episodic course.
    E. None of the above.

The correct response is option C.

AIDS mania seems to have a clinical profile somewhat different from that of primary mania. Irritable mood is often a prominent feature, but elevated mood can be observed. Sometimes prominent psychomotor slowing accompanying the cognitive slowing of AIDS dementia will replace the expected hyperactivity of mania, which complicates the differential diagnosis. AIDS mania is usually quite severe in its presentation and malignant in its course. AIDS mania seems to be more chronic than episodic, with infrequent spontaneous remissions, and usually relapses with cessation of treatment. Because of their cognitive deficits, patients have little functional reserve to begin with and are less able to pursue treatment independently or consistently. **(p. 216)**

5. Which of the following personality characteristics *best* describes the majority of patients who would be seen in an AIDS clinic in a metropolitan area?

    A. Unstable extravert.

    B. Stable extravert.

    C. Unstable introvert.

    D. Stable introvert.

    E. None of the above.

The correct response is option A.

Unstable extraverts are the most prone to engage in practices that place them at risk for HIV. In the psychiatry service of the Johns Hopkins AIDS clinic (a referral-biased sample), about 60% of patients present with this blend of extraversion and emotional instability (Lyketsos et al. 1994). Unstable extraverts are more likely to engage in behavior that places them at risk for HIV infection and are more likely to pursue sex promiscuously. The second most common personality type is that of the stable extravert. Introverted personalities appear to be less common. Their focus on the future, avoidance of negative consequences, and preference for cognition over feeling render them more likely to engage in protective and preventative behaviors. Unstable introverts are anxious, moody, and pessimistic. Typically, they seek drugs and/or sex not for pleasure, but for relief or distraction from pain. Stable introverts are least likely to engage in risky or hedonistic behaviors. They are HIV-positive, typically, as a result of a blood transfusion or an occupational needle stick. **(p. 219)**

References

Chiesi A, Agresti MG, Dally LG, et al: Decrease in notifications of AIDS dementia complex in 1989–1990 in Italy: possible role of the early treatment with zidovudine. Medicina (Firenze) 10:415–416, 1990

Chiesi A, Vella S, Dally LG, et al: Epidemiology of AIDS dementia complex in Europe. AIDS in Europe Study Group. J Acquir Immune Defic Syndr Hum Retrovirol 11:39–44, 1996

Lyketsos CG, Hanson A, Fishman M, et al: Screening for psychiatric morbidity in a medical outpatient clinic for HIV infection: the need for a psychiatric presence. Int J Psychiatry Med 24:103–113, 1994

Lyketsos CG, Hoover DR, Guccione M, et al: Changes in depressive symptoms as AIDS develops. Am J Psychiatry 153:1430–1437, 1996

Portegies P, De Gans J, Lange JM, et al: Declining incidence of AIDS dementia complex after introduction of zidovudine treatment. BMJ 299:819–821, 1989 (published erratum appears in BMJ 299:1141, 1989)

Sidtis JJ, Gatsonis C, Price RW, et al (for the AIDS Clinical Trials Group): Zidovudine treatment of the AIDS dementia complex: results of a placebo-controlled trial. Ann Neurol 33:343–349, 1993

Chapter 12—Dermatology

Select the single best response for each question.

1. Atopic dermatitis is an often-chronic clinical problem with meaningful psychiatric co-morbidity. Which of the following statements is *not* true?

   A. Stressful life events often precede the onset or exacerbation of atopic dermatitis.
   B. Stress may have an effect on atopic dermatitis through an interaction between the central nervous system (CNS) and the immune system.
   C. Various behavioral therapy models have been shown to reduce anxiety and depression in patients with atopic dermatitis.
   D. Topical doxepin cream has been shown to decrease itching in atopic dermatitis.
   E. Trimipramine has been shown to reduce nighttime scratching by increasing the time spent in Stage I sleep.

   The correct response is option E.

   Trimipramine, an antidepressant with histamine receptor antagonism, decreases the fragmentation of sleep and reduces the time spent in Stage I sleep, which in turn diminishes the amount of scratching that occurs during the night (Savin et al. 1979). **(p. 239)**

2. Psoriasis is a chronic and relapsing dermatological disease of major importance to the psychiatrist, both because the disease is associated with significant psychiatric comorbidity and because it can occur as a side effect of psychiatric treatment. Which of the following statements is *true?*

   A. Lithium-induced psoriasis typically persists after lithium is discontinued.
   B. Lithium-induced psoriasis typically occurs after several years of lithium treatment and rarely during the first few years of treatment.
   C. Psoriasis patients have been shown to be at high risk for comorbid personality disorders, including schizoid and avoidant personality disorders.
   D. Disability from psoriasis is more strongly correlated with disease severity and location than with psychosocial variables.
   E. Psoriasis is much more common in men (2:1) than in women.

   The correct response is option C.

   Patients with psoriasis have been shown to have high levels of anxiety and depression and significant comorbidity with several personality disorders, including schizoid, avoidant, passive-aggressive, and compulsive personality disorders. Lithium-induced psoriasis typically occurs within the first few years of treatment, and resolves after the lithium is discontinued. Psychological factors are stronger determinants of disability in patients with psoriasis than are disease severity, location, and duration. Common triggers of psoriasis include cold weather, physical trauma, acute bacterial and viral infections, corticosteroid withdrawal, beta-adrenergic blockers, and lithium. Psoriasis affects about 2% of the U.S. population and is equally common in women and men. **(pp. 239–240)**

3. Delusional parasitosis is an unusual syndrome in which the patient believes that he or she is infested with living organisms. Which of the following is *not* true?

A. Patients typically have experienced a specific precipitating event.
B. Patients typically have had actual exposure to parasites.
C. Delusional parasitosis typically occurs with other delusions and with other impairment of thought or thought processes.
D. Affected patients often respond to treatment with pimozide.
E. Delusional parasitosis has a female-to-male ratio of 3:1 in patients age 50 years and older.

The correct response is option C.

Delusional parasitosis typically occurs as a single somatic delusion with no other impairment of thought or thought processes. A specific precipitant and "actual" exposure to contagious organisms or infestation are common. Delusional parasitosis has an equal sex distribution in patients younger than 50 years and a female-to-male ratio of 3:1 in patients age 50 years and older (Lyell 1983). **(pp. 243–244)**

4. Psychogenic excoriation may lead to substantial dermatological problems. Depressive and anxiety disorders are common in patients with this condition. Case reports and small open trials have shown some efficacy for psychotropic medications in psychogenic excoriation. Which two tricyclic antidepressants (TCAs) have been shown to be effective?

A. Nortriptyline and doxepin.
B. Doxepin and clomipramine.
C. Nortriptyline and desipramine.
D. Imipramine and doxepin.
E. Imipramine and desipramine.

The correct response is option B.

The TCAs doxepin (Harris et al. 1987) and clomipramine (Gupta et al. 1986) have been shown to be effective for psychogenic excoriation, as have several selective serotonin reuptake inhibitors and antipsychotics. **(p. 245)**

5. Which of the following is *not* true of trichotillomania or its psychiatric comorbidity?

A. The mean age at onset of trichotillomania is after age 15 years.
B. Anxiety, mood, and substance use disorders are commonly comorbid with trichotillomania.
C. The lifetime prevalence of trichotillomania is 0.6% for both men and women.
D. The behavioral treatment of habit reversal has been reported to be effective in trichotillomania.
E. Clomipramine has been shown to be superior to desipramine for treatment, supporting an "obsessive-compulsive spectrum" construct for trichotillomania.

The correct response is option A.

The mean age at onset of trichotillomania is 13 years, and the lifetime prevalence of trichotillomania is 0.6% when strict criteria are used. Comorbid psychiatric disorders in patients with trichotillomania include anxiety, mood, substance abuse, and eating disorders. A family history of obsessive-compulsive disorder and trichotillomania is common (Swedo and Leonard 1992). In one study, trichotillomania showed a better response to clomipramine than to desipramine (Swedo et al. 1989). The behavioral treatment of habit reversal has been reported to be effective in trichotillomania and involves awareness of situations or stressors associated with hair pulling; relaxation training; and competing response training (Azrin et al. 1980). **(p. 246)**

References

Azrin NH, Nunn RG, Frantz SE: Treatment of hairpulling (trichotillomania): a comparative study of habit reversal and negative practice training. J Behav Ther Exp Psychiatry 11:13–20, 1980

Harris BA, Sherertz EF, Flowers FP: Improvement of chronic neurotic excoriations with oral doxepin therapy. Int J Dermatol 26:541–543, 1987

Gupta MA, Gupta AK, Haberman HF: Neurotic excoriations: a review and some new perspectives. Compr Psychiatry 27:381–386, 1986

Lyell A: Delusions of parasitosis. Br J Dermatol 108:485–499, 1983

Savin JA, Paterson WD, Adam K, et al: Effects of trimeprazine and trimipramine on nocturnal scratching in patients with atopic eczema. Arch Dermatol 115:313–315, 1979

Swedo SE, Leonard HL: Trichotillomania: an obsessive compulsive spectrum disorder? Psychiatr Clin North Am 15:777–790, 1992

Swedo SE, Leonard HL, Rapoport JL, et al: A double-blind comparison of clomipramine and desipramine in the treatment of trichotillomania (hair pulling). N Engl J Med 321:497–501, 1989

Chapter 13—Surgery

Select the single best response for each question.

1. Which of the following are the elements of informed consent that a surgeon should include in his or her discussion with a patient about a proposed surgery?

    A. Diagnosis.
    B. Why the surgery is the treatment of choice.
    C. Expected risks and benefits.
    D. Alternatives and their consequences.
    E. All of the above.

    The correct response is option E.

    The communication of factual information understandable to the patient is the responsibility of the surgeon. It should include diagnosis, reasons that the operation is thought to be the treatment of choice, and expected risks and benefits and their probabilities. Alternatives and their consequences, as well as financial costs, also should be discussed. Competent patients have a right to decide whether to accept or reject a proposed surgery. Although the psychiatric consultant cannot legally declare a patient incompetent, he or she can evaluate the medicolegal elements of the patient's decision-making capacity. **(p. 262)**

2. What percentage of patients experience significant preoperative anxiety?

    A. Less than 10%.
    B. 10%–20%.
    C. 40%–60%.
    D. 80%–90%.
    E. None of the above.

The correct response is option C.

Nearly 20 years ago, Regal and colleagues (1985) systematically assessed 150 patients before surgery and found that 54% were anxious. Many patients were anxious about the anesthesia; patients often feared that the anesthetic would prematurely wear off or feared they would not wake up from the anesthesia. Nearly one-third of patients are afraid of anesthesia, as distinct from the operation itself (van Wijk and Smalhout 1990). **(p. 263)**

3. Risk factors for developing postoperative delirium include all of the following *except*

    A. Older age.
    B. Alcohol use.
    C. Cognitive impairment.
    D. Male gender.
    E. Type of surgery.

The correct response is option D.

Multiple preoperative risk factors for postoperative delirium have been identified and include older age, alcohol use, cognitive impairment (especially the dementias), chronic comorbid illnesses and medications used to treat these illnesses, severity of the acute illness, and type of surgery. Postoperative changes in the sleep–wake cycle, inadequately treated pain, and use of medications such as benzodiazepines increase the likelihood of delirium. **(p. 266)**

4. Delirium is common in burn patients. All of the following are common causes of delirium in burn patients *except*

    A. Hypernatremia.
    B. Hypophosphatemia.
    C. Fluid shifts.
    D. Opioids.
    E. Sepsis.

The correct response is option A.

Hyponatremia (not hypernatremia) and hypophosphatemia, fluid shifts and electrolytes imbalance, as well as sepsis and the use of opioids to treat pain, are common causes of delirium in burn patients. **(p. 271)**

5. Bariatric surgery is usually performed for patients with extreme or morbid obesity. According to the National Heart, Lung, and Blood Institute guidelines, *extreme obesity* is a body mass index (BMI) of

    A. >15 kg/m^2.
    B. >20 kg/m^2.
    C. >25 kg/m^2.
    D. >30 kg/m^2.
    E. >40 kg/m^2.

The correct response is option E.

The National Heart, Lung, and Blood Institute (1998) clinical guidelines define extreme obesity as a BMI greater than 40 kg/m². BMI is a calculated number attained by dividing weight in kilograms by height in meters squared. Extreme obesity is also called morbid obesity because it is associated with high premature morbidity and mortality, most commonly as a result of complications of type 2 diabetes mellitus, hypertension, hyperlipidemia, or sleep apnea. **(p. 274)**

References

National Heart, Lung, and Blood Institute: Clinical Guidelines on the Identification, Evaluation, and Treatment of Overweight and Obesity in Adults. Bethesda, MD, National Institutes of Health, National Heart, Lung, and Blood Institute, June 1998Regal H, Rose W, Hahnel S, et al: Evaluation of psychological stress before general anesthesia. Psychiatr Neurol Med Psychol (Leipz) 37:151–155, 1985

van Wijk MG, Smalhout B: A postoperative analysis of the patient's view of anaesthesia in a Netherlands' teaching hospital. Anaesthesia 45:679–682, 1990

Chapter 14—Organ Transplantation

Select the single best response for each question.

1. Which of the following organ transplantations has the highest percentage of patient survival at 10 years posttransplant?

    A. Lung.
    B. Kidney.
    C. Pancreas.
    D. Heart.
    E. Liver.

    The correct response is option C.

    Pancreas transplant recipients have the highest percentage of survival at 10 years posttransplant, a survival rate of approximately 70%. **(p. 286, Figure 14–1)**

2. Psychosocial rating instruments may be of value in assessing patients' psychological preparation for and adaptation to transplant surgery. All of the following are true *except*

    A. The Psychosocial Assessment of Candidates for Transplantation (PACT) provides both an overall score and a series of subscale scores.
    B. The PACT can be quickly completed but requires scoring by a skilled and experienced clinician.
    C. The Transplant Evaluation Rating Scale (TERS) rates 10 discrete areas of psychological functioning.
    D. The TERS summary score is derived from a mathematical formula.
    E. The TERS is a self-administered instrument and does not require a skilled clinician to administer it.

    The correct response is option E.

The TERS and the PACT both require administration by a skilled clinician to maintain accuracy. **(p. 290)**

3. Factors that increase the risk of posttransplantation psychiatric illness include all of the following *except*

    A. Pretransplant history of psychiatric illness.
    B. Longer hospitalization.
    C. Male gender.
    D. Greater physical impairment.
    E. Fewer social supports.

The correct response is option C.

Female gender, not male gender, is one of the factors that increases the risk of posttransplantation psychiatric illness. **(p. 291)**

4. Because of the complexity of posttransplant immunosuppressive and other ongoing medical therapy, treatment compliance is crucial to the ongoing well-being of these patients. Which of the following statements is *not* true?

    A. Medical noncompliance in posttransplant patients is estimated at 20%–50%.
    B. Noncompliance is a major risk factor for graft rejection and may account for 25% of deaths after the initial recovery period.
    C. In the Dew study of compliance in heart transplant recipients (Dew et al. 1996), nonadherence to immunosuppressive medication regimens was the most frequent area of noncompliance.
    D. Persisting psychiatric illness after transplantation is associated with medical noncompliance.
    E. In an extensive literature review of posttransplant compliance for all organ types, one research team found that anxiety disorders were significantly associated with noncompliance.

The correct response is option C.

Medical noncompliance in posttransplant patients is estimated at 20%–50%. Dew and colleagues (1996) examined compliance in eight domains of posttransplant care. The degree of noncompliance varied, but noncompliance was most persistent in the domains of exercise (37%), blood pressure monitoring (34%), immunosuppressive medication (20%), smoking (19%), diet (18%), blood work completion (15%), clinic attendance (9%), and heavy drinking (6%). **(p. 293)**

5. As is true in other areas of medical practice in which a high degree of personal investment in care is required for a successful sense of physician–patient collaboration, patients with personality disorders present special challenges for the multidisciplinary transplant team. Which of the following personality disorders is associated with the highest rate of posttransplant noncompliance?

    A. Obsessive-compulsive.
    B. Borderline.
    C. Antisocial.
    D. Narcissistic.
    E. Avoidant.

The correct response is option B.

Borderline personality disorder is considered to represent the highest risk for post-transplant noncompliance. **(p. 297)**

Reference

Dew MA, Roth LH, Thompson ME, et al: Medical compliance and its predictors in the first year after heart transplantation. J Heart Lung Transplant 15:631–645, 1996

Chapter 15—Neurology and Neurosurgery

Select the single best response for each question.

1. Which of the following statements concerning a cerebrovascular accident or stroke is *false?*

    A. The survival rate 1 year after cerebral hemorrhage is 33%.
    B. Cerebral hemorrhage is four times more common than cerebral infarction.
    C. The survival rate 1 year after cerbral infarction is 75%.
    D. Strokes are the third most common cause of death in the Western world.
    E. Stroke occurs more commonly in men than in women.

    The correct response is option B.

    Cerebral infarction is four times more common than cerebral hemorrhage. **(pp. 313–314)**

2. Which of the following is a category or type of vascular dementia?

    A. Subcortical ischemic dementia.
    B. Multi-infarct dementia.
    C. Dementia due to focal "strategic" infarction.
    D. A and B.
    E. A, B, and C.

    The correct response is option E.

    Vascular dementia is an imprecise term referring to a heterogeneous group of dementing disorders caused by impairment of the brain's blood supply. These disorders fall into three principal categories: subcortical ischemic dementia, multi-infarct dementia, and dementia due to focal "strategic" infarction. **(p. 314)**

3. Which of the following statements concerning psychiatric symptoms in Parkinson's disease (PD) is *true?*

    A. Hallucinations and delusions occur in 29%–54% of cases of PD without dementia.
    B. Hallucinations in PD are usually auditory and occur without insight.
    C. Depression has a prevalence rate of 40%–50% in PD.
    D. High-potency typical antipsychotics are preferred in PD because of fewer anticholinergic side effects.
    E. Anxiety is uncommon in PD and usually occurs earlier in the disease process.

    The correct response is option C.

Hallucinations and delusions occur in 29%–54% of cases of PD with dementia and in 7%–14% of cases of PD without dementia. Hallucinations usually occur in the presence of intact insight and frequently are visual. The prevalence rate of depression in PD is 40%–50%. Atypical antipsychotic medications are preferred in PD, and high-potency typical antipsychotic agents should be avoided. Anxiety is common in PD and tends to occur later in the disease process. **(pp. 316–317)**

4. Which of the following statements about psychiatric symptoms in multiple sclerosis (MS) is *false?*

   A. More than half of MS patients report depressive symptoms.
   B. Cortical syndromes such as aphasia, apraxia, and agnosia are relatively rare.
   C. Cognitive impairment is rare, affecting less than 10% of MS patients.
   D. Fatigue is the most common single symptom in MS.
   E. Acute and chronic pain are common and disabling complications of MS.

   The correct response is option C.

   Cognitive impairment affects at least half of all patients with MS. Although depression and cognitive impairment are common, cortical syndromes are rare. Pain is common and disabling in MS patients. **(p. 318)**

5. Which of the following statements concerning Huntington's disease is *true?*

   A. Has a prevalence rate of 5–7 per 100,000 population.
   B. Affects men more than women.
   C. The most common age at onset is in young or middle adulthood.
   D. A and C.
   E. A, B, and C.

   The correct response is option D.

   Huntington's disease occurs at a prevalence of 5–7 per 100,000 population in the United States, with wide regional variations. Onset can be at any age but most commonly is in young or middle adulthood. The sexes are affected equally. The disorder exhibits the phenomenon of anticipation, in which the age at onset tends to decrease over the generations, especially with paternal transmission. **(p. 320)**

Chapter 16—Obstetrics and Gynecology

Select the single best response for each question.

1. Infertility is a common clinical problem in obstetric/gynecological practice that is often fraught with psychosocial distress. Attention to and management of comorbid psychiatric illness may be an important part of infertility treatment. All of the following statements are true *except*

   A. The prevalence of infertility has increased steadily since 1965.
   B. Generalized anxiety disorder (GAD) is associated with lower rates of fecundity.
   C. Comorbid depression is associated with lower pregnancy rates in women undergoing in vitro fertilization.
   D. Restrictive or purging eating behaviors are often undisclosed and result in poor fecundity.

E. The majority of infertility problems are attributable to the male or are of unknown etiology.

The correct response is option A.

The rate of infertility has remained relatively stable since 1965, although the popular impression is that it has risen. GAD is associated with lower rates of fertility (King 2003). Depression is associated with lower pregnancy rates after in vitro fertilization (Demyttenaere et al. 1998). Eating disorders are associated with poor fecundity. **(p. 344)**

2. The pharmacological interactions between psychotropic medications and contraceptives may result in unwelcome clinical events. All of the following statements are true *except*

A. Implanted levonorgestrel metabolism can be enhanced by phenobarbital, decreasing contraceptive effectiveness.
B. Oral contraceptives inhibit the metabolism of tricyclic antidepressants, thus increasing serum levels.
C. Oral contraceptives enhance the metabolism of benzodiazepines, decreasing their effectiveness.
D. Modafinil increases the metabolism of oral contraceptives.
E. Carbamazepine and oxcarbazepine both enhance the metabolism of oral contraceptives.

The correct response is option C.

Oral contraceptives inhibit the hepatic oxidation of benzodiazepines and tricyclic antidepressants, thus enhancing their effectiveness. By contrast, modafinil, carbamazepine, and oxcarbazepine enhance the metabolism of oral contraceptives, thereby decreasing their effectiveness. **(p. 346)**

3. Hysterectomy is a common gynecological procedure that frequently involves significant psychiatric factors. Which of the following statements is *true?*

A. The mean age of women undergoing hysterectomy is the early to mid-50s, when menopause normally occurs.
B. Among women who undergo hysterectomy, African American women have the procedure at an older age than do other American women, on the average.
C. Women who undergo hysterectomy for chronic pelvic pain have better psychological outcomes than do women who undergo hysterectomy for bleeding.
D. Women undergoing surgical hysterectomy with oophorectomy are at risk for depression, especially if they have a history of depression associated with reproductive events.
E. Most studies show a decrease in sexuality in women following hysterectomy.

The correct response is option D.

The mean age of women undergoing hysterectomy is the mid-40s, or an average of 6–7 years before the mean age at natural menopause. Women undergoing hysterectomy with oophorectomy are subject to sudden surgical menopause and are at risk for depression, especially if they have a history of depression associated with reproductive events. Although vaginal hysterectomies are associated with less surgical mortality and shorter lengths of stay, abdominal hysterectomies are still more commonly performed. African American women, on the average, undergo hysterectomy at a younger age. Women who have hysterectomy for chronic pelvic pain have worse psychological outcomes than do women who have the procedure because of bleeding. Most studies have found no change in sexuality in women following hysterectomy. **(pp. 347–348)**

4. Psychiatric disorders that occur during pregnancy can be of great concern because of the challenges of managing a pregnant psychiatric patient. Which of the following statements is *true?*

   A. Panic disorder patients who become pregnant should continue on medication throughout pregnancy.
   B. Obsessive-compulsive disorder is likely to worsen postpartum but not prepartum.
   C. Electroconvulsive therapy (ECT) for acute psychosis during pregnancy can be effective and is generally safe for the fetus.
   D. Despite the later-appearing cognitive impairments, the perinatal mortality for fetal alcohol syndrome is less than 5%.
   E. In "crack babies," the cognitive impairments are usually due to the toxic exposure to cocaine in utero rather than to social factors.

   The correct response is option C.

   ECT for acute affective psychotic episodes can be effective and is relatively safe for the fetus. Patients with panic disorder should be tapered off medication gradually and treated with cognitive-behavioral therapy. Obsessive-compulsive disorder is likely to worsen both pre- and postpartum. The perinatal mortality for fetal alcohol syndrome is 17%. Most of the negative cognitive and behavioral findings in "crack babies" appear to result from the environment in which they grow up rather than from intrauterine exposure to cocaine. **(pp. 352–353)**

5. Postpartum depression and psychosis are among the most serious and potentially dangerous conditions in psychiatry because of their threat to infant safety. Which of the following statements is *true?*

   A. Miscarriage increases the risk of depression in subsequent pregnancies, but stillbirth does not.
   B. Postpartum depression incidence in North America is 30%–40% of pregnancies.
   C. Symptoms of depression begin about the same time as "baby blues," normally within a few days after birth.
   D. Antecedent anxiety disorder is an important risk factor for postpartum depression.
   E. Relatives of a patient with postpartum depression should typically offer to assume total care of the newborn.

   The correct response is option D.

   Antecedent anxiety disorder may be a more important risk factor for postpartum depression than is antecedent depression (Matthey et al. 2003). Symptoms of depression typically begin later than "baby blues" and range from 4 weeks to 12 months postpartum. Stillbirths, as well as miscarriages, increase the risk of posttraumatic stress, anxiety, and depression in a subsequent pregnancy. Postpartum depression occurs in up to 10%–20% of mothers in North America. Thyroxine administration does not appear to reduce the risk of postpartum depression. Relatives should not offer to assume total care of the newborn, because doing so would only exacerbate the mother's sense of failure and deprivation; rather, they should offer to help with household tasks, allow her to care for the infant, and reinforce her sense of maternal adequacy. **(p. 355)**

References

Demyttenaere K, Bonte L, Gheldof M, et al: Coping style and depression level influence outcome in vitro fertilization. Fertil Steril 69:1026–1033, 1998

King R: Subfecundity and anxiety in a nationally representative sample. Soc Sci Med 56:739–751, 2003

Matthey S, Barnett B, Howie P, et al: Diagnosing postpartum depression in mothers and fathers: whatever happened to anxiety? J Affect Disord 74:139–147, 2003

Chapter 17—Pediatrics

Select the single best response for each question.

1. Which of the following is *not* one of Piaget's stages of cognitive development?

    A. Concrete operations.
    B. Informal operations.
    C. Sensorimotor operations.
    D. Preoperational thought.
    E. Formal operations.

The correct response is option B.

Informal operations is not a Piagetian stage. Children appear to follow a developmental path of understanding their bodies that roughly corresponds to Piaget's stages of cognitive development. *Sensorimotor* children (birth to approximately 2 years) are largely preverbal and do not have the capacity to create narratives to explain their experiences. Their perception of their bodies and of illness is therefore primarily built on sensory experiences and does not involve any formal reasoning. *Preoperational* children (approximately 2–7 years) also understand through perception, but they are able to use words and some very basic concepts of cause and effect. They tend to be most aware of parts of the body that they can directly sense, such as bones and heart (which they can feel) and blood (which they have seen come out of their bodies). They also have no real sense of organs, but instead conceptualize blood and food as going into or coming out of their bodies as though the body were itself the container. This leads to many humorous but confusing assumptions and misunderstandings. *Concrete operational* children (approximately 7–11 years) are able to apply logic to their perceptions. However, the logic is quite literal or concrete and allows for only one cause for an effect. Children tend to be eager to learn factual information about the body and illness at this age, but they will have difficulty with any concepts that require abstract reasoning. *Formal operational* children (11+ years) are able to use a level of abstract reasoning that allows discussion of systems rather than simple organs and can incorporate multiple causations of illness. It should not be assumed, however, that all adolescents approach the understanding of illness and their bodies at this level of cognition. **(p. 375)**

2. Which of the following statements concerning failure to thrive (FTT) children is *incorrect?*

    A. Feeding problems and growth deficiencies can occur.
    B. Mothers of FTT children are reported to have experienced high rates of physical abuse.
    C. If a FTT child gains weight in the hospital, a psychosocial cause of the FTT should be presumed.
    D. Former FTT children have more behavioral problems than do children without a history of FTT.
    E. None of the above.

    The correct response is option C.

    Some FTT children who have an inadequate caregiver will still lose weight in the hospital, simply because they are separated from the caregiver. In one study of FTT children (who had no identifiable biological contributors), 80% of the mothers reported a history of physical abuse (Weston et al. 1993). Former FTT children have been found to be smaller, less cognitively able, and more behaviorally disturbed than children without a history of FTT, especially if their mothers are poorly educated (Drewett et al. 1999; Dykman et al. 2001). **(p. 382)**

3. Which of the following statements about cystic fibrosis is *correct?*

    A. Rates of psychiatric disorders among patients with cystic fibrosis are twice that of the general population.
    B. Approximately 250,000 children and adults in the United States have cystic fibrosis.
    C. Less than 10% of patients with cystic fibrosis are adults.
    D. More than 80% of patients with cystic fibrosis are diagnosed by age 3 years.
    E. The median age of survival is 15 years.

    The correct response is option D.

    More than 80% of cystic fibrosis patients are diagnosed by age 3 years; however, almost 10% are diagnosed at age 18 years or older. Nearly 40% of individuals with cystic fibrosis are adults. A defective gene causes the body to produce a thick, sticky mucus that clogs the lungs and leads to life-threatening lung infections. These secretions also obstruct the pancreas, preventing digestive enzymes from reaching the intestines. Cystic fibrosis affects approximately 30,000 children and adults in the United States and is the most common hereditary disease in white children. The median age of survival is 33.4 years. Rates of psychiatric disorders among patients with cystic fibrosis do not appear to be greater than the prevalence reported in the general population. **(p. 387)**

4. Vocal cord dysfunction

    A. Commonly occurs comorbidly with asthma.
    B. Is often associated with anxiety.
    C. Can mimic asthma.
    D. Is associated with chronic stress.
    E. All of the above.

    The correct response is option E.

Vocal cord dysfunction can mimic asthma and commonly occurs comorbidly with asthma. It is a condition of involuntary paradoxical adduction of the vocal cords during the inspiratory phase of the respiratory cycle. It is often associated with anxiety or chronic stress; however, sexual abuse in this population is not as prevalent as was previously believed (Brugman et al. 1994; Gavin et al. 1998). Patients with vocal cord dysfunction frequently present with stridulous breathing, experience tightness in their throats, and feel short of breath. It can be quite worrisome that the symptoms are unrelieved by asthma medications. **(p. 388)**

5. Which of the following statements concerning juvenile-onset diabetes is *incorrect?*

    A. Puberty can lead to increased insulin resistance.
    B. Poor control commonly occurs during adolescence.
    C. Children at higher risk for developing psychiatric comorbidity are those 5–10 years after diagnosis.
    D. Beta-blockers should not be used to treat anxiety because they mask the early warning signs of hypoglycemia.
    E. Self-efficacy types of behavioral interventions have been shown to be particularly effective in fostering adherence to treatment.

    The correct response is option C.

    Children at higher risk of developing psychiatric comorbidity appear to be those in the first year after diagnosis. All the other statements are true. **(pp. 390–391)**

References

Brugman SM, Howell JH, Mahler JL, et al: The spectrum of pediatric vocal cord dysfunction. Am Rev Respir Dis 149:A353, 1994

Drewett RF, Corbett SS, Wright CM: Cognitive and educational attainments at school age of children who failed to thrive in infancy: a population-based study. J Child Psychol Psychiatry 40:551–561, 1999

Dykman RA, Casey PH, Ackerman PT, et al: Behavioral and cognitive status in school-aged children with a history of failure to thrive during early childhood. Clin Pediatr (Phila) 40:63–70, 2001

Gavin LA, Wamboldt M, Brugman S, et al: Psychological and family characteristics of adolescents with vocal cord dysfunction. J Asthma 35:409–417, 1998

Weston JA, Colloton M, Halsey S, et al: A legacy of violence in nonorganic failure to thrive. Child Abuse Negl 17:709–714, 1993

Chapter 18—Physical Medicine and Rehabilitation

Select the single best response for each question.

1. Which of the following is considered a *less* significant risk factor for psychiatric illness following traumatic brain injury (TBI)?

    A. Poor neuropsychological functioning.
    B. Preinjury psychiatric history.
    C. Preinjury social impairment.
    D. Increased age.
    E. Alcohol abuse.

The correct response is option A.

Poor neuropsychological functioning is a less significant risk factor for psychiatric illness following TBI, whereas preinjury psychiatric history, preinjury social impairment, increased age, alcohol abuse, and arteriosclerosis are highly significant risk factors. **(pp. 408–409, Table 18–2)**

2. Regarding post-TBI psychosis, which of the following statements is *true?*

    A. In TBI-associated psychosis, hallucinations are more commonly reported than are delusions.
    B. Right hemisphere lesions are more common than left-sided lesions in TBI-associated psychosis.
    C. Seizure disorder rates in patients with post-TBI psychosis are higher than estimates for rates of post-TBI seizure disorders in general.
    D. The onset of psychotic symptoms is typically within 3 months of injury, with delayed onset after 1 year rarely reported.
    E. Negative symptoms are more common in post-TBI psychosis than are positive symptoms.

The correct response is option C.

Rates of seizure disorders in patients with psychosis after TBI have been found to be much higher than estimates for rates of seizure disorders after TBI in general (Fujii and Ahmed 2002). Delusions, most commonly persecutory, are much more common than hallucinations. Risk factors for psychosis include left hemisphere and temporal lobe lesions, closed head injury, and increasing severity of TBI. The onset of psychotic symptoms is typically gradual and delayed, often occurring more than 1 year after injury. Auditory hallucinations and paranoid delusions are more common than negative symptoms. **(p. 413)**

3. All of the following are considered risk factors for postconcussive syndrome *except*

    A. Older age.
    B. Previous TBI.
    C. Psychosocial stress.
    D. Male gender.
    E. Ongoing litigation.

The correct response is option D.

Male gender is not a risk factor for postconcussive syndrome. The more common risk factors are female gender, older age, history of previous TBI, psychosocial stress, poor social support, low socioeconomic status, and presence of ongoing litigation. **(p. 416)**

4. Numerous psychotropic medications can be used to treat the symptoms of apathy and fatigue in central nervous system injury. Which of the following medications used for this purpose carries a risk of inducing seizures at usual doses?

    A. Modafinil.
    B. Methylphenidate.
    C. Dextroamphetamine.
    D. Bromocriptine.
    E. Amantadine.

The correct response is option E.

Amantadine has been associated with an increased risk of seizures, but methylphenidate, dextroamphetamine, and bromocriptine do not seem to lower the seizure threshold at typical doses. **(p. 426)**

5. Which anticonvulsant/mood stabilizer has been associated with paradoxical agitation in TBI and should thus be used with some caution and careful monitoring?

    A. Oxcarbazepine.
    B. Topiramate.
    C. Valproate.
    D. Lithium.
    E. Gabapentin.

The correct response is option E.

Some TBI patients may experience paradoxical agitation with gabapentin (Childers and Holland 1997). This side effect has not been reported with any other medications. **(p. 429)**

6. The use of atypical antipsychotic agents in TBI may be helpful in controlling problematic psychotic and agitation symptoms. However, TBI patients are prone to delirium from anticholinergic drug effects and may also have an increased risk of seizures. For these reasons, which of the following antipsychotics should be used only with extreme caution in this population?

    A. Clozapine.
    B. Olanzapine.
    C. Risperidone.
    D. Quetiapine.
    E. Ziprasidone.

The correct response is option A.

Clozapine carries a risk of seizures and should be used with extreme caution in TBI patients, particularly when compliance is in question. **(pp. 428, 430)**

References

Childers MK, Holland D: Psychomotor agitation following gabapentin use in brain injury. Brain Inj 11:537–540, 1997

Fujii D, Ahmed I: Characteristics of psychotic disorder due to traumatic brain injury: an analysis of case studies in the literature. J Neuropsychiatry Clin Neurosci 14:130–140, 2002

Chapter 19—Pain

Select the single best response for each question.

1. The International Association for the Study of Pain (IASP) has defined *pain* as

    A. An unpleasant, abnormal sensation that can be spontaneous or evoked.
    B. An increased response to a stimulus that is normally painful.

C. An unpleasant sensory and emotional experience associated with actual or potential tissue damage.

D. An abnormal sensation, spontaneous or evoked, that is not unpleasant.

E. None of the above.

The correct response is option C.

Pain has been defined by the IASP as "an unpleasant sensory and emotional experience associated with actual or potential tissue damage, or described in terms of such damage" (Merskey et al. 1986, p. S217). **(p. 451)**

2. Visual prodromal symptoms, such as scintillating scotomata, are indicative of what type of headache?

A. Classic migraine.

B. Complicated migraine.

C. Chronic daily headache.

D. Common migraine.

E. Hemicrania continua.

The correct response is option A.

Common migraine is defined as a unilateral pulsatile headache, which may be associated with other symptoms such as nausea, vomiting, photophobia, and phonophobia (Szirmai 1997). The classic form of migraine adds visual prodromal symptoms such as scintillating scotomata. Complicated migraine includes focal neurological signs such as cranial nerve palsies and is often described by the name of the primary deficit (e.g., hemiplegic, vestibular, or basilar migraine). Chronic daily headache affects about 5% of the population and encompasses constant (transformed) migraine, chronic tension-type headaches, new-onset daily persistent headache, and hemicrania continua (Lake and Saper 2002). **(p. 454)**

3. Which of the following statements concerning low back pain is *true?*

A. Nearly 25% percent of patients with acute low back pain will go on to develop chronic symptoms.

B. The least powerful predictor of chronicity is poor functional status 4 weeks after seeking treatment.

C. Economic and social rewards are not associated with higher levels of disability and depression in patients with chronic back pain.

D. Psychological factors highly correlated with low back pain include distress, depressed mood, and somatization.

E. The presence of an anxiety disorder has been demonstrated to increase the risk of developing chronic musculoskeletal pain 3 years later.

The correct response is option D.

Psychological factors are highly correlated with low back pain; these factors include distress, depressed mood, and somatization, which predict the transition from acute to chronic low back pain. A minority of patients (about 8%) with acute low back pain will go on to develop chronic low back pain, with disproportionate distress and disability (Carey et al. 2000). The most powerful predictor of chronicity is poor functional status 4 weeks after seeking treatment. In a study of secondary gain, both economic and social rewards were associated with higher levels of disability and depression in patients with chronic nonmalignant back pain (Ciccone et al. 1999). The presence of a depressive disorder has been demonstrated to increase the risk of developing chronic musculoskeletal pain 3 years later. **(p. 455)**

4. Using DSM-IV diagnostic criteria for pain disorder, researchers have estimated the lifetime prevalence of somatoform pain disorder to be

    A. 5%.
    B. 12%.
    C. 17%.
    D. 22%.
    E. 34%.

    The correct response is option B.

    The lifetime prevalence of somatoform pain disorder (as defined by DSM-III-R [American Psychiatric Association 1987] criteria) in the general population was 34%, with a 6-month prevalence of 17% (Grabe et al. 2003). However, when the DSM-IV (American Psychiatric Association 1994) requirement of significant distress or psychosocial impairment was added to make the diagnosis, the lifetime prevalence was only 12%, and the 6-month prevalence decreased to 5%, with the female-to-male ratio remaining 2:1. **(p. 458)**

5. During the first 5 years after the onset of chronic pain, patients are at increased risk of developing new substance use disorders and experiencing additional physical injuries. This risk is highest in patients with a history of

    A. Substance abuse or dependence.
    B. Childhood physical abuse.
    C. Psychiatric comorbidity.
    D. Childhood sexual abuse.
    E. All of the above.

    The correct response is option E.

    During the first 5 years after the onset of chronic pain, patients are at increased risk for developing new substance use disorders and incurring additional physical injuries (Brown et al. 1996; Savage 1993). This risk is highest in patients with a history of substance abuse or dependence, childhood physical or sexual abuse, and psychiatric comorbidity (Aronoff 2000; Fishbain et al. 1998; Miotto et al. 1996). **(p. 459)**

References

American Psychiatric Association: Diagnostic and Statistical Manual of Mental Disorders, 3rd Edition, Revised. Washington, DC, American Psychiatric Association, 1987

American Psychiatric Association: Diagnostic and Statistical Manual of Mental Disorders, 4th Edition. Washington, DC, American Psychiatric Association, 1994

Aronoff GM: Opioids in chronic pain management: is there a significant risk of addiction? Curr Rev Pain 4:112–121, 2000

Brown RL, Patterson JJ, Rounds LA, et al: Substance use among patients with chronic pain. J Fam Pract 43:152–160, 1996

Carey TS, Garrett JM, Jackman AM: Beyond the good prognosis: examination of an inception cohort of patients with chronic low back pain. Spine 25:115–120, 2000

Ciccone DS, Just N, Bandilla EB: A comparison of economic and social reward in patients with chronic nonmalignant back pain. Psychosom Med 61:552–563, 1999

Fishbain D, Cutler R, Rosomoff H: Comorbid psychiatric disorders in chronic pain patients. Pain Clin 11:79–87, 1998

Grabe HJ, Meyer C, Hapke U, et al: Somatoform pain disorder in the general population. Psychother Psychosom 72:88–94, 2003

Lake AE 3rd, Saper JR: Chronic headache: new advances in treatment strategies. Neurology 59 (suppl 2):S8–S13, 2002

Merskey H, Lindblom U, Mumford JM, et al: Pain terms: a current list with definitions and notes on usage. Pain Suppl 3:S215–S221, 1986

Miotto K, Compton P, Ling W, et al: Diagnosing addictive disease in chronic pain patients. Psychosomatics 37:223–235, 1996

Savage SR: Addiction in the treatment of pain: significance, recognition and management. J Pain Symptom Manage 8:265–278, 1993

Szirmai A: Vestibular disorders in patients with migraine. Eur Arch Otorhinolaryngol Suppl 1:S55–S57, 1997

Index

*Page numbers printed in **boldface** type refer to tables or figures.*